MANAGEMENT GUIDELINES

FOR GERONTOLOGICAL

NURSE PRACTITIONERS

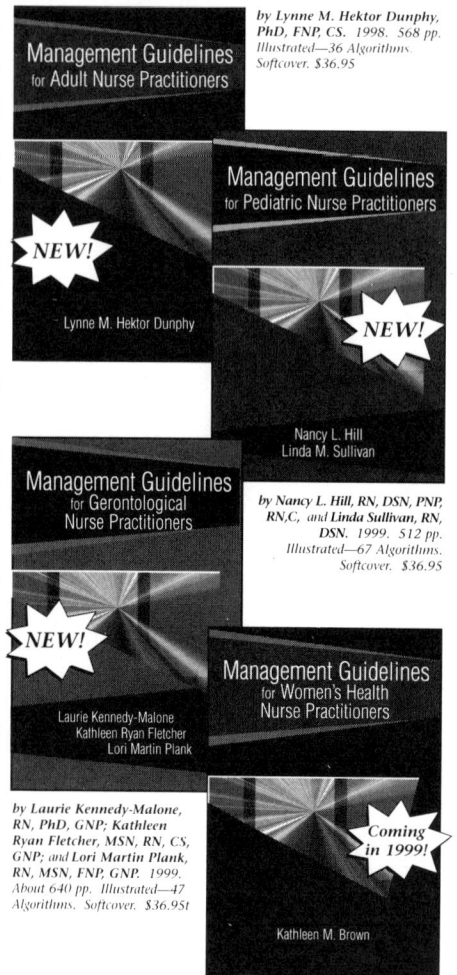
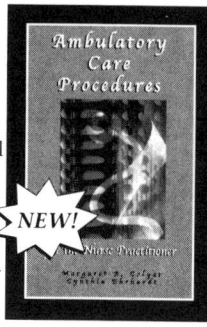

MANAGEMENT GUIDELINES FOR GERONTOLOGICAL NURSE PRACTITIONERS

Laurie Kennedy-Malone, PhD, RN, CS
Associate Professor, School of Nursing
Director of Adult/Gerontological Nurse Practitioner Program
University of North Carolina at Greensboro
Greensboro, North Carolina

Kathleen Ryan Fletcher, MSN, RN, CS
Gerontological Nurse Practitioner
Director of Geriatric Services
University of Virginia Health System
Charlottesville, Virginia

Lori Martin Plank, MSPH, MSN, RN, CS, FNP, GNP
Nurse Practitioner, Palisades Family Health Center
St. Luke's Health Services
Bethlehem, Pennsylvania
Adjunct Faculty
Allentown College of Saint Francis de Sales
Allentown, Pennsylvania
Rutgers University
Newark, New Jersey
Doctoral Student
Duquesne University
Pittsburgh, Pennsylvania

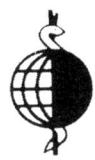 F. A. DAVIS COMPANY • Philadelphia

F. A. Davis Company
1915 Arch Street
Philadelphia, PA 19103

Printed in the United States of America

Last digit indicates print number: 10 9 8 7 6 5 4 3 2 1

Acquisitions Editor: Joanne P. DaCunha, RN, MSN
Production Editor: Michael Schnee
Cover Designer: Louis J. Forgione

As new scientific information becomes available through basic and clinical research, recommended treatments and drug therapies undergo changes. The authors and publisher have done everything possible to make this book accurate, up to date, and in accord with accepted standards at the time of publication. The authors, editors, and publisher are not responsible for errors or omissions or for consequences from application of the book, and make no warranty, expressed or implied, with regard to the contents of the book. Any practice described in this book should be applied by the reader in accordance with professional standards of care used with regard to the unique circumstances that may apply in each situation. The reader is advised always to check product information (package inserts) for changes and new information regarding dose and contraindications before administering any drug. Caution is especially urged when using new or infrequently ordered drugs.

Library of Congress Cataloging-in-Publication Data

Management guidelines for gerontological nurse practitioners / [edited
   by] Laurie Kennedy-Malone, Kathleen Ryan Fletcher, Lori Martin
   Plank.
       p.   cm.
   Includes bibliographical references and index.
   ISBN 0-8036-0297-9 (alk. paper)
     1. Geriatrics.   2. Nurse practitioners.   3. Aged—Diseases-
-Treatment.   I. Kennedy-Malone, Laurie, 1957–   II. Fletcher,
Kathleen Ryan, 1951–   . III. Plank, Lori Martin.
     [DNLM: 1. Geriatric Nursing—methods. 2. Geriatrics.   WY 152
M2655   1999]
RC954.M356   1999
610.73′65—dc21
DNLM/DLC
for Library of Congress
                                                         99-15302
                                                            CIP

I would like to dedicate this book to Chris; Brendan; and my parents, Edward and Nancy Kennedy.

L.K.-M.

I dedicate this work to Steve and Ian, who understand my professional commitments and provide unfailing support and encouragement.

K.R.F.

I dedicate this book to my husband, Rick, and my daughter, Erin.
L.M.P.

PREFACE

Because of the recent rapid increase in the growth of our older adult population, there will be an increased need for primary-care providers to deliver age-specific care and direct disease management. *Management Guidelines for Gerontological Nurse Practitioners* will serve as a guide for advanced practice nurses and students who are privileged to provide primary care to these older adults. This book will also serve as a helpful guide for clinical nurse specialists, nurse case managers, and registered nurses who are caring for older adults in ambulatory-care settings.

Unit I, "The Healthy Older Adult," covers a review of normal aging changes, including important—but often overlooked—psychosocial issues, pharmacological guidelines for prescribing medications, current recommendations for health-promotion and disease-prevention strategies for older adults, components of nutritional assessment, and requirements for a healthy diet for older adults. Because older adults are often at risk for nutritional deficiencies, the unit also covers the unique signs and symptoms of this condition in older adults.

Unit II, "Assessment," presents an overview of history-taking techniques that are useful when acquiring information from older adults. A presentation of common geriatric symptoms and guidance for functional assessment is also presented, and a selection of assessment instruments is provided. A review of critical elements needed for an effective physical examination and selection of diagnostics is included as a guide for the reader.

Unit III, "Treating Illness," provides 12 chapters of concise information on disease management of illnesses common in older adults. Each chapter opens with an assessment section that provides the reader with a focused review of systems and physical examination needed to obtain pertinent information from the older adult. One chapter presents common symptoms found in the older adult population. Throughout this unit, diagnostic decision trees are provided to aid the reader to establish differential diagnosis and derive treatment plans. Additional charts and tables are provided in the Appendixes for quick reference. Also included in this unit is a listing of national organizations, with telephone numbers, that can be used to locate resources for the older adult.

ACKNOWLEDGMENTS

This book would not have become a reality if not for the kind asistance of some wonderful people whom we would like to thank. To Joanne DaCunha, our editor, who continued to encourage us to complete this task; to Terry A. Purnell and Karen Beard, for information retrieval; to Chris A. Malone, who assisted with the figure designs; and to Robert V. Buccini, MD, for review of Chapter 10—Abdominal Disorders.

L.K.-M.

Knowledge development in gerontology is a wonderful thing, and I acknowledge the contributions of my mentors and colleagues who continue to inspire me to know more.

K.R.F.

My heartfelt thanks to my husband, Rick, and daughter, Erin.

L.M.P.

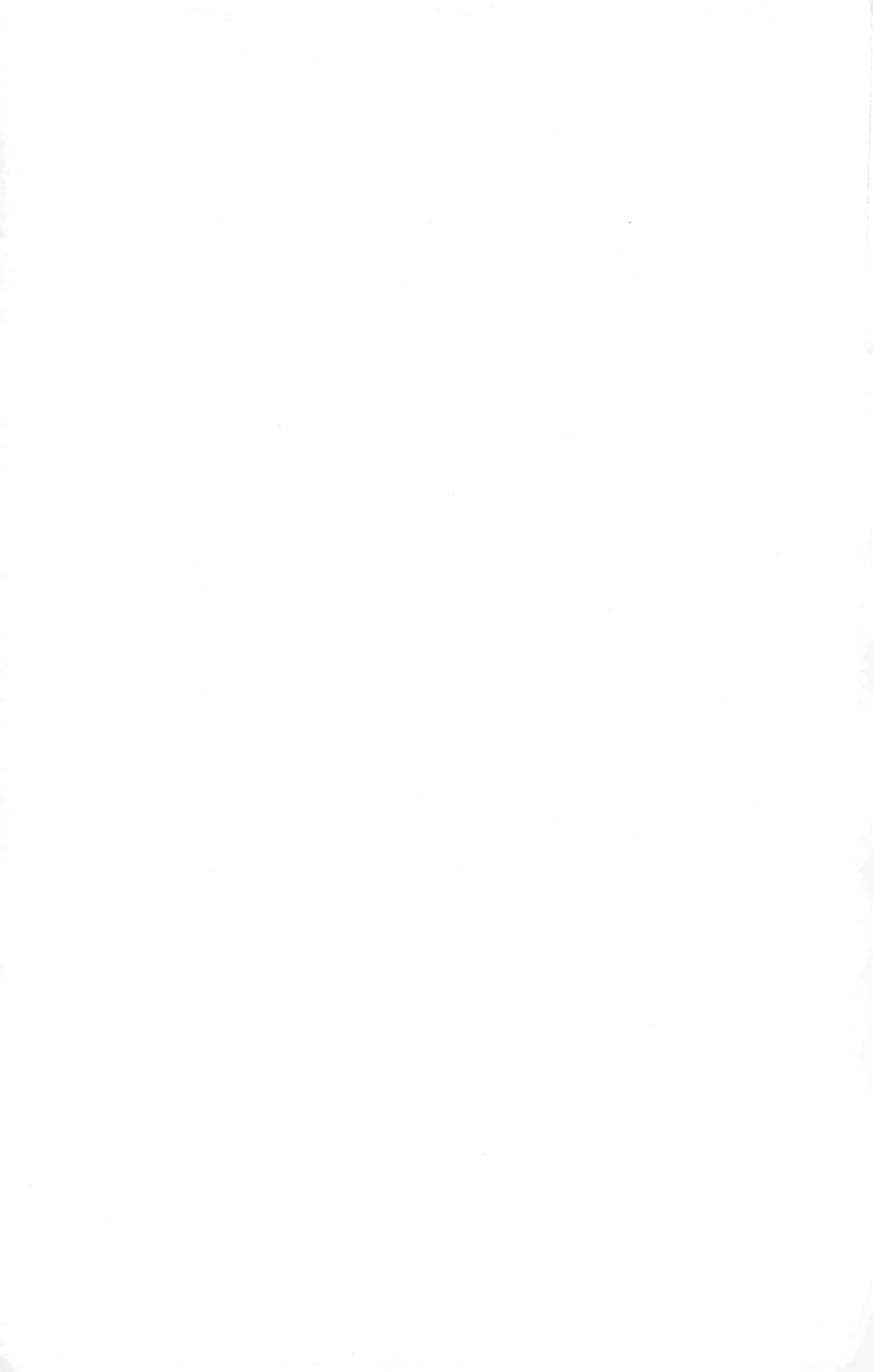

CONTRIBUTORS

Shelley L. Africa-Floyd, MSN, RN, CS
Gerontological Nurse Practitioner
Salisbury Veterans Affairs Medical
  Center
Salisbury, North Carolina
  Fatigue

Kim Bahnsen, BSN, RN
Staff Nurse
JFK Medical Center
Royal Palm Beach, Florida
  Upper Respiratory Infection

Tracy M. Ballard, MSN, RN, CS
Gerontological Nurse Practitioner
Greensboro Medical Associates
Greensboro, North Carolina
  *Chapter 9—"Peripheral Vascular
  Disorders"*

Beth E. Barba, PhD, RN
Associate Professor, School of Nursing
University of North Carolina at
  Greensboro
Greensboro, North Carolina
  Chapter 1—"Changes with Aging"

Karen Beard, MSN, RN, CS
Gerontological Nurse Practitioner
Hematology and Oncology
  Department
Wake Forest University Baptist
  Medical Center
Winston-Salem, North Carolina
  *Insect Bites and Stings, Oral
  Cancer, Rhinitis, Lung Cancer,
  Breast Cancer, Endometrial
  Cancer, Prostatic Cancer, Brain
  Cancer*

Susan Hill Craven, MSN, RN, CS
Gerontological Nurse Practitioner
Hamlet Hospital
Hamlet, North Carolina
  Hyperlipidemia, Obesity

Kathleen Ryan Fletcher, MSN, RN, CS
Gerontological Nurse Practitioner
Director of Geriatric Services
University of Virginia Health System
Charlottesville, Virginia
  *Chapter 1—"Changes with Aging";
  Chapter 3—"Nutrition"; Chapter
  4—"History Taking"; Chapter
  5—"Review of Systems"; Cardiac
  Assessment; Cardiac Arrhythmias;
  Hypertension; Ischemic Heart
  Disease; Valvular Heart Failure;
  Peripheral Edema; Syncope*

Lynne M. Dunphy, PhD, RN, FNP, CS
Associate Professor, College of
  Nursing
Florida Atlantic University
Boca Raton, Florida
  Vomiting

Joan Iannone Galbraith, MSN, RN, CS
Gerontological Nurse Practitioner
  Spinal Care Team
Durham Veterans Administration
  Medical Center
Durham, North Carolina
  Involuntary Weight Loss

Lisa J. Granville, MD
GRECC Investigator
Miami Veterans Administration
  Medical Center
Miami, Florida
Associate Professor of Clinical
  Medicine
University of Miami, School of
  Medicine
Miami, Florida
  Hoarseness

Kenneth W. Hazell, MSN, RN, FNP
Nurse Practitioner, Emergency
  Department
West Palm Beach Veterans
  Administration Medical Center
West Palm Beach, Florida
Faculty School of Nursing
Palm Beach Community College
Lakeworth, Florida
  Hearing Loss

Tomasita Riveria Jacubowitz, MSN, RN, CS
Adult/Gerontological Nurse
  Practitioner
Clinical Assistant Professor
School of Nursing
University of North Carolina at
  Greensboro
Greensboro, North Carolina
  Skin and Lymphatics Assessment, Diabetes Mellitus

Kay Jenkins, MSN, RN, CS
Geriatric Nurse Practitioner—Long
  Term Care
Veterans Administration Medical
  Center
Fayetteville, North Carolina
  Herpes Zoster

Laurie M. Kennedy-Malone, PhD, RN, CS
Associate Professor, School of Nursing
Director of Adult/Gerontological
  Nurse Practitioner Program
University of North Carolina at
  Greensboro
Greensboro, North Carolina
  Burns; Cellulitis; Skin Cancer; Chapter 10—"Abdominal Disorders"; Prostatitis; Chapter 11—"Reproductive Disorders"; Alzheimer's Disease; Parkinson's Disease; Depression, Endocrine, Metabolic, and Nutritional Assessment; Chronic Pancreatitis; Hyperthyroidism; Hypothyroidism; Malnutrition; Pancreatic Cancer

Tracy Kientz, BSN, RN, CCRN
Director of Nursing
Fort Union Nursing Home
Fort Union, Virginia
  Congestive Heart Failure, Myocardial Infarction

Gail Kimball, MSN, RN, CS
Gerontological Nurse Practitioner
Yadkin Medical Associates
Yadkinville, North Carolina
  Atropic Vaginitis

Sandra Klug, MSN, RN, CS
Gerontological Nurse Practitioner
Alamance Regional Hospital Skilled
  Nursing Facility
Burlington, North Carolina
  Epistaxis, Pharyngitis

Ruth Krissak, MSN, RN, CS
Gerontological Nurse Practitioner
J. Paul Sticht Center on Aging and
  Rehabilitation
Wake Forest University Baptist
  Medical Center
Winston-Salem, North Carolina
  *Corns and Calluses, Fungal
  Infections*

Sheree L. Loftus, MSN, RN, CS
Gerontological Nurse Practitioner/
  Nurse Manager
The Alan and Barbara Miken
  Department of Neurology
Coordinator, National Parkinson
  Foundation Clinic Offices
Beth Israel Medical Center
New York, New York
  Parkinson's Disease

Teresa A. Macon, MSN, RN, CS
Gerontological Nurse Practitioner
Southeastern Eye Center
Greensboro, North Carolina
  Dysphagia

Sheila A. McDermott, RN, MSN,
  ANP
Adult Nurse Practitioner
Beth Israel Medical Center
New York, New York
  *Head, Neck, and Face Assessment;
  Retinopathy; Hematological and
  Immune Assessment; Hematuria;
  Hemoptysis, Joint Pain*

Laurie A. Lovejoy McNichol, MSN,
  RN, CS, CWOCN
Gerontological Nurse Practitioner
Advanced Home Care
Greensboro, North Carolina
  Pressure Ulcers

Rita Napier, MSN, ARNP, FNP-C,
  ANP-C
Adult Nurse Practitioner, Primary
  Care Medicine
West Palm Beach Veterans
  Administration Medical Center
West Palm Beach, Florida
  Chalazion

Margo Packheiser, MSN, RN, CS
Adult/Gerontological Nurse
  Practitioner
Clinical Assistant Professor
School of Nursing
University of North Carolina at
  Greensboro
Greensboro, North Carolina
  Depression, Tremor

Lori Martin Plank, MSPH, MSN,
   RN, CS, FNP, GNP
Nurse Practitioner, Palisades Family
   Health Center
St. Luke's Health Services
Bethlehem, Pennsylvania
Adjunct Faculty
Allentown College of Saint Francis de
   Sales
Allentown, Pennsylvania
Rutgers University
Newark, New Jersey
Doctoral Student
Duquesne University
Pittsburgh, Pennsylvania
   Chapter 2—"Health Promotion";
   Acute Glaucoma, Cataracts,
   Chronic Glaucoma, Respiratory
   Assessment, Chronic Obstructive
   Pulmonary Disease, Pneumonia,
   Pulmonary Embolism, Pulmonary
   Tuberculosis, Restrictive Lung
   Disease, Reproductive Assessment,
   Benign Prostatic Hypertrophy,
   Drug-Induced Impotence, Gait
   Disorders, Human
   Immunodeficiency Virus, Iron
   Deficiency Anemia, Agitation,
   Delirium, Symptom Assessment,
   Bowel Incontinence, Chest Pain,
   Constipation, Dehydration,
   Diarrhea, Headache, Urinary
   Incontinence

Luanne Sadowsky, MSN, RN, CS
Gerontological Nurse Practitioner/
   Psychiatric Clinical Nurse Specialist
Beaufort Psychiatry
Beaufort, South Carolina
   Depression

Marianne Shaughnessy, PhD, RN,
   CS
Adult/Gerontological Nurse
   Practitioner
Assistant Professor
University of Maryland at Baltimore
Baltimore, Maryland
   Central and Peripheral Nervous
   System Disorders, Cerebrovascular
   Accident, Transient Ischemic Attack

Kathleen Stauffer, MSN, RN, CS
Gerontological Nurse Practitioner
Assistant Professor, College of
   Applied Sciences
Western Carolina University
Cullowhee, North Carolina
   Psychological Assessment, Alcohol
   Abuse, Anxiety, Elder Abuse, Grief,
   Insomnia, Wandering

Ladsine Taylor, RN, MSN
Gerontological Nurse Practitioner
Veterans Administration Medical
   Center
Salisbury, North Carolina
   Chronic Bronchitis

Tamara Tripp, MSN, RN, CS
Adult/Gerontological Nurse
   Practitioner
Nalle Clinic
School of Nursing
UNC–Charlotte Adjunct Faculty
Charlotte, North Carolina
   Dizziness

CONSULTANTS

Kathleen C. Buckwalter, PhD, RN, FAAN
Professor, Graduate and Doctoral Programs
University of Iowa College of Nursing
Iowa City, Iowa

Geraldine F. Marroco, RN, MSN, EdD
Professor, Chair of Continuing Education
St. Vincent's College of Nursing
Bridgeport, Connecticut

B. Joan McDowell, PhD, CRNP, FAAN
Associate Professor of Nursing
University of Pittsburgh School of Nursing
Pittsburgh, Pennsylvania

Christine M. Sheehy, PhD, RN
Former Associate Professor
Arizona State University
Tempe, Arizona

CONTENTS

UNIT **I**

THE

HEALTHY

OLDER ADULT

CHAPTER 1

CHANGES WITH

AGING

Today the aged population is incredibly diverse; it includes some individuals who are nearly twice as old as others, yet all are considered to be within the same cohort. Determining what is expected in aging, what is disease in aging, and what constitutes successful aging is an immense challenge even for the most skillful advanced clinician. When assessing the aging individual, the clinician should be familiar with the range of normal and expected changes associated with aging so that older persons falling outside this range may be identified and interventions taken appropriately and expeditiously.

In the past, wellness was considered the mere absence of disease, but with more information from longitudinal studies of aging we are learning a great deal about the characteristics of successful physiologic and psychosocial agers and about those who not only defy disease but also may not experience the expected normal aging changes (Rowe, 1987). A profile of successful agers is beginning to emerge, with the illness-health continuum expanding to include them. The implications for the gerontological nurse are significant: finally, some targetable criteria exist with which to direct efforts "to develop, offer, and evaluate services in a variety of institutional and community settings that promote healthy aging, prevent development or exacerbation of health problems, and support the strengths of the older person" (ANA, 1987).

Physiologic Aging

PHYSIOLOGIC CHANGES WITH AGING

The physiologic changes associated with the usual aging process are listed by system in Appendix A. The clinician must appreciate that some processes previously considered normal age-related changes are now being refuted. Historically, normal aging studies were conducted using a cross-sectional study method. Today, results are becoming increasingly available from longitudinal studies of aged populations, some of which began in the 1930s. This more reliable methodology provides some challenges to previously held conclusions; for example, the notion that cardiac output declines with aging. Results from the Framingham studies demonstrate that cardiac output declines with disease but not with age alone (Schulman, 1994). The clinician is encouraged to keep informed of the research in the area of expected and successful aging so that this information may be carefully considered and interpreted and applied to the clinical setting. During the clinical decision-making process, the informed clinician will be less likely to undertreat a treatable condition. For example, the astute clinician will use the diagnostic process to differentiate the more benign seborrheic keratosis from the more serious actinic keratosis in the aged individual. While educating the older patient, the informed professional will be less likely to attribute a finding to the aging process alone. When clinicians attribute findings to aging alone, the older person may conclude that there is no point in changing behavior because the process is inevitable.

In addition to detailing the expected physiologic changes of aging, Appendix A also includes the related functional changes and implications. Although this appendix uses a systems approach, all the systems interact. For example, the risk of respiratory infection in the geriatric population is considerable and the physiologic influences on development may include limited chest wall expansion as well as alterations in the immune system functioning. In reviewing the physiologic changes, the clinician should consider that the primary impact involves the following:

- Reduced physiologic reserve of most body systems: particularly cardiac, respiratory, and renal.
- Reduced homeostatic mechanisms that fail to adjust regulatory systems: such as temperature control and fluid and electrolyte balance.
- Impaired immunologic function: infection risk is greater, autoimmune diseases more prevalent.

LABORATORY VALUES AND AGING

Healthy individuals of all ages often have asymmetric distribution of tests results. Normality in a statistical sense may be extrapolated incorrectly to normality in terms of health.

In addition, the standards previously available to the health-care worker with which to compare laboratory values have been based on collected samples typically from young, college-age men. Fortunately, we are beginning to use "reference ranges," usually the middle 95% of all values provided by the sample population +2 standard deviations (SDs). Reference intervals such as age, sex, or race can be defined demographically. These may be further defined physiologically (e.g., fasting, ambulatory status) or pharmacologically (e.g., medication usage, tobacco or alcohol use). Even this more precise method does not ensure a "healthy" sampled population as the standard. The reference values presented for the older adult cohort (Appendix B) are not necessarily desirable ones. Longitudinal chemical studies support the concept of biochemical individuality; that is, each individual's variation is often much smaller than that of the larger group as a whole. Biochemical individuality is of particular importance in detecting asymptomatic abnormalities in older adults. Significant homeostatic disturbances in the same individual may be detected through serial laboratory tests, even though all individual test results may lie within normal limits of the reference interval for the entire group.

The clinician must determine whether a value obtained reflects a normal aging change, a disease, or the potential for disease. Although abnormal laboratory findings are often attributed to "old age," rarely are they true aging changes. Misinterpretation of an abnormal laboratory value as an aging change can lead to underdiagnosis and undertreatment in some situations (e.g., anemia or urinary tract infection) and overdiagnosis and overtreatment in others (e.g., hyperglycemia, asymptomatic bacteriuria).

One value of particular significance to the practitioner with prescriptive privileges is the calculation of creatinine clearance in the estimation of renal function. Measured creatinine clearance provides an index of renal function for use in choosing doses of renally eliminated or nephrotoxic drugs (such as digoxin, H2 blockers, most antibiotics, and salicylates) or in the general assessment of renal stability.

CROCKCROFT-GAULT FORMULA FOR ESTIMATED CREATININE CLEARANCE

$$\text{Creatinine clearance (mL/min)} = \frac{(140 - \text{age (yr)}) \times \text{body weight (kg)}}{72 \times \text{serum creatinine (mg/dL)}}$$

In women, the calculated value is multiplied by 0.85.

Accurate creatinine clearance estimates are critical in dosing drugs with low toxicity thresholds or narrow therapeutic indices. More recent research is challenging this estimated method of categorizing older individuals according to renal function (Malmrose, 1993). Malmrose demonstrated that current equations provide unacceptable predictions of creatinine clearance in normal aging individuals. Researchers cautioned that overestimation of creatinine clearance might result in nephrotoxicity when administering certain drugs. Underestimation, on the other hand, risks the underdosing of certain medications such as antibiotics, which may cause severe consequences in a compromised individual. The use of serum drug concentration measurements (where these are available) or timed urine specimens is recommended until more acceptable methods of calculating renal function in this population become available.

Finally, when considering which laboratory tests to order, it is worth remembering the doctrine "primum non nocere," to do no harm. Excessive blood sampling may lower the hematocrit, repeated fasting tests may provoke nutritional compromise, and extensive use of tests often require drugs that may cause adverse drug reactions. Any risks involved in laboratory testing must be considered with respect to the patient's clinical condition and weighed against the test's expected benefits. The clinician should plan in advance the use for each test result value obtained, especially for less specific or less sensitive tests such as sedimentation rate and serum alkaline phosphatase levels.

MEDICATIONS AND AGING

Polypharmacy and Adverse Drug Reaction

Polypharmacy is a major concern in geriatric health care. Although older adults represent 12% of the population, they consume 30% of all prescription drugs and approximately 40% of all over-the-counter medications. Polypharmacy is a primary predictor for an adverse drug reaction (ADR), which is any undesired or unwanted consequence that occurs as a result of taking medications.

The magnitude of the problem is reflected in some current statistics. Three of every five visits to the emergency department by older adults are the result of an ADR, and 10.5% of all acute care admissions of the elderly are precipitated by medication problems. More than 50% of all fatalities from ADRs occur in elderly persons. The most significant factor contributing to the risk of an ADR in older individuals is the number of drugs taken.

ESTIMATES OF THE ADR RISK WITH NUMBER OF DRUGS TAKEN

6% if two drugs are used.
50% if five drugs are used.
100% if eight drugs are used.

(From Sloan, RW: Practical Geriatric Therapeutics. Medical Economics Books, Oradell, NJ, 1986, p. 39.)

Factors contributing to the increased ADR risk in elderly people include not only polypharmacy but also pharmacokinetics and pharmacodynamics that are altered with aging, adherence problems, and inappropriate health-care provider and self prescribing. In general, the therapeutic window narrows with age, so that the potential for benefiting the patient measured against the risk of doing harm becomes more significant for the prescribing professional (Fig. 1–1).

Pharmacokinetics and Pharmacodynamics

Certain changes occurring with the aging process alter the dynamic processes that drugs undergo to produce therapeutic effects. These changes involve the processes of pharmacokinetics (what the body does to the drug) and pharmacodynamics (what the drug does to the body). Table 1–1 shows the age-related changes that are relevant to drug pharmacology.

Drug absorption is generally thought to have a less significant impact on pharmacokinetics than does drug distribution, biotransformation, or excretions.

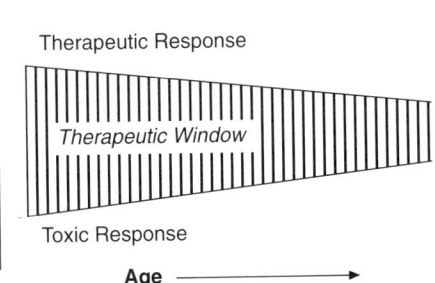

FIGURE 1–1 Narrowing of the therapeutic window. (From Kane, R, Ouslander, J, and Abrass, I: Essentials of Clinical Geriatrics. McGraw-Hill, New York, 1994.)

Gastric acidity declines with age because of decreased intestinal blood flow and fewer absorbing cells in the gastrointestinal (GI) tract. These changes appear to be offset, however, by the longer contact time that occurs as transit time slows (in aging, this slowing is more functional than physiologic).

Another factor that affects drug absorption is the presence of food and other drugs in the stomach at the same time. Antacids and iron, for example, inhibit the absorption of tetracycline; antacids can significantly decrease the bioavailability of digoxin. Anticholinergic medications cause a slowing of colonic motility and can result in greater absorption rates. Metabolic diseases such as thyroid disease

TABLE 1–1 AGE-RELATED CHANGES
RELEVANT TO DRUG PHARMACOLOGY

Parameter	Age-related Change
Absorption	Decreases in: absorptive surface, splanchnic blood flow Increased gastric pH Altered gastrointestinal motility Other influencing factors: Pain, anticholinergic response, metabolic disease, adequate fluid intake with the drug
Distribution	Decreases in total body water, lean body mass, serum albumin level Increased body fat Altered protein binding Other influencing factors: Bioavailability depends on the route of administration, solubility of the drug, blood flow to site
Biotransformation	Decreases in liver blood flow, liver enzyme activity Other influencing factors: Smoking, activity level, gender (men biotransform faster)
Excretion	Decreases in glomerular filtration rate, renal size, renal blood flow Other influencing factors: Hydration status, competition for excretion sites
Tissue responsiveness	Alterations in receptor number and receptor affinity

or diabetes can cause an increase or decrease in transit time and therefore can cause either increased or decreased drug absorption.

Still another consideration is whether an oral medication actually passes through the esophagus before it is absorbed. Many older adults take medications without adequate fluid, increasing the potential for esophageal damage from the dissolution of drugs in the esophagus. Esophageal erosions have been noted with the more caustic drugs alendronate potassium and tetracycline.

Drug distribution is affected by aging, particularly individuals of smaller body size, those who have decreased body water, and those with higher body fat. Drugs distributed in water (such as alcohol and lithium) have higher concentration in elderly persons, thereby exerting a more profound effect. Drugs distributed in fat (such as most psychoactive drugs) have a wider distribution and less intense effect but a more prolonged action, particularly in those individuals with greater adipose tissue. Medications with a higher protein-binding rate (digoxin, warfarin, meperidine) have a greater potential to cause an ADR in those with less lean body mass. Because these individuals have fewer receptor sites and less albumin for binding, plasma concentration is greater and more free drug is available for tissue distribution, pharmacologic activity, and elimination. Protein-bound drugs in particular may reach toxic levels if the patient is not monitored closely. Distribution influences are marked in the patient who is malnourished and dehydrated.

Drug distribution also relies on the bioavailability of the drug. The amount of the drug that reaches the systemic circulation may be increased or decreased, depending on certain influencing factors:

1. The **route of administration** is important to consider because inhalants and drugs given intravenously and topically are usually more readily available than drugs administered intramuscularly, subcutaneously, orally, or rectally.
2. The **solubility of the drug** is influential, as aqueous solutions are available more quickly than oily ones.
3. **General circulation to the site of drug administration** has an impact; blood flow increases with massage, heat, or presence of an occlusive dressing, and decreases during shock or during the administration of vasoconstrictors.

Biotransformation occurs in all body tissues but primarily in the liver, where enzymatic activity (cytochrome P-450 system) alters and detoxifies the drug and prepares it for excretion. With advancing age, the ability of the liver to metabolize drugs does not decline similarly for all pharmacological agents. Although liver size and blood flow do decline with age, routine liver function test results are typically normal when no disease exists. Decreased liver size and blood flow can result in a decreased first-pass metabolism; drug activity for some medications is prolonged, as drugs are metabolized and eliminated more slowly.

Being familiar with the age-related pharmacokinetics of drugs is of utmost importance when determining the initial and maintenance dosages. One example of a dosage consideration is seen with theophylline. Elderly individuals usually need 25%–50% less theophylline, as a result of decreased metabolism by the liver. Other drugs known to have reduced hepatic metabolism are listed in Table 1–2.

Other factors influence biotransformation also. For example, smoking may slow it. Men have faster and more efficient biotransformation, presumably because of serum testosterone. Conditions of increased or decreased liver perfusion alter the overall level of the drug.

The most profound pharmacokinetic change is reduced elimination of drugs. Most drugs are excreted in the urine via the renal system, although some are excreted in the feces via the biliary system. Water-soluble drugs are excreted directly by the kidneys, and fat-soluble drugs are converted to water-soluble drugs by the liver first. Changes in kidney function begin in the fourth decade of life, with a 6%–10% reduction in the glomerular filtration rate and renal plasma flow every 10 years. Therefore, by age 70, an individual might reasonably have a 40%–50% decrease in renal function, even in the absence of disease. These kidney function changes may prolong the half-lives of drugs. This is particularly important

TABLE 1–2 MEDICATIONS WITH REDUCED HEPATIC METABOLISM WITH AGE

Psychoactive Drugs	
Alprazolam (Xanax)	Chlordiazepoxide (Librium)
Imipramine (Tofranil)	Diazepam (Valium)
Desipramine (Norpramine)	Flurazepam (Dalmane)
Amitriptyline (Elavil)	Nortriptyline (Aventyl)

Cardiovascular Drugs	
Amlodipine	Propranolol (Inderal)
Diltiazem	Quinidine
Lidocaine	Verapamil

Analgesics and Anti-inflammatory Drugs	
Morphine	Meperidine (Demerol)
Propoxyphene	Ibuprofen (Advil)
Naproxen	

Other	
Theophylline	Tolbutamide (Orinase)
Diphenhydramine (Benadryl)	Levodopa

Adapted from The Merck Manual of Geriatrics, 2nd Edition, edited by William B. Abrams, Mark H. Beers, and Robert Berkow. Copyright 1995 by Merck & Co., Inc., Whitehouse Station, NJ, with permission.

for drugs that are excreted unchanged in the urine (i.e., digitalis, lithium). Estimated or actual creatinine clearance may be used to determine drug dosage. Drug categories known to be particularly nephrotoxic in older persons include radiocontrast material, aminoglycosides, ACE inhibitors, and nonsteroidal anti-inflammatory drugs (NSAIDs).

It is important to know the pharmacodynamic influences of the drug as well. Furosemide offers a good example. Generally, drug accumulation increases the pharmacological effect; however, although furosemide accumulates as renal function falls, its efficacy decreases. Because furosemide and other diuretics act on the luminal side of the renal tubule, their access to this site of action decreases as renal function declines. Therefore, more furosemide may be required to produce the desired diuretic response.

Finally, consideration must be given to the pharmacodynamic process: what the body does to the drug. The older adult tends to exhibit enhanced responses to drugs affecting the central nervous system, and this is attributed to greater tissue sensitivity caused by aging. Older adults given opiates are more likely to experience ataxia and those taking haloperidol are more likely to experience extrapyramidal symptoms. Some studies demonstrate that older individuals may have an increased tissue sensitivity for oral anticoagulants. In certain instances, patients may exhibit a decreased rather than an exaggerated response at this tissue level; this appears to be the case with beta-blockers, in which an increased dosage may be required to have a desired effect.

Drug responsiveness may vary depending on the patient's activity and stress levels and on the environment. These factors have not yet been adequately studied, however.

NONADHERENCE

In the 1930s drugs were mystical; in the 1950s labeling of medications began, but even today the consumer is too often unfamiliar with why and how to take the medication. Perhaps the term "noncompliance" is outdated in this day when the consumer and the health-care professional share in the decision-making process. Because some "noncompliant" older adults are in fact quite knowledgeable, the term "nonadherence" may be more appropriate when describing a situation in which the patient is not taking the drug as directed.

Studies have shown that the prevalence of nonadherence in the aged population is between 26% and 59% (Col, 1990). The factors that influence adherence are consumer related, therapy related, prescriber related, and socioeconomically related.

Consumer-related Factors

The patient may fail to understand the medication instructions. Understanding the level of education and the reading and comprehension levels of the patient is critical to medication instruction. The physical ability to read labels or to hear the instruction and the manual dexterity to administer, apply, or inhale a medication must be determined and validated. Cognitive abilities must be (sufficiently) intact for the patient to understand why he or she has been prescribed the medication and how to take it. The consumer must be able to process the instruction, execute the series of steps necessary to administer the drug, and to recognize potential reactions to the medication and the appropriate actions to take should they occur. Poor recall ability has been a statistically significant factor associated with a higher risk of hospitalization in patients who have been nonadherent. The nonadherent patient may require assessment for depression, as nonadherence may be an indirect self-destructive behavior (ISDB).

The trend of consumers making more choices in the self-management of illness will certainly continue, with an increasing array of over-the-counter drugs including nonsteroidal anti-inflammatories, antihistamines, antifungal agents, steroid creams, and H2 blockers. Alcohol, also an over-the-counter drug, interferes with more than 50% of all medications. Access to these drugs poses a high risk in patients lacking understanding of the indications and appropriate dosing.

Therapy-related Factors

The most significant therapy-related predictors of nonadherence include the number of drugs taken and the complexity of the regimen. The greater the number of medications taken and the more difficult the process, the less likely the patient will adhere. Additionally, patients are unlikely to take medications that they believe are causing adverse or unpleasant symptoms. Those drugs known to cause the most adverse drug reactions in elderly persons are listed in Table 1–3.

Prescriber-related Factors

The potential for a new drug to cause an ADR may be unknown to the elderly patient. New drugs on the market have not been tested in the representative elderly population because many in this group (those in poor health or who are taking other medications) are specifically excluded from the clinical trials required by the Food and Drug Administration (FDA). Consequently, some geriatricians avoid prescribing a new drug for several years, waiting for these ADRs to surface.

TABLE 1–3 DRUGS MOST COMMONLY ASSOCIATED WITH ADVERSE DRUG REACTIONS IN ELDERLY PERSONS

Analgesics: nonsteroidal anti-inflammatories, nonnarcotic analgesics, some narcotics
Psychotropics: neuroleptics, antidepressants, anxiolytics, sedatives/hypnotics
Cardiovascular: antiarrhythmics, antihypertensives, diuretics, potassium supplements
Others: H2 blockers, antibiotics, anticoagulants, antiparkinsonians, hypoglycemics, bronchodilators

Because the FDA's system designed to facilitate reporting by health professionals (MedWatch) continues to be a voluntary program, prescribers do not necessarily report all adverse reactions.

Drugs are taken less often also when they cause the patient distress. Drugs known to cause the most unpleasant symptoms include those with anticholinergic side effects causing constipation, dry mouth, blurred vision, and sometimes mental impairment.

The relationship between the prescriber and the patient may also influence adherence to therapy. The provider may lack a complete profile of prescribed and over-the-counter medications taken by the patient. Often the aged individual sees more than one health-care provider and may obtain drugs at more than one pharmacy. Efficient links enabling connections among the many points of medication delivery process would facilitate better case management in the individual patient. These links, however, have not been established.

The patient may be hesitant to inform the provider of the lack of effectiveness of a prescribed drug. A trusting and open relationship can develop over time, as information is shared and problems are addressed.

The provider does not always recognize the value of teaching the patient about their prescribed medications. Teaching materials specific to this age group are just beginning to be developed and used.

Physicians prescribe potentially dangerous "inappropriate" medications for nearly one-quarter (23.5%) of all Americans age 65 and older. A panel of experts from the National Medical Expenditure Survey in 1987 identified 23 potentially inappropriate drugs for use in elderly patients (Beers, 1991) (Table 1–4).

Inappropriate prescribing includes not just that done by the provider (as when the wrong diagnosis is made and therefore the wrong drug is prescribed) but also that done by the consumer. In the self-management of symptoms, patients have applied Monostat to atrophic vaginitis and used Pepcid for the pain of a myocardial infarction. Diuretics and digitalis have been prescribed to patients thought to be in congestive heart failure whose edema and dyspnea were later attributed to anemia and malnutrition.

COMMON PRESCRIBING PROBLEMS

- Lack of a complete inventory of medications.
- Lack of use of alternatives to medication management.
- Wrong diagnosis made and wrong drug prescribed.
- Failure to reevaluate drugs when condition changes or at periodic intervals.
- Failure to monitor therapeutic levels of drugs.
- Lack of patient follow-up to monitor for ADRs and adherence.

The clinician may fail to reevaluate drugs when the patient's condition changes or when the drug is no longer indicated. The provider often lacks a comprehensive profile of all the medications the patient is taking including those bought over the counter, such as transdermal patches, eyedrops and eardrops, and herbal remedies. More than one patient has taken simultaneously both a prescribed and

TABLE 1–4 INAPPROPRIATE DRUGS
FOR ELDERLY PATIENTS

Drug Type	Generic Drug Name
Sedatives or hypnotics	Diazepam
	Chlordiazepoxide
	Flurazepam
	Meprobamate
	Pentobarbital
	Secobarbital
Antidepressants	Amitriptyline
NSAIDs	Indomethacin
	Phenylbutazone
Oral hypoglycemics	Chlorpropamide
Analgesics	Propoxyphene
	Pentazocine
Dementia treatments	Isoxsuprine
	Cyclandelate
Platelet inhibitors	Dipyridamole
Muscle relaxants or antispasmodics	Cyclobenzaprine
	Methocarbamol
	Carisoprodol
	Orphenadrine
Antihypertensives	Propranolol
	Methyldopa
	Reserpine
Antiemetic agents	Trimethobenzamide

Adapted from Beers, MH, et al: Explicit criteria for determining inappropriate medication use in nursing home residents. Archives of Internal Medicine 151:1829, 1991.

an over-the-counter anti-inflammatory drug unbeknownst to the provider and the consumer.

Sometimes inappropriate prescribing occurs when there is a lack of appreciation for and familiarity with alternatives to medication management or in the value of low-dosing over-the-counter drugs. The consumer expects to get more than Tylenol or bran; and neither consumer nor provider may appreciate the value of massage, heat or cold applications, relaxation or therapeutic exercises, or the addition of water to the treatment plan.

Procedures may overlook the fact that certain drugs (i.e., digoxin, phenytoin, heparin, theophylline, lithium) require testing of therapeutic levels at regular intervals. Too often providers do not follow up in the monitoring of patients for ADRs and adherence issues.

Socioeconomically Related Factors

Socioeconomic constraints also influence adherence. The availability of and ease of access to a prescribed drug certainly affects how quickly the patient initiates therapy. Not all medications are available at all pharmacies; combination drug products are not always covered by insurance programs that help defray the cost of medications. The expense of a particular medication or in combination with other medications has a negative impact on adherence. Finally, the existence of family and social support systems to monitor medication adherence is a significant socioeconomic factor.

Safe Prescribing

Some suggested principles for safe prescribing of medications for the elderly are listed in Table 1–5; the key principle is "Less is more." Decision making regarding drug therapy is always made within the context of the individual patient and his or her diagnosed disease and/or illness. A complete inventory of all medications is essential. The provider and consumer must weigh the potential benefit against the potential harm with any therapeutic agent. Drugs are compared to select the best one for the individual patient within the familiar repertoire of the provider. When a new drug is initiated, the lowest possible dosage should be used to achieve the therapeutic purpose with the least potential for negative effects. When more of the drug is needed, it should be added slowly. The complexity of the treatment and any factors that may influence patient adherence should be reviewed on an ongoing basis. Optimally, the provider should have the patient demonstrate medication administration techniques and explain why each drug is being taken. After initiation, all medications are reviewed regularly, and those no longer indicated discontinued.

TABLE 1–5   PRINCIPLES OF SAFE PRESCRIBING
FOR ELDERLY PATIENTS

Consider nondrug therapy first.
Accurately diagnose the disease or illness.
Inventory all drugs and therapeutic measures taken.
Less is more.
Keep it simple.
Teach the patient about the drug.
Review medications regularly and when a change in condition occurs.
Monitor therapeutic drug levels as indicated.
Discontinue drugs no longer indicated.
Determine adherence and acceptability.

Psychosocial Issues

The aging process is inextricably linked to changes in psychosocial functioning. Theories of aging provide links between psychosocial functioning and physical behaviors, such as stress and lowered immunity. Outcomes of these psychosocial stressors may be undesirable behavioral alterations, loss of function, loss of independence, powerlessness, anxiety, depression, and even suicide. Certainly most older adults use past experiences to help them develop and grow toward full and satisfying older years. Interventions that consider the individual's whole person and promote a sense of belonging and physical and psychological well-being help the person reach a higher quality of life.

This section of the text reviews a few relevant psychosocial issues important to aging adults. The problems associated with these issues can affect the well-being of older persons and their families.

DEATH AND DYING

Although unique to each individual, birth, dying, and death are normal and necessary experiences of living. Early in the century, most deaths occurred in individuals under age 50. Today most deaths occur in the over-65 population, particularly among those in institutional settings. Health-care institutions may be the least suitable places for the dying older person. Physicians and nurses often experience discomfort and guilt when faced with people who are dying despite their efforts.

The most common cause of death and disability in older adults in the United States is cardiovascular disease, coronary artery disease being responsible for 85% of deaths attributed to heart disease. Cancer is the second most frequent cause, with colorectal, breast, lung, pancreatic, and ovarian cancers found most commonly in women, and lung, colorectal, prostate, pancreas, and stomach cancers most common in men. Cardiovascular accidents rank third in persons between age 55 and 75 and Alzheimer's type dementia ranks fourth most common cause of death in the United States and Canada for individuals over age 65. Accidents or unintentional injury ranks eighth among those over 75 years; falls account for approximately 59% of home-related accidental deaths. Renal disease ranks ninth for those over age 65, and intestinal obstruction and diverticular disease cause most GI-related deaths.

Although no two people react to death and dying in the same way, the psychological and physiologic characteristics of grief have been described by many significant theorists such as Bolby, Kübler-Ross, and Parkes. Grief is a normal response to the pain of loss. Older people experience loss of health, friends, relatives, roles, and financial security, and these losses accumulate over time. Many experience grief over imminent loss of their own lives. Each individual passes through the process of grieving differently, but all are helped by sharing thoughts, feelings, and silence. Normal grieving should resolve over several months; unresolved grief suggests the need for special help. An extreme depressive reaction leading to suicide is not common but needs to be assessed. Acceptance of the inevitable losses associated with the dying process can lead to acceptance of death itself.

Some elderly persons consider death as a welcome alternative, an experience to be desired if not actively sought. Death may be seen as a natural ending to life, preferred to more feared alternatives such as becoming cognitively impaired, dependent, or seriously ill. This attitude toward death may be a major difference between the young-old and the old-old.

Older persons confronting the dying experience may be concerned about the surrounding events such as rejection, loneliness, loss of self-determination, and isolation more than with death itself. As the older person faces death, decisions often involve whether or not to withhold treatment or resuscitation and admission to acute-care facilities. Attempting to make these decisions with few guidelines can cause anxiety among older people, their families, and their health-care providers.

A variety of fears are experienced by the dying person, especially the fear of pain. Pain should be managed to provide relief from suffering while continuing to allow the patient's emotional participation with others The dying elderly person should be assured that narcotic addiction is not a concern, and that symptoms contributing to suffering will be treated aggressively.

Other concerns of the dying elderly person include fear of being abandoned, loss of independence, and fear of the unknown. The emotional and physical presence of caregivers helps alleviate feelings of abandonment. Loss of independence occurs with loss of function. Keeping the person in control of personal and financial affairs as long as possible helps to build a sense of control. Fear of the unknown can be somewhat ameliorated by the presence of family and other caregivers.

Because each dying elderly person is human, dignity is considered a right. Promoting dignity means preserving a person's right to self-determination and personal and moral worth. It has been suggested that the dying person be informed about what is happening and be able to discuss his or her concerns, have the opportunity to make decisions regarding the dying process, and experience dying in an open and caring environment.

LOSS OF FUNCTION

Activities of daily living (ADLs) include activities people do as part of daily living relevant to the situation in which they function. Functional ADLs encompass activities necesary for self-care such as bathing, toileting, dressing, and tranferring, whereas instrumental activities of daily living (IADLs) include activities that facilitate independent living in the community such as shopping, transportation, and meal preparation.

Many losses affect function as one ages. Older people hardly realize the gradual slowing down of physical functioning, such as decreases in hearing and sight, until they are deaf in one ear or, after cataract surgery, they realize how minimal their operative vision was. The same thing can occur with ability to perform ADLs. Many functional losses in older adults reflect normal physiological changes of aging. Elderly persons must manage the requirements of daily living need with decreased agility, balance, strength, endurance, and sensual acuity. People adjust to decreased abilities. Adaptations may be needed in the approaches for meeting the demands of daily living, particularly in the environment.

The National Health Survey on Aging shows that 67.5% of people over 65 report good to excellent health. In a sample of 27,909, researchers found that the older people get, the more difficulty they have performing ADLs. In 1987, 3.6 million of the 28 million adults over 65 had difficulty performing one or more ADL tasks; about 17.5% had difficulty with one or more IADL tasks. African-American and Hispanic noninstitutionalized elderly persons have more difficulty with ADLs than white elderly persons. More older African-Americans and lower-income older Americans report their health as poor or fair, compared with white older Americans and those with higher incomes. Functional ability seems to have more to do with self-assessment of health than with the number of diagnosed chronic conditions. Because chronic illess is common in elderly individuals, the medical diagnoses do not provide accurate information about self-care ability. A comprehensive functional assessment is necessary to achieve appropriate diagnosis of functional abilities.

Aspects of the physical environment that may infringe on an older person's health include housing and the neighborhood, which interact with the social aspects of the environment. For example, some housing arrangements provide more challenges than others, and some neighborhoods encourage more social interaction than others. Environmental modifications can enhance function. Varying certain aspects as lighting intensity, glare, and background noise to compensate for normal age-related sensory changes are simple interventions that affect the older person's immediate environment. These alterations may even affect the person's perceptions of the larger environment.

Family and social groups are important environmental considerations for older adults. They influence the person's responses to aging and illness because social support has been strongly related to people's health and well-being. Family members may help with ADLs and provide emotional support. Social groups such as friends, religious groups, and neighborhood acquaintances may provide assistance, particularly during illness. Religious affiliation influences attitudes toward aging, illness, and dying.

NURSING HOME PLACEMENT

Long-term care (LTC) facilities serve older adults in need of treatment for chronic disease and disability when it is impossible or impractical to provide this care in the home or other setting. Nursing home placement is an option for older adults who need more help managing their personal care than is possible by family and community members. In 1990, approximately 7 million older adults needed LTC; by the year 2005, the number will increase to an estimated 9 million. By the year 2020, the estimates are that 12 million people over 65 will need LTC in the private home, the community, or the nursing home.

The difficult decision to relocate for LTC is often based on loss of functional ability, social support, and adequate financial support. Occasionally, relocating to a nursing home, where competition is not as acute, and where the stress of deciding on self-care or caregiver is removed, may relieve a person's burden. Institutionalization does, however, require a patient's adjustment to lack of privacy, to staff and roommates who are strangers and of different backgrounds, to new rules and mores, and to isolation from familiar surroundings and social contacts.

Ideally, an LTC facility should provide excellent medical and nursing care in a homelike atmosphere. Skilled care services should be available 24 hours a day and should include nursing, recreational, rehabilitative, pharmaceutical, and medical services, as well as others. Intermediate care services are less extensive and are for persons who need less assistance. The administrator, who should be educated in health-care administration, must recognize the need for older adults as individuals and make provisions for them. Nurses play a critical role in providing comprehensive health care for nursing home residents. They are responsible for the plan of care, utilization of resources, and advocacy within the facility and community.

Two types of residents are found in nursing homes. The long-term stay resident is often older, with one or more chronic illnesses, and has more functional and cognitive impairments. These people generally remain in the facility until they die. Short-term residents, who are usually younger, with more physical than cognitive problems, stay from 3 to 6 months. Women are residents of LTC facilities about 1½ times more often than men; the older people more than likely will be institutionalized. Eighty percent of residents of LTC facilities die in the facility or in acute care institutions; the other 20% return to a community dwelling.

It is commonly believed that institutional environments have deleterious effects on physical, psychological, and social function. There has been discussion of transplantation shock, transfer trauma, and other terms to indicate the dangers of relocating for older adults. For newly admitted nursing home residents, the relocation may be quite stressful because the move connotes significant negative changes in lifestyle. Relocation has effects on behavior, health, and mortality. Nursing home relocation has been associated with indifference, abdication, depression, psychological withdrawal, and physical decline.

Quality of life of the residents can be improved by having them dressed and out of bed; encouraging participation in varied activities; providing interaction with all-aged visitors; including animal therapy, gardening, and travel films in activities; providing for resident governance; and involving residents in outdoor activities. Residents of nursing homes who are given personal control over their environments are physically and mentally healthier and live longer than those given less control who have similar physical health, mental health, and prior socioeconomic status.

Wives whose spouses are admitted to nursing homes pass through the first stage of widowhood, complaining of symptoms of depression and poor health, even though their caregiver burden is lightened. Deleterious effects of nursing home placement can be effectively managed by predictability of the move, by preplanning, and by giving the resident some degree of control over the decision-making process. Preadmission family visits, opportunities for ventilation of concerns, and realistic appraisal of options can be offered. For outcomes that are unavoidable, thoughtful nursing assessment and intervention can minimize or reverse consequences.

RETIREMENT ISSUES

Retirement is frequently the first role change to occur in later life. For many, this period encompasses one-third of their life. For some, retirement is a welcome event, an active, independent, healthy time of life. For others, it is a source of unhappiness, associated with loss of role, collegial relationships, self-esteem, and identity. Retirement can be particularly stressful for the person who has not developed leisure pursuits.

It would be erroneous to assume that retirement necessarily means a complete cessation of work, as many people work part-time, become self-employed, or become volunteer workers. Decisions about whether people should retire at age 65, or earlier or later, usually depend on expected income. A set mandatory retirement age is gradually being eliminated for all but a few jobs. More often the individual decides.

During retirement, spouses become increasingly aware of their partners' faults, and couples do not increase time spent together or with their children during this period. Men seem to be happier in retirement than women. Women who were homemakers lose a sense of freedom and control by the desire to accommodate their spouses' presence. Retired persons who are unhappy in this new role manifest signs of boredom, apathy, and lack of meaning in life. Self-esteem disturbance and social isolation are common problems if the person enters retirement with unrealistic goals and expectations. People whose lives have been dominated by their work and identities shaped by their jobs have these patterns deeply ingrained in their lives. In retirement, they see themselves as no longer capable, significant, or useful, which causes them to feel a profound loss. More retirement anxiety is reported among persons who usually have difficulty in life transitions.

Retirement requires preplanning and realistic perceptions of the changes that occur. Counseling is suggested to assist couples to identify what new roles might be and to organize their new lifestyle to define how these roles fit.

Retirement often means reduced income for many older persons. Problems from reduced income depend on the amount of preplanning necessary and the lifestyle adjustments the family must make to meet current financial actualities. Drastic lifestyle changes brought about by changes in finances can lead to fear, disturbances in self-esteem, social isolation, loss of independence and control, and anxiety. Preplanning, even as late as the middle years, could lead to an increased sense of autonomy and power.

LEGAL ISSUES

Legal issues for older adults involve government policies affecting health care, including those concerned with health maintenance, access to care, funding, and standards of care. With passage of the Social Security Act of 1935, the federal government became intimately involved in services to the elderly population. From 1935 to the mid-1970s, expansion of Social Security benefits continued; then the focus changed to reduction of federal expenditures and shift of financial responsibility to the states. Medicare, Medicaid, Social Services Block Grants, the Older Americans Act of 1965, and the Omnibus Budget Reconciliation Act of 1981 (OBRA) are the major pieces of legislation affecting the older population. As reform of the health-care delivery system progresses, the effects on the older population will be astounding. Gerontological health-care providers should be familiar with newly enacted legal provisions, regulations, rules, and guidelines.

Legal issues surrounding older adults concern the areas of specific physical problems, competency, negligence, rights of elderly persons, and abuse. The physical problems that most concern health-care personnel and older clients today involve skin breakdown, falls, and use of restraints. Assessment and documentation of potential and actual occurrences are the best defense against liability.

For skin breakdown, the nurse should record detailed assessment findings along with care and treatment given to the patient. Because falls among older people are common, fall potential needs to be assessed and preventive measures implemented. If a fall occurs, the person's physical and mental condition must be evaluated. Lack of documentation of prefall conditions is the most common cause for liability. Restraints can be used only under very specific conditions. Chemical restraints are particularly regulated because of their potential in older people to cause serious side effects leading to serious consequences. Recording of circumstances surrounding application of physical and chemical restraints must be detailed and include continuous assessment.

Competency issues are complex because competency is difficult to define. The courts define a competent person as one who is aware of the situation, understands the issues, and makes a decision based on this awareness and under-standing. Competency may be thought of as a continuum, with someone capable of being competent in one area and not in another. For example, an older person may not be able to manage ADLs but can probably understand moral issues associated with specific treatment options. A competent older person has the right to make health-care decisions and even to refuse treatment. Incompetency is decided by the courts.

The Patient Self-Determination Act of 1990 was a legal effort to ensure that a person's health-care wishes are carried out if the person becomes incompetent. This act encourages competent people to decide future health-care situations by using advanced directives. The right to die has become a conscious decision for patients, families, and health-care providers; however, it is superceded by the presumed right to treatment. To resolve any complications, people are not advised to indicate before the situation arises whether they would wish to have medical interventions aimed at circumventing death. A "living will" indicates the type of future treatment preferred, and a durable power of attorney for health care designates a person to carry out health-care wishes if the person becomes unable to decide. Because states differ in specific definitions of health-care interventions, people must be aware of pertinent requirements.

Elder abuse and neglect can take many forms. Defined as intense and frequent behavior harmful toward an older adult, producing psychological, physical, financial, or social harm, the signs and symptoms include undermedication or overmedication, poor nutritional status, poor hygiene, withdrawal, and unexplained injuries. Up to 1.2 million older adults are victims of some type of abuse or mistreatment each year. Health-care professionals must report any suspicions of elder mistreatment without fear of libel, as most states provide for anonymity of reporter and protection against such suits.

As the population ages, more legal issues involving older adults will pervade the courts. Health-care providers must be aware of government policies, rules, and regulations affecting care of the older population. As advocates for elderly persons, we can make a difference in health care.

ETHICAL ISSUES

Ethical dilemmas involving older adults can be categorized into societal, family, and individual issues. Societal issues include standard of care for older people versus younger people, rationing of health-care resources, and rights of patients in institutions. Individual and family issues include limitation of care, autonomy of decision making, and conflicts among family members about treatment decisions. Almost daily gerontological nurses feel the effects of ethical dilemmas surrounding quality of life of older adults.

Standard of care issues center on whether the government should expand reimbursement of community-based services, or limit institutional services, or do both. Should support be given to the prevailing LTC model or should increased reimbursement for community-based services be increased at the expense of the institutional model?

Rationing certain health-care services on the basis of age becomes more likely as changes in Medicare force continued cost-containment measures. Suggested approaches to decision making include selection committees and lotteries. Gerontologists generally concur that rationing of health-care decisions based on chronological age is inappropriate, and that functional capacity may be a more reasonable criterion. The central question is whether advanced age reduces one's ability to benefit from advanced health-care interventions. Some services are already being rationed for the elderly, based on regulatory policy. For example, Medicare reimburses for home health care only during unstable episodes of chronic diseases, even though older people would benefit from these services also during remissions.

In LTC institutions, the dilemma of protecting the rights of older residents has been partially addressed by the Nursing Home Patients' Bill of Rights, required for certification by Medicare/Medicaid procedures. One of the rights identified in this document is privacy. Institutionalized persons have a right to private conversation during visits, without someone intruding, and to private telephone conversations. The right of a person to select health-care providers tends to be limited in institutional settings; indeed, complaints about services may engender reprisal. Rights can be curtailed in the name of efficiency or paternalism. The right of an older person to be autonomous can be compromised when the person is forgetful or shows evidence of cognitive impairment. At what level of cognitive impairment is an individual no longer able to make decisions regarding his or her medical treatment? It is generally agreed that once the patient understands the goals of therapy and the side effects of treatment or lack of treatment, he or she can make decisions regarding that treatment.

Limitation of care activities based on chronological age and presence of chronic conditions and/or cognitive impairment involves anyone who has an interest in the older person. Questions center on the principle of beneficence, on respect for individual rights and values, and on respect for self-determination. Potential courses of action include continuing current level of treatment, providing no treatment, or seeking further assessment and evaluation. Consideration of the consequences of each option is essential to the debate. Differences of opinion about treatment alternatives often occur among family members and pose further dilemmas for health-care providers.

Ethical dilemmas by nature involve choosing among equally unacceptable alternatives. The first step in resolving these dilemmas is to identify the issue and the ethical principles involved. Thorough assessment of the situation and all ramifications must be undertaken by all parties involved and a decision made after consideration of options.

Societal perceptions of aging and of aging persons influence the resolution of ethical issues in gerontological nursing. Ageism is discrimination by one age group toward another. With urbanization and industralization, greater emphasis has been placed on the negative effects of aging, characterizing older people as useless and incapable of adapting to rapid societal change. On the other hand, cultural and religious tradition tends to underscore respect and honor for older adults. Assumptions about old age are not uniform or applied equally. Gerontological health-care personnel are responsible for repudiating negative perceptions and basing ethical decisions on unbiased reasoning. Although the rights of older adults to participate actively in their own health-care decisions are recognized in ethical principle, in actual health-care situations these rights may be overruled.

BIBLIOGRAPHY

Physiologic Aging

Abrams, B, et al (eds): The Merck Manual of Geriatrics, ed 2. Merck Research Laboratories, Whitehouse Station, NJ, 1995.

American Nurses' Association: Standards and the Scope of Gerontological Nursing Practice. ANA, Washington, DC, 1991.

Baum, C, et al: Drug use in the United States in 1981. JAMA 241:1293, 1984.

Beers, MH, et al: Explicit criteria for determining inappropriate medication use in nursing homes. Arch Intern Med 151:1825, 1991.

Berkman, LF, et al: High, usual, and impaired functioning in community-dwelling older men and women. J Clin Epidemiol 46:10, 1129–1140, 1993.

Col, A, Fanale, JE, and Kronholm, P: The role of medication noncompliance and adverse drug reactions in hospitalizations of the elderly. Arch Intern Med 150:841, 1990.

Kahl, A, et al: Geriatric education centers address medication issues affecting older adults. Public Health Rep 107:1, 38, 1992.

Kane, R, Ouslander, J, and Abrass, I (eds): Essentials of Clinical Geriatrics. McGraw-Hill, New York, 1994.

Lamy, PP: Adverse drug effects. Clin Geriatr Med 6:293, 1990.

Malmrose, LC, et al: Measured versus estimated creatinine clearance in a high-functioning elderly sample: MacArthur foundation study of successful aging. J Am Geriatr Soc 41:715, 1993.

MedWatch: The FDA's Desk Guide for Adverse Event and Product Problem Reporting. Food and Drug Administration, Rockville, MD.

Meisekothen, L: Noncompliance in the elderly: A pathway to suicide. Journal of the American Academy of Nurse Practitioners 5:2, 67, 1993.

Melillo, K: Interpretation of laboratory values in older adults. Nurse Pract 18:7, 59, 1993.

Nell Di Lima, S, and Hildebrandt, U (eds): Geriatric Patient Education Resource Manual. Aspen Publishers, Gaithersburg, MD, 1995.

Nolan, L: Prescribing for the elderly: Sensitivity of the elderly to ADR. J Am Geriatr Soc 36:2, 142, 1988.

Ray, W, Friffin, MR, and Shorr, RI: Adverse drug reactions and the elderly. Health Affairs 114, Fall 1990.

Rowe, JW, and Kahn, RL: Human aging: Usual and successful. Science 237:4811, 143, 1987.

Schulman, SP: Normal aging changes of the cardiovascular system. In Tresch, DD, and Aronow, WS (eds): Cardiovascular Disease in the Elderly Patient. Marcel Dekker, New York, 1994.

Sloan, RW: Practical Geriatric Therapeutics. Medical Economics Books, Oradell, NJ, 1986.

Stein, B: Avoiding drug reactions: Seven steps to writing safe prescriptions. Geriatrics 49:9, 28, 1994.

Wilcox, SM, Himmelstein, DU, and Woolhandler, S: Inappropriate drug prescribing for the community-dwelling elderly. JAMA 272:4, 292, 1994.

Psychosocial Issues

Aiken, TD: Legal issues affecting the elderly. In Stanley, M, and Beare, PG (eds): Gerontological Nursing. FA Davis, Philadelphia, 1995, pp 37–50.

American Cancer Society: Cancer Facts & Figures. American Cancer Society, Atlanta, 1994.

Benoliel, JQ: Care, communication and human dignity. In Garfield, C (ed): Psychosocial Care of the Dying Patient. McGraw-Hill, New York, 1978.

Berman, PM, and Kirsner, JB: Gastrointestinal problems. In Steinberg, FU (ed): Care of the Geriatric Patient, ed 6. CV Mosby, St. Louis, 1983.

Black, HC: Black's Law Dictionary, ed 5. West, St. Paul, MN, 1979.

Burnside, I: Nursing and the Aged: A Self-Care Approach, ed 3. McGraw-Hill, New York, 1988.

Butler, RN: Age-Ism: Another form of bigotry. Annals of the American Academy of Political and Social Science 503:138, 1969.

Calne, OB: Normal aging of the nervous system. In Anders, R, Bierman, E, and Hazzard, W (eds): Handbook of Geriatric Medicine. McGaw-Hill, New York, 1985.

Cutler, NE, and Gregg, DW: The human wealth span and financial well-being in older age. Generations 15:45, 1991.

Fletcher, WL, and Hansson, RO: Assessing the social components of retirement anxiety. Psychol Aging 6:76, 1991.

Gerber, RM: Coronary artery disease in the elderly. J Cardiovascular Nurs 4:23, 1990.

Henderson, ML, and McConnell, ES: Ethical considerations. In Matteson, MA, and McConnell, ES (eds): Gerontological Nursing: Concepts and Practice. WB Saunders, Philadelphia, 1988, pp 93–121.

Houldin, AD, et al: Psychoneuroimmunology: A review of the literature, Holistic Nurs Practice 5:16, 1991.

Johnston, T: Retirement: What happens to the marriage? Mental Health Nursing 11:347, 1990.

Kane, RL: Long-term care resources. In Kane RL, Ouslander, JG, and Abrass I (eds): Essentials of Clinical Geriatrics. McGraw-Hill, New York, 1989, p 397.

Kemper, P, and Murtaugh, CM: Lifetime use of nursing home care. N Engl J Med 324: 595, 1991.

Langer, E, and Rodin, J: The effects of choice and enhanced personal responsibility for the aged: A field experiment in an institutional setting. J Pers Soc Psychol 34:191, 1976.

Leon, J, and Lair, T: Functional status of the non-institutionalized elderly: Estimates of ADL and IADL difficulties. (DHHS publication no. 90-3462). National Medical Expenditure Survey Research Findings 4, Agency for Health Care Policy and Research. Public Health Service, Rockville, MD, 1990.

Melcher, J: Advances in aging research. US Senate Special Committee on Aging, US Government Printing Office, Washington, DC, 1988, pp 3–7.

Pillemer, KA, and Finkelhor, D: The prevalence of elder abuse. A random sample survey. Gerontologist 28:51, 1988.

Riffle, KL: Falls: Kinds, causes, and prevention. Geriatr Nurs 3:165, 1982.

Rodin, J, and Langer, E: Long-term effects of a control-relevant intervention with the institutionalized aged. J Pers Soc Psychol 35:897, 1977.

Rosenthal, CJ, and Dawson, P: Wives of institutionalized elderly men. Journal of Aging and Health 3:315, 1991.

Rosswurm, MA: Relocation and the elderly. J Gerontol Nurs 9:632, 1983.

US Bureau of the Census: Projections of the population of the US by age, sex and race 1988 to 2080 (Current population. Report series, p 23, no. 138). US Government Printing Office, Washington, DC, 1984.

US Senate Special Committee on Aging: Aging America: Trends and Projections (Serial No. 101-J). US Government Printing Office, Washington, DC, 1990.

US Senate Special Committee on Aging, the American Association of Retired Persons, The Federal Council on the Aging, and the US Administration on Aging: Aging America: Trends and Projections. US Department of Health and Human Services, Washington, DC, 1991.

Yancik, R, Kessler, L, and Yates, JW: The elderly population: Opportunities for cancer prevention and detection. Cancer 62:1823, 1988.

CHAPTER **2**

HEALTH PROMOTION

The concept of health promotion includes activities to which an individual is committed and performs proactively to further his or her health and well-being. This includes not only preventive and health-protective measures but also actualization of one's health potential. The broadest definition, identified by the World Health Organization, includes healthy lifestyle promotion, creation of supportive environments for health, community action, redirection of health services, and healthy public policy formulation. All these measures are within the scope of the nurse practitioner and enhance the visibility of the role while advancing the needs of patients. Additionally, nurse practitioners are in a unique and pivotal position to guide and encourage health-promotion programs and individual efforts. From our nursing background, we bring a holistic orientation to health and wellness, knowledge of developmental tasks, and the wellness-illness continuum. Our advanced practice education helps us to diagnose and treat patients in a way that supports their return to optimal level of function and/or maximizes their coping abilities within the limits of their existing function.

This particular blend of competencies is especially valuable in working with older patients. Heterogeneity increases with aging, presenting the gerontological nurse practitioner with the challenge of individualizing health-promotion recommendations for each patient. Additionally, clear, age-specific preventive health guidelines for the older population are scarce. Primary health-care providers who are not oriented toward the potential of healthy aging often discount the importance of health promotion in this age group. This, combined with ageist attitudes in our youth-oriented society, has a spillover effect on older patients, sending the message that lifestyle changes are without value in late adulthood. The current health insurance climate also decries financial expenditures for aggressive medical interventions in older patients. Some elders already have a misguided belief that retirement gives them permission to "take it easy" and indulge themselves in sedentary lifestyles and unhealthy food choices. They mistakenly identify morbidity as a natural consequence of the aging process.

Given that life expectancy exceeds 75 years in both men and women, with a potential to live to 120 years, it behooves us to focus on prevention and health promotion in our older patients to maximize the quality of these years. A collaborative plan should include:

- Consideration of the patient's health beliefs and goals.
- Present and anticipated level of function.
- Risks and benefits of proposed interventions.
- Effectiveness of specific preventive interventions for older adults.

Health-promotion activities should be incorporated into every patient encounter, as opposed to being addressed selectively.

Health promotion for older patients may be approached in several ways. The Health Risk Appraisal, a self-reported questionnaire completed by the patient, uses age, sex, health behaviors, risk factor history, and selected, epidemiologically sound, physiologic indices to estimate risk of dying within a certain time period. It also pinpoints disease-causing "hazards" that can be the focus of preventive health interventions. Studies have demonstrated that health-risk appraisal, combined with education and health-promotion interventions, can result in positive behavioral changes over a 1-year period in older adults (Uriri and Thatcher-Winger, 1995).

The guidelines of the United States Preventive Services Task Force (USPSTF) and other authorities can be used to provide a framework and timeline for health promotion and preventive activities. These guidelines represent the best effort to date to identify screenings and interventions that have scientific merit and efficacy. Many of these items do not specifically target the older age group, but they may be adapted as clinical judgment permits. Primary and secondary prevention in the areas of immunizations, screening, and counseling is addressed; the active role of the primary health-care provider is emphasized.

Several nurse practitioners have expanded on these approaches by including social and financial assessment, wellness spirituality, tertiary prevention, rehabilitation, and even a health-promotion diary for patients (Kotthoff-Burrell, 1992; Leetun, 1996; Pizzi and Wolf, 1998). The discussion of health-promotion recommendations that follows incorporates all these sources.

Immunizations

Unless contraindicated, influenza vaccine is recommended annually for all older adults. Persons with a history of anaphylactic reaction to eggs or documented IgE-mediated sensitivity to eggs should not receive the vaccine. Patients in febrile states should be deferred until symptoms have ceased. Optimal timing for vaccine administration is mid-October through November, before the peak flu season. Medicare and other insurance carriers cover the vaccine. Community-dwelling older adults can avail themselves of opportunities to receive the vaccine at senior centers, grocery stores, or physician offices. It is especially important that residents of long-term care facilities receive the vaccine, since they are often in a frail state and environmental factors in these facilities may favor rapid spread of influenza. Many patients are reluctant to be immunized because of a respiratory infection that occurred coincidentally after receiving the vaccine in the past. Education of the patient may reverse this resistance. Caregivers of frail elderly persons should also receive the vaccine. Elderly patients account for 80%–90% of flu-related deaths.

Pneumococcal vaccine is recommended for all immunocompetent older adults and other high-risk groups, including:

Institutionalized persons age 50 and over.

Those age 2 or over with certain chronic conditions including diabetes mellitus, chronic cardiac or pulmonary disease, and anatomic asplenia without sickle-cell disease.

Those living in environments or social settings associated with increased risk of pneumococcal illness, including Native-Alaskan and Native-American people.

Immunocompromised individuals with alcoholism, cirrhosis, chronic renal failure, nephrotic syndrome, sickle-cell disease, acquired or congenital immunodeficiency, metastatic or hematologic malignancy, or multiple myeloma, or organ transplant recipients should be considered for the vaccine also, although the proof of efficacy in these populations has not been established. Revaccination is not routinely advised; however, in those populations at highest risk for pneumococcal-related morbidity or mortality (those over age 75 or those with severe chronic disease), a repeat vaccination may be warranted after 5 years.

The tetanus-diphtheria (Td) vaccine should be given every 10 years to those who have completed their primary childhood immunization series. The American College of Physicians recommends less-frequent boosters, stating that one booster in mid-adulthood is sufficient. When a patient sustains a dirty wound, tetanus vaccine is repeated if the interval since the last booster is more than 5 years. Patients who never received the primary tetanus series need three Td vaccinations. The second dose can be administered 4–8 weeks after the first, and the third dose is given 6–12 months after the second. Contraindications include prior history of reaction or hypersensitivity to components of the vaccine. Adults over age 60 account for 60% of the cases of tetanus annually.

In addition to the foregoing immunizations, the use of aspirin prophylaxis for men with risk factors for coronary heart disease, in whom aspirin is not contraindicated, can be considered on an individual basis by patient and provider, weighing its risks and benefits. For women, the use of postmenopausal hormone replacement therapy (HRT) and its available options, benefits, and risks should be discussed during the patient's perimenopausal stage. Studies by the USPSTF have shown a positive response to HRT even when instituted in the postmenopausal period; providers can individualize the timing and frequency of discussion (Table 2–1).

TABLE 2-1   SUMMARY OF PREVENTIVE SERVICES TO CONSIDER

Immunizations and Chemoprophylaxis

Tetanus-diphtheria booster
Influenza vaccine
Pneumococcal vaccine
Hepatitis B vaccine (high-risk only)

Discussion of aspirin prophylaxis in high-risk group
Discussion of hormone replacement therapy for women

Conditions and Factors to Remain Alert For

Depression symptoms
Suicide risk factors
Abnormal bereavement
Medications that increase risk for falls
Change in functional status

Signs of physical abuse or neglect
Malignant skin lesions
Peripheral arterial disease
Tooth decay, gingivitis, loose teeth
Change in mental or cognitive status

Screening/Counseling

History
  Dietary intake
  Physical activity
  Tobacco, alcohol, or drug use
  Functional status in normal environment
  Social supports
  Financial supports
  Spiritual supports
Physical Examination
  Clinical breast examination
  Blood pressure
  Height and weight
  Visual acuity
  Hearing screening
  Multisystem examination
    Skin: premalignant/malignant changes, dietary fiber and sodium, lymphadenopathy
    Cardiovascular: arrhythmias, murmurs, bruits, peripheral vascular disease (PVD), ulcers
    Pulmonary: adventitious sounds
    Oral/dental: denture fit, lesions (examination by dental professional every 6 months)
    Abdomen: organomegaly, masses
    Genitourinary/Rectal: prostate, incontinence, cystocele, rectocele, atrophic vaginitis, lesions or masses
    Neuromuscular: gait, balance, strength, mobility

Laboratory/Diagnostic Tests
  Cholesterol
  Mammogram
  Fecal occult blood test and/or sigmoidoscopy
  Papanicolaou smear
High-Risk Groups
  Human immunodeficiency virus (HIV) screen
  Prior history of transient ischemic attacks (TIAs)
  Tuberculin skin test (PPD)
  Electrocardiogram
  Complete blood count
  Cholesterol profile
  Ophthalmoscopic examination
  Thyroid-stimulating hormone (TSH) level
Counseling
  Diet: Fat, cholesterol, calcium (women), caloric balance
  Substance use: smoking cessation, alcohol, other drugs including prescription, drinking and driving, treatment for substance abuse
  Injury prevention: falls, seatbelts, smoke detectors, hot water heater
  Dental health: daily brushing with fluoridated toothpaste, flossing, regular checkups, denture fit
  Skin: protection from ultraviolet light
  Physical activity: exercise prescription

Screening

Sensory losses, common in older patients, have serious implications for functional living, safety, and socialization. Periodic otoscopic examination and questioning regarding hearing changes are recommended. If you suspect a hearing deficit, refer the patient to a hearing specialist for further evaluation instead of directing him or her to a hearing aid vendor. Eye examination and visual acuity testing using the Snellen chart is recommended every 2 years. Refer individuals with vision problems or questionable findings and those with risk factors for glaucoma to an eye health specialist for examination.

Height and weight should be measured periodically, with optimal frequency determined by the health-care provider. Increases in morbidity and mortality are noted with even a 10% increase over ideal body weight. An increase of 20% is associated with higher risk of coronary artery disease, hypertension, and non–insulin-dependent diabetes mellitus. Counseling regarding nutrition and physical activity benefits should accompany screening for patients who weigh 20% more than their desirable weight.

Blood pressure should be measured at least every 2 years in asymptomatic older adults. Initial measurement should include both arms, performed in both a sitting and a lying position. According to the Sixth Report of the Joint National Committee on Prevention, Detection, Evaluation, and Treatment of High Blood Pressure (JNC VI), gains against hypertension are declining. The same report shows that even modest increases in blood pressure into the high-normal range of 130–139 mmHg systolic or 85–89 mmHg diastolic are associated with target organ damage. On the positive side, losing weight, increasing physical activity, and making dietary modifications have been effective in reducing mild to moderate hypertension. If blood pressure is elevated on more than one successive measurement, the overall health status of the patient should be evaluated and counseling provided. Other factors to consider for these patients include:

Preexisting conditions.
Medications.
Alcohol and tobacco use.
Stress factors.

Cholesterol screening may be prudent in this population and in those with other cardiovascular risk factors. The USPSTF recommends cholesterol screening every 5 years up to age 65. It found insufficient evidence to recommend routine cholesterol testing in the older adult, especially over age 75 years; however, provider discretion is advised.

Mammography and clinical breast examination for cancer screening are advised every 1–2 years at age 50 and over, with provider discretion regarding frequency of screening after age 70. A gynecologic examination, including a Papanicolaou (PAP) smear for cervical cancer, is recommended every 1–3 years. After age 65, the continuation and frequency of PAP smear testing in patients with previously normal results is left to the provider's discretion.

Fecal occult blood testing (FOBT) or sigmoidoscopy to screen for colorectal cancer is recommended for all persons age 50 or over, although experts disagree on the frequency of such testing; suggestions range from annually to every 3–5 years. FOBT instructions should follow guidelines for dietary restrictions, sample collection, and storage. If sigmoidoscopy is performed, longer, flexible sigmoidoscopes offer greater patient comfort and yield more sensitive results. Patients at high risk for colorectal cancer, those with symptoms, and those with positive test results require further testing or referral to a specialist.

Screening to identify problem drinking is advisable for all patients over 65 who have access to alcohol. Obtain a thorough history of alcohol use, quantity, frequency, type, and effects (intoxication, driving under the influence [DUI] offenses, motor vehicle accident [MVA], abusive behavior). Hidden alcohol abuse in older adults is a documented problem, particularly in those who live alone, have experienced a recent loss, or have a prior history of substance abuse or depression. Problem drinking in older patients may be complicated by functional or safety issues, medication interactions, or incipient mental status decline. Use of the Michigan Alcoholism Screening Test (MAST), Alcohol Use Disorders Identification Test (AUDIT), or CAGE questionnaire may be helpful in establishing the existence of an alcohol problem. Family members, neighbors, or caregivers may also provide pertinent information. Counseling and intervention strategies specific to the patient and situation are indicated.

In addition to the screening procedures mentioned here and recommended by major authorities, individual primary health-care providers may deem other screening tests prudent after evaluating the risk factors, depending on the patient's state of health, functional status, motivation, and potential. Also, patients in long-term care settings may be required to undergo certain screenings, such as that for tuberculosis, to detect infectious diseases that can be spread to other patients. During periodic physical examinations, always be alert to evidence of neoplastic disease. The USPSTF report indicates a paucity of research on the effectiveness of or necessity for certain screening tests in the older adult population. Gerontological nurse practitioners are well positioned to conduct this research and to carve out more specific guidelines for older adults (see Table 2–1).

Older adults should receive a complete functional status assessment as part of the health-promotion plan. Specific mental status screening for the presence of dementia or depression is frequently indicated as well. To complete the screening portion of the health-promotion plan, assess the patient's social support system, access to health-promotion resources, financial support, home environment (for community-dwelling older adults), and spiritual support. Although the importance of appropriate screening and ensuring current immunizations cannot be under-rated, counseling patients for positive lifestyle changes is most critical in promoting health. Studies also show the receptiveness of older adults to health-promotion strategies and their willingness to modify current behaviors in this direction (Uriri and Thatcher-Winger, 1996). Counseling about substance use (tobacco, alcohol, drugs) and injury prevention can be combined naturally within the issue of safety. Smoking is the leading preventable cause of death in the United States. Smoking cessation also yields many benefits to former smokers in terms of reduction of risk for several chronic illnesses and stabilization of pulmonary status. Clear and specific guidelines are available to help health-care providers advise tobacco users to quit and to provide them with follow-up encouragement and relapse prevention management (Agency for Health Care Policy and Research, 1996). Quitting smoking may not be a choice for the institutionalized older adult but rather dictated by the policy of the institution. Health-care providers can offer support and encouragement, emphasizing the positive health changes that will result.

Counseling regarding alcohol or other drug use can be preventive or interventional, depending on the initial assessment. Emphasize the dangers of drinking and driving and/or the increased risk of falling while under the influence of alcohol or any drug that acts on the central nervous system. Teach patients about the coincidental interactions between alcohol and many prescription drugs, over-the-counter (OTC) preparations such as acetaminophen, and herbal remedies. The contribution of alcohol abuse to problems such as insomnia, depression, aggressive behaviors, and deteriorating social relationships should be addressed. Likewise, the problem of dependence on prescription drugs such as analgesics, hypnotics, tranquilizers, or anxiolytics should be assessed and addressed. Counseling in the form of individual follow-up sessions, group support, outpatient or inpatient rehabilitation may be indicated. In a group-living situation, the governing body (i.e., resident council) may become involved if the patient's behavior threatens the safety or well-being of the other group members. Monitoring for depression and/or suicidal ideation may be indicated during and after substance withdrawal.

Before initiating counseling on diet and exercise, obtain baseline information on current dietary intake and activity pattern and combine this with height and weight data and other health status information. For patients in the long-term care setting this information is easily obtained from chart documentation. For community-dwelling older adults, the Nutrition Screening Initiative tools are most specific and easily administered (Table 2–2). The initial, self-administered questionnaire can be given to patients waiting to see their health-care provider. After scoring the questionnaire, refer at-risk patients for additional screening, using the mnemonic DETERMINE to identify risk for nutritional deficiencies:

Disease.
Eating poorly.
Tooth loss or mouth pain.
Economic hardship.
Reduced social contact and interaction.
Multiple medications.
Involuntary weight loss or gain.
Need for assistance with self-care.
Elder at an advanced age.

Further screening using the mnemonic ABCDEF gathers more information to complete the assessment and pinpoint interventions:

Anthropometric: Height and weight.

Biochemical: Serum albumin less than 3.5 mg/dL is a nonspecific indicator of poor nutrition. Hemoglobin determination for anemia, hematocrit for hemoconcentration with dehydration, serum cholesterol for elevation, and serum B_{12} to rule out deficiencies complete the screen.

Clinical, physical, and medical history (self-explanatory).

Dietary history: Food diary of a normal 24- to 48-hour period, listing all food and drink, supplements, food sources, storage, and cooking facilities, as well as any cultural and religious preferences and taboos.

Empathy: Active listening, inquiring about diet and giving the patient time to share any problems.

Functional assessment: Assessment of activities of daily living (ADL) and instrumental activities of daily living (IADL) abilities related to meal planning, shopping, preparation, and storage.

Although this approach may seem redundant, it yields more specific information for designing individualized interventions and is therefore more likely to be successful.

General guidelines for dietary counseling include:

Limiting fat and cholesterol.

Maintaining a balanced caloric intake.

Emphasizing the inclusion of grains.

Fruits and vegetables daily.

Ensuring an adequate calcium intake, especially for women.

A modified version of the food pyramid for older adults can serve as a guide. It is important to include information on portion size when using this, to avoid confusion and overfeeding (Fig. 2–1).

A plethora of information exists regarding the benefits and risks of exercise for older adults. Regular physical activity reduces morbidity and mortality resulting from coronary heart disease, hypertension, and obesity. It also helps to decrease the risk of developing non–insulin-dependent diabetes mellitus, retard the progress of bone loss, and improve mild to moderate affect disorders. Other benefits include increased muscle strength, flexibility, and balance; socialization potential; prevention of falls and fractures; and extension and enhancement of self-care capabilities and independence. These advantages are not limited to the community-dwelling elderly person; they have demonstrated efficacy in the long-term care setting as well.

From 40%–60% of older adults are sedentary. This inertia, combined with normal aging changes, results in deconditioning and impaired functioning. It also presents the health-care provider with the challenge of motivating patients to exercise. Individualizing counseling to the situation of the patient is helpful in this respect, as is writing a personal exercise prescription. Using the resources available via managed-care programs can provide subscribers with fitness center benefits and the services of a personal fitness trainer. For other, nonsubscribing,

TABLE 2-2 DETERMINE YOUR NUTRITIONAL HEALTH (NSI)

	YES
I have an illness or condition that made me change the kind and/or amount of food I eat.	2
I eat fewer than 2 meals per day.	3
I eat few fruits or vegetables, or milk products.	2
I have 3 or more drinks of beer, liquor or wine almost every day.	2
I have tooth or mouth problems that make it hard for me to eat.	2
I don't always have enough money to buy the food I need.	4
I eat alone most of the time.	1
I take 3 or more different prescribed or over-the-counter drugs a day.	1
Without wanting to, I have lost or gained 10 pounds in the last 6 months.	2
I am not always physically able to shop, cook and/or feed myself.	2
	TOTAL

Total Your Nutritional Score. If it's—

These materials developed and distributed by the Nutrition Screening Initiative, a project of:

0–2   Good! Recheck your nutritional score in 6 months.

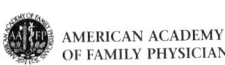 AMERICAN ACADEMY OF FAMILY PHYSICIANS

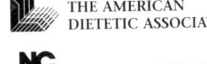 THE AMERICAN DIETETIC ASSOCIATION

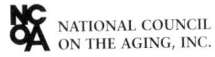 NATIONAL COUNCIL ON THE AGING, INC.

3–5   **You are at moderate nutritional risk.** See what can be done to improve your eating habits and lifestyle. Your office on aging, senior nutrition program, senior citizens center or health department can help. Recheck your nutritional score in 3 months.

6 or more   **You are at high nutritional risk.** Bring this checklist the next time you see your doctor, dietitian or other qualified health or social service professional. Talk with them about any problems you may have. Ask for help to improve your nutritional health.

Remember that warning signs suggest risk, but do not represent diagnosis of any condition.

Reprinted with permission by the Nutrition Screening Initiative, a project of the American Academy of Family Physicians, the American Dietetic Association, and the National Council on the Aging, Inc., and funded in part by a grant from Ross Products Division, Abbott Laboratories.

A Guide to Daily Food Choices

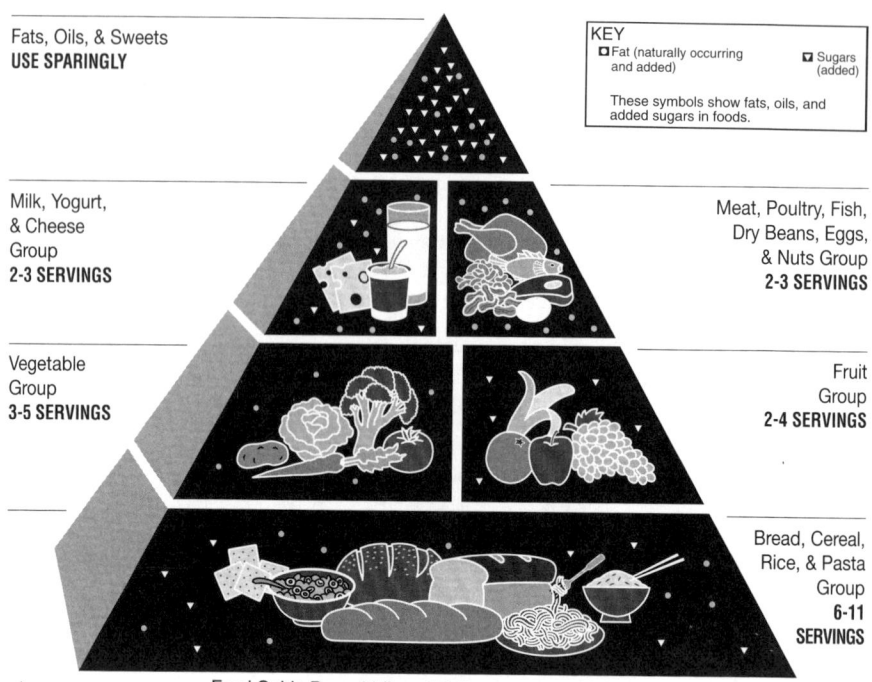

Food Guide Pyramid (from US Department of Agriculture).

FIGURE 2–1 Guide to daily food choices. Adapted from *Food Facts for Older Adults,* US Department of Agriculture, Human Nutrition Information Service, Home and Garden Bulletin #251.

patients, tailoring the plan to their health needs, interests, lifestyle, and available resources may achieve success. Group programs at community sites offer peer support and encouragement. Local schools or malls are often open before or after regular hours to provide indoor walking access. Knowledge of available resources is key in maximizing the moment of opportunity. Recent studies have demonstrated comparable benefits from a regimen of brief exercise periods spread throughout the day and longer periods at one time during the day. Research has also shown that any sustained increase in physical activity, even mild to moderate, is advantageous.

Before prescribing a personalized exercise plan, assess physical strength and weakness, using the history and physical examination. Table 2–3, Initial Evaluation of the Elderly Patient for Physical Activity Prescription, summarizes salient considerations. Authorities disagree on how much of a workup, if any, is needed before starting an exercise program. The American College of Sports Medicine advises

TABLE 2-3 INITIAL EVALUATION OF THE ELDERLY PATIENT FOR PHYSICAL ACTIVITY PRESCRIPTION

Objectives/Principles	Interventions	Tips to Suggest to Patients
Identify chronic disease or physical limitations that could affect exercise capabilities. Modified exercise is generally safe and will help maintain independence and quality of life.	Individualize the exercise program within the safety guidelines or physical limitations.	Monitor blood pressure and heart rate before, during, and after exercise. Exercise only when feeling well. Exercise 2 hours after eating a meal.
Modify physical activities to provide enjoyable and practical exercises so that exercise is more likely to be maintained.	Help the patient choose low- to moderate-impact exercises such as walking or swimming. Incorporate a variety of activities into the routine.	Begin slowly and increase duration gradually. Adjust exercise to the weather. Dress in comfortable clothes.
Set realistic program goals that the patient is likely to attain and continue.	Determine the elder's willingness to include exercise.	Walk with the Senior Citizens group three times a week.
Evaluate dietary history with emphasis on dietary inadequacies. Dietary inadequacies are common and may be compounded by modest increases in caloric expenditure due to increased activity.	Encourage patient to eat a regular balanced diet high in protein, minerals, and vitamins.	Stop exercising if faintness, upper body discomfort, and/or bone/joint pain occur.
Evaluate for potential injury. Degenerative joint disease is common in this age group. Neuropathy, gait disturbance, impaired equilibrium, orthostatic hypotension, and cardiovascular symptoms may be present.	Use assistive devices such as walkers with wheels to provide stability. Include range of motion and resistance training to increase stability.	
Review medications to avoid adverse interactions with activity program, in particular, note whether patient is taking: diuretics (can cause hypercalcemia, hypokalemia, arrhythmias, and volume depletion) beta blockers (can reduce exercise tolerance) tranquilizers (can cause orthostatic hypotension and dizziness and can impair thermoregulation) insulin (may require dose adjustment).	Teach the patient self-monitoring of HR, BP, respirations.	Monitor HR, BP, respirations. Drink enough water before and after exercise. Eat foods high in calcium and potassium. Take prescribed calcium and potassium supplements. Reduce the intensity of exercise. Take extra time for warming up and cooling down. Get up and down slowly. Eat high-carbohydrate snacks before exercising. Keep hard candy readily available.

Used with permission from M. Allison and C. Keller: Physical activity in the elderly: Benefits and intervention strategies, *The Nurse Practitioner* 22 (8): 53–69. © Springhouse Corporation.

an exercise stress test for anyone over age 60 who is beginning an exericise program. When the program consists of a gradual increase in activity, such as progressive walking, treadmill testing is usually unnecessary.

Healthy elderly individuals can follow a balanced exercise program comparable to that of younger adults, including aerobic, endurance, and strength training. To prevent injury, include warm-up and cool-down periods. The exercise prescription should have four components: intensity, frequency, duration, and mode of activity. Once the pattern of exercise has been established, your encouragement and the support from significant others are vital to its continuance.

Exercise in the frail elderly person should focus initially on muscle strengthening and flexibility. Premature attempts to mobilize without this could result in injury and sabotage the program altogether. Success of such a program also depends on the education of family and facility caregivers, changing their mindset from one of dependency to one of potential.

Counseling regarding dental health in the older patient includes the need for regular visits to the dental-care provider, daily flossing, and brushing with a fluoride toothpaste. Many elders have dentures and assume that dental checkups are no longer necessary. Oral screening for cancer is still indicated, as is periodic assessment of denture fit and functionality. Another concern is for the condition of the remaining teeth of some older adults. Periodontal disease, erosion of dentin, or other problems may render the teeth nonfunctional for chewing and a potential source for infection. Dependence on others for transportation or lack of availability of dental resources for those in long-term care settings further complicate the problem. Caregivers may simply overlook this aspect of preventive health, or financial considerations may preclude treatment. Patient and family education regarding dental health is essential.

Counsel older adults regarding safe sex and avoidance of high-risk behavior. Assumptions regarding lack of sexual expression in the healthy older adult are unfounded. With the possibility of pregnancy eliminated, many mature adults feel

TABLE 2–4 RISK FACTORS FOR FALLS IN THE ELDERLY

Physiologic	Environmental
Gait disturbances	Stairs
Poor vision	Pavement irregularities
Decreased muscle strength	Slippery surfaces (loose rugs)
Postural instability	Incorrect footwear
Cognitive impairment	Low chairs
Number of medications	Inadequate lighting
Psychoactive drugs	Unexpected objects
Antihypertensive drugs	
Multiple physiologic problems	

TABLE 2-5 HOME SAFETY CHECKLIST

Place a check mark next to each question if the answer is yes. Use this checklist to correct all hazards in the home.

Housekeeping

____ Do you clean up spills as soon as they occur?
____ Do you keep floors and stairways clean and free of clutter?
____ Do you put away books, magazines, sewing supplies, and other objects as soon as you are through with them and never leave them on floors or stairways?
____ Do you store frequently used items on shelves that are within easy reach?

Floors

____ Do you keep everyone from walking on freshly washed floors before they are dry?
____ If you wax floors, do you apply 2 thin coats and buff each thoroughly or use self-polishing wax?
____ Do all area rugs have nonslip backings?
____ Have you eliminated small rugs at the tops and bottoms of stairways?
____ Are all carpet edges tacked down?
____ Are rugs and carpets free of curled edges, worn spots, and rips?
____ Have you chosen rugs and carpets with short, dense pile?
____ Are rugs and carpets installed over good quality, medium-thick pads?

Lighting

____ Do you have light switches near every doorway?
____ Do you have enough good lighting to eliminate shadowy areas?
____ Do you have a lamp or light switch within easy reach of every bed?
____ Do you have night lights in your bathrooms and in hallways leading from bedrooms to bathrooms?
____ Are all stairways well lit with light switches at both top and bottom?

Bathrooms

____ Do you use a rubber mat or nonslip decals in tubs and showers?
____ Do you have a grab bar securely anchored over each tub and shower?
____ Do you have a nonslip rug on all bathroom floors?
____ Do you keep soap in easy-to-reach receptacles?

Traffic Lanes

____ Can you walk across every room in your home, and from one room to another, without detouring around furniture?
____ Is the traffic lane from your bedroom to the bathroom free of obstacles?
____ Are telephone and appliance cords kept away from areas where people walk?

(continued)

TABLE 2–5 (Continued)

Stairways

_____ Do securely fastened handrails extend the full length of the stairs on each side of the stairways?

_____ Do the handrails stand out from the walls so you can get a good grip?

_____ Are handrails distinctly shaped so you are alerted when you reach the end of a stairway?

_____ Are all stairways in good condition, with no broken, sagging, or sloping steps?

_____ Are all stairway carpeting and metal edges securely fastened and in good condition?

_____ Have you replaced any single-level steps with gradually rising ramps or made sure such steps are well lighted?

Ladders and Step Stools

_____ Do you always use a step stool or ladder that is tall enough for the job?

_____ Do you always set up your ladder or step stool on a firm, level base that is free of clutter?

_____ Before you climb a ladder or step stool, do you always make sure it is fully open and that the stepladder spreaders are locked?

_____ When you use a ladder or step stool, do you face the steps and keep your body between the side rails?

_____ Do you avoid standing on the top step of a step stool or climbing beyond the second step from the top on a stepladder?

Outdoor Areas

_____ Are walks and driveways in your yard and other areas free of breaks?

_____ Are lawns and gardens free of holes?

_____ Do you put away garden tools and hoses when they are not in use?

_____ Are outdoor areas kept free of rocks, loose boards, and other tripping hazards?

_____ Do you keep outdoor walkways, steps, and porches free of wet leaves and snow?

_____ Do you sprinkle icy outdoor areas with de-icers as soon as possible after a snowfall or freeze?

_____ Do you have mats at doorways for people to wipe their feet on?

_____ Do you know the safest way of walking when you can't avoid walking on a slippery surface?

Footwear

_____ Do your shoes have soles and heels that provide good traction?

_____ Do you avoid walking in stocking feet and wear house slippers that fit well and don't fall off?

_____ Do you wear low-heeled oxfords, loafers, or good-quality sneakers when you work in your house or yard?

_____ Do you replace boots or galoshes when their soles or heels are worn too smooth to keep you from slipping on wet or ice surfaces?

Personal Precautions

_____ Are you always alert for unexpected hazards, such as out-of-place furniture?

_____ If young children visit or live in your home, are you alert for children playing on the floor and toys left in your path?

_____ If you have pets, are you alert for sudden movements across your path and pets getting underfoot?

_____ When you carry packages, do you divide them into smaller loads and make sure they do not obstruct your vision?

_____ When you reach or bend, do you hold onto a firm support and avoid throwing your head back or turning it too far?

_____ Do you always move deliberately and avoid rushing to answer the phone or doorbell?

_____ Do you take time to get your balance when you change position from lying down to sitting and from sitting to standing?

_____ Do you keep yourself in good condition with moderate exercise, good diet, adequate rest, and regular medical checkups?

_____ If you wear glasses, is your prescription up to date?

_____ Do you know how to reduce injury in a fall?

_____ If you live alone, do you have daily contact with a friend or neighbor?

Adapted from: National Safety Council, _Falling—The Unexpected Trip: A Safety Program for Older Adults_ (Program Leader's Guide). Chicago: National Safety Council; 1982. Used with permission of the National Safety Council; copyright © 1982.

less restraint. Because of divorce or widowhood, they may seek satisfaction with new partners. Teach the patient about methods for safe sex, use of a barrier to avoid sexually transmitted diseases (STDs), including HIV and hepatitis B. Using the patient's sexual history, explore patient needs, preferences, and medical or psychological obstacles to sexual expression. This facilitates counseling and interventions to promote healthy sexuality.

Prevention of injury in the older patient is of paramount importance to continuing functionality and quality of life. Part of this counseling involves reinforcement of extant recommendations, including wearing lap and shoulder seatbelts in a motor vehicle, avoiding drinking and driving, having working smoke detectors in the residence, and keeping hot water set at less than 120°–130°F. For older adults who operate a motor vehicle, periodic assessment of their ongoing ability to perform this task safely is vital to the patient and the public at large. The largest number of accidents are those that involve the very young drivers and older drivers.

Two other recommendations are especially significant for the older adult. The first involves the safe storage and removal of firearms. Possession of a firearm combined with depression, caregiver stress, irreversible illness, or decline in functional abilities can invite self-inflicted injury, suicide pacts, or other acts of violence. Counsel patients to avoid firearms in the home and to use alternative means for self-protection such as alarm systems, pepper mace spray, and the like. Falls are the leading cause of nonfatal injuries and unintentional death from injury in older persons. Certain combinations of physiological and environmental factors place some patients at increased risk. About 85% of falls occur at home, in the later part of the day. Table 2–4 lists the known risk factors.

TABLE 2-6   WELLNESS SPIRITUALITY PROTOCOL

 I. Clinical Presentation:
   A. The extent and direction of the wellness spirituality assessment and spiritual wellness care is directed by how aging clients are responding to conditions in life or illness. These responses are, overtly or covertly, identified partly in the interview process as the clinician inquires about an aging client's chief complaint, present problem, and data about his or her personal and social history other than spirituality.
     1. Actively involved in life
     2. Heightened awareness of aging changes
     3. Separation from religious and cultural ties
     4. Challenges in beliefs and value system
     5. Disfigurement or altered body image
     6. Disability or loss of function
     7. Chronic pain
     8. Anger toward others or God
     9. Change in meaningful relationships
    10. Limitations imposed by situations or others
    11. Hospitalization or institutionalization
    12. Isolation or confinement
    13. Opposition or interference by caregivers or family caregiver
    14. Cognitive regression
II. Diagnosis/Evaluation
   A. History; Self-Actualization Activities
     1. What are the good things about growing older?
     2. What are the difficult things about growing older?
     3. On a scale of 0 to 10 (0 = very closely related; 10 = only slightly related), how do you feel about your life at the present time?

Boring	Rewarding	Hopeless
Lonely	Useless	Many friends
Hopeful	Interesting	Disappointing
Filled with guilt	Free from guilt	
Filled with worry	Free from worry	
Brings out the best in me—the worst in me		

     4. What are your plans for the future?
     5. Tell me about some of your personal achievements and other significant life experiences.
     6. What were the achievements that make (made) you feel proud?
     7. What is your role in the family now?
     8. What bothers you most about your present circumstances?
     9. What are you doing to cope with your present circumstances?
   B. History: Connectedness Activities
     1. What helps you keep in touch with nature and the world?
     2. What do you hope to leave to your family or this world?
     3. Who or what do you turn to for help?
     4. Have you had the opportunity to help a family member, close relative, or disabled or elderly person in the past 12 months?
     5. Have you had the opportunity to visit a sick or shut-in person who is not a family member?
   C. History: Healing and New Life Activities
     1. What else is going on in your life?
     2. What about being sick has been most troublesome?

3. Have you found a meaning for your life? How does it make you feel?
4. Is there anything particularly frightening or meaningful to you now?
5. What are some of the things you look forward to each day?
6. In what way do you enjoy the people in your life?
7. What do you like about being alone?
8. In what way do others show they care for you?
9. What do you do to show you care for them?
10. Do you have a role in saving our environment?
11. What are some of the things that give you a strong sense of fulfillment?
12. What in your daily life brings you a sense of closeness to God or a sense of relationship with a higher being?
13. What is God's role in all of this?

D. History: Religious or Humanistic Activities
1. In what or who do you find hope and strength?
2. Who or what brings you joy and laughter?
3. Who or what gives you a sense of peace and harmony?
4. How would you describe your current relationship with a church or spiritual community?
5. In what way is prayer, Scripture, meditation, religious reading, or music helpful to you?
6. Does your relationship with God or a higher being contribute to your sense of well-being?
7. Do religious rituals or sacraments improve your well-being?
8. Is God or your religion helpful to you at this time in your life?

III. Plan/Management
A. Consult or refer when clinician recognizes that the activities or work of the spirit would be served better through contact with clergy, a spiritual leader, or a parish nurse.
B. Treatment to support or restore self-actualization.
1. Listen, encourage, affirm, and support.
2. Respect habits of personal hygiene or attire that have special significance.
3. Discuss anxieties and concerns about the future.
4. Obtain life history to assist creative expression of aging clients' experiences.
5. Arrange visits from those who appreciate them.
6. Recommend assistive mobility aids to support independence.
7. Arrange for guidance in taping their memories and autobiography.
8. Review life accomplishments through reminiscence.
9. Teach and practice methods of visual imagery of life accomplishments.
C. Treatment to support or restore connectedness
1. Suggest ways for sharing self with others (e.g., a meal with another).
2. Promote awareness of the world around them (e.g., sitting and observing traffic or pigeons on the roof carry on their wooing).
3. Arrange for mentorships, bartering activities, and sharing their talents.
4. Encourage reminiscence through music, pictures, and religious symbols (e.g., crosses, rosaries, menorahs).
5. Encourage storytelling with adults and children.
6. Suggest letter "writing" by tape to grandchildren and friends.
7. Facilitate regular contacts with nearby neighbors, clubs, and social groups.
8. Recommend calling others who need help.
9. Arrange for converting a legacy into some tangible form (i.e., photograph albums, taped memories).

(continued)

TABLE 2–6   (*Continued*)

10. Stimulate interest in writing letters to politicians.
11. Advise serving in volunteer capacities.
D. Treatment to support or restore healing and new life
  1. Encourage dialogue and sharing painful memories and events with another.
  2. Perform or arrange for therapeutic touch.
  3. Encourage discussion of anxieties and uncertainties.
  4. Inquire about future plans.
  5. Foster anticipation of enjoyment from everyday events.
E. Treatment to support or restore religious and humanistic activities orientation
  1. Promote the possibility of gardening with what is available to them (i.e., garden spot, windowsill, flowerpot).
  2. Identify avenues for them to participate in recycling.
  3. Support prayer or meditation.
  4. Advise journal keeping.
  5. Advocate time alone.
  6. Arrange for access to religious or spiritual articles and religious ceremonies.

Used with permission from M.C. Leetun: Wellness spirituality in the older adult, *The Nurse Practitioner* 22 (8):60–70, © Springhouse Corporation.

Evaluation of risk factors and a home safety assessment by a home health nurse or a geriatric assessment team can provide direction for preventive intervention and education (Table 2–5). Potential recommendations include exercise programs to build strength, modification of environmental hazards, monitoring and adjusting of medications, external protection against falling on hard surfaces, and measures to increase bone density. If urinary incontinence is a contributing factor, a urologic workup may be indicated. Falls are often alarming to patients and families; in some cases, family members may desire nursing home placement for the patient because of a fall. In other cases, patients may be fearful of ambulation as a result of a fall. Falls also pose a challenge in the long-term care environment. The use of active restraining devices does not prevent falls; in fact, some patients are injured further because of the restraints. However, families may insist on restraining the patient for safety. Education and counseling combined with an assessment of the patient environment is helpful. Keeping water, call bell, telephone, and other necessities available, and toileting regularly, can minimize the potential for falling.

Health promotion in older adults can be expanded to include presence or absence of social and financial support systems, completion of an advanced directive, and evaluation of spiritual needs. The latter area, wellness spirituality, has recently been discussed in detail by one of our own colleagues (Leetun, 1996), who identified four key domains for assesssment: self-actualization activities, connectedness activities, healing and new life activities, and religious and humanistic orientation activities. A wellness spirituality protocol is organized around these domains to promote spiritual health and wholeness (Table 2–6).

BIBLIOGRAPHY

Alessi, CA, et al: The process of care in preventive in-home comprehensive geriatric assessment. J Am Geriatr Soc 45(9):1044–1050, 1997.

Allison, M, and Keller, C: Physical activity in the elderly: Benefits and intervention strategies. Nurse Pract 22(8):53–69, 1997.

Buchner, DM, et al: Effects of physical activity on health status in older adults. Annu Rev Public Health 13:469–488, 1992.

Fiatarone, MA, O'Brien, K, and Rich, BSE: Exercise Rx for a healthier old age. Patient Care 30(16):145–158, 1996.

Frenn, M: Older adults' experience of health promotion: A theory for nursing practice. Public Health Nurs 13(1):65–71, 1996.

Johnson, RM, Kaiser, FE, Kerstetter, JE, and Reuben, DB: Maintaining good nutrition in the elderly. Patient Care 29(21):46–60.

Kolcaba, K, and Wykle, M: Health promotion in long-term care facilities. Geriatr Nurs 15:266–270, 1994.

Kotthoff-Burrell, E: Health promotion and disease prevention for the older adult: An overview of the current recommendations and a practical application. Nurse Pract Forum 3(4):195–209, 1992.

Leetun, MC: Wellness spirituality in the older adult: Assessment and intervention protocol. Nurse Pract 21(8):60–70, 1996.

Pender, NJ: Health Promotion in Nursing Practice, ed 3. Appleton & Lange, Stamford, CT, 1996.

Pizzi, ER, and Wolf, ZR: Health risks and health promotion for older women: Utility of a health promotion diary. Holistic Nurs Practice 12(2):62–72, 1998.

Steiner, JP: Preventive medicine. In Jahnigen, DW, and Schrier, RW (eds): Geriatric Medicine, ed 2. Blackwell Science, Cambridge, MA, 1997.

Uriri, JT, and Thatcher-Winger, R: Health risk appraisal and the older adult. J Gerontol Nurs 21(5):25–31, 1995.

US Department of Health and Human Services, Public Health Service: Clinician's Handbook of Preventive Services, ed 2. Government Printing Office, Washington, DC, 1996.

US Department of Health and Human Services, Public Health Service, Agency for Health Care Policy and Research: Clinical Practice Guideline Number 18: Smoking Cessation, AHCPR Publication No 96-0692, Rockville, MD, 1996.

US Preventive Services Task Force: US Task Force Guide to Clinical Preventive Services, ed 2. Williams & Wilkins, Baltimore, 1996.

CHAPTER **3**

NUTRITION

Few advanced-practice nurses and physicians believe they have been adequately prepared to assess, identify, and manage nutritional problems in elderly individuals. Fortunately, more emphasis has been placed on researching the nutritional needs and concerns in the older age group. A major effort to facilitate use of this new information in clinical practice is the Nutritional Screening Initiative (NSI). A collaborative project of the American Dietetic Association, the American Academy of Family Physicians, and the National Council on Aging, the NSI was started in 1990 in response to the Healthy People 2000 goals. The tools of the NSI provide the clinician with a systematic approach to identify and treat nutritional problems. This initiative represents a major step in addressing this growing issue.

Reasons for older adults' being at higher risk for poor nutrition include physical, functional, social, and environmental factors. Nutritional deficiency and excessive calorie intake contribute to disease and disability in elderly persons. Dietary factors are associated with five of the ten leading causes of death in older adults: coronary artery disease, some types of cancer, stroke, non–insulin-dependent diabetes, and atherosclerosis. Diet is also associated with risk factors of obesity and hypertension. Teaching the elderly good nutritional practices does not begin at the tertiary level, when poor nutrition is evident. Screening for and early detection of nutritional inadequacies and teaching elderly persons primary preventative nutritional strategies remain important. The goals for nutritional health may need to be modified for the aged population. Certainly the strategies used to achieve these goals must address the multifactorial issues involved.

Principles of a Healthy Diet

The U.S. Department of Agriculture and the U.S. Department of Health and Human Services provide seven guidelines for meal planning and eating that are intended to guide healthy Americans in their food choices.

DIETARY GUIDELINES FOR AMERICANS

- Eat a variety of foods.
- Maintain healthy weight.
- Choose a diet low in fat, saturated fat, and cholesterol.
- Choose a diet with plenty of vegetables, fruits, and grain products.
- Use sugars only in moderation.
- Use salt and sodium only in moderation.
- If you drink alcoholic beverages, do so in moderation.

In 1992, the U.S. Department of Agriculture replaced "food groups" with the "food pyramid," which serves as another educational tool for the food consumer (see Fig. 2–1).

Although these tools may seem simplistic, they target what is known about the common deficiencies and excesses in the typical American diet. Dietary patterns for old adults are usually similar to those of younger adults: intake of total fat, saturated fat, refined carbohydrates, and sodium is generally higher than recommended, and intake of complex carbohydrate and fiber is lower than recommended.

Risk Factors Influencing Nutritional Health

Poor nutritional status is not inevitable with the process of aging. Many factors, including the prevalence of diseases and medications taken for these diseases, as well as social and environmental changes, have a greater impact on nutritional habits and status than does aging itself. Physiological aging, however, can influence nutritional health. With aging, body composition changes, resulting in a decrease in lean body mass and an increase in total body fat. As the lean body mass decreases, the basic metabolic rate also decreases. Total body fluid level declines with age, and older individuals exhibit less thirst than do younger adults. A loss of taste buds and, to a greater extent, loss of sense of smell have been documented. The functional impact of these age-related sensory changes on nutrition is thought to be minor, however.

A relationship between low income and poor nutritional status has consistently been demonstrated. Reasons for this relationship include the lack of appropriate variety and nutrient density in foods selected, insufficient calorie intake to meet energy needs, and an excessive intake of refined carbohydrates, fat, and cholesterol among elderly persons of low income. Living alone, especially for men, appears to be associated with a low intake of calories. In some studies lifestyle was the most important predictor of dietary intake in old age (Horwath, 1991). Encouraging elderly individuals to participate in various activities and clubs and to share meals with friends or neighbors may be far more effective in improving dietary intake than giving simple dietary advice.

Alcoholism, estimated at a prevalence of 10% in older adults, can contribute to nutritional deficiencies. Malnutrition associated with alcoholism comes from displacement by alcohol of nutrient-dense foods, alcohol-induced appetite changes, limited access to food, and increased nutrient requirements caused by alcohol's metabolic effects. Alcohol-associated malnutrition may be more problematic in low-income elderly persons because higher-income alcohol users tend to add alcohol to nutrients in the diet, whereas lower-income alcohol users tend to replace the nutrients with alcohol. Medical and surgical conditions most often associated with poor nutrition are listed in Table 3–1. Remember: sometimes the disease affects the appetite and sometimes it affects the person's functional ability to obtain and eat proper foods.

Physical impairments such as decreased mobility, blindness, and poor dentition are also important risk factors for malnutrition. Nearly half of individuals over age 65 have no teeth and those individuals wearing dentures may have problems with them as bone loss occurs. With better dental care and fluoride in the water systems, older adults are keeping their teeth longer but with increasing rates of periodontal disease and root caries over time.

Lack of physical exercise contributes to body fat accumulation, and body fat accumulation contributes to the lack of physical exercise. Sarcopenia, the age-related loss of skeletal muscle mass, results in decreased strength, aerobic capacity, and thus, functional capacity. Sarcopenia is closely linked to elevated body fat content, as well as to age-related losses in bone mineral and decreased basal metabolic rate and to inadequate dietary protein intake. This process is not inevitable. Nutritional benefit derived from regular exercise includes reduced body fat, increased basal metabolic rate, and increased caloric intake, which increases the likelihood that essential nutrients will be consumed. Even up to age 96, men and women can respond to resistance training with a substantial (>200%) increase in strength and muscle size.

Medications often taken by elderly persons such as corticosteroids, immunosuppressants, hypercholesterolemics, antihypertensives, and anticonvulsants can affect nutrition. Many prescribed and over-the-counter (OTC) medications taken by older individuals have anticholinergic side effects, including dry mouth and constipation, which can influence nutritional status. Anorexia is a side effect of

TABLE 3–1   MEDICAL AND SURGICAL CONDITIONS ASSOCIATED WITH POOR NUTRITION IN ELDERLY PERSONS

Burns	Neurologic impairments
Cancer	Respiratory diseases
Arthritis	Congestive heart failure
Dementias	Renal or hepatic failure
Depression	Gastrointestinal disorders
Metabolic diseases (diabetes, thyroid)	Surgical procedures

some drugs commonly prescribed for elderly persons, including the cardiac drug digitalis and the new selective serotonin reuptake inhibitors (SSRIs) often given for depression. Drugs known to stimulate the appetite include chlorpromazine, insulin, lithium carbonate, thioridazine, and prednisone. More than 60% of elderly persons take laxatives, the majority of which are OTC medications that can lead to malabsorption, potassium deficiency, and cathartic bowel.

Hospitalization often has a negative impact on nutritional status. The patient who is slightly compromised on admission may become acutely malnourished as metabolic needs increase and intake often decreases. Protein energy malnutrition is the most underdiagnosed nutritional disorder worldwide, and the individual at highest risk is the older adult who has been hospitalized 2 weeks or longer. If nutritional needs are not met 2 to 3 days of the onset of acute illness, the declines in immune, hepatic, and gastrointestinal function appear to contribute significantly to increased morbidity, mortality, and prolonged hospital stays.

In nursing homes, most residents are at risk nutritionally. More than two-thirds of older people in nursing homes have dementia; they may forget to eat, be unable to make good choices in food selection, or become too impaired to feed themselves. It is estimated that nearly half of elderly individuals in nursing homes are depressed, another contributor to inadequate intake. Although only 2% of older people living in the community cannot feed themselves when food is placed in front of them, more than one-third of institutionalized residents require feeding assistance. Malnutrition has been documented in as many as 55% of nursing home residents.

Nutritional Needs

Food-energy requirements are related more to energy expenditure than to age. Much information regarding nutrient requirements for elderly people is still unknown. The nutritional needs of 70-year-olds vary considerably more than those of 3-year-olds; therefore, establishing definitive guidelines for this more diverse cohort remains a challenge.

Recommended daily allowances (RDAs) are the level of intake of essential nutrients that are adequate to meet the nutrient needs of most healthy adults. RDAs were established primarily to evaluate the nutritional status of groups of individuals rather than a single individual. The most recent update was in 1989 by the National Research Council Subcommittee. The guidelines are both age- and gender-specific; the adult categories currently include 25- to 50-year-olds and those age 51 and older. The Subcommittee considered an over-70 age group category, but there remained insufficient support at the time to include specific guidelines for elderly individuals.

RDAs are provided for energy, protein, 11 vitamins, and seven minerals. These daily nutritional allowances are neither minimal requirements nor ideal standards. The margins for each level (except energy) were set at +2 standard deviation (SD) higher than average, to meet the needs of 98% of the defined population. The RDAs do not take into account disease or disability states or other problems that might influence the individual's ability to obtain, consume, and use nutrients.

ENERGY

Energy requirements decline with age because lean body mass, resting energy expenditure, and general activity level decrease. The average reduction in energy is about 12 cal/m^2 per hr between ages 20 and 90. The current RDA for energy allowance for persons over age 51 is 1.5 multiplied by resting energy expenditure (REE), assuming a moderate amount of physical activity is maintained. The energy allowance for an average-size man is 2300 kcal/day; for a woman 1900 kcal/day. Representing a 20% reduction for the over-50 man and a 15% reduction for the over-50 woman. No specific guidelines exist for how these calories ought to be distributed, but general consensus, based on the RDA for protein and need for sufficient vitamins and minerals, is that 12% to 15% are in the form of protein, 55% to 60% carbohydrates, and a maximum of 30% fats.

Greater physical activity increases the thermic exercise response and therefore increases the energy needs. Exercise training not only increases thermogenesis of activity but also may increase the REE levels. The energy needs of active elderly persons may not be any less than those of their younger colleagues.

PROTEIN

Although the 1989 RDA recommends 0.8 g protein per kilogram of body weight, studies of nitrogen balance show that protein needs may be greater in elderly persons. Efficiency of protein use is diminished in older adults, and 0.9 to 1.0 g/kg of body weight has been proposed instead.

CARBOHYDRATES

An RDA is not defined for carbohydrate intake. Sufficient glucose is needed to prevent ketosis. Typical recommendations are that carbohydrates make up 55% to 60% of total calorie intake, with the majority in the form of complex carbohydrates that contain the necessary vitamins and minerals. Older adults with insulin resistance or diabetes should limit their intake of simple carbohydrates. Intake of more complex carbohydrates, particularly those containing soluble fiber, should be encouraged.

FATS

Fats provide the most efficient energy source, with twice the energy content per gram of carbohydrates or proteins. The RDAs for essential fatty acids can be met with 2% of calorie intake, but general recommendations are that total fat be limited to 30%. Recommendations for cholesterol intake are determined on an individual basis because extremely high or extremely low cholesterol intake is associated with an increased risk of death. Age-related increases in serum total cholesterol and low-density lipoprotein are seen after the fourth decade and then level off after age 70. High-density lipoprotein levels remain constant over time.

FIBER

Because fiber is not a nutrient, it has no RDA for intake. For good gastrointestinal function, the American Cancer Society recommends a daily intake range from 25 to 35 g from both soluble and insoluble sources. Insolubles (e.g., bread, cereal, skins of fruit, vegetables) include cellulose and lignin that bind with water and cause bulkier, larger stools. Solubles (e.g., fruits, legumes, oat bran) dissolve and thicken in water; they contain pectin and gums that are broken down by bacteria in the large intestine, which results in increased fecal mass caused by bacterial growth. The solubles also decrease blood glucose and plasma cholesterol levels. Because fiber can impair bioavailability of the minerals zinc, calcium, and iron, specific instructions should be given to the patient to include foods that cause less mineral impairment (i.e., carrots, peas, turnips, cabbage, potatoes).

WATER

Fluid requirements do not change with age, but older adults are less likely to take in the necessary amount of water. Dehydration is common in this age group. Older individuals should take a minimum of 1.5 to 2 L of fluids daily, or an amount sufficient to maintain urine osmolarity below 800 mOsm/L, at which the urine will be a clear light yellow. Past habits also influence water intake. Some elderly individuals, fearing leakage of urine, take in insufficient quantities of fluids.

VITAMINS

No vitamin requirements are established specific to the elderly; however, vitamin deficiencies are common. Often subclinical deficiencies occur in ill and debilitated older adults, those taking medications that interfere with vitamin absorption, and those ingesting limited amounts of fruits and vegetables. More than one-half of the elderly population take vitamin supplements. Because these may be toxic when taken in high doses and may interfere with nutrients or medications, vitamin supplements should be carefully reviewed by the clinician.

The fat-soluble vitamins include vitamins A, D, K, and E. Vitamin A levels are rarely deficient in elderly persons. Although surveys show that many older people take less than the RDA for vitamin A, few studied participants had low serum levels of vitamin A. Vitamin A, an antioxidant known as retinol, helps maintain vision and tissue growth. The carotenoids (vitamin A food groups) have also been shown to reduce cancer risk.

Vitamin D RDA levels may be too low for elderly persons. Lack of sunlight and impaired skin synthesis of precholecalciferol caused by advanced age, along with low serum parathyroid hormone (PTH) levels and related bone loss, suggest that the recommended 5 μg/day may be too low for the many older adults who are not exposed to sunlight. To reduce age-related bone loss, the housebound or institutionalized older person may need low-dose (10 μg/day) vitamin D supplements. Adequate vitamin D can be obtained from 15 minutes of sun exposure daily, or longer in cloudy or polluted environments.

Vitamin K is required for the synthesis of prothrombin. Although the incidence of an abnormal prothrombin time increases with age, it is not necessary to increase the amount of vitamin K beyond 1 μg/day currently recommended. Because absorption of vitamin K is affected by mineral oil ingestion, the clinician should consider this when the patient takes this laxative regularly.

The interest in vitamin E has grown, this vitamin has been touted as one retarding the aging process. Although studies have shown that as many as 40% of elderly individuals do not meet the RDA for vitamin E, few have low serum levels of this vitamin. There is growing evidence that there may be some cardiovascular protective effect to vitamin E supplementation beyond that suggested by the current RDA. A protective effect against Alzheimer's disease is also being studied. Controlled clinical trials in both of these areas are under way, so it is premature to suggest a change in RDAs at this time.

The water-soluble vitamins include the B vitamins, vitamin C, niacin, and folate. Vitamin B_1 (thiamine) has a role in the metabolism of glucose and fatty acids. Thiamine intake for most healthy older adults appears to be adequate. Elderly individuals in the community and in geriatric facilities, whose food intake is low or alcohol intake is high, however, may be thiamine deficient.

Vitamin B_2 (riboflavin) is required for oxidation-reduction reactions of metabolism. Age-related changes in the need for riboflavin are unfounded, although low dietary intake of this vitamin is common in elderly individuals. Because exercisers may have a greater vitamin B_2 requirement, adequate intake in the athletic older adult should be ensured.

Vitamin B_6 (pyridoxine) is essential for maintaining the production of antibodies and for nerve functioning. Many older adults have low intakes of vitamin B_6 that may not resolve completely with replacement. Research in this area is needed. Riboflavin needs may be greater in the smoker, those who consume large amounts of alcohol or protein, or those taking estrogens.

Vitamin B_{12} (cobalamin) is needed for hemopoiesis, DNA synthesis, and nerve function. Even though serum vitamin B_{12} levels decline with age, they still appear to remain within normal limits. Patients who are strict vegetarians, and those with pernicious anemia, atrophic gastritis, and pancreatic disease are at greater risk for vitamin B_{12} deficiency.

Vitamin C (ascorbic acid) is important in forming collagen and cartilage. Additional vitamin C intake is not necessary for the healthy older individual. Smoking, stress, and certain medications can increase the risk of deficiency.

Niacin deficiency is rare in those who consume adequate animal protein. Low-income and sick elderly persons may be at higher risk for niacin insufficiency. Niacin may also help reduce blood lipid levels.

Folate intake varies widely, and deficiency is rare except in patients consuming alcohol or medications that alter folate absorption and use. The role of folate in maintaining normal serum homocysteine levels is being investigated and a possible cardiovascular protective effect is being explored.

MINERALS

The mineral RDAs generally ensure adequate intake for older persons. There may be reason for concern in three areas of mineral RDAs; iron, calcium, and zinc. Inadequacies of these minerals should be reviewed.

Because iron stores tend to increase with age, when iron deficiency occurs it is most often due to bleeding or inflammatory disease. Older individuals with low caloric intake, low animal protein intake, or high tea intake (which reduces iron absorption), as well as those with acchlorhydria, may have iron deficits.

Calcium is the nutrient most often found inadequate in the diet. The primary source of calcium is dairy products. Elderly men and women often take less than the RDA for calcium. The requirements may be greater among elderly individuals, owing to decreased calcium absorption, decreased physical activity, and significant bone loss. Calcium intakes of 1200 to 1500 g/day have been recommended. Lactose intolerance is often overlooked as a potential contributor to inadequate calcium intake.

Zinc intakes decline with advanced age. Little is known about zinc except that impaired cellular immune response and wound healing may be related to zinc deficiency. Hospitalized patients have shown 27% lower zinc levels than healthy elderly persons. Individuals who consume alcohol, take diuretics, or have wound healing problems may need zinc supplements.

Nutritional Screening and Assessment

The purpose of nutritional screening is to determine the adequacy of intake. The nutritional screen includes a history and a physical examination and an evaluation of social and environmental factors that might influence nutritional status. For persons whose initial screens generate an index of suspicion, nutritional assessment is conducted. The NSI developed a checklist (see Table 2–2) to help the older adult or the caregiver determine if the older person is at nutritional risk. The checklist gathers information about illness and function, medications, weight change, and influencing social factors. This self-scored screen encourages those at moderate to high nutritional risk to seek appropriate counseling.

If nutritional risk is apparent, a nutritional assessment should be completed. The nutritional assessment includes a clinical assessment and more detailed dietary intake review along with anthropometric measurements, and a biochemical profile. During the physical examination, the clinician should be alert to the potential for nutritional problems (Table 3–2). Developed by the NSI, Table 3–2 assists the clinician in completing a more comprehensive risk profile. During the clinical examination, the clinician should evaluate the impact of disease, function, and social changes on food intake.

DIETARY INTAKE

A detailed record of dietary intake is the cornerstone of nutritional assessment. Assessing dietary intake by patient recall can pose a problem in geriatric patients with cognitive or communication impairments. A 24-hour diet recall is not as valuable as a 3-day dietary intake record. The patient should be asked specifically about intake at each meal, any dietary supplements taken, food preferences, intolerances, and allergies. Asking the patient if any foods are being avoided, and if so, why and for how long, can provide the clues to identify specific vitamin, mineral, or protein deficiency. The dietary intake record should also include questions about alcohol and caffeine consumption. The completed dietary intake record should be reviewed, interpreted, and analyzed by a registered dietitian.

ANTHROPOMETRICS

Anthropometry is the measurement of the body's physical dimensions and gross composition. Repeated anthropometric measurements provide information on the variations in nutritional status over time. These measurements and procedures must be standardized, and the clinician completing these must be skilled in the implementation of these standards.

Weight, the most common anthropometric measurement, is not always the best indicator of nutritional status in the elderly. Body weight measurement alone does not distinguish between body size and body composition. Weight should be measured, preferably on a calibrated scale, weekly if the patient is at risk nutritionally and every few months if the patient is nutritionally stable. The body mass index (BMI, Fig. 3–1), a weight-stature index, is used in the diagnosis of obesity and protein energy malnutrition. For healthy adults, most assessment standards look for a range of between 22 and 27. Controversy exists on BMI ranges for older persons; however, studies show an increase in relative mortality with BMI below 20 and above 30.

Height is more difficult to measure in older adults because height decreases as much as 3 inches by age 85, primarily as a result of shortening of the spinal column. Older adults often report their height as it was in their youth, and studies show that elderly men and women overestimate their height (Mohs, 1994). Therefore, the clinician must obtain an exact current height measurement. For those unable to stand erect, alternative methods for estimating the individual's height include measurements of arm span, total arm length, and knee-ankle ratios;

TABLE 3–2   KEY CLINICAL, DIETARY, AND ANTHROPOMETRIC
DATA REQUIRED TO EVALUATE A PATIENT'S
RISK OF NUTRITIONAL PROBLEMS

Height (inches)
Weight (lb)
% Desirable body weight
Body mass index
Weight loss/gain in 6 months
Clinical features
  Difficulty chewing or swallowing
  Problems with mouth, teeth, or gums
  Skin changes suggest malnutrition
  Angular stomatitis
  Glossitis
  History of bone pain
  Bone fractures
Living environment
  Annual income less than $6000/
    person
  Lives alone
  Concerned about home security
  Inadequate heating or cooling
  No stove or refrigerator
  Unable or prefers not to spend money
    on food
Functional status: Needs assistance with
  Bathing
  Dressing
  Continence
  Toileting
  Eating
  Ambulation
  Transportation
  Food preparation
  Shopping
Mental/cognitive status
  Mini-mental examination indicates
    impairment (score <26)
  Depression scale suggests depression
    (Beck <15, GDS >5)

Drug use
  More than 3 prescription drugs
  More than 3 nonprescription drugs
  Vitamin and mineral supplements
Dietary data
  Does not have enough food each day
  Number of days per month without any food
  Poor appetite
  Usually eats alone
  Special dietary needs
    Self-defined
    Prescribed
    Problems with compliance/meeting special
      needs
  Multiple diet prescriptions
  Other unusual dietary practices
Usual daily food intake
  Fewer than 2 servings of milk or dairy products
  Fewer than 2 servings of meat/poultry/fish/eggs
  Fewer than 2 servings of fruit/juice
  Fewer than 3 servings of vegetables
  Fewer than 6 servings of bread/cereals/grains
  More than 2 ounces of alcohol for men
  More than 1 ounce of alcohol for women
Laboratory and anthropometric data
  Serum albumin less than 3.5 g/dL
  Serum cholesterol less than 160 mg/dL
  Serum cholesterol greater than 240 mg/dL
  Triceps skinfold thickness below 10% of desirable
  Mid-arm muscle circumference below 10% of
    desirable

Source: *Adapted from* Nutrition Screening Initiative: Nutrition Interventions Manual for Professionals Caring for Older Americans. Washington, DC, Nutrition Screening Initiative, 1992; with permission of the Nutrition Screening Initiative, a project of the American Academy of Family Physicians, The American Dietetic Association, and the National Council on the Aging, and funded in part by a grant from Ross Laboratories, a division of Abbott Laboratories; with permission.

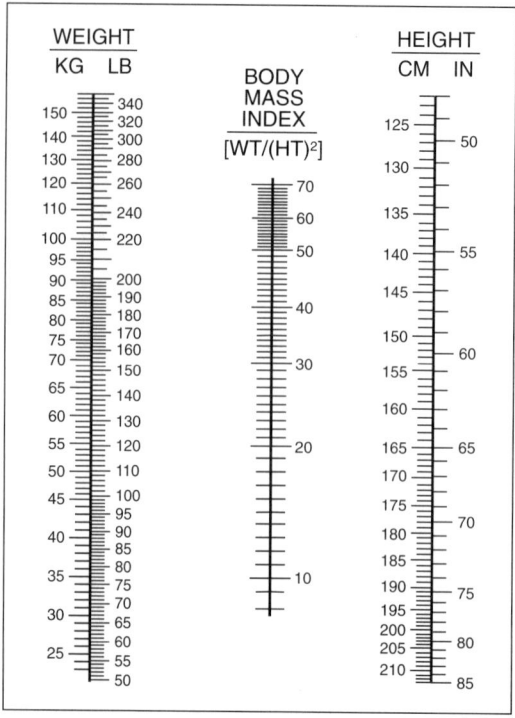

WEIGHT
KG   LB

BODY
MASS
INDEX
[WT/(HT)²]

HEIGHT
CM   IN

FIGURE 3–1 Nomogram for body mass index.

nomograms have been developed for these calculations. Bony chest breadth as measured by radiography may be a useful indicator of frame size, fat-free mass, and relative fatness.

Skinfold thickness provides a simple measure to assess muscle and fat mass. The triceps skinfold (TSF) measurement and mid-arm circumference (MAC) are the tools used the most; standards have been established for these. The TSF, measured by calipers, indirectly measures adipose tissue stores. MAC, measured in centimeters using a flexible tape measure, reflects somatic protein stores. For skinfold measurements to have validity and reliability, initial and subsequent readings should be obtained by the same clinician. Because this is often not possible, skinfold thickness may not be a practical measure.

BIOCHEMICAL PROFILE

Laboratory data are the most objective of nutritional information. The nutritional status changes reflected in laboratory data are seen earlier than with any other measurement method. The creatinine height index (CHI) compares the value of urinary creatinine with a standard based on an ideal excretion value for a person of the same height. In the absence of renal impairment, the CHI provides some prediction of muscle protein status. The 24-hour urinary creatinine excretion test is used to reflect lean body mass. The creatinine arm index (CAI) takes into account ideal body weight based on wrist circumferences and total arm length and has been used as an alternative to CHI.

Blood parameters include albumin, prealbumin, transferrin, and retinol-binding protein. Supplementary values include the blood urea nitrogen (BUN) creatinine, hemoglobin, hematocrit, iron, iron-binding capacity and sometimes cholesterol and total lymphocyte count. Albumin reflects the decline in protein status caused by a decline in the rate of protein synthesis. Albumin, a protein that is included in routine blood panels, is sensitive to changes in nutritional status and is consequently a good initial screening test of protein stores. It has a long half-life (17 to 21 days), it is not sensitive to acute malnutrition and should not be used to monitor the early effectiveness of protein supplementation. Table 3–3 includes the normal ranges of these values and the level of significance of abnormality.

Measuring transferrin, with its shorter half-life (8 to 10 days), is a better monitoring tool than measuring albumin. Albumin and transferrin readings may be affected by hydration status, renal failure, heart failure, bedrest, inflammation, or infection. Measurement of prealbumin (2-day half-life) and retinol-binding protein (12-hour half-life) are more sensitive indices of recent dietary protein deficiency than are transferrin or albumin. Prealbumin levels might be checked weekly if the clinician is monitoring the response to nutritional intervention.

Additional blood testing may be conducted if indicated. Hematologic tests measuring values for hemoglobin, hematocrit, iron, iron binding capacity may reflect anemia. A low cholesterol level, which may indicate a malnourished state, is a significant predictor of morbidity and mortality. A high cholesterol level should alert the clinician to the potential for heart disease. A lymphocyte count is available on a complete blood count (CBC) with differential. Low lymphocyte values, which can indicate immune suppression, should be evaluated. An anergy panel, to look for cell-mediated immunity, may be needed.

A single abnormal index does not constitute a diagnosis of nutritional deficiency. The clinical examination, along with the history of food intake and anthropometric and biochemical measures, provides the screening and assessment pa-

TABLE 3–3 PROTEIN LABORATORY VALUES AND SIGNIFICANCE

Lab Screened	Estimated Half-Life	Normal Value	Deficit: Mild	Deficit: Moderate	Deficit: Severe
Albumin (g/dL)	7–21 days	3.5–5.0	3.5–3.2	3.2–2.8	<2.8
Transferrin (mg/dL)	8–10 days	180–369	200–180	180–160	<160

rameters needed to determine if the patient has or is at risk for developing a nutritional disorder. The patient's level of physical activity must be assessed to determine his or her energy requirements.

Indicators of Poor Nutritional Health

During the nutritional screening and assessment, the clinician should check if any symptoms or signs of a nutritional deficit are present (Tables 3–4, 3–5).

In individuals over age 65, a BMI of less than 20 or greater than 30 is a significant indicator of poor nutrition. Both obesity and malnutrition are concerns. An estimated 25% of all older men and 33% of all older women are obese.

Protein-energy malnutrition (PEM) occurs when the intake of calories and protein is insufficient or when sufficient carbohydrate carlories are taken at the expense of protein calories. The usual indicators of PEM are weight loss, loss of muscle mass, and hypoproteinemia (if long-standing PEM exists). Anemia and cutaneous anergy may also be present. Weight loss is also common in elderly individuals. A high level of concern exists if the weight loss is involuntary and if it is greater than 10% of total body weight in 6 months, 7.5% in 3 months, or 5% in 1 month. Table 3–6 defines parameters associated with common nutritional problems in institutionalized older persons.

TABLE 3–4   SYMPTOMS AND SIGNS OF A NUTRITIONAL DEFICIT IN ELDERLY PERSONS

Symptoms	Signs
Weight loss or gain	Underweight or overweight
Decrease or loss in appetite	Low serum albumin
Nausea	Mid-arm muscle circumference
Heartburn	Less than 10th percentile
Constipation or diarrhea	Triceps skinfold
Swallowing problem	Less than 10th percentile
Changes in taste or smell	Greater than 95th percentile
Decrease in salivation	Anergy
Change in functional status	Edema
	Cheilosis or poor dentition
	Poorly healing wounds
	Dehydration
	Cognitive impairment
	Alcoholism
	Neuropathy

TABLE 3–5 SYMPTOMS AND SIGNS OF NUTRITIONAL
DEFICIENCIES IN ELDERLY PERSONS

Protein-Calorie Malnutrition

—Low body weight
—Diminished subcutaneous fat
—Pallor and fatigue
—Temporal wasting

—Dermatitis
—Impaired immunity with increased risk of infection
—Hypoproteinemia and edema

Vitamin Deficiency

B_1
—Anorexia
—Malaise
—Weakness of legs
—Pins and needles
  (burning feet syndrome)
—Sluggish or absent reflexes
—Palpitations
—Heart failure
—Encephalopathy

B_2
—Cheilosis
—Angular stomatitis
—Misty vision with
  burning sensation in the eyes
—Orogenital syndrome
—Excessive hair loss

B_3
—Depression and mood
  changes
—Irritability and forgetfulness
—Peripheral neuropathy
—Altered reflexes
—Spinal ataxia
—Anemia
—Easily fatigued

Folate
—Anorexia
—Irritability, forgetfulness, paranoid behavior
—Anemia
—Malabsorption

C
—Loss of energy
—Spontaneous bruising
—Arthralgia
—Gingivitis
—Bleeding gums

D
—Bone pains
—Waddling gait
—Spontaneous fractures
—Accelerated loss of vertical height
—Loss of mobility
—Muscle weakness

A
—Poor night vision
—Dermatitis

B_{12}
—Megaloblastic anemia
—Glossitis
—Neurologic damage
—Malabsorption

Mineral Deficiency

Calcium, phosphorus
—Aches and pains
—Osteoporosis
—Repeated fractures

Zinc
—Loss of taste and smell
—Excessive hair loss
—Prostatism
—Impaired night vision
—Poor wound healing
—Anorexia

Iodine
—Goiter

(continued)

TABLE 3–5   *(Continued)*

	Mineral Deficiency
Fluoride	—Dental caries
Copper	—Hypochronic, microcytic anemia —Neutropenia —Bony abnormalities
Chromium	—Glucose intolerance
Selenium	—Cardiomyopathy —Myositis —Hemolytic anemia

Source: From Gupta, KL, Dworkin, B, and Gambert, SR: Common nutritional disorders in the elderly: Atypical manifestations. Geriatrics 43(2):96, 1988, with permission.

Vitamin and mineral deficiencies are often associated with vague symptoms including anorexia, fatigue, and subtle changes in pigmentation, skin, mouth, hair, and sensation. Because these signs are often subclinical and nonspecific, they are often missed or attributed to the aging process. Well-controlled studies about needs and levels of vitamins and minerals in older persons are lacking. In spite of supplementation, many patients fail to normalize their blood levels of vitamins and minerals. The most critically important nutrient that is inadequate in most diets is calcium. The lack of sufficient calcium contributes to the high prevalence of osteoporosis and risk of fracture in older women and men. Vitamin D deficiency is also quite prevalent. More than half of institutionalized elderly persons are vitamin D deficient and may require a supplement.

TABLE 3–6   NUTRITIONAL PARAMETERS AND COMPATIBLE ICD-9 CODES

ICD-9 Code:

—260 Kwashiorkor (hypoalbuminemia): alb. ≤ 3.0 g/dL with hx of poor protein intake.
—261 Marasmus: wt. loss ≥ 10% or ≤ 60% of ideal; alb. ≥ 3.0 g/dL.
—262 Malnutrition of severe degree: alb. < 2.2; wt. loss ≥ 20% of pre-illness wt. or < 60% of ideal.
—263 Malnutrition of moderate degree: alb. 2.3–2.6; wt. loss of 15% of pre-illness wt. or < 70% of ideal.
—263.1 Malnutrition of mild degree: alb. 2.7–2.9; wt. loss of 10% pre-illness wt.
—278 Obesity: BMI > 30.

Source: University of Virginia, Manual for Clinical Nutrition Management.

Summary

Older adults are susceptible to nutritional deficiences for a variety of reasons. The Dietary Guidelines for Americans offer the older adult strategies for maintaining nutritional health. In addition to using these general guidelines, the clinician should emphasize to elderly individuals the importance of getting regular exercise, maintaining adequate fluid intake, and sharing meals. Because dietary supplements, including those for vitamins and fiber, are not always necessary, the clinician should advise the patient on when and how to self-prescribe these supplements.

Nutritional health status screening should be a routine part of the review of health of every older adult. Individuals with risk indicators should have a thorough nutritional assessment initially, followed by periodic monitoring of nutritional status. A registered dietitian should be consulted for the patient who needs a nutritional assessment, and asked to collaborate in the design of individualized strategies to address nutritional problems. Disease prevention and health promotion advice for older individuals should become routine with each health-care encounter. The long-range patient goal is to attain or maintain nutritional health, to maximize function and reduce the risk of morbidity and premature death.

BIBLIOGRAPHY

Nutrition

Bartlett, S, Marian, M, Taren, D, and Muramoto, ML: Geriatric Nutrition Handbook. Chapman & Hall, New York, 1997.

Bidlack, WR, and Wang, W: Chapter 4: Nutrition requirements of the elderly. In Morley, JE, Glick, Z, Rubenstein, LZ (eds): Geriatric Nutrition: A Comprehensive Review, ed. 2. Raven Press, New York, 1995.

Carter, WJ: Chapter 2: Macronutrient requirements for elderly persons. In Chernoff, R: Geriatric Nutrition: The Health Professional's Handbook. Aspen Publications, Gaithersburg, MD, 1991.

Chernoff, R: Baby boomers come of age: Nutrition in the 21st century. J Am Diet Assoc 95(6):650–654, 1995.

Evans, WJ: Exercise, nutrition, and aging. Clin Geriatr Med 11(4):725–734, 1995.

Evans, WJ: Exercise, nutrition, and aging. J Nutr 122:796–801, 1992.

Fogot, EJ, Bell, SJ, and Blackburn, GL: Chapter 5: Nutrition assessment of the elderly. In Morley, JE, Glick, Z, and Rubenstein, LZ (eds.): Geriatric Nutrition: A Comprehensive Review, ed. 2. Raven Press, New York, 1995.

Gupta, KL, Dworkin, B, and Gambert, SR: Common nutritional disorders in the elderly: Atypical manifestations. Geriatrics 43(2):87–97, 1988.

Ham, RJ: The signs and symptoms of poor nutritional status. Primary Care: Nutrition in Old Age 21(1):33–35, 1994.

Horwath, C: Nutritional goals for older adults: A review. Gerontologist 31(6):811–821, 1991.

Kendrick, ZV, Nelson-Steen, S, and Scafidi, K: Exercise, aging, and nutrition. South Med J 87(5):s50–s60.

Kerstetter, J, et al: Nutrition and nutritional requirements for the older adult. Dysphagia 8:51–18, 1993.

Lipschitz, DA: Screening for nutritional status in the elderly. Primary Care: Nutrition in Old Age 21(1):55–67, 1994.

Miller, DK, Morely, JE, and Rubenstein, LZ: Chapter 1: An overview of international aging and nutrition. In Morley, EI, Glick, Z, and Rubenstein, LZ (eds): Geriatric Nutrition: A Comprehensive Review, ed. 2. Raven Press, New York, 1995.

Mohs, ME: Chapter 9: Assessment of nutritional status in the aged. In Watson, RR (ed): Handbook of Nutrition in the Aged, ed. 2. CRC Press, Boca Raton, FL, 1994.

National Research Council Subcommittee: Recommended Dietary Allowances, ed. 10. National Academy Press, Washington, DC, 1989.

Roe, D: Geriatric Nutrition, ed. 3. Prentice-Hall, Englewood Cliffs, NJ, 1992.

Roe, DA: Medications and nutrition in the elderly. Primary Care: Nutrition in Old Age: 21(1):135–147, 1994.

US Department of Agriculture and US Department of Health and Human Services: Nutrition and Your Health. Dietary Guidelines for Americans, ed. 3. Home and Garden Bulletin No. 252. US Government Printing Office, Washington, DC, 1990.

US Department of Agriculture: The Food Guide Pyramid. Home and Garden Bulletin No. 252. US Government Printing Office, Washington, DC, 1992.

Wellman, NS: Dietary guidance and nutrient requirements of the elderly. Primary Care: Nutrition in Old Age 21(1):1–18, 1994.

White, J: Risk factors for poor nutritional status. Primary Care: Nutrition in Old Age 21(1):19–31, 1994.

UNIT **II**

ASSESSMENT

CHAPTER **4**

HISTORY TAKING

The primary goals in the problem-identification process are to recognize the disease that the patient has and to describe its impact on the patient. This fluid process involves both collecting relevant information from the patient or significant other and performing the indicated physical and functional examination. The data sources in geriatric assessment are interrelated. The symptom of pruritus, for example, leads the clinician to look for evidence of a rash. The sign of crackles alerts the clinician to ask about dyspnea and changes in respiratory function. After the subjective and objective details are obtained, they are analyzed together to determine any significant threat or potential threat to the patient's health status. The assessment includes the diagnosis(es) made, which then leads to a therapeutic plan. The ongoing evaluation of the effectiveness of the defined interventions is the impetus for additional data collection.

Most encounters between the geriatric patient and the practitioner are triggered by an episodic change in health status, in which the patient has experienced new or changed symptoms of illness or has developed some physical signs of disease. During the evaluation of a complaint, it helps to put the complaint into the context of the patient's previous health and illness. Ideally, a detailed health history of the patient is already available addressing the information in Table 4–1.

Comprehensive Health History

A comprehensive health history provides the best data, but it is quite time consuming, frequently requiring several lengthy visits to complete. To save time, some professionals send a geriatric history-taking form to the able patient in advance so that the completed details may be reviewed and expanded on during the visit. For older persons, the format for history taking (with certain modifications) is similar to that for younger adults. Less emphasis may be placed on family medical

TABLE 4–1 COMPONENTS OF A COMPREHENSIVE HEALTH HISTORY

A. Chief Complaint
   The patient's purpose for requesting health care at this time
B. Patient Profile
   Identifying information
   The source of referral, usual source of health care
   The source and reliability of information
C. History of Present Illness
   Clear, chronological narrative account of the problem(s) for which the patient is seeking care
   Description of symptoms using the dimensions of symptomatology
D. Past Health History
   General state of health
   Birth history
   Growth and development
   Childhood illnesses, injuries, hospitalizations
   Immunizations
   Adult illnesses, injuries, hospitalizations
   Operations
   Hazardous exposures
   Allergies
   Medications (including over-the-counter drugs, homeopathic remedies)
   Diet
   Sleep patterns
   Habits (alcohol, tobacco, drug intake; seatbelt use; exercise)
E. Family History
   Age and health, or age and cause of death, of each immediate family member (grandparents,
     parents, siblings, aunts, uncles, spouse, children)
   Occurrences within the family of: similar symptomatology, diabetes, tuberculosis, heart disease,
     hypertension, allergies, neurological disorders (stroke, seizure, migraine), kidney disease,
     bleeding disorders, cancer (type), anemia, genetic disorders, mental illness, suicide, alcohol-
     ism, obesity, musculoskeletal disorder (arthritis, bone disease)
F. Psychosocial History: Outline or narrative description capturing the most important things
     about the patient as a person
   Patient profile: relationships, occupational history, economic status and resources, educational
     level
   Living circumstances: typical day, environmental factors
   Mental health: coping, adaptation, cognitive abilities, depression, mood swings, memory
     changes, concentration abilities
   View of the present and future outlook: relevant religious beliefs, spiritual practices
G. Review of Systems
   General review
   Specific review of each body system: head to toe

history and more on family support; little time is spent on childhood illness but greater attention is given to chronic illness and functional impairment. Too often, without a comprehensive health history, abbreviated versions of the history and sketchy details of past illnesses are all that is available to the clinician during episodic patient evaluations.

Taking the health history of an older adult poses some challenges because of an expectation that the significant elements of the patient's prior health status can be obtained in an unrealistically short time. This is because what the patient considers significant often differs from what the clinician considers significant. A good strategy is to begin with an open-ended question and then target the relevant data by asking the patient specific questions. The narrative should be directed without risking the therapeutic relationship by bruskly interrupting the patient's discourse.

The chief complaint is the main reason the patient has requested the visit. In the older adult, a number of symptoms rather than a single complaint or symptom may give the clinician clues to the diagnosis. Symptom assessment of the older adult has some special considerations. Underreporting of symptoms, particularly of pain, is common because the older adult may attribute the symptom to the aging process itself. In addition, the individual may not be able to distinguish a new pain from an old one. Some patients may be reluctant to report a symptom for various reasons. They may fear the finding, not trust the professional or health-care system, be fearful of retaliation (i.e., abuse), or be uncertain of the consequences (i.e., nursing home placement for the patient who falls). If the clinician is concerned that the patient is underreporting, even a quick review of common geriatric symptoms may uncover a problem (Table 4–2). Recent research demonstrates the screening value of the review of systems in detected unsuspected diseases.

It is common for the older adult to complain of multiple symptoms when the patient has several chronic diseases or a multisystem acute disease. Clustering the presenting symptoms can help to identify the problem. For example, joint pain accompanied by fever may reflect an inflammatory process, and dyspnea and edema may indicate heart failure. Always consider the possibility of depression in older adults with frequent, multiple symptoms. Because somatic manifestations of depression are most common in elderly persons, geriatric depression often goes unrecognized and untreated.

The symptoms of the older patient may be vague and atypical. For nonspecific complaints, a more thorough physical assessment and functional assessment is indicated, with greater use of diagnostic and laboratory tests to aid in the diagnosis. Functional assessment, considered by many to be the cornerstone of assessment of older adults, may be accomplished prior to the visit by use of a checklist form (Table 4–3).

Older adults are most likely to experience vision, hearing, speech, and cognition deficits, impairing their ability to communicate. These impairments must be recognized and measures taken to maximally correct or accommodate for them at the onset of the visit. Although the mental status examination, if performed early in the history-taking process, may reveal the "unreliable historian," it may also pose a threat to the patient with early-onset dementia. When feeling threatened, the patient might be reluctant to answer further questions or might resort to "cover-up" strategies in attempts to hide the cognitive deficit. The clinician

TABLE 4-2 COMMON GERIATRIC SYMPTOMS

Body System	Symptom
Skin	Itching
	Lesions
	Dryness
Respiratory	Difficulty breathing
	Cough
Cardiovascular	Chest pain
	Swelling
	Pain in legs with walking
	Palpitations
	Loss of consciousness
Gastrointestinal	Difficulty chewing or swallowing
	Heartburn
	Abdominal pain
	Change in bowel habits or characteristics
Genitourinary	Frequency
	Urgency
	Nocturia
	Dysuria
	Hesitancy, intermittent stream, straining to void
	Incontinence
	Hematuria
	Vaginal bleeding or discharge
	Change in sexual functioning
Musculoskeletal	Restricted motion
	Pain
	Stiffness
	Weakness
	Joint swelling
Neurologic	Numbness or tingling of extremities
	Loss of sensation in extremities
	Sleep disorders
	Dizziness
	Balance problems
	Changes in memory
	Transient focal symptoms
Psychiatric	Depression
	Panic or anxiety
	Alcoholism
Sensory	Visual changes
	Changes in hearing
	Altered taste or smell

TABLE 4–3   GERIATRIC FUNCTIONAL ASSESSMENT

	ADL Scale
Bathing	I: Able to bathe completely or needs help with only a single body part
	A: Needs help with more than one body part, getting in/out of the tub or special tub attachments
	D: Completely unable to bathe self
Dressing/Undressing	I: Able to pick out clothes, dress/undress self, manage fasteners/braces
	A: Needs assistance or remains partially undressed
	D: Completely unable to dress/undress self
Grooming	I: Able to comb hair, shave self without help
	A: Needs help to comb hair, shave
	D: Completely unable to care for appearance
Toileting	I: Able to get to, on and off the toilet, cleans self after toileting, uses bedpan only at night
	A: Needs help getting to and using toilet, uses bedpan regularly
	D: Completely unable to use toilet
Continence	I: Urination/defecation self-controlled
	A: Partial or total urine/stool incontinence or control by enemas, catheters, regulated use of urinals/bedpans
	D: Uses catheter or colostomy
Transferring	I: Able to get in and out of bed or chair without assistance from humans or mechanical aids
	A: Needs human assistance/mechanical aids
	D: Completely unable to transfer, needs lifting
Walking	I: Able to walk without help except from cane
	A: Needs human assistance/walker or crutches
	D: Completely unable to walk, needs lifting
Eating	I: Able to feed self
	A: Needs help with cutting food, buttering bread
	D: Completely unable to feed self or needs parenteral feeding

(Continued)

should not underestimate the patient's abilities to give relevant information. This low expectation of abilities can be avoided by eliciting details of the symptom from the patient first and then supplementing the information with contributions from the caregiver. The clinician should use short one-dimensional questions and recognize nonverbal signs of discomfort so as not to provoke an anxiety response common in cognitively impaired individuals when excess demand is placed on them. The caregiver can provide valuable information about the patient's behavioral or functional changes, which may reflect a change in the patient's overall health status. Attention to sleep and appetite problems may unearth information about the patient's physical and mental health.

Once a list of the symptoms and signs has been obtained, the clinician should prioritize the assessment and the treatment of symptoms and signs. To do this, one should first determine if anything is life threatening or potentially life threaten-

TABLE 4–3   (*Continued*)

Instrumental ADL Scale	
Using the telephone	I: Able to look up numbers, dial, receive, and make calls without help
	A: Able to answer phone or dial operator in an emergency but needs special phone or help in getting the number or dialing
	D: Unable to use the telephone
Traveling	I: Able to drive own car or travel alone on buses or taxis
	A: Able to travel but needs someone to travel with
	D: Unable to travel without a special vehicle
Shopping	I: Able to take care of all food/clothes shopping with transportation provided
	A: Able to shop but needs someone to shop with
	D: Unable to shop
Preparing meals	I: Able to plan and cook full meals
	A: Able to prepare light meals but unable to cook full meals alone
	D: Unable to prepare any meals
Managing money	I: Able to manage buying needs, write checks, pay bills
	A: Able to manage daily buying needs, but needs help
	D: Unable to handle any day to day buying
Taking medicine	I: Able to prepare/take meds in the right dose at the right time
	A: Able to take meds but needs reminding or someone to prepare it
	D: Unable to take or self-administer

I = Independent   **A = Assisted**   **D = Dependent**

Source: Adapted from the Duke Center for the Study of Aging and Human Development. Eric Pfeiffer, M.D., Project Director: Older Americans Resources & Services (OARS) Program, 1975.

ing. Next it is necessary to determine the worst possible condition the patient might be experiencing. The novice clinician, who actually has an advantage here, often assumes the worst (e.g., a headache signals an aneurysm or chest pain signals myocardial infarction). Having more experience and greater familiarity with the most common conditions, the advanced clinician is more likely to base priorities on the most likely cause of the patient's symptoms. For example, a patient's complaint of headache is most likely attributable to stress or tension, and chest pain is more likely to be indigestion. This prioritization method is riskier with elderly individuals, who often present atypically. For example, research studies show that after age 85 the most common symptoms of myocardial infarction are acute confusion and dyspnea rather than chest pain and diaphoresis (Bayer, et al., 1986). Therefore, the clinician is advised always to err on the side of caution when determining relative significance. The secondary assessment necessary to rule in or rule out the "worst case scenario" usually requires some additional time and resources but minimizes the risk of underestimating the significance of a symptom.

Episodic Health History

With the list of symptoms prioritized, the episodic history is guided by seven dimensions of the present illness.

PARAMETERS OF A SYMPTOM

- Location and radiation.
- Quantity and quality.
- Aggravating and alleviating factors.
- Associated symptoms and signs.
- Absence of associated symptoms and signs.
- Evolution and course of the symptom.
- Effect of the symptom on normal daily activities.

These parameters can be applied to any symptom, placing greater emphasis on selected components in the presentation. For example, if the patient complains of chest pain, the clinician can have the patient point to the location of the discomfort and trace how it radiates. Quantifying pain can be accomplished in various ways (Fig. 4–1), although older adults may prefer verbally descriptive scales. Cognitively impaired individuals may be more responsive to the "fear faces" as a visual representation of their pain experience.

Qualification refers to the characteristics of the symptom. Chest pain, for example, may be qualified by adding more descriptive terms such as sharp, dull, aching, boring, burning, cramping, or stabbing. Some pain assessment tools provide this type of "laundry list" for the patient to use. Such tools should be used discriminately, however, because they may lead the patient to provide less accurate information. Eliciting what aggravates and what relieves the discomfort provides more information. Factors that aggravate and relieve chest pain may include position change, activity, coughing, or food or antacid use.

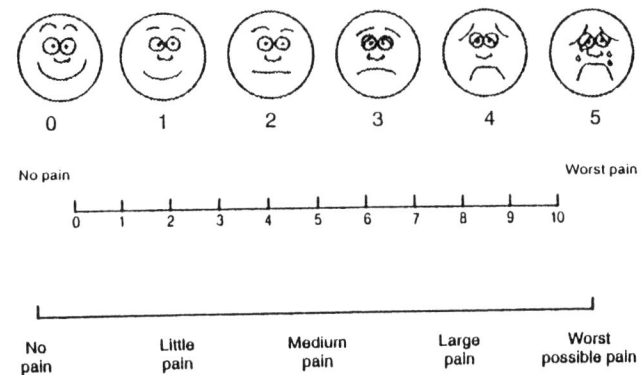

FIGURE 4–1   Rating scales for pain. Wong-Baker FACES Pain Rating Scale. From Wong DL, Hockenberry-Eaton M, Wilson D, Winkelstein E, DiVito-Thomas PA: Whaley & Wong's Nursing Care of Infants and Children, ed 6, St. Louis, 1999, Mosby.

Psychosocial and environmental relationships may be explored. For example, does the symptom occur when the patient is in a certain location or is with certain individuals? How has the patient attempted to relieve the symptoms and what effect has it had? This should include self- and provider-prescribed medications, home remedies, or other therapeutic measures (e.g., heat, movement, relaxation exercises).

Exploration of the presence or absence of associated symptoms and signs is important: a symptom does not usually occur in isolation. In the example of chest pain, the relationship of the pain with symptoms such as dyspnea, cough, palpitations, edema, and fever may provide the clinical portrait necessary to determine the diagnosis. Documenting the absence of symptoms and signs is just as important as documenting their presence. Negative documentation reflects the clinician's search for evidence at the time and supports the judgment used to define the course of treatment or nontreatment.

Emergency History Taking

When the patient is in distress, limited information is available. As the physical examination proceeds relevant details of the patient's symptoms can be elicited. The clinician should give priority to the aspects of the history that are most relevant to the immediate situation. Here, direct questions are preferred to open-ended ones, as this saves time. When it is necessary to modify the interview because of the patient's distress, information might be obtained from other sources such as family, friends, or hospital records. Regardless of the circumstances, adherence to the general order of the interview, followed by the physical examination, will increase accuracy and save time.

Documenting the History

Recording the history of present illness should begin with the current experience, followed by its chronological evolution. The chief complaint is always stated in the patient's own terms and written in quotes. The history of present illness is recorded using the seven dimensions listed earlier as a guide; this is followed by recording the relevant past history and family history. The complete inventory of the patient's medications must be listed because drugs are frequently the cause or contributing factor to a new symptom. Using the SOAP (Subjective, Objective, Assessment, Plan) format may help to organize the database for record keeping. The main principle is KISS: Keep It Short and Simple. The use of sentence fragments, line drawings, and diagrams makes the narrative more interesting and keeps it concise.

Summarizing

After taking the history of an older adult, the clinician should summarize for the patient what was heard. This gives the patient the opportunity to clarify or deny any parts of the discussion. Summarization is a most important step in the history-taking process, particularly when the interview has been conducted very quickly. It also helps to establish the trusting relationship that is necessary to the assessment process. This is the time when the patient may reveal any "hidden agenda": The chief complaint is not always the reason the patient is seeking help. After a more trusting relationship has been established, the patient is more likely to reveal any underlying concerns.

BIBLIOGRAPHY

Bayer, AJ, et al: Changing presentation of myocardial infarction with increasing old age. J Am Geriatr Soc 34:4, 1986.

Boland, BJ, Wollan, PC, and Silverstein, MD: Review of systems, physical examination, and routine tests for case-finding in ambulatory patients. Am J Med Sci 309:4, 194, 1995.

Herr, K, and Mobily, P: Comparison of selected pain assessment tools for use with the elderly. Appl Nurs Res 6:1, 39, 1993.

Wasson, J, et al: The Common Symptom Guide, ed 4. McGraw-Hill, New York, 1997.

CHAPTER **5**

REVIEW OF SYSTEMS

Assessment Parameters

Because older individuals represent a richly diverse population, the components of assessment may vary from person to person. We all age at different rates, and body organ failure, psychosocial adaptations, environmental supports, and functional ability evident over time can differ dramatically among individuals of the same chronological age. Figure 5–1 illustrates the multidimensional assessment processes in elderly persons. The advanced-practice clinician working with the geriatric patient must have a repertoire of assessment skills and access to and familiarity with appropriate instruments and screening tools. The types and variety of skills, instruments, and screening tools used by the gerontological nurse practitioner are listed in Tables 5–1, 5–2, and 5–3.

Of greatest value is the availability of clinicians with specialized geriatric knowledge in problem areas that are particularly difficult to assess and manage using standardized approaches. For example, the skin care specialist might be consulted about proper treatment of the complicated stage 3 decubitus ulcer; the geropsychiatrist, to help manage the patient with combined delirium, dementia, and/or depression; the retirement counselor, for anticipatory guidance in role transition; and the substance abuse counselor, for the patient determined to change addictive behavior.

Familiarity with community resources available to geriatric patients is important in ensuring quality care management. Because often no single source for this information exists most clinicians over time form a "mental file" of these individuals and organizations. The process of finding care experts continues to be limited. Very few board-certified geropsychiatrists exist in this country, so finding one in rural areas is unlikely. It frequently works best to share in the assessment, having

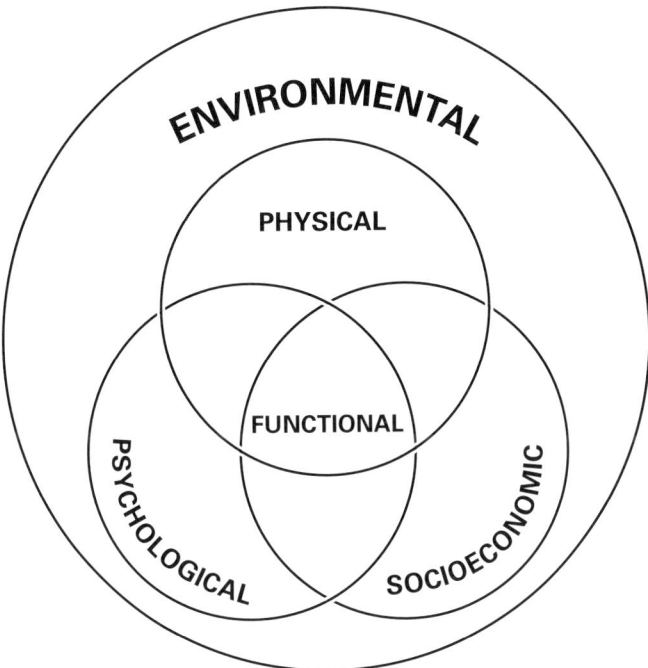

FIGURE 5–1 Components of assessment in elderly persons.

the geriatric expert contribute the "age perspective" and the psychiatric expert the "mental perspective."

With an increasing trend toward streamlined care that includes more exclusive assessment and management by the generalist and less emphasis on specialized care, leaders in gerontological care would be remiss in suggesting that all older individuals must be assessed by a team of geriatric professionals. Multidimensional assessment skills are critical for the primary care practitioner to have; using standardized approaches with simple and valuable tools such as those described in this book is generally the best way to accomplish this. As it is beyond the scope

TABLE 5–1
ASSESSMENT SKILLS

Communication	Social
Physical	Family
Functional	Environmental
Mental status	Spiritual
Psychological	Financial

TABLE 5-2 ASSESSMENT INSTRUMENTS

Otoscope/ophthalmoscope: eye/ear examination
Eye charts: near, far, color, illiterate
Hand-held audiometer: hearing examination
Tuning fork: vibratory sense
Reflex hammer: deep tendon reflexes
Needles and cotton: sensory testing
10 g monofilament: protective sensation of the feet
Goniometer: range of motion
Stethoscope (diaphragm, bell): cardiopulmonary and abdominal examinations
Scale: height, weight
Calipers: anthropometrics
Tape measure: lesion and edema assessment
Pocket magnifying glass: lesion assessment
Various scents: testing smell
Skin marking pencil: diaphragmatic movement, liver size, edema
Availability of: portable Doppler scanner, pulse oximeter, glucometer, cholesterol screening, ECG, punch biopsy, examination light, examination table, speculums

---

of this text to give detailed information in multidimensional domains, readers are referred to other sources for comprehensive information.

Overview of Screening, Comprehensive, and Problem-Focused Examinations

The patient history provides the clues necessary for determining the approach to and method of the physical examination. Several tiers to this investigation include:

TABLE 5-3
ASSESSMENT TOOLS

Mental status	Dementia assessments
Depression scale	Caregiver burden
Skin risk assessment scale	Gait/balance
Decubitus staging	Incontinence assessment
Dyspnea index rating	Pain assessment
Cardiac functional rating	BPH assessment
Involuntary movement scale	Home safety checklist
Functional assessment tool	Values assessment
Alcohol questionnaire	Elder abuse

Screening examination, often chosen when the purpose is early case finding (i.e., breast examination).

Comprehensive examination, selected when determining care requirements (i.e., minimum data set for long-term care).

Problem-focused examination, conducted when the patient experiences a new sign or symptom of disease or illness.

How detailed the physical examination should be is controversial. Primary care professionals have recognized the need to perform a focused physical examination rather than the exhaustive complete examination taught in schools. In the symptomatic patient, the physical assessment is guided by the symptom(s) or sign(s). The screening criteria for those asymptomatic patients over age 65 are summarized in the "Guide to Clinical Preventive Services" by the U.S. Preventive Services Task Force (1996). When deciding to abbreviate the physical examination, remember that touch has therapeutic value and that teaching the patient may be as important as the therapeutic intent of diagnosing disease or illness.

The novice advanced-practice clinician needs to concentrate first on mastering the techniques of examining individuals experiencing healthy or expected aging. After the novice becomes more confident in the content and has memorized the sequencing, the skills in identifying disease and formulation of diagnostic hypotheses become more refined. Students in advanced-practice programs are encouraged to master the comprehensive approach to assessment while the opportunity is available. Then, in clinical practice, the practitioner can use his or her procedural memory when performing the contextual examination. In a crisis situation, for example, when evaluating a patient experiencing chest pain, the essential components of cardiopulmonary, peripheral vascular, and vital signs will automatically be included in the examination. This regional approach to the physical examination makes more sense than the systems approach because it is faster, more comfortable, and most useful in addressing the patient's problems. Unlike the screening examination, the regional problem-focused examination is used to investigate those symptoms and signs that are of the highest concern and to begin diagnosing, treating, and managing the disease or illness.

Integrating the Components of the Examination

Regardless of how detailed the investigation process is, critical elements must be included for effective examination (Table 5–4). Adequate preparation of the environment, the equipment, and the patient is an essential preliminary step that is most often overlooked.

Clinicians sometimes assume that the patient is available for examination at the time most convenient for the examiner. During a scheduled office visit, this is usually a legitimate assumption; however, in the acute care or nursing home

TABLE 5–4
CRITICAL ELEMENTS TO
EFFECTIVE EXAMINATION

Pre-examination preparations
   Timing arranged with patient
   Conductive physical space
   Uninterrupted time
   Available and operational supplies/equipment/tools
Conducting the examination
   Organized
   Efficient
   Sequential
   Comfortable
   Documented
Postexamination procedures
   Summarization of findings with patient
   Patient teaching

setting, the patient may have other commitments. To avoid potential conflicts, coordinate the scheduling of the examination with the patient and the staff. Consider the physical space in determining a suitable environment. Pay attention to privacy, comfort, and quiet and ask permission to turn off the TV or radio, pull the curtain, and/or close the door. Allow for uninterrupted time for the examination. Turn beepers to "vibration mode" or hold calls; staff should be alert to the importance of minimizing disruption of the examiner and the patient. Ask the geriatric patient specifically whether he or she needs to void, so that he or she may be more comfortable and undisturbed during the examination. Finally, the prepreparations should include a check to ensure that all the equipment is available and in working order.

The examination should be conducted in an organized fashion; once a suitable sequencing has been established the examiner is encouraged to follow this method each time. Once committed to memory, the examination sequence flows better and saves times. A new clinician often spends an hour conducting a complete examination, whereas a more experienced one can complete the same examination in approximately half the time. There is no "standardized" way of organizing the examination. The most important considerations are patient comfort and the efficiency and effectiveness of the examination. Always consider the efficiency of motion of both yourself and the patient (see Table 5–5).

After completing the examination, discuss the general findings with the patient. The patient might be commended for positive behaviors taken to improve or maintain health. This is also an opportune time to teach the patient self-assessment and self-care management strategies.

TABLE 5–5
EXAMINATION SEQUENCING IN THE GERIATRIC PATIENT

Pre-exam: Patient completes self-rated health instruments.
  Examiner reviews the completed self-rated health instruments.
Prior to undressing: History, mental status, distant vision, height, weight, vital signs with blood
  pressure positionally, psychosocial assessment.

Examination Process	Examination Position
General appearance	Patient seated
Skin on exposed surfaces	Examiner facing patient
Arthritic changes of upper body	
Range of motion/strength upper extremities and neck	
Facial symmetry, mobility, sensation	
Temporal artery	
Conjunctivae and sclerae	
Ocular movements and field testing	
Cerebellar testing (finger-nose, nystagmus)	
Near/color vision	
Pupil responsiveness	
Fundiscopic examination	
Ear examination	
Hearing testing	
Nose	
Oral cavity examination	
Swallowing function	
Head and neck nodes	
Pulses: radial, carotid, brachial	
Thyroid anterior	
Thyroid posterior	Patient seated
Curvature/protrusions of spine	Examiner behind patient
Palpation of spine	
CVA tenderness	
Diaphragmatic excursion/movement	
Tactile fremitus	
Posterior lung assessment	
Anterior lung assessment	Patient seated
Breast inspection	Examiner in front of patient
Axillary and epitrocholear nodes	
Cardiac (sitting)	
Cardiac (supine and left lateral)	Patient supine (30-degree angle for JVD)
Carotid bruit	
Jugular venous distension	Examiner on right side of patient
Palpate breasts	
Abdominal aorta, renal, femoral, iliac bruit	
Abdomen	
Lymph nodes: inguinal, popliteal	
Arteries: femoral, popliteal, pedal	

(continued)

TABLE 5–5   (*Continued*)

Examination Process	Examination Position
Vascular assessment lower extremities	
Arthritic changes in lower extremities	
Range of motion/strength of lower extremities	
Cerebellar testing (RAM, heel to shin)	
Sensation (light touch/pain/vibration)	
Deep tendon reflexes	Patient seated
Plantar reflex	Examiner facing patient
Clonus	
Gynecologic examination	Patient lithotomy position
Rectal examination	Patient side-lying position
Romberg maneuver	Patient standing
Gait assessment	Examiner in front of patient
Range of motion spine	Examiner behind patient
Prostate examination	

JVD = jugular venous distension; RAM = rapid alternating movement.

Selective Use of Laboratory and Diagnostic Tests: Screening and Diagnosing

Chapter 1 discusses the changes associated with aging that are reflected in laboratory values. This section provides some general guidelines on when to order testing. The reader is referred to the disease sections of this text for more specific guidelines and to Appendix C for diseases and disorders associated with abnormal results of some common laboratory tests. The objective differs when tests are used to screen geriatric patients than when used to aid in the diagnosis. Screening can be defined as "the presumptive identification of unrecognized disease or defect by the application of tests, examinations, or other procedures which can be applied rapidly to sort out apparently well persons who probably have a disease from those who probably do not" (Magenheim, 1992). The screening test is not intended to be diagnostic. The U.S. Preventive Services Task Force (1996) has defined screening parameters for those over age 65, which includes laboratory and diagnostic testing (Table 5–6).

The overall validity of the test helps determine the value in screening a patient. Validity refers to the degree to which the test correctly identifies individuals with the condition (sensitivity) and the degree to which the test correctly identifies those without the condition (specificity). The guidelines for laboratory screening for the over-65 group were developed by a consensus group. The clinician is advised to use these only as a guide and to use clinical discretion for final determination as to the appropriateness of a screening test.

TABLE 5–6 GUIDELINES FOR HEALTH EVALUATION—AGE 65 AND OVER

Interventions Considered and Recommended for the Periodic Health Examination	Leading Causes of Death
	Heart diseases
	Malignant neoplasms (lung, colorectal, breast)
	Cerebrovascular disease
	Chronic obstructive pulmonary disease
	Pneumonia and influenza

Interventions for the General Population

Screening

Blood pressure
Height and weight
Fecal occult blood test[1] and/or sigmoidoscopy
Mammogram ± clinical breast exam[2] (women ≤69 yr)
Papanicolaou (Pap) test (women)[3]
Vision screening
Assess for hearing impairment
Assess for problem drinking

Counseling

Substance Use
Tobacco cessation
Avoid alcohol/drug use while driving, swimming, boating, etc.°

Diet and Exercise
Limit fat and cholesterol; maintain caloric balance; emphasize grains, fruits, vegetables
Adequate calcium intake (women)
Regular physical activity°

Injury Prevention
Lap/shoulder belts
Motorcycle and bicycle helmets°
Fall prevention°
Safe storage/removal of firearms°
Smoke detector°
Set hot water heater to <120–130°F°
CPR training for household members

Dental Health
Regular visits to dental care provider°
Floss, brush with fluoride toothpaste daily°

Sexual Behavior
STD prevention: avoid high-risk sexual behavior°; use condoms°

Immunizations

Pneumococcal vaccine
Influenza[1]
Tetanus-diphtheria (Td) boosters

Chemoprophylaxis

Discuss hormone prophylaxis (women)

Interventions for High-Risk Populations

Population	*Potential Interventions*
	(See detailed high-risk definitions)
Institutionalized persons	PPD (HR1); hepatitis A vaccine (HR2); amantadine/rimantadine (HR4)
Chronic medical conditions; TB contacts; low income; immigrants; alcoholics	PPD (HR1)
Persons ≥75 yr; or ≥ 70 yr with risk factors for falls	Fall prevention intervention (HR5)
Cardiovascular disease risk factors	Consider cholesterol screening (HR6)
Family history of skin cancer; nevi; fair skin, eyes, hair	Avoid excess/midday sun, use protective clothing° (HR7)

(continued)

TABLE 5–6   (*Continued*)

Interventions for High-Risk Populations

Native Americans/Alaska Natives	PPD (HR1); hepatitis A vaccine (HR2)
Travelers to developing countries	Hepatitis A vaccine (HR2); hepatitis B vaccine (HR8)
Blood product recipients	HIV screen (HR3); hepatitis B vaccine (HR8)
High-risk sexual behavior	Hepatitis A vaccine (HR2); HIV screen (HR3); hepatitis B vaccine (HR8); RPR/VDRL (HR9)
Injection or street drug use	PPD (HR1); hepatitis A vaccine (HR2); HIV screen (HR3); hepatitis B vaccine (HR8); RPR/VDRL (HR9); advice to reduce infection risk (HR10)
Health care/lab workers	PPD (HR1); hepatitis A vaccine (HR2); amantadine/rimantadine (HR4); hepatitis B vaccine (HR8)
Persons susceptible to varicella	Varicella vaccine (HR11)

High-Risk Categories

HR1 = HIV-positive, close contacts of persons with known or suspected TB, health-care workers, persons with medical risk factors associated with TB, immigrants from countries with high TB prevalence, medically underserved low-income populations (including homeless), alcoholics, injection drug users, and residents of long-term care facilities.

HR2 = Persons living in, traveling to, or working in areas where the disease is endemic and where periodic outbreaks occur (e.g., countries with high or intermediate endemicity; certain Alaska Native, Pacific Island, Native American, and religious communities); men who have sex with men; injection or street drug users. Consider for institutionalized persons and workers in these institutions, and day-care, hospital, and laboratory workers. Clinicians should also consider local epidemiology.

HR3 = Men who had sex with men after 1975; past or present injection drug use; persons who exchange sex for money or drugs, and their sex partners; injection drug-using, bisexual, or HIV-positive sex partner currently or in the past; blood transfusion during 1978–1985; persons seeking treatment for STDs. Clinicians should also consider local epidemiology.

HR4 = Consider for persons who have not received influenza vaccine or are vaccinated late; when the vaccine may be ineffective due to major antigenic changes in the virus; for unvaccinated persons who provide home care for high-risk persons; to supplement protection provided by vaccine in persons who are expected to have a poor antibody response; and for high-risk persons in whom the vaccine is contraindicated.

TABLE 5-6 *(Continued)*

High-Risk Categories

HR5 = Persons aged 75 years and older; or aged 70–74 with one or more additional risk factors including: use of certain psychoactive and cardiac medications (e.g., benzodiazepines, antihypertensives); use of ≥4 prescription medications; impaired cognition, strength, balance, or gait. Intensive individualized home-based multifactorial fall prevention intervention is recommended in settings where adequate resources are available to deliver such services.

HR6 = Although evidence is insufficient to recommend routine screening in elderly persons, clinicians should consider cholesterol screening on a case-by-case basis for persons ages 65–75 with additional risk factors (e.g., smoking, diabetes, or hypertension).

HR7 = Persons with a family or personal history of skin cancer, a large number of moles, atypical moles, poor tanning ability, or light skin, hair, and eye color.

HR8 = Blood product recipients (including hemodialysis patients), persons with frequent occupational exposure to blood or blood products, men who have sex with men, injection drug users and their sex partners, persons with multiple recent sex partners, persons with other STDs (including HIV), travelers to countries with endemic hepatitis B.

HR9 = Persons who exchange sex for money or drugs and their sex partners; persons with other STDs (including HIV); and sexual contacts of persons with active syphilis. Clinicians should also consider local epidemiology.

HR10 = Persons who continue to inject drugs.

HR11 = Healthy adults without a history of chickenpox or previous immunization. Consider serologic testing for presumed susceptible adults.

[1]Annually. [2]Mammogram q1–2 yr, or mammogram q1–2 yr with annual clinical breast exam. [3]All women who are or have been sexually active and who have a cervix: q ≤ 3 yr. Consider discontinuation of testing after age 65 yr if previous regular screening with consistently normal results.
°The ability of clinician counseling to influence this behavior is unproven.

One of the considerations in ordering tests for diagnostic purposes is whether the test result will alter the diagnosis, prognosis, or management of a condition.

DECISION-MAKING GUIDELINES FOR DIAGNOSTICS
- Is the test necessary to make the diagnosis?
- Will the test be accepted and tolerated by the patient?
- Does the benefit of the test outweigh the risk?
- Is it the least invasive test available?
- Can the results be interpreted?
- Will the results change the treatment of the patient?

For example, will the positive Pap smear in the 78-year-old affect the plan of care? If the answer is no, then the risk (i.e., cost and discomfort of the procedure)

TABLE 5–7 DEFINITIONS OF STANDARD
LABORATORY TEST TERMINOLOGY

Sensitivity	The number of diseased patients with a positive test, divided by the number of diseased patients
	OR
	The likelihood of a positive test result in a person with the disease
Specificity	The number of patients without disease with a negative test, divided by the number of patients without disease
	OR
	The likelihood of a negative test result in a person without the disease
Pretest probability of disease "D"	The likelihood that "D" is present before the test result is obtained
Posttest probability of disease, given a positive test result	The number of true positives divided by the sum of all true positives and false positives
Posttest probability of disease, given a negative test result	The number of false negatives divided by the sum of false negatives and true negatives

Source: Wernick, R: Avoiding laboratory test misinterpretation in geriatric rheumatology. Geriatrics 44(Feb):61–80, 1989.

outweighs the benefits and testing is not indicated. To be of diagnostic value, a test for a given disease must produce patient results that differ substantially from normal results as well as from results in patients with other diseases that may be mistaken for that disease. Even highly accurate tests produce false results when applied inappropriately and without a firm understanding of the concepts (Table 5–7).

Another consideration is cost and risk. Are there simpler, less-expensive, less-invasive ways to make the same diagnosis? Will the computerized axial tomography (CAT) give adequate information, or is the magnetic resonance imaging (MRI) essential? For example, endoscopy and biopsy are not cost-effective first steps in managing a suspected peptic ulcer. Empirical antisecretory therapy, along with antibiotics for those who test serologically positive for *Helicobacter pylori*, is more cost effective than more invasive and costly procedures.

Most importantly, consider the test's acceptability to the patient. This is perhaps most significant in the patient who cannot make a choice and give consent. In such individuals, a proxy is needed to gain permission to give the test. Although some patients may be unable to express themselves clearly verbally, their behavior may give nonverbal expression to their feelings toward the test's acceptability.

Follow-up Assessment

Older adults are expected to decline in health and develop some disease or illness over time. They are also the most susceptible to the adverse effects of the diagnostic procedures and therapeutic measures used to identify and treat the problems once they are detected. Be alert to these changes early in their development and carefully monitor the patient's responsiveness to treatment over time. Because the person closest to the patient (i.e., family, nurse aide) is the one most likely to note these changes, he or she needs to realize the significance of reporting these observations. Subtle changes in function are often the first signs of a disease or may represent the adverse effects of treatment. A flowchart may be helpful in identifying what to look for in these circumstances. The data selected should reflect both the most significant and the most likely changes to occur and should be capable of detecting small but meaningful changes. This flowchart method is much more valuable than relying on a fixed plan of periodic examinations to determine change and identfiy disease.

The "benchmarking" approach requires some type of prediction of the patient's expected course. As the patient alters from this course, a reevaluation is triggered, and interventions can be performed early in the course to get the patient back on track. The Minimum Data Set (MDS) (Appendix D) is a standardized form designed for assessing problems initially and reassessing for changes in functional levels over time.

Summary

Assessment of the older individual is a forensic process. The advanced-practice clinician has equipment, tools, and skills to help identify actual or potential disease or illness. Proper use of individuals with specialized geriatric knowledge helps when assessing and managing the more complex older individual who is not responsive to traditional approaches or strategies.

Regardless of the detail or the brevity of the examination process, the skilled clinician uses an integrated, organized, and familiar approach, so that the examination is efficient and effective and the critical elements are consistently included. Diagnostics and therapeutics are selectively used to identify and manage the patient's problems. Once a baseline of health status has been established, care must be taken so that a patient's new signs and symptoms or changes in function trigger a problem-focused examination.

BIBLIOGRAPHY

Fendrick, AM, et al: Cost effectiveness of initial management strategies for patients with suspected peptic ulcer disease. Ann Intern Med 123(4):260–268, 1995.

Frank, S, Stange, K, Moore, P, and Smith, CK: The focused physical examination: Should checkups be tailor-made? Postgraduate Medicine 92(2):171–186, 1992.

Gallo, J, Reichel, W, and Andersen, L: Handbook of Geriatric Assessment, ed 2. Aspen, 1995.

Kane, R, Ouslander, J, and Abrass, I: Essentials of Clinical Geriatrics, ed 3. McGraw-Hill, New York, 1994.

Magenheim, MJ: Chapter 13: Preventive Assessment. In Calkins, E, Ford, AB, and Katz, PR (eds): Practice of Geriatrics, ed 2, 1992.

US Preventive Services Task Force: Guide to Clinical Preventive Services, ed 2. International Medical Publishing, Alexandria, VA, 1996.

Wernick, R: Avoiding laboratory test misinterpretation in geriatric rheumatology. Geriatrics 44(Feb):61–80, 1989.

Willms, J, Schneiderman, H, and Algranati, P: Physical Diagnosis: Bedside Evaluation of Diagnosis and Function. Williams & Wilkins, Baltimore, 1994.

TREATING

ILLNESS

CHAPTER **6**

SKIN AND

LYMPHATICS

The skin tells a story. Proper assessment of an older adult's skin, hair, and nails reveals the patient's history of sun exposure, nutrition, socioeconomic status, and education, as well as his or her surgical and medical history. The largest organ of the body, the skin, undergoes certain normal changes with age. The number of cells in the epidermis, such as Langerhans' cells, which are responsible for immune surveillance, begin to decline. Melanocytes also decrease, thereby reducing the skin's natural protection from the sun.

Skin renewal turnover time increases to approximately 87 days in elderly adults, compared with 20 days during youth. This fact becomes an important consideration in surgical and dermatologic healing. With aging, the collagen and fibroblasts in the dermis decrease in number and become tangled and ropelike, resulting in thicker, less elastic skin.

Walls of blood vessels in the dermis weaken during aging, and capillary microcirculation becomes disorganized. This results in decreased absorption and clearance, and delayed wound healing. The subcutaneous tissue that houses the eccrine, sebaceous, and apocrine glands thins, thereby providing less protection from heat exposure and less insulation, energy storage, and shock absorption. Secretions aiding temperature control, moisturization, and odor production are also reduced. Fat is generally redistributed to the abdomen and thighs, leaving bony surfaces such as the face, hands, and sacrum exposed to potential injury. The skin's repair system becomes impaired, with delayed cell regeneration and poor circulation.

All of these tissue changes represent a near-catastrophic scenario of aged skin poorly protected from the environment (especially the sun, heat, and cold) and that is slow to respond to immunologic challenges, producing minimal or delayed urticaria and swelling.

87

Assessment of the skin begins with the chief complaint and history, including the skin problem's onset, duration, location, size, color, and change.

1. Investigate associated symptoms such as wheezing, loss of appetite, fever, and malaise.
2. Question current and chronic medication history, nutritional history, and childhood diseases (especially asthma, atopic dermatitis, and chickenpox).
3. Ask about contact with chemicals, lifetime occupation, level of lifetime sun exposure, family history of skin cancer, contact with animals, change in environmental or internal habits (e.g., change in soap or laundry detergent, or in cereal or cooking product).
4. Ask whether the person has been treated for a similar situation in the past, and if so, as about the result.
5. Note whether the patient appears uncomfortable or pruritic.
6. Observe overall hygiene and grooming.

Proper equipment for inspection includes good overhead and tangential lighting, a magnifying glass, and blades and collection devices for biopsies and microscopic study. Gloves should be readily available. Inspect the skin for any signs of possible abuse, neglect, or decreased function. Bruises at different levels of healing indicate ongoing insults to the skin. Poorly healing wounds or chronic pressure ulcers may signal a problem not only with the patient but with the caregiver. Welts, lacerations, burns, and distinctive markings from an iron, brush, or teeth may all indicate a need for intervention.

Inspect the hair and nails. The hair may be graying and thinner than in youth. Normally, nails start to form ridges after age 80. A recent (in the past year) change in quality of hair and nails is a significant finding. For example, the hair may have become dryer, duller, and thinner, or the nails pitted or brittle.

Inspection of the skin for even color and overall quality and care is important. Lesions require close scrutiny, description, and classification. Description by type, shape, arrangement, and distribution is a widely accepted and usable format.

Type: Is the lesion a macule or papule? Is it eroded, excoriated, hyperpigmented, or hypopigmented?

Shape: Is the periphery of the lesion round, ulcerated, or linear?

Arrangement: Are multiple lesions grouped, serpiginous, with or without definable borders?

Distribution: Is the extent of the lesion isolated, region, or generalized? Is the pattern symmetrical or over pressure sites, hairline, or sun-exposed areas? Is the distribution characteristic of scabies, seborrheic dermatitis, contact dermatitis, lupus?

The lesion may be classified as primary or secondary. Primary lesions (vesicles, tumors, burrows) arise from normal tissue. Secondary lesions (infections, crusts, lichenification) arise from changes to the primary lesion. Palpate for moisture, temperature, mobility, and turgor. Lax skin may indicate weight loss, whereas fixed skin may be associated with sclerotic or scarred tissue. Lesions should also be palpated to check whether they are fluctuant, hard, or fixed.

At the end of the examination, consider associated pathology, especially thyroid disorders, diabetes, autoimmune conditions, and anemia. Provide wellness instructions, including those concerning proper nutrition, moisturizing, and sun protection. Awareness of the high susceptibility of the elderly to hyperthermia and hypothermia secondary to reduced thermoregulation in the skin should be emphasized. Review the ABCDEs of malignant melanoma:

A: Asymmetry.
B: Border is irregular, notched.
C: Color is mixed, haphazard.
D: Diameter is 6 mm (pencil eraser).
E. Elevation (except for malignant lentigines, which is flatter).

Lesions that concern you or the patient should be examined through biopsy. Lesions that warrant biopsy are those that have changed, bleed, or are painful. Treatment for skin lesions must take impaired absorption, duration, dosage, and delivery method (e.g., cream, powder, ointment) into consideration. Patients for whom treatment plans fail initially should be referred to a dermatologist.

Burns

Burns are injuries to tissues, caused by thermal, chemical, or electrical contact. They may be classified by severity of injury to the body surface area (BSA), as follows:

- Small (less than 15% BSA).
- Moderate (15%–49% BSA).
- Large (50%–69% BSA).
- Massive (greater than or equal to 70% BSA).

The depth of the burn is described as first, second, or third degree.

- **First-degree burns:** Erythema of the tissue; burns are sensitive to touch.
- **Second-degree burns:** Partial-thickness burn; may or may not have blisters.
- **Third-degree burns:** Skin is tough and leathery, wound may appear pale or charred or ulcerated with extensive tissue necrosis.

Etiology: With a burn injury wound edema and loss of intravascular volume, caused by increased vascular permeability, occur. Because of the normal aging changes of the skin, the older adult who suffers from a burn injury is at increased risk for morbidity and mortality. The decreased vascular response of skin in older adults contributes to poor wound healing and increased risk of infection.

Occurrence: An estimated 2 million injuries, 60,000 requiring hospitalization, and 6000 deaths occur annually in the United States from burns.

Age: Burns occur in all age groups, but the rate of fatal burns is much greater among persons age 75 and older. Ninety percent of fatal burns result from residential fires.

Ethnicity: Injuries from burns are more common in non-Caucasian populations.

Gender: Burns occur equally in men and women.

Contributing Factor: Poverty is one of the strongest risk factors for fatality in a residential fire because of the overall poor living conditions. Cigarettes cause almost 50% of all residential fires. The use of space and kerosene heaters, fireplaces, faulty electrical wires, lack of smoke detectors and fire extinguishers, scalding liquids, heating pads, and prolonged exposure to the sun all contribute to burn injuries in older adults.

Signs and Symptoms: A detailed history of the incident should be obtained from the patient or significant other, including any substances involved, duration of exposure, emergency treatment (if any), overall condition of the patient before the incident (including medications, mental status, prior history of any burn injuries, and medical diagnosis). Physical examination should include assessment of vital signs and of the burn area and surrounding tissues. For patients with a suspected respiratory ventilation injury, conduct a nasal and oropharyngeal examination to discover any singed nasal hairs and a chest examination. In determining the extent of the burn injury, the "rule of nines" helps to assess the body surface area; however, only second- and third-degree burns are included when calculating the total burn surface (Table 6–1). Of concern during an assessment of the patient with a burn is the likelihood of local edema. Remove any objects such as clothing or jewelry as soon as possible to avoid constriction of the area surrounding the burned tissue and to promote circulation to the wound.

TABLE 6–1   RULE OF NINES

Area	%*
Head and neck	9
Right upper extremity	9
Left upper extremity	9
Anterior chest and abdomen	18
Posterior chest and abdomen	18
Genitals	1
Right lower extremity	18
Left lower extremity	18
Total	100

*The percentages are added to determine the extent of burn injury in the patient.

Diagnostic Tests: General laboratory tests for the patient with an extensive burn injury include electrolytes, urinalysis, blood urea nitrogen (BUN), complete blood count (CBC), and type and cross-matching for blood products. Chest x-ray examination and electrocardiogram (ECG) are also ordered. For patients with suspected respiratory inhalation injury, obtain arterial blood gas and carboxyhemoglobin levels, to determine respiratory function. A xenon lung scan is also beneficial in diagnosing inhalation damage. For those with electrical burns, urine myoglobin and creatine phosphokinase (CPK) levels are measured to determine if there has been muscle swelling and evidence of myoglobinuria. A bronchoscopy may be ordered to assess the extent of smoke inhalation damage.

Differential Diagnosis: Toxic epidermal necrolysis or scalded skin syndrome can mimic the presentation of a burn injury.

Treatment: Immediate treatment for a burn is to apply wet towels soaked in ice water or cold water to the burn or, if possible, to immerse the burned area in cold tap water. The burned area should be kept moist with cold water until the burn is free of pain both in and out of the water. Depending on the extent of the burn, it may take 30 minutes for this analgesic effect to occur. To guard against potential hypothermia in patients with large-BSA burns being treated with ice water or cold water, the unaffected part of the body should be covered with a blanket. Patients with superficial small-BSA burns and without inhalation injury may be treated on an outpatient basis; however, in older adults, the patient's overall health condition must be considered when determining the treatment plan. Generally, patients are hospitalized if the face, hands, perineum, or feet are injured. Refer any patient with a burn associated with electrical current. A burned area exceeding 10%–15% of the BSA, or a full-thickness burn exceeding 3% of the BSA needs to be referred for hospitalization.

First-degree burns can be treated with cold compress applications and analgesics such as aspirin or acetaminophen as needed. A moisturizer can be applied to areas of intact burned skin to promote healing; no dressing is required. After the cold compresses have relieved the initial pain of a second-degree burn, cleanse the wound with a gentle irrigation of sterile saline, apply a topical antibiotic such as silver sulfadiazine, and wrap the wound in a sterile occlusive dressing. An oral analgesic may be administered to the patient prior to the irrigation of the wound. For patients with second- or third-degree burns and an infection at the burn site, a sample of the wound should be cultured and the appropriate antibiotic prescribed. Prophylactic systemic antibiotics are no longer advocated.

Follow-up: Outpatients should be reevaluated 72 hr after the burn injury. Examine the condition of the wound and surrounding tissues for signs of healing or impending infection. Re-examine respiratory status of patients with an inhalation injury to detect diffuse wheezing and rhonchi. Have the patient or significant

other demonstrate proper dressing techniques. Depending on the severity of
the burn, the patient may be asked to return once a week until progressive
healing is noted.

Sequelae: Immediate complications from a burn injury can include burn wound
sepsis, pneumonia, decreased mobility and function of an affected extremity,
and gastrointestinal ulcer. Long-term complications from a burn can include
squamous cell carcinoma developing at the scar site of the original injury.

Persons age 70 and older have a poor prognosis for recovery from a burn
injury. The survival rate from a burn injury is related to the severity of the
burn, especially if respiratory ventilation injury accompanied the burn.

Prevention/Prophylaxis: Antibiotic prophylaxis was discussed earlier. Tetanus
prophylaxis is recommended for second- and third-degree burns because these
wounds are tetanus-prone. A booster injection of tetanus toxoid should be
administered intramuscularly (IM) to those patients who have had been immunized in the past but have not received a booster injection within the past 5
years. If the patient has not been actively immunized, then give antitetanus
globulin, 250–500 units IM in addition to the tetanus toxoid, depending on the
severity of the burn.

Scalding injuries can often be prevented. Older adults should be instructed
to set the hot water heater temperature at 43°–49°C (110°–120°F).

All homes should have an evacuation plan, in case of an emergency. If the
emergency phone number 911 is not available in the area, then the numbers
for all local emergency services should be either programmed on the telephone
or listed within easy access. Encourage the use of functioning smoke detectors
and home fire extinguishers. Although the use of a heating unit or fireplace in a
home may be unavoidable, older adults should be rehearsed in safety precautions
needed for these heating systems. Any home assessment should include an
evaluation of fire prevention measures. Residents of long-term care facilities
should be permitted to smoke only when supervised. A sunscreen with a sun
protection factor (SPF) of at least 15 should be used and protective clothing
worn during episodes of prolonged sun exposure. Anyone with a healed burn
site should cover that area with a sunscreen throughout the year.

Referral: Outpatients being treated for a burn may require referral to a physical
therapist for wound therapy. Older adults who have suffered a moderate or
major burn injury require hospitalization and possibly admission to a specialized
burn care unit. Anyone experiencing smoke inhalation should be referred to a
respiratory physician specialist.

Education: Following treatment for a burn, patients should:

- Keep the wound clean and dry.
- Keep the wound elevated, if applicable.
- Change the dressing as directed.
- Take antibiotics as directed.

Patients should be informed that using home remedies such as butter and mayonnaise are not effective for wound healing; in fact, these products may actually promote bacterial growth.

Cellulitis

Cellulitis is a deep infection of the skin, most commonly caused by group A streptococci, by *Staphylococcus aureus,* or occasionally by a gram-negative organism. Cellulitis can also be caused by specific pathogens from human or animal bites.

Etiology: Although cellulitis usually occurs when an organism enters the skin through an open area, it can also occur in intact but edematous skin. Cellulitis involves the dermis and subcutaneous tissue. A clear site of entry may not be evident in patients with obesity, edema, or alcoholism.

Occurrence: The occurrence of cellulitis is unknown.

Age: Cellulitis can occur at any age. Facial cellulitis is more common in people age 50 or older.

Ethnicity: No known predominant ethnic group is associated with cellulitis incidence.

Gender: Cellulitis occurs equally among men and women.

Contributing Factor: Cellulitis can occur in patients who have arterial insufficiency, diabetes mellitus, lacerations, lower extremity edema, human or animal bites, tinea infections, recurring cellulitis, burns, trauma, stasis ulceration, ischemia, and puncture wounds. It is associated also with certain surgical procedures and environmental and occupational hazards. Intravenous (IV) drug use is another factor contributing to the development of cellulitis. Acute and chronic sinusitis can lead to periorbital or orbital cellulitis. Patients with history of a coronary artery bypass with removal of the saphenous vein are also susceptible to cellulitis.

Signs and Symptoms: Patients may complain of fever, chills, malaise, anorexia, nausea, or headache, and, in severe cases, patients may have tachycardia, hypotension, and delirium. Cellulitis most often appears on the lower extremities following a skin aberration such as dermatitis, ulceration, trauma, or tinea pedis. Scars from previous cardiovascular surgery are common sites for recurrent cellulitis. Examine for skin temperature, note any breaks in the skin and ulcerations, and determine presence of pulses and sensation. Local erythema with edema and tenderness elicited by palpation are presenting signs of cellulitis. The affected area may take on the appearance of an orange peel when the surface is infiltrated. Because lymphangiitis and regional lymphadenopathy may also occur with cellulitis, the clinician should examine for red streaks extending proximally to the infected area. If gas gangrene (anaerobic cellulitis) is suspected, the skin should be inspected for crepitus and foul-smelling exudate and the surrounding area palpated for muscle tenderness. A cardiac examination is warranted to assess for a heart murmur (Fig. 6–1).

Diagnostic Tests: Unless pus has formed in the wound, a tissue culture is usually not necessary. In cases of extensive infection or suspected systemic toxicity, blood cultures and a complete blood count (CBC) with differential should be obtained to determine the severity of illness. Leukocytosis is present in patients with anaerobic cellulitis, and the Gram's stain smear shows gram-positive encapsulated bacilli. Patients with diabetes mellitus should have a radiograph of the area to rule out the presence of osteomyelitis.

Differential Diagnosis: The conditions that can mimic cellulitis include lipodermatosclerosis, acute severe contact dermatitis, acute gout, fasciitis, thrombophlebitis, and pseudogout.

Treatment: Patients with an open wound should initially be asked when their last tetanus toxoid booster was given; if the most recent booster was 10 or more years ago, 0.5 mL of tetanus toxoid should be administered immediately. If the wound is grossly contaminated and the patient's last tetanus booster was 5–10 years ago, the clinician should consider giving another booster at this time. An older adult who has not had primary immunization requires tetanus toxoid and tetanus immune globulin.

Patients with mild cellulitis may be given oral antibiotics. The drugs of choice include erythromycin, amoxicillin-clavulanate, azithromycin, clarithromycin, clindamycin, and a first-generation cephalosporin such as cephalexin. For streptococcal cellulitis, penicillin is the drug of choice. Oxacillin is also effective for both streptococcus and staphylococcus. Oral therapy should be prescribed for a 7- to 10-day period. Patients with underlying tinea should be treated with topical antifungal medications as well as antibiotics. Consider the patient's renal function before prescribing any medication. Tell the patient to elevate the affected area, keep the area as clean as possible, and avoid any trauma to the area. Moist warm soaks can be applied to the affected area. Patients may require analgesics in appropriate dosages for pain. Patients with edema should take measures to control the edema by elevating the extremity(ies). Blood glucose levels need to be carefully monitored if the patient has diabetes. Patients with complications (see referral section) should be hospitalized for monitoring and to receive IV antibiotics.

Follow-up: Outpatients should be requested to contact their health-care providers within a week if no improvement is noted or within 48 hr if fever or inflammation continues. On their return visit, patients should be examined for evidence of thrombophlebitis or recurrence of the cellulitis.

Sequelae: In patients with cellulitis of the lower extremities, thrombophlebitis is a potential complication. Additional problems arising from cellulitis include bacteremia and lymphangiitis, especially in people with recurrent cellulitis.

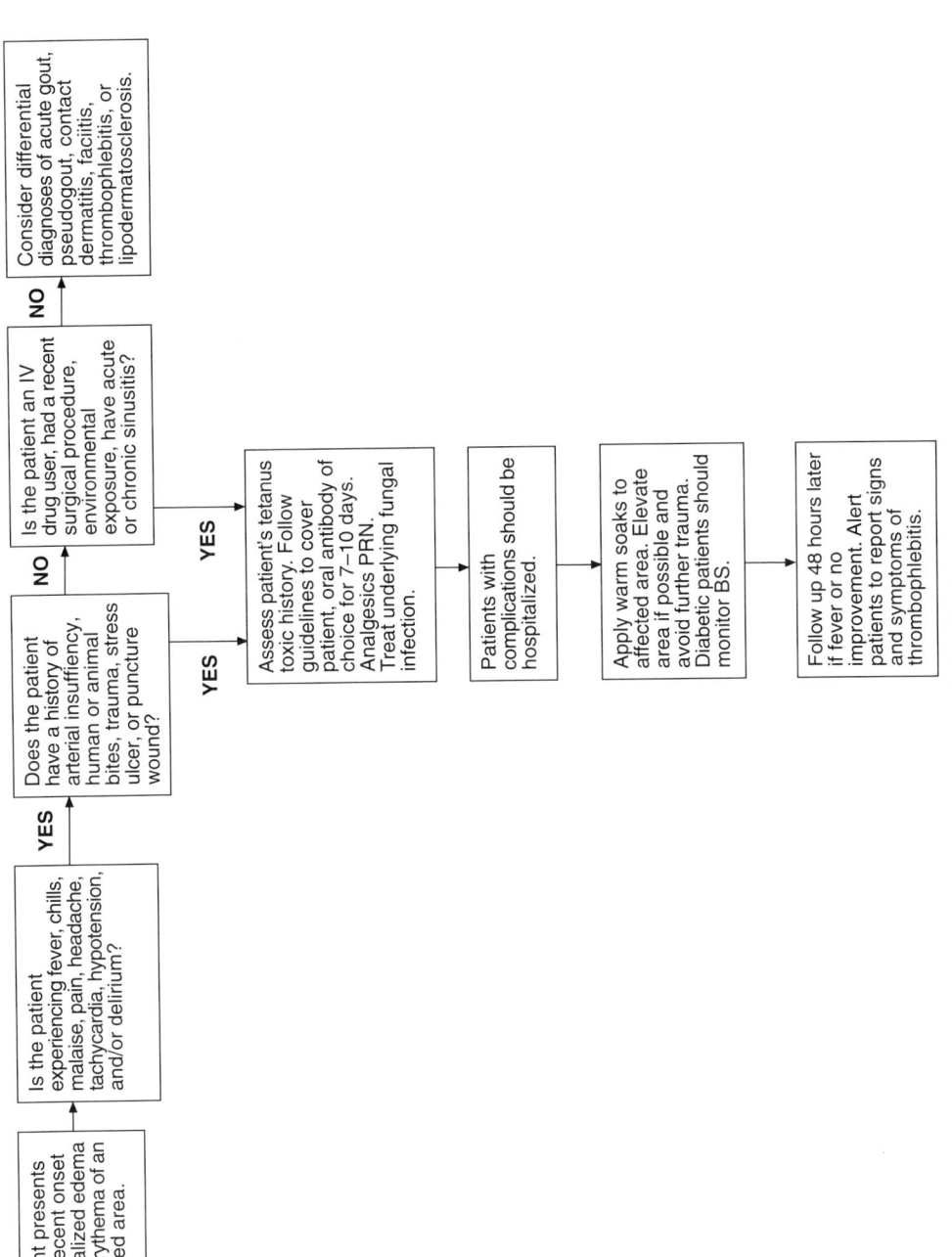

FIGURE 6–1 Cellulitis.

Prevention/Prophylaxis: Some preventative measures for cellulitis include reduction of chronic edema in patients with peripheral vascular disease, control of blood glucose in those with diabetes, and meticulous hand-washing. Wheelchair-bound patients should have protective measures to avoid trauma to their extremities.

Referral: Patients should be hospitalized if they have high fever, diabetes, alcoholism, human immunodeficiency virus (HIV), anaerobic cellulitis, necrotizing fasciitis, or cellulitis of the orbit or face, or if they are experiencing extreme pain. Consultation with an infectious disease specialist may be necessary. Order a surgical consultation for patients who require incision and drainage of abscesses and debridement of necrotic tissue. Home IV treatment may also be indicated to shorten hospital stay.

Education: Patients with cellulitis must be informed that completion of the antibiotic regimen is mandatory. They should not attempt to scratch the affected area but should keep the site meticulously clean to avoid superinfection. Advise patients with lower extremity involvement to maintain bedrest with bathroom privileges and elevate the limb. Apprise them of the signs and symptoms of thrombophlebitis.

Corns and Calluses

Corns and calluses are aggregations of hyperkeratotic skin on the foot.

Etiology: Corns and calluses are caused by increased rubbing of, pressure on, or friction to the foot. The most common cause is poorly fitting shoes. Individuals with foot deformities, or gait disturbances, or both, are also at high risk for developing calluses, especially over bony prominences.

Age: Individuals over age 65 most commonly develop corns and calluses.

Gender: More common in women secondary to restrictive footwear.

Contributing Factors: Gait disturbance and/or imbalance secondary to weakness, arthritis, normal aging changes of the foot, foot deformities, and use of improper footwear.

Signs and Symptoms: Usually corns and calluses are asymptomatic. Thick calluses may cause a burning sensation in the foot. Depending on the location of the callus, tight-fitting shoes may cause severe pain (Fig. 6–2).

Diagnostic Test: An x-ray examination of the foot may be warranted, to rule out abnormal bone structure.

Differential Diagnosis: Plantar ulcers and plantar warts (verrucae) may mimic corns and calluses.

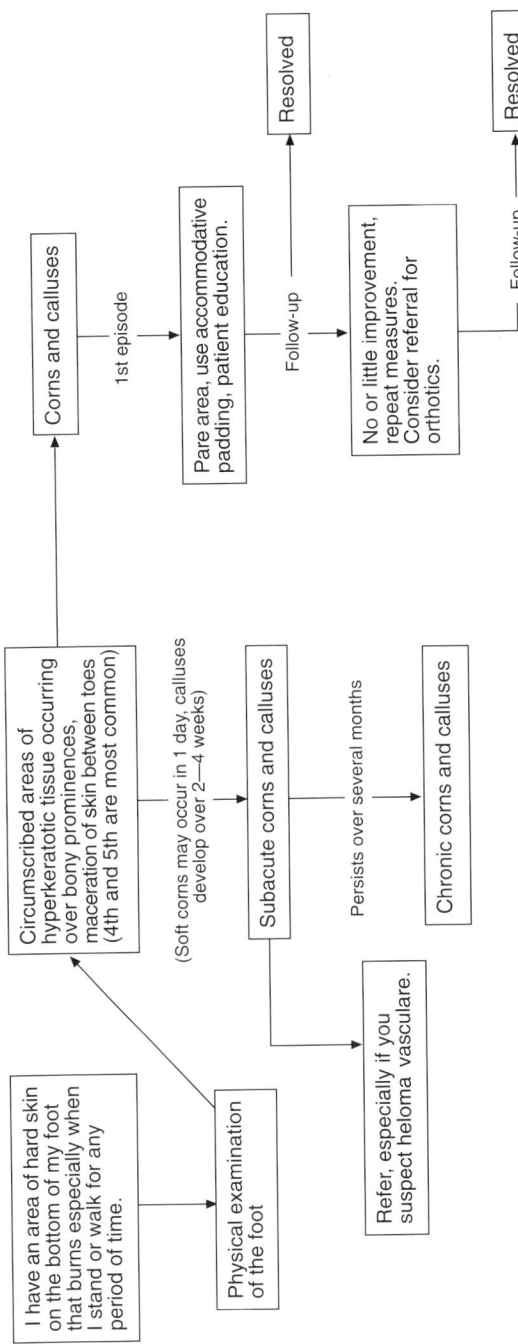

FIGURE 6–2 Corns and calluses.

Treatment: Mechanical paring of the corn, callus, or both, is recommended. Improper footwear should be avoided. Use of accommodative padding such as a metatarsal pad helps to relieve pressure.

Follow-up: Periodic physical examination of the foot is needed, to assess the status.

Prevention/Prophylaxis: Relief of the pressure on the affected area can prevent development of corns and calluses. Shoes should be wide enough at the toe to allow the toes to extend straight ahead. Encourage women to avoid wearing shoes with high heels.

Referral: Refer patients with complicated management to a podiatrist.

Education: Teach patients the importance of avoiding improper footwear. To prevent injury to the toes, ½ inch extra should be allowed in the toe box.

Fungal Infection of the Skin and Nails

The skin, nails, or both, may be infected by fungal organisms called dermatophytes, which have the ability to utilize keratin to maintain their physiologic requirements.

Etiology: The most common dermatophytes are *Trichophyton unguium* and *T. mentagrophytes.*

Occurrence: This type of infection affects approximately 4% of the general population. In elderly persons, tinea pedis and tinea unguium (onychomycosis) are the most prevalent skin and nail fungal infections.

Ethnicity: Incidence of fungal infection has no ethnic significance.

Gender: Fungal infection occurs equally in men and women.

Contributing Factors: Factors contributing to fungal infection of the skin and nails are increased susceptibility to infection, diabetes mellitus, hyperkeratosis of the feet, use of socks or stockings that do not wick away moisture, residual fungal spores present in the patient's footwear.

Signs and Symptoms: Chronic tinea pedis, which may have been present for most of the patient's adult life, may be asymptomatic. The toenails affected by this type of fungal infection are thick, discolored, and hypertrophic, with debris beneath the nail plate. Inflammatory forms of tinea pedis may exhibit interdigital maceration, diffuse scaling of the soles in a "moccasin"-type fashion, and vesicles and pustules on the instep of the feet (Fig. 6–3).

Diagnostic Tests: A potassium hydroxide (KOH) preparation as skin and nail plate scrapings, in addition to fungal cultures, is used in diagnosis of fungal infections.

Differential Diagnosis: Contact dermatitis, dyshidrotic eczema, trauma to the area, psoriasis, and normal aging may cause symptoms that mimick fungal infections.

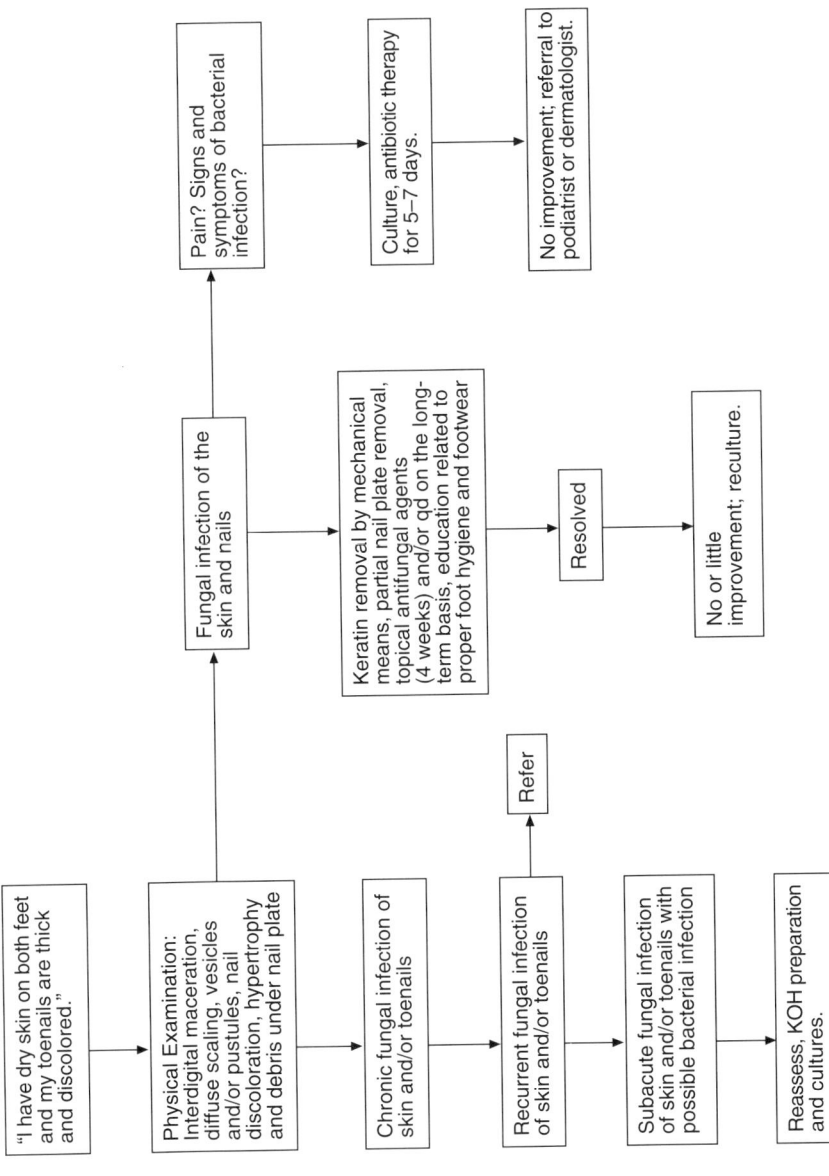

FIGURE 6–3 Fungal infection of the skin and nails.

Treatment: In general, no treatment is required if the patient is asymptomatic. Topical antifungal agents are ineffective in the management of onychomycosis because of their poor penetration of the nail plate. Prolonged use of oral antifungal agents should be approached cautiously in elderly persons because of age-related physiological changes and the effect these agents may have on renal, hepatic, and hematopoietic function. In managing tinea pedis, measures to decrease sweating, such as use of cotton socks, are most beneficial. Daily use of antifungal powders, sprays, or both, may help relieve burning and itching of the feet.

Follow-up: Fungal infections can be chronic. In patients who develop diffuse plantar scaling, vesiculopustular eruptions, or evidence of secondary infection, both KOH preparation and culture should be repeated to rule out other differential diagnoses and determine appropriate treatment regimens.

Prevention/Prophylaxis: Proper cleansing and drying of the feet (especially between the toes) by patient, caregiver, or both, helps to prevent maceration. Avoid use of socks or stockings made of synthetic materials.

Referral: Refer to a podiatrist or dermatologist any patient exhibiting signs and symptoms of bacterial infection or experiencing moderate to severe pain, especially of the nailbed and surrounding nail margins.

Education: Teach proper foot hygiene to reduce risk of an environment that encourages fungal growth. Emphasize the importance of using appropriate socks and stockings and of avoiding damp or wet footwear.

Herpes Zoster

Herpes zoster is an acute vesicular eruption caused by a virus histologically identical to the varicella (chickenpox virus). Herpes zoster is human (alpha) herpes virus 3 (varicella-zoster virus, V-Z virus, or VZV), a member of the herpesvirus group.

Etiology: Recurrent VZV infection causes herpes zoster. The patient has initial contact with VZV in the form of chickenpox. The DNA virus resides within the neurons. During reactivation, the virus spreads across the ganglion to other neurons, which causes a cutaneous eruption of a dermatome distribution. Herpes zoster is self-limited. Although chickenpox is one of the most readily communicable diseases, herpes zoster has a much lower rate of transmission. Nonimmune persons are considered contagious 8–21 days after exposure to VZV. Mode of transmission is coming into contact with the vesicle fluid. Patients with herpes zoster may be sources of infection for a week after the appearance of vesicle lesions. Nonimmune individuals can transmit infection and should avoid content with patients with herpes zoster.

Occurrence: Herpes zoster occurs worldwide, more commonly in older adults. An estimated half of the population will be affected by age 85.

Age: This infection is most common in those over age 55.

Ethnicity: No ethnic preference exists for herpes zoster.

Gender: Herpes zoster occurs equally in men and women.

Contributing Factors: Individuals are more likely to develop herpes zoster if they are over age 55, immunosuppressed (e.g., HIV-infected patients), or have a malignancy. Physiologic or psychological stressors can precipitate the development of herpes zoster.

Signs and Symptoms: Patients usually experience burning or tingling pain at the site 4 to 5 days before the eruption appears. The eruption is maculopapular for a few hours, then becomes characterized as grouped vesicles on an erythematous base over one dermatome (usually). As vesicles age, they become pustular and then crust over after 3–4 days, finally healing in 2–4 weeks. Lesions may appear in irregular crops and are typically unilateral. Most common distributions are on the trunk or face, in elderly persons. Regional lymph nodes may or may not be swollen and tender. Pain can last 6–12 months after disappearance of the rash (postherpetic neuralgia) (Fig. 6–4).

Diagnostic Tests: Diagnosis is usually based on clinical appearance and distribution of the eruption and careful history of when the rash appeared. The laboratory tests listed here are useful in complicated cases and epidemiological studies.

- Tzanck test results may be positive. Scrape the roof and base of a vesicle with a scalpel blade, smearing material on a glass slide and staining it with Wright's, Giemsa, or Papanicolaou stain. This reveals the presence of multinucleated giant cells, which indicates herpesvirus but not specifically herpes zoster.
- Viral cultures may be performed, but these viruses are slow growing and do not aid in timely treatment.
- A recently developed fluorescein antibody test, which can identify VZV within 2 hours, is not readily available.

Differential Diagnosis: When the pain of pre-eruptive herpes occurs, zoster, migraine, myocardial infarction, and acute abdomen, to name a few, depending on the dermatome involved, must be ruled out. Once the rash or eruption appears, contact dermatitis, cellulitis, and poison oak and ivy should be ruled out (linear vesicles are more typical of contact allergic dermatitis and grouped vesicles are more typical of viral infection).

Treatment: Antiviral agents are recommended in the presence of significant pain, serious herpes zoster, or involvement near the eye. Postherpetic neuralgia is not reduced by antiviral therapy, but these agents may help with healing in the acute phase. Dosage is acyclovir 800 mg five times a day for 7 days, famciclovir 500 mg PO every 8 hr for 7 days, or valacyclovir 1000 mg PO every 8 hr for 7 days. These drugs must be given within 48–96 hr after onset of rash to be

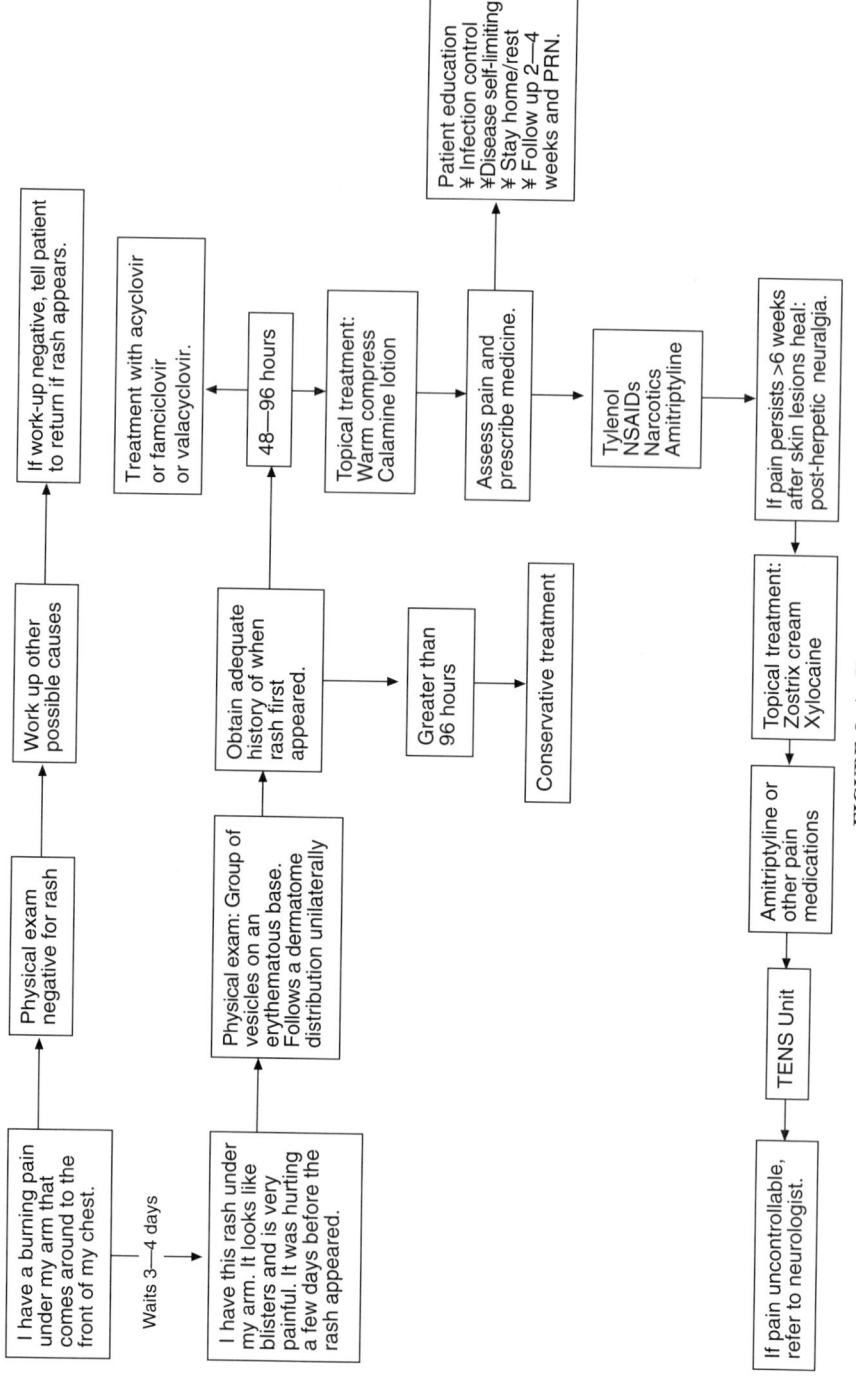

FIGURE 6–4 Herpes zoster.

effective, and their use must be monitored in patients with reduced renal function.

Topical agents are also effective in treating Herpes zoster. The use of cool compresses with 1 : 20 Burrow's solution, calamine lotion, and topical xylocaine is recommended for the soothing local effect.

Analgesics may be necessary for the initial pain associated with herpes zoster. Acetaminophen is recommended initially. Opiates, such as codeine and oxycodone-acetaminophen (Percocett) can be used for severe pain but are not generally recommended for elderly individuals.

For postherpetic neuralgia pain, capsaicin (Zostrix cream) can be applied topically. Also, amitriptyline 25 mg PO tid or doxepin 25–50 mg tid is helpful. In cases of severe pain, a transcutaneous electrical nerve stimulator (TENS) unit may be tried.

Follow-up: Patients should be reexamined in 2–4 weeks to monitor progression of rash, and as needed for follow-up of postherpetic neuralgia.

Sequelae: Postherpetic neuralgia is the primary complication, occurring almost exclusively in persons over age 60. This pain persists at least 6 weeks after skin lesions. The pain, characterized as constant, severe, sharp, or burning, may develop into a longstanding and debilitating problem. Postherpetic neuralgia usually lasts no longer than a year.

Another consequence of herpes zoster is secondary bacterial infection leading to cellulitis, caused by staphyllococci group A or group A beta-hemolytic streptococci. Cutaneous or visceral dissemination, the appearance of numerous varicella-like lesions in extradermatomal sites, may cause pneumonitis or encephalitis.

Prevention/Prophylaxis: The only effective prevention for herpes zoster is prevention of primary varicella infection (chickenpox) because latent varicella virus cannot be cleared from the sensory ganglia. The varicella vaccine now available to prevent chickenpox in children may logically be expected to decrease the incidence of herpes zoster if it comes into widespread use. High-risk individuals such as immunosuppressed patients as well as those who have not had chickenpox, should be kept from exposure. In varicella-nonimmune individuals who have been exposed, passive immune treatment with varicella-zoster immune (VZI) globulin should be used to modify the infection.

Referral: Refer to an ophthalmologist patients with lesions on the nose or in the eye area because of probable ocular involvement. Patients with disseminated herpes zoster should be referred to a specialist. Refer those with severe uncontrollable postherpetic neuralgia to a neurologist.

Education: Emphasize to the patient the need to stay home and get plenty of rest. Teach patients proper infection control measures and proper disposal of dressings of clothing that contain vesicle fluid. Patients should avoid contact with immunosuppressed individuals, pregnant women, or those who have not had chickenpox. Emphasize that herpes zoster is self-limited.

Insect Stings and Bites

Insect stings and bites are skin punctures or wounds caused by contact with an insect. Venom may be secreted into tissues or a stinger left imbedded in the skin.

Etiology: In North America, the black widow or show button, red-legged widow, and brown recluse spiders cause the most serious spider bites. Found throughout this continent, the black widow or show button spider is identified by a characteristic red "hourglass" on the abdomen. The red-legged widow is usually found in Florida. The brown recluse spider is found in the southern, midwestern, and southwestern United States. Stings or bites from bees, wasps, hornets, yellowjackets, or fire ants, occurring throughout North America, may have local or systemic effects. Fire ants, which may be red or black, are found in the southern United States and in states bordering Mexico. Ticks can act as vectors for bacterial or viral infections but usually cause only local irritation. Disease-causing ticks are most common in the southeastern and northeastern United States and in Western Canada. Flea, centipede, chigger, horsefly and deerfly bites may cause local irritation or initiate bacterial skin infections such as cellulitis. The bite of the nocturnal kissing bug, found throughout the southern United States, causes lesions on the extremities.

Occurrence: Insect bites and stings usually occur between April and October in North America.

Age: Insect bites and stings can affect individuals of any age.

Ethnicity: There is no known prevalence among ethnic groups.

Gender: Occurs equally in men and women.

Contributing Factors: People involved in outdoor activities are most likely to experience insect bites or stings. Outdoor activities involving food, such as picnics, increase the risk of sting from bees, hornets, wasps, or fire ants. Coming in contact with animals and engaging in activities in thickly forested areas predisposes individuals to tick bites. Spiders are found in wood piles, sheds, basements, and outdoor toilets.

Signs and Symptoms: Individuals who have been stung by a bee, hornet, wasp, or fire ant usually complain of a pinprick, then a stinging or burning sensation, followed after several minutes by local pruritus. A red papule is present at the site, and sometimes the stinger may be seen imbedded in the skin. Multiple stings may produce nausea, vomiting, or diarrhea. Local or systemic allergic reactions occur within 2–60 min in 10%–15% of the population. Urticarial reactions may remain local or progress to life-threatening anaphylaxis, with symptoms of nausea, abdominal and uterine cramps, bronchospasm, angioedema, edema of the glottis with wheezing and stridor, dyspnea, cyanosis, and hypotension.

Spider bites usually produce a sharp, intense pain at the site. Black widow or show button spider bites may be followed in 15–60 min by complaints of cramping in the extremities or trunk. The abdomen becomes boardlike but is nontender on examination, despite waves of pain. Respiration may be labored, and the patient may experience nausea, vomiting, headache, diaphoresis, excessive salivation, tremor, twitching, and parasthesias of the distal extremities. Hyperreflexia and elevated systolic blood pressure may be present, and leukocytosis can accompany fever. Serious complications such as respiratory distress, respiratory arrest, coma, or death occur most often in children or elderly persons.

Brown recluse spider bites initially produce minor localized pain and erythema, progressing to intense local pain within 2–8 hr. Necrosis of tissue at the site of the bite may begin within 4 hr. These spider bites resemble a pustule, vesicle, or bullae with a sunken middle and necrosis at the base of the wound. Fever, chills, nausea, vomiting, myalgias, and weakness can begin 12 hr after the bite.

Most other insect bites produce localized pruritus with erythematous papules or nodules. Centipede bites are very painful and can produce lymphangiitis in addition to erythema and local edema. Kissing bug bites, which occur at night, resemble hemorrhagic bullous lesions on the extremities and may be confused with brown recluse spider bites. Kissing bug bites occur in groups, however, rather than singly as spider bites do.

The history of patients who complain of insect bite or sting should include any previous allergic reactions to bites or stings because 40% of persons who develop anaphylaxis have a history of a severe allergic reaction to an insect attack. Ask the patient to describe the insect and to tell the type of insect and when and where the bite occurred, if possible.

Diagnostic Tests No diagnostic tests are indicated, unless systemic sequelae are suspected.

Differential Diagnosis: Puncture wounds, cellulitis, bacterial or fungal skin infection, superficial phlebitis, vasovagal episodes, and hyperventilation may mimic anaphylaxis.

Treatment: Anaphylaxis or suspected progression to anaphylaxis (based on patient's history) should be treated with epinephrine 1:1000 aqueous solution 0.3 to 0.5 mL subcutaneously every 20–30 min. When symptoms are mild, with urticaria and pruritus, epinephrine injection is continued and an intramuscular antihistamine such as diphenhydramine 50–80 mg is administered. These patients must be observed for a minimum of 6–8 hr, must take oral antihistamines for the next 24 hr, and should be seen for follow-up the next day. On follow-up, the provider should prescribe EpiPen and teach the patient how and when to use it. Referral to an allergist for testing and desensitization is recommended. If symptoms such as angioedema, bronchospasm, and hypotension are severe, additional measures and transport to an emergency department are indicated. Begin an IV infusion of D5W. Administer oxygen via nasal cannula and isoproterenol via nebulizer, when possible. Application of a tourniquet above the site of the bite or sting may decrease the spread of the toxin; removal of the stinger, while avoiding compression over the site, is recommended.

When a black widow spider bite is suspected and symptoms confirm it, administration of antivenin and pain relief are the goals of therapy. Transport to a hospital emergency department is recommended. Treatment may include the administration of 10% calcium gluconate and 10% methocarbomal to relieve cramping.

Treatment of brown recluse spider bite varies, depending on the severity of symptoms. Apply ice to and elevate the affected area. Bullae formation with increasing erythema within 8 hr usually indicates a severe bite, and transfer to the hospital for parenteral glucocorticoids is recommended. The patient should be seen for follow-up in 24–48 hr to assess for necrosis at the site of the bite.

Most insect bites require minimal care. Wash the bite or sting with soap and water. The stinger or tick should be removed using sterile forceps, being careful not to leave any pieces embedded in the skin. For patients with tick bites, educate the patient about the signs and symptoms of Lyme disease and Rocky Mountain spotted fever which require immediate follow-up. Ice, rather than heat, should be applied to the area. An oral antihistamine, diphenhydramine 25 mg every 6 hr (every 8 hr for older adult patients) or hydroxyzine hydrochloride 25 mg every 6 hr (10 mg every 6 hr for older adult patients), as needed, can be prescribed to relieve pruritus. Occasionally, for severe local reactions, oral steroid therapy, such as a prednisone 5-mg dose pack, may be prescribed. Antibiotics may be prescribed to prevent secondary infection, especially in the case of spider bites. Erythromycin 500 mg bid or cephalexin 250 mg every 6 hr is recommended. Obtain the patient's tetanus toxoid immunization history and consider administration of tetanus toxoid if it has been more than 5 yr since the last dose (Fig. 6–5).

Follow-up: Follow-up is indicated only if the patient develops anaphylaxis or a brown recluse spider bite is suspected, as noted previously.

Sequelae: Consequences of insect bites include anaphylaxis or hypersensitivity reaction and, rarely, secondary bacterial infection.

Prevention: Caution patients to avoid wearing bright clothing or perfumes during outdoor activities. Shoes should always be worn for outdoor activities. Wearing long sleeves and pants that fit snugly reduces the chance of getting insect bites and stings. The use of insect repellents is recommended during outdoor activities.

Referral: Patients who develop anaphylaxis should be transported to a hospital emergency department. Later referral to an allergist is recommended if the patient has a hypersensitivity reaction. A dermatologist may be consulted for insect bites or stings that do not respond to the treatments described earlier. A surgeon may be necessary in the case of a severe brown recluse spider bite.

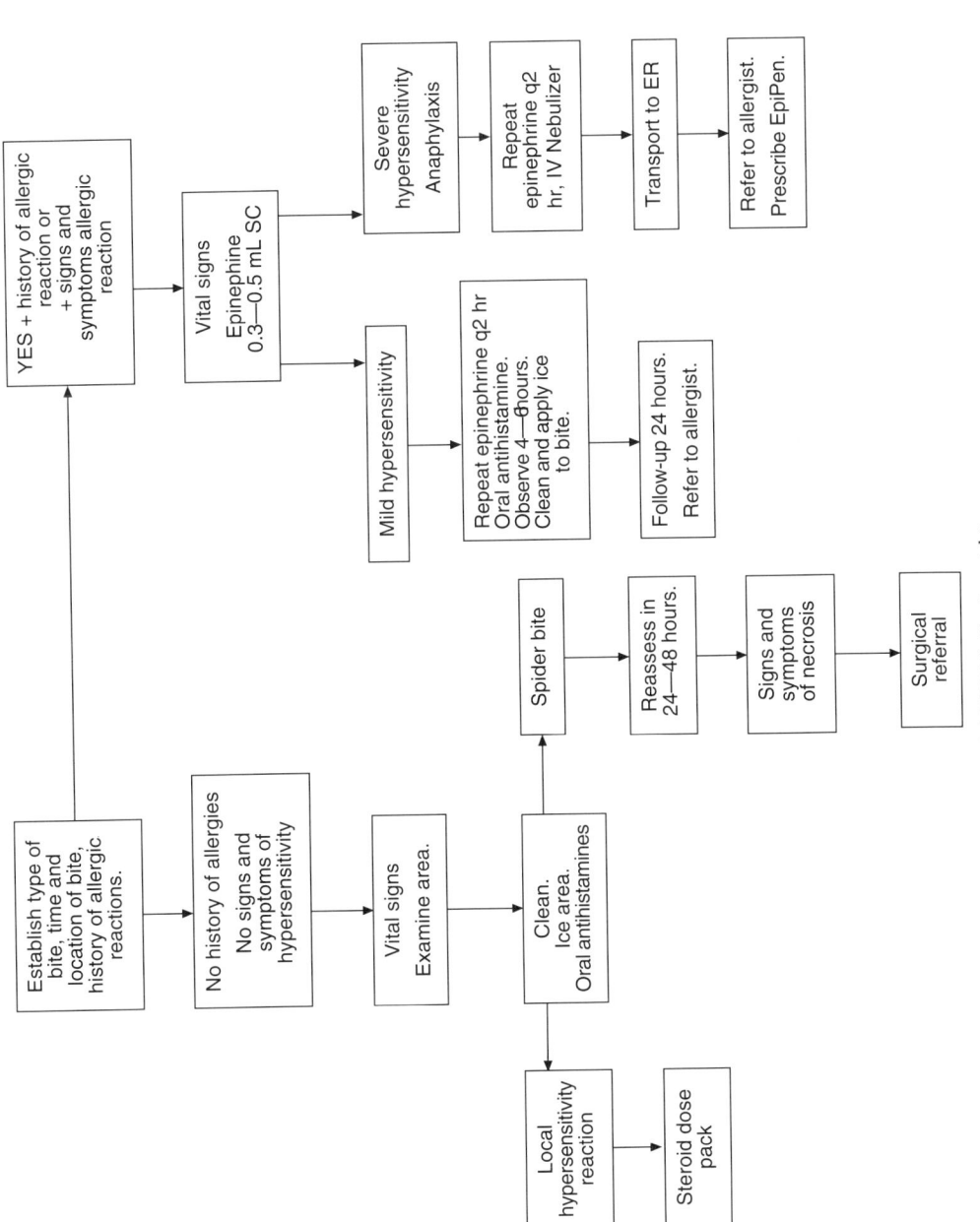

FIGURE 6–5 Insect bites.

Education: Review with patients strategies for the prevention of spider bites and stings. Teach patients with a history of anaphylaxis or hypersensitivity reactions how to use the EpiPen.

Pressure Ulcers

Pressure ulcers are localized areas of tissue necrosis that tend to develop when soft tissue is compressed between a bony prominence and an external surface for a prolonged period.

Etiology: Pressure is the major causative factor in pressure ulcer formation. However, several factors play a role in determining whether pressure is sufficient to create an ulcer. The pathological effect of excessive pressure on soft tissue can be attributed to:

- Intensity of pressure.
- Duration of pressure.
- Tissue tolerance (the ability of both the skin and its supporting structures to endure pressure without adverse sequelae).

Occurrence: The prevalence of pressure ulcers among patients in acute-care settings is 3%–14%, whereas that among patients admitted to nursing homes is 15%–25%. Patients admitted to a hospital geriatric unit have a similarly high prevalence rate, 24%.

Age: The generalized prevalence of pressure ulcers in the elderly population is 11.6%–27.5%, with an increased risk assigned to advancing age. Of patients under age 70 years, only 6% have pressure ulcers, whereas for those age 70 or older, the prevalence almost doubles to 11.6%.

Ethnicity: There is no known prevalence among ethnic groups.

Gender: Pressure ulcers occur equally in men and women.

Contributing Factors: The three major contributing factors to pressure ulcer development are friction, shear, and nutritional debilitation. Moisture, specifically incontinence, is frequently cited as a related condition because moisture alters the resiliency of the epidermis to external forces. Other predisposing factors include advanced age, low blood pressure, smoking, elevated body temperature, and dehydration.

Signs and Symptoms: Clinical presentation can vary from nonblanching erythema to ecchymosis, and then to frank necrosis. Nonblanching erythema results from damage to blood vessels and extravasation of blood into the tissues. Its presence suggests that tissue damage is imminent or has already occurred. The color of the skin can be an intense bright red to a dark red or purple; pressure-induced nonblanching erythema is often misdiagnosed as a hematoma or ecchymosis.

When deep tissue damage is also present, the area is often either indurated or boggy when palpated. Note ulcer size, depth, presence of exudate, epithelialization, granulation tissue, and findings such as necrotic tissue, sinus tracts, undermining, tunneling, and purulent drainage or other signs of infection.

Diagnostic Tests
- Wound cultures are not indicated routinely because, although all dermal wounds are contaminated, not all are infected.
- Wound culture and sensitivity is indicated for any of the following: signs of local infection (erythema, edema, induration, purulent or very foul smelling drainage, pain, crepitus); signs of systemic infection (fever, leukocytosis); bone involvement (because of risk for osteomyelitis); and nonhealing wound.
- Staging of pressure ulcers is done to classify the degree of tissue damage observed. Numerical identification of stages does not necessarily imply a progression in ulcer severity.

Differential Diagnosis: Skin cancers, fungal and yeast infections, venous or arterial leg ulcers, and neuropathic ulcers may mimic pressure ulcers.

Treatment: An effective ulcer treatment plan should have three components:
1. Nutritional assessment and support.
2. Management of tissue loads (pressure, friction, and shear).
3. Ulcer care and management of bacterial colonization and infection (debridement, wound cleansing, application of dressings, and measures to control bacterial colonization and treat infection).

These components are equally important, so they should be addressed simultaneously. If an ulcer is complicated by infection, the antibiotic program should include anaerobic as well as aerobic coverage (Fig. 6–6).

Follow-up: Caregivers should evaluate the patient's progress toward healing at least weekly. If signs of ulcer deterioration are observed sooner, steps to reverse them should be taken immediately. If the patient's general condition deteriorates, the ulcer should be reassessed promptly. Caregivers should monitor the individual's general health, nutritional adequacy, psychosocial support, and pain level and should be alert to signs of complications. Frequency of monitoring should be determined by the clinician, based on the condition of the patient, the condition of the ulcer, the ulcer's healing rate, and the type of the patient's health-care setting.

Sequelae: Cellulitis, bacteremia, osteomyelitis, and meningitis may occur secondary to pressure ulcers.

Prevention/Prophylaxis: Screening tests and risk assessment tools are critical to any pressure ulcer prevention program. The specific deficits contributing to a score must be considered, to implement a treatment plan. The negative effects of risk factors may be minimized by correct positioning, providing pressure-

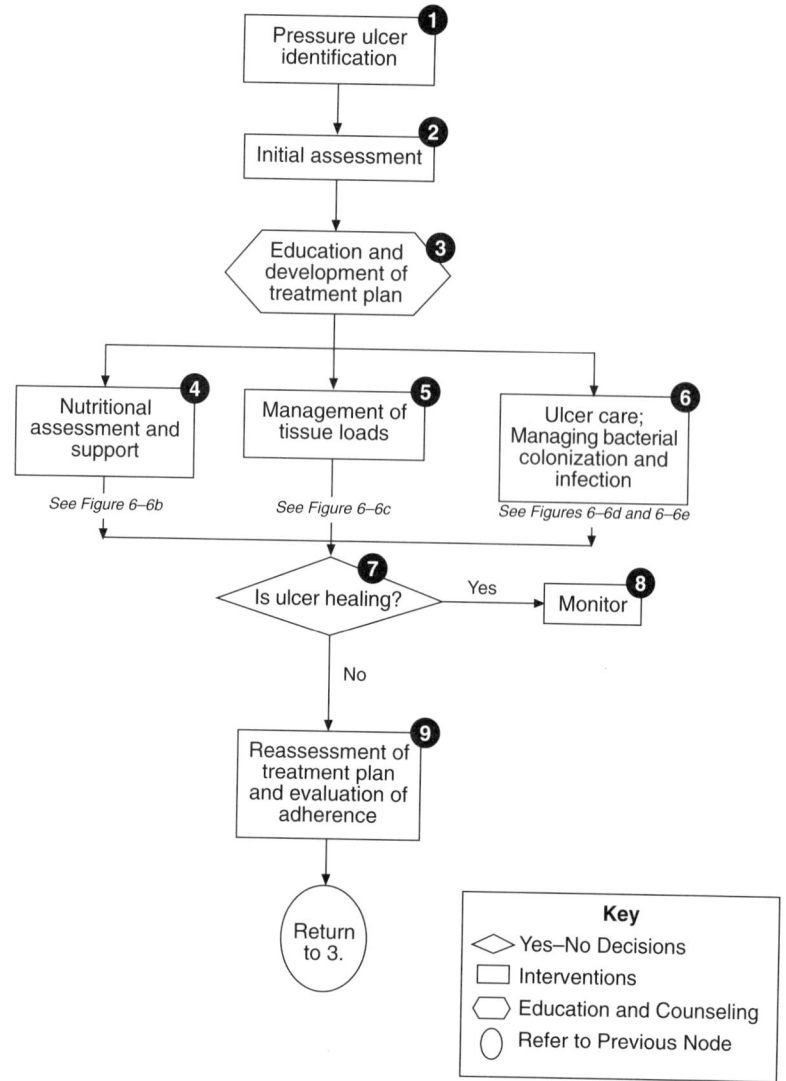

FIGURE 6–6a Treatment of pressure ulcers: Management of pressure ulcers.

reduction sleep or sitting surfaces, improving the nutritional status of the individual, and managing incontinence.

Referral: Refer the patient to a specialist (endostomal therapist nurse, plastic surgeon, dermatologist) if the wound does not respond to therapy or for product recommendation, debridement, biopsy, or surgical intervention (i.e., graft or myocutaneous flap).

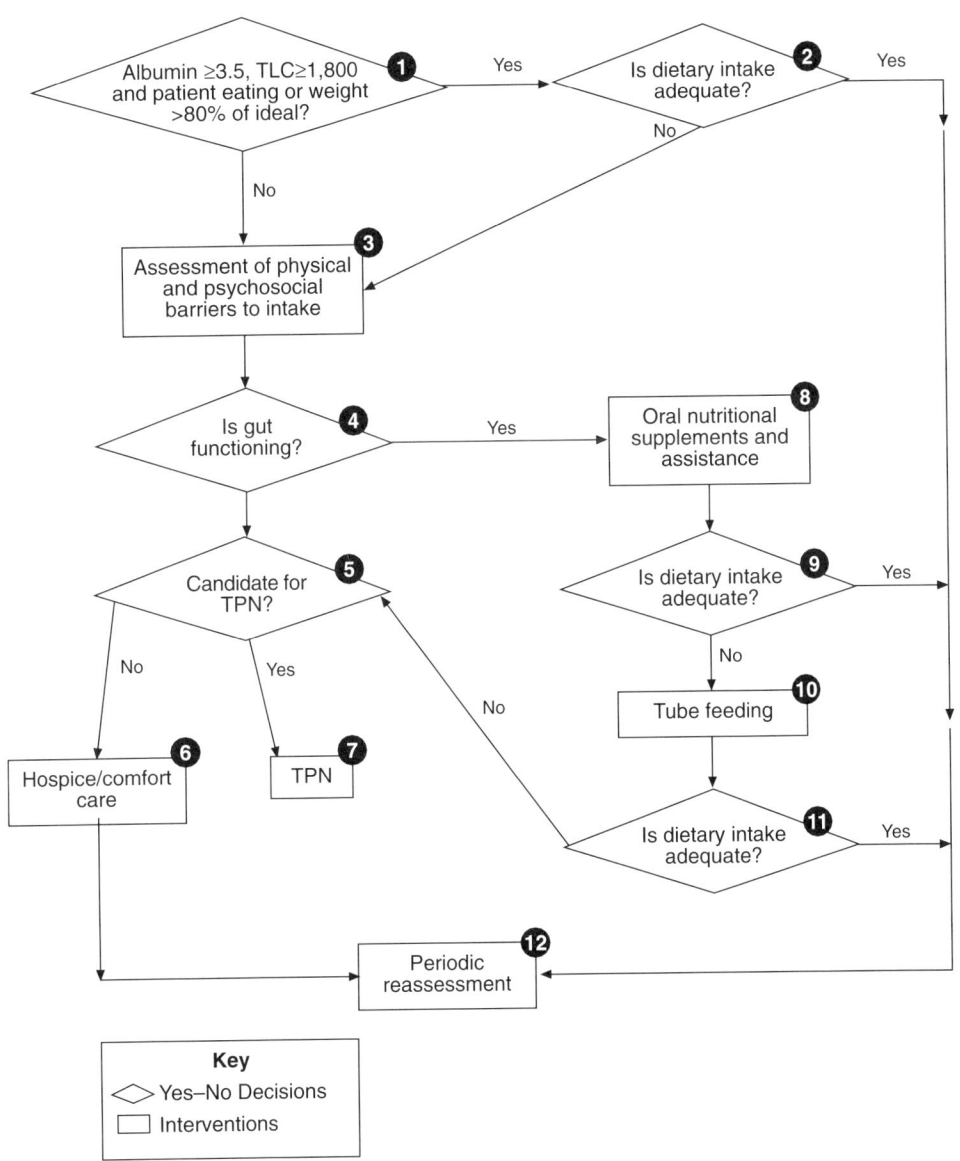

Key
◇ Yes–No Decisions
▢ Interventions

Note: TLC = total lymphocyte count; TPN = total parenteral nutrition.

FIGURE 6–6b Treatment of pressure ulcers: Nutritional assessment and support.

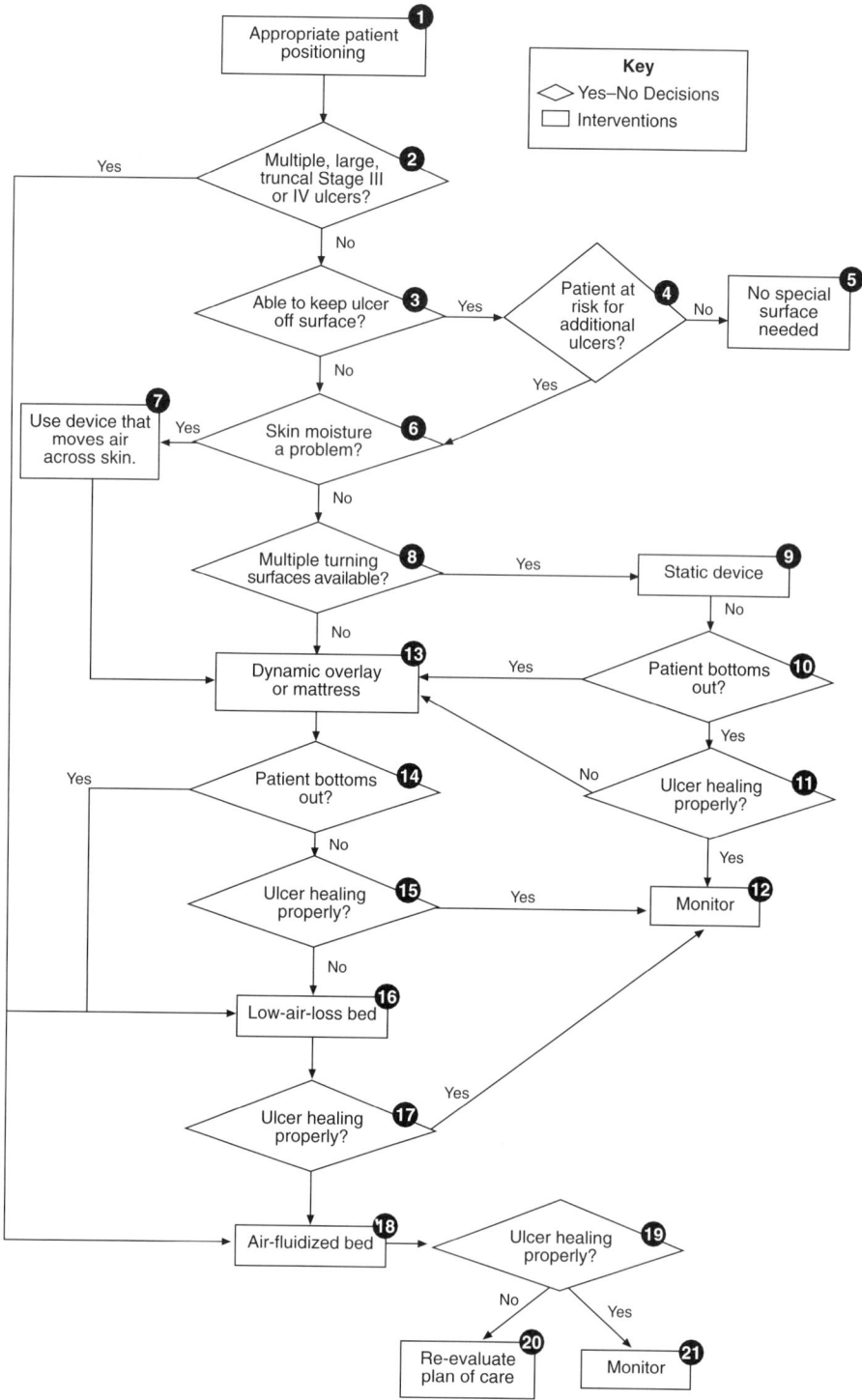

FIGURE 6–6c Treatment of pressure ulcers: Management of tissue loads.

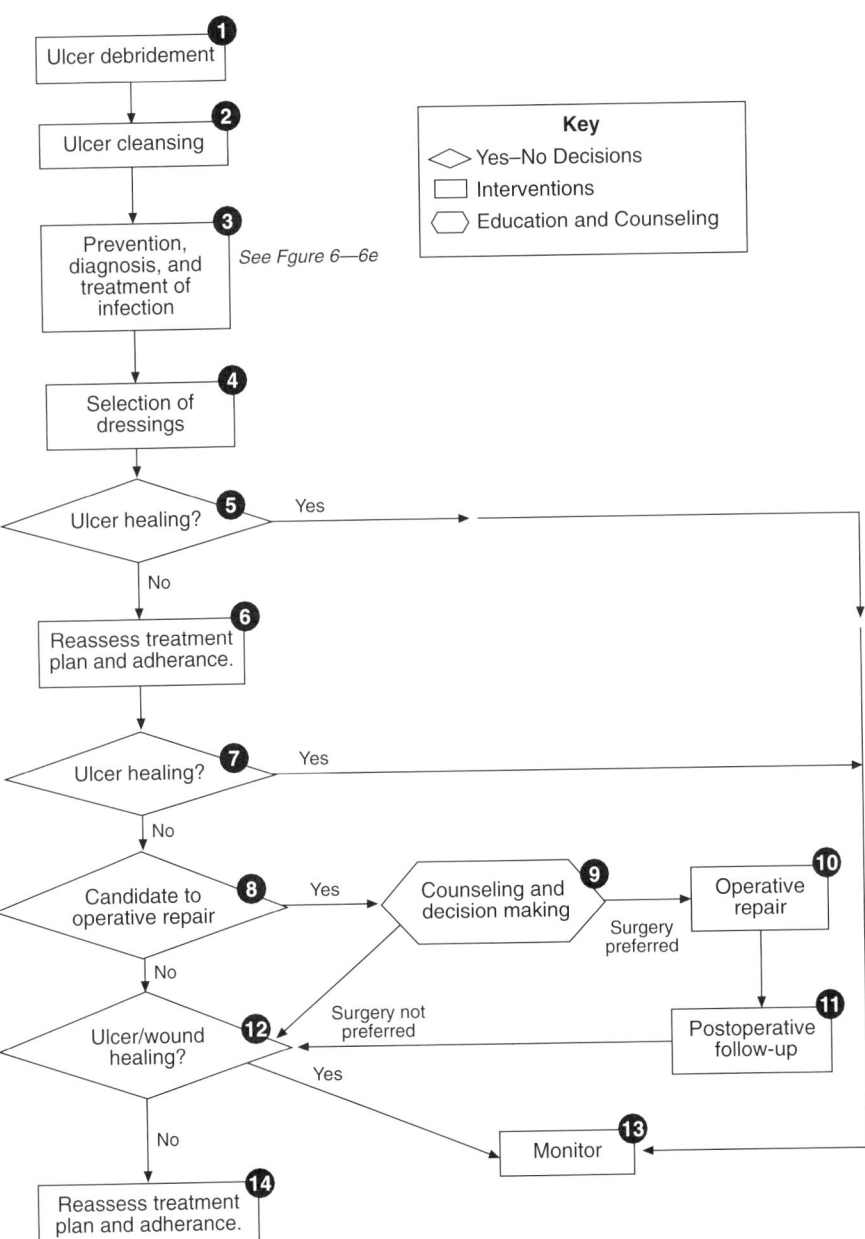

FIGURE 6–6d Treatment of pressure ulcers: Ulcer care.

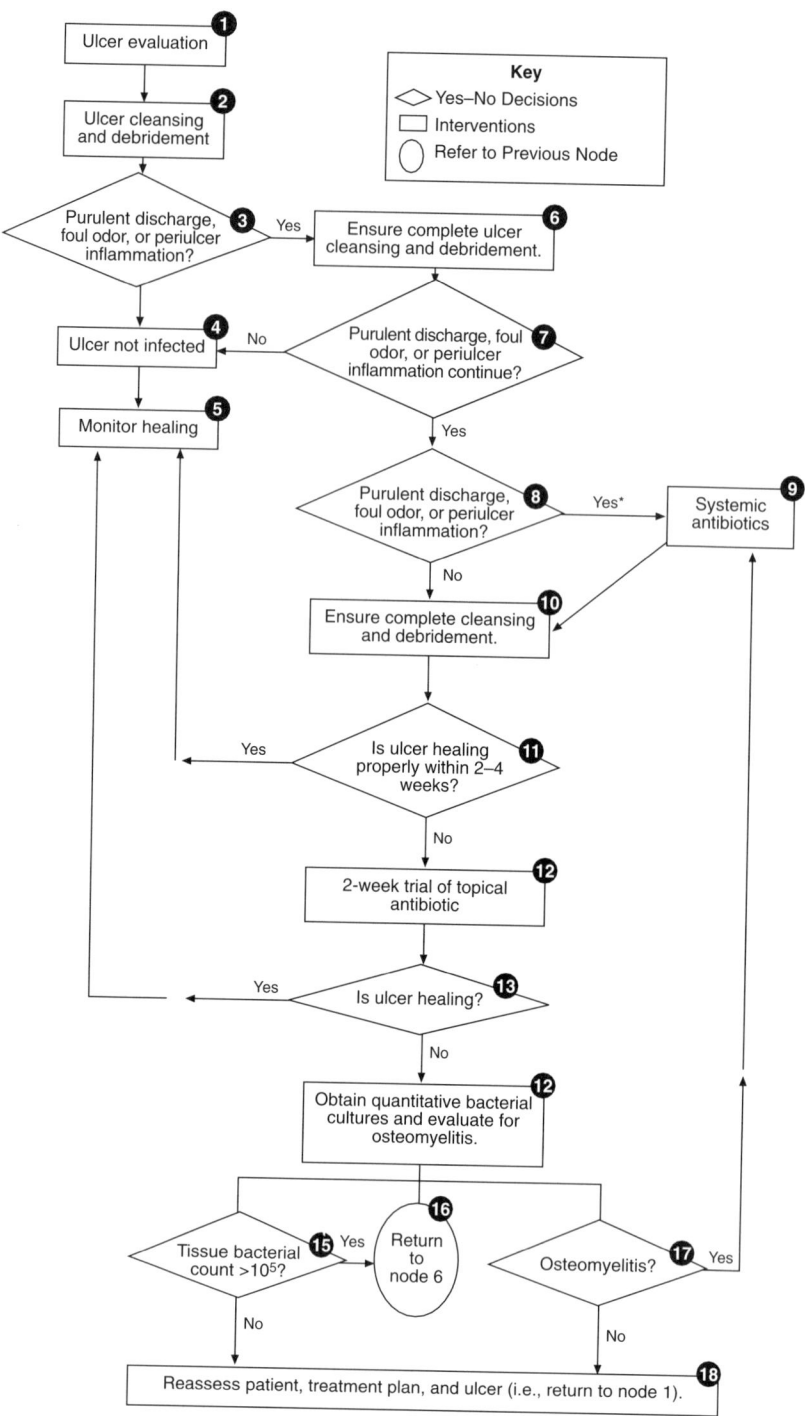

FIGURE 6–6e Treatment of pressure ulcers: Managing bacterial colonization and infection.

Education: Patients and family caregivers should be given enough information to enable them to understand the contributing factors of pressure ulcer formation, treatment modalities, and expected outcomes. Proper handwashing technique should be taught.

Skin Cancer

Neoplasms of the skin are the most common type of cancers in humans. Three main types of skin cancer are:

Basal cell carcinoma (BCC), which arises from the basal cell layer of the epidermis.

Squamous cell carcinoma (SCC), which originates in the squamous cells of the epithelium.

Malignant melanoma (MM), which is a tumor arising in a pigmented area.

Etiology: The major risk factor for the development of skin cancers is exposure to ultraviolet (UV) sunlight. Patients who have or had an occupation requiring them to spend extensive time outdoors are susceptible to the development of skin cancer. There is a high recurrence rate for basal cell carcinoma.

Occurrence: More than 500,000 new cases of skin cancer are diagnosed in the United States each year. BCC, the most common type of skin cancer, represents 65%–80% of these cases. SCC constitutes 10%–25% of all skin cancers; malignant melanomas account for the remainder of skin cancers.

Age: The incidence of all types of skin cancers increases with age, owing to sun exposure over an extended period.

Ethnicity: All skin cancers are more prevalent in fair-skinned persons, especially those people with blonde or red hair. SCC is more common than BCC in African-Americans.

Gender: Currently, more men than women are found to have BCC, but the number of women with BCC is increasing. SCC and MM are equally prevalent in both men and women.

Contributing Factors: Besides sun exposure as a contributing factor, skin cancer may also occur as a late sequela to burns, scars, chronic ulcers, or radiodermatitis. Inorganic arsenic exposure has also been linked to the development of BCC. Patients who have had a renal transplant and immunosuppression are also at risk for developing skin cancer. Human papillomavirus may play a role in the development of SCC. A familial tendency to develop melanoma exists.

Signs and Symptoms: Patients need to be questioned regarding their history of sun exposure, severe sunburn, burns, scars, ulcers, radiation dermatitis, previous skin cancer, prior occupation, and family history of skin cancer.

The presentation of the skin cancer depends on the type of tumor. BCC generally presents first as a dome-shaped white-to-pink papule or nodule having a raised pearly border with prominent telangiectasia. Patients may describe this lesion as a pimple that did not heal. As the nodule enlarges, scaling, crusting, or central ulceration may become noticeable. More than 90% of BCC occurs on the head and neck.

SCC often originates at the site of chronic inflammation or old scars. Actinic keratoses, which appear as round or irregular-shaped erythematous or tan plaques with a scaly or rough surface, are a precursor to SCC. Signs of malignancy include elevation, ulceration, or inflammation of the lesion; the original lesion may also have enlarged in size. In later stages of SCC, the surface may appear crusted and a horn of keratin forms. SCC appears on sun-exposed as well as on non–sun-exposed areas of the body. These tumors may be tender to touch owing to their rapid growth and inflammatory process. Examine the scalp, ears, lower lip, and dorsa of the hands for squamous cell carcinoma.

The clinical features of a lesion suspected to be MM (the ABCDEs of melanoma) are:

*A*symmetry.
*B*order irregularity.
*C*olor variation.
*D*iameter greater than 6 mm.
*E*levation of a previously flat lesion.

Patients may be concerned about a new pigmented lesion or a change in an already existing one. Patients may report associated itching, burning, or pain in a mole. Superficial spreading melanoma is a flat to slightly raised pigmented lesion with irregular borders, commonly found on the backs of men and the lower legs of women. Lentigo maligna melanoma, an irregularly pigmented macule with notched borders, occurs on sun-exposed areas, especially on the face of older adults. Nodular melanoma, brown or black papules usually located on the trunk, head, and neck, is characterized by rapid growth. Acral lentiginous melanomas, the most common type of melanoma in African-Americans, occur on the palms, soles, fingers, and toes; a pigmented streak of the cuticle is diagnostic (Hutchinson's sign) of this type of melanoma.

Clinical evaluation for skin cancer also includes a total body skin examination and palpation of regional lymph nodes, liver, and spleen.

Diagnostic Tests: Biopsy of the suspected lesion is necessary to confirm the diagnosis via histological examination of the tissue; an adequate tissue sample should be excised.

Differential Diagnosis: Actinic keratoses, seborrheic keratosis, keratoacanthoma, atypical nevi, blue nevus, dermatofibroma, venous lakes, and pyogenic granulomas all may be mistaken for skin cancer.

Treatment: Several factors need to be considered before skin cancer therapy begins: patient's age and general health, size and location of the tumor, the pathology of the tumor, and the cosmetic concerns of the patient. BCC may be treated by excisional surgery, electrodesiccation and curettage, cryotherapy, ionizing radiation, and Mohs' micrographic surgery. A chemotherapeutic agent such as 5-fluorouracil is used as a topical agent for superficial or small BCCs.

SCC may be treated the same as BCC; however, because of its more truculent growth pattern, wider excision and Mohs' micrographic surgery are the preferred methods of treatment.

Treatment of MM is surgical. An excisional margin surrounding the tumor will be made, depending on the thickness of the tumor. Chemotherapy and radiation are used for palliative measures in the treatment of metastatic disease.

Follow-up: Follow-up for a patient with diagnosed skin carcinoma is essential, as the recurrence rate of skin cancer is high; 50% of persons with BCC and SCC will have a reappearance of a cancerous lesion within 5 yr. A person that is susceptible to skin cancer may develop another cancerous lesion at any time. Precancerous lesions should be examined regularly every 6–12 months.

Sequelae: BCC rarely metastasizes; however, if it is not treated early, the carcinoma may invade the surrounding tissue and bone. Advanced SCC lesions of the lips, pinna, and genitalia often metastasize. Prognosis for MM is determined by the thickness of the tumor.

- Tumors less than 0.75 mm are associated with a 95% 10-year survival rate.
- Tumors 0.76–1.5 mm, with an 85% 10-year survival rate.
- Tumors 1.50–2.49 mm, with a 75% 10-year survival rate.
- Tumors greater than 4.0 mm, with a 25%–40% 10-year survival rate.

Prevention/Prophylaxis: All older adults, especially those who are fair-skinned, should wear sunscreen with an SPF of at least 15 throughout the year. The yearly physical examination should include assessment of the head, scalp, and skin, and an accurate recording of descriptions of any suspicious lesions. All precancerous lesions should be evaluated by a dermatologist. Lesions that have variegated colors, irregular elevations, or irregular borders should be examined by biopsy.

Referral: When a suspicious lesion is found, referral to a dermatologist for evaluation and possibly biopsy is necessary.

Education: Advise older patients that skin cancers are a common occurrence as one ages, especially for patients at risk. Older adults should perform a monthly self-evaluation of the skin; suggest the use of mirrors to examine lesions on the back. Any suspicious open lesion that does not heal in a reasonable time needs to be examined by a primary care provider. Patients also need to report any slow-growing flesh-colored or pigmented lesion, noting if the lesion has irregular borders, changes in color, ulceration, bleeding, or horn formation. Sun exposure, especially during the hours of 11:00 AM–2:30 PM, should be avoided. Year-round broad-spectrum sunscreen that blocks both ultraviolet A (UVA) and B (UVB) light is recommended. Vulnerable areas such as the head and neck should be covered with protective clothing.

Patients can obtain written information from American Cancer Society, 1599 Clifton Road NE, Atlanta, GA 30329 and The Skin Cancer Foundation, 245 Fifth Avenue, Suite 2402, New York, NY 10016.

BIBLIOGRAPHY

Assessment

Fitzpatrick, TB: Color Atlas and Synopsis of Clinical Dermatology. Common and Serious Disease, ed 2. McGraw-Hill, New York, 1992.

Burns

Allwood, JS: The primary care management of burns. Nurse Pract 20:74, 1992.

Dietch, EA: The management of burns. N Engl J Med 323:1249, 1990.

Gillespie, RW, et al: Advanced Burn Life Support Course Instructors Manual. National Burn Institute, Lincoln, NE, 1994.

Grisso, JA, and Mezey, MD: Preventing dependence and injury: An approach to sensory changes. In Lavizzo-Mourey (ed): Practicing Prevention for the Elderly. Hanley and Belfus, Philadelphia, 1989.

Hirsch, EF: Burns and nuclear. In Noble, J (ed): Textbook of Primary Care Medicine. CV Mosby, St. Louis, 1996.

Peate, WF: Outpatient management of burns. Am Fam Physician 45:1321, 1992.

Cellulitis

Bartlett, J: Infection of skin, soft tissue, and bone. In Stobo, J, et al (eds): The Principles and Practice of Medicine, ed 23. Appleton & Lange, Stamford, CT, 1996.

Berg, D: Handbook of Primary Care Medicine. JB Lippincott, Philadelphia, 1993.

Elder, DM, and Greer, KE: Venous disease: How to heal and prevent chronic leg ulcers. Geriatrics 50:30, 1995.

DeGowin, RL: DeGowin & DeGowin's Bedside Diagnostic Examination, ed 5. McGraw-Hill, New York, 1987.

Goldstein, EJ, and Shellow, WR: Approaches to bacterial skin infections. In Goroll, AH, May, LA, and Mulley, AG (eds): Primary Care Medicine: Office Evaluation of the Adult Patient, ed 3. JB Lippincott, Philadelphia, 1995.

Middleton, DB: Cellulitis and other bacterial skin infections. In Mengel, MB and Schwiebert, LP (eds): Ambulatory Medicine: The Primary Care of Families, ed 2, Appleton & Lange, Stamford, CT, 1996.

Corns and Calluses

Gordon, GM, and Cuttic, MM: Exercise and the aging foot. South Med J 87:36, 1994.

Richards, RN: Calluses, corns and shoes. Semin Dermatol 10:112, 1991.

Fungal Infections of the Skin and Nails

Leyden, JL: Tinea pedis pathophysiology and treatment. J Am Acad Dermatol 31:31, 1994.

Lookingbill, DP, and Marks, JG: Principles of Dermatology. WB Saunders, Philadelphia, 1993.

Newcomer, VD, and Young, EM: Geriatric Dermatology. Igaku-Shoin Medical Publishers, New York, 1989.

Herpes Zoster

Abrams, WB, Beers, MH, and Berkow, R: The Merck Manual of Geriatrics, ed 2. Merck Research Laboratories, Whitehouse Station, NJ, 1995.

Benenson, AS (ed): Control of Communicable Diseases in Man, ed 15. American Public Health Association, Washington, DC, 1990.

Chenitz, WC, Stone, JT, and Salisbury, SA: Clinical Gerontological Nursing. WB Saunders, Philadelphia, 1991.

Donahue, JG, and Manson, JE: The incidence of herpes zoster. Arch Intern Med 155:1605, 1995.

Dornbrand, L, Hoole, AJ, and Pickard, CG (eds): Manual of Clinical Problems in Adult Ambulatory Care. Little, Brown, Boston, 1992.

Nursing 95 Drug Handbook. Springhouse, Corp, Springhouse, PA, 1995.

Rakel, RE (ed): Conn's Current Therapy. WB Saunders, Philadelphia, 1991.

Seller, RH: Differential Diagnosis of Common Complaints, ed 2. WB Saunders, Philadelphia, 1993.

Woeltje, KF, and Fraser, JV: Infection control and isolation recommendations. In Carey, CF, Lee, HH, and Woeltje, KF (eds): The Washington Manual of Medical Therapeutics, ed 3. Lippincott-Raven, Philadelphia, 1998.

Woeltje, KF, and Ritchie, DJ: Antimicrobials. In Carey, CF, Lee, HH, and Woeltje, KF (eds): The Washington Manual of Medical Therapeutics, ed 3. Lippincott-Raven, Philadelphia, 1998.

Wood, MJ, et al: A randomized trial of acyclovir for 7 days or 21 days with and without prednisolone for treatment of acute herpes zoster. N Engl J Med 330:896, 1994.

Yoshikawa, TT, Cobb, E, and Brummel-Smith, K: Ambulatory Geriatric Care. CV Mosby, Boston, 1993.

Insect Bites and Stings

Austen, KF: Diseases of immediate type hypersensitivity. In Isselbacher, KJ et al (eds): Harrison's Principles of Internal Medicine, ed 13. McGraw-Hill, New York, 1994.

Goldstein, EJ, and Shellow, WV: Approach to bacterial skin infections. In Goroll, AH, May, LA, and Mulley, AG (eds): Primary Care Medicine Office Evaluation and Management of the Adult Patient, ed 3. JB Lippincott, Philadelphia, 1995.

Jerrard, DA (ed): Management of insect stings. Am J Emerg Med 14:429, 1996.

Semia, TP, Beizer, JL, and Higbee, MD: Geriatric Dosage Handbook. Lexi-Comp, Cleveland, 1995.

Uphold, CR, and Graham, MV: Clinical Guidelines in Adult Health. Barmarrae Books, Gainesville, FL, 1994.

Wallace, JF: Disorders caused by venoms, bites, and stings. In Isselbacher, KJ, et al (ed): Harrison's Principles of Internal Medicine, ed 13. McGraw-Hill, New York, 1994.

Pressure Ulcers

Baranoski, S: Wound assessment and dressing selection. Ostomy and Wound Management 41(7A):7, 1995.

Bergstrom, N, et al: Treatment of Pressure Ulcers. Clinical Practice Guidelines, No. 15. AHCPR Publication No. 95-0652. US Department of Health and Human Services. Public Health Service, Agency for Health Care Policy and Research. Rockville, MD, December 1994.

Bryant, RA: Acute and Chronic Wounds. CV Mosby Year Book, Philadelphia, 1992.

Friedman, SJ: Management of skin ulceration. In Goroll, AH, May, LA, and Mulley, AG (eds): Primary Care Medicine: Office Evaluation of the Adult Patient, ed 3. JB Lippincott, Philadelphia, 1995.

Panel for the Prediction and Prevention of Pressure Ulcers in Adults: Pressure Ulcers in Adults: Prediction and Prevention. Clinical Practice Guideline, No. 3. AHCPR Publication no. 92-0047. US Department of Health and Human Services, Public Health Service, Rockville, MD, Agency for Health Care Policy and Research, May 1992.

Skin Cancer

Friedman, RJ, Rigel, DS, and Kopf, AW: Early detection of malignant melanoma: The role of physician examination of self-examination of the skin. CA Cancer J Clin 25:130–151, 1985.

Goldstein, BG, and Goldstein, AO: Practical Dermatology. Mosby Year Book, St. Louis, 1992.

Ho, VC, and Sober, AJ: Therapy for cutaneous melanoma: An update. J Am Acad Dermatol 22:159–176, 1990.

NIH Consensus Development Conference. Melanoma consensus statement. 10:1–25, 1992.

Shaw, JC, Roberston, MH, and Parker, F: Common skin disorders. In Noble, J (ed): Textbook of Primary Care Medicine. CV Mosby, St. Louis, 1996.

Stadler R, and Garbe C: Disseminated malignant melanoma: New therapeutic approachs. Int J Dermatol 30:239, 1991.

CHAPTER **7**

HEAD, NECK, AND

FACE DISORDERS

A systematic and thorough examination of the head and neck begins with the inspection of the face, head, and scalp. Assess the shape, size, and symmetry of the patient's features. Examine the shape of the skull palpating the bones of the head for any anatomic irregularities, masses, or areas of tenderness. Inspect the hair for distribution, quantity, and any balding patterns, noting any uniform alopecia, nits, or seborrhea. The scalp should be carefully inspected for any skin lesions on sun-exposed areas, noting pigment changes, tenderness, scales, or lumps. Assess for scars or bruising patterns. Be careful to note normal changes in skin that have other manifestations of serious skin disease. Note the symmetry of the patient's features, facial expressions, the presence of involuntary tics or tremors, periorbital edema, or facial drooping: palpate over the temples for any abnormality or tenderness in the temporal arteries. The presence of pain and nodules upon palpation is not a normal finding even in very old individuals. Cranial nerve VII (facial nerve) should also be assessed at this time, noting any facial asymmetry, weakness, drooping of the lower eyelid, and unilateral paralysis.

Eyes

Begin the inspection of the eyes by noting the position and symmetry of the surrounding skin and tissue, as well as the presence and position of eyebrows and eyelashes. Screen visual acuity before proceeding with any other examination of the eye. Using a Snellen chart from 20 feet or a handheld chart approximately 12 inches from the patient, assess cranial nerve I for acuity. Note the condition of the skin around the eyes, check the sclera, and note the color of the conjunctiva. Assess the presence of exophthalmos, xanthelasma, pinguecula, ptosis, edema, and skin lesions. The lids should be carefully examined for the presence of hordeolum, chalazion, ectropion, and entropion, which is most common among elderly persons. Examine the cornea for any scarring, presence of pterygium, corneal arcus and opacities. Note that basal and squamous cell carcinomas are common around the eye. Palpate for any tenderness over the lacrimal gland and assess the patency of the lacrimal duct. Examine the extraocular motions of the eye (cranial nerves III, IV, VI). Check the visual fields (cranial nerve II), corneal reflexes (cranial nerve V), and pupillary reactions (cranial nerves II, III), with direct and consensual reactions. Carefully perform a fundoscopic examination; most elderly patients need dilation for accurate assessment of the fundi. If you see the fundi, note the narrow, pale appearance of the arterioles common in elderly persons. Be careful to note any abnormalities in blinking (Parkinson's disease), dull or blank staring (hypothyroidism), residual facial paralysis (Bells' palsy or cerebrovascular accident [CVA]), and skin changes. Decreased elasticity and turgor is a normal aging pattern; the skin around the eyes becomes thin and wrinkles appear. This is a normal change in the older adults and makes skin turgor a poor determinant of hydration status.

Sinus

Inspect and palpate over the frontal and maxillary sinus areas. Using light to transilluminate the sinus cavity can be helpful in the examination for sinusitis. Note any gross tenderness or inflammation in the sinus area or around the eyes. Palpate the posterior portion of the neck under the skull for the presence of occipital lymphadenopathy.

Nose

Inspect the external nose for any asymmetry, inflammation, gross septal deviation, or deformities. If applicable, assess the function of the olfactory nerve (cranial nerve I) by having the patient identify a familiar-smelling item with the eyes closed. The olfactory sense greatly diminishes as a normal part of aging. Assess for patency of each nostril. Examine the internal nose, noting any discharge, bleeding, or edema. Check the status of the turbinates and position of the septum. The color and consistency of the inferior and middle turbinates, as well as the presence of any polyp, should be noted.

Ears

Carefully examine the external ears, noting their position and symmetry on the head, as well as any abnormal lesions, deformities, and the presence of tophi, keloids, or cysts. Estimate auditory acuity (cranial nerve VIII) by using the whisper test, testing each ear separately. Use the Weber and Rinne tests to assess for any conductive or sensorineural hearing loss. Palpate the tragus for any tenderness as well as for any preauricular or postauricular adenopathy. When examining the middle ear, note any inflammation, discharge, erythema, or cerumen in the canal. If visible, inspect the tympanic membranes and surrounding landmarks for abnormalities. Note any foreign bodies, dull membranes, alterations in the cone of light reflex, as well as presence of fluid or scarring. Be careful to inspect the posterior ear and helix for any skin lesions or carcinomas.

Oral Cavity

Perform a complete assessment of the lips, mouth, oral mucosa, and pharynx, noting the color, moisture, and presence of any abnormal lesions on and around the lips. Assess for any herpes simplex I, chancres, angular stomatitis, mucous retention cysts, angioedema, and fissures. Check the color and pigmentation of the buccal mucosa. If the patient has dentures, these should be removed to do a complete oral examination. Examine the fit of the dentures and assess the consistency of the gums under the dentures. If natural teeth are present, note any loose or broken teeth, as well as caries. Because periodontal disease is the primary cause of tooth loss in the adult, do a careful oral and gum examination. Examine the gums for bleeding, discoloration, swelling, and retractions. Note the attrition of the teeth (exposed dentin) and enamel loss from years of chewing. Note the condition of the hard palate and the presence of torus palatinus, thrush, or other lesions. Assess the gag reflex and rise of the palate (cranial nerves IX, X). Carefully examine the tongue for symmetry, enlargement (hypothyroidism), growths, protrusions, or abnormal movements (cranial nerve XII) and dorsum for any papillary atrophy. A swollen, red painful tongue may indicate vitamin B or riboflavin deficiency. Note any inflammation or obstruction in the parotid (Stensen) or submaxillary (Warton) ducts. Thoroughly examine the area underneath the tongue, the floor of the mouth, and the tonsils, soft palate, uvula, and posterior pharynx, noting any lesions, inflammation, or exudate, and the color. Examine the strength and movement of the temporal and masseter muscles (cranial nerve V), as well as any crepitus in the mandible junction. Complete assessment would also include evaluation of the voice (cranial nerve X) and speech (cranial nerves V, VII, X, XII).

Neck

Inspect the neck for symmetry, masses, scars, tracheal position, and deviation. Look for the presence of thyroid inflammation of goiters. Carefully palpate for any lymphadenopathy noting that loss of lean muscle makes it easier to feel nodes in the cervical region of elderly persons. Assess supraclavicular, tonsilar, superficial, deep and posterior cervical chains, tonsilar, submaxillary, submental, occipital and preauricular and postauricular nodes, noting any inflammation, tenderness, or change in size, position, or shape. Gently palpate and ausculate the carotid arteries bilaterally for any nodularity or bruits. Note any jugular vein distention that occurs when the patient is seated. Check to see if the patient uses any neck muscles to breath. Carefully inspect and palpate the thyroid gland, noting any inflammation or nodules (unilateral). Examination of the range of motion of the neck should include flexion, extension, rotation, and lateral bending. Check the strength of the trapezius and sternomastoid muscles (cranial nerve XI).

A complete and thorough detailed examination of the head and neck has the potential to allow the examiner to discover multiple variants from the normal. Develop a clear and concise pattern of examination to ensure appropriate evaluation of these areas. Keep in mind the normal variants of the older person and how these differ from pathological or abnormal findings.

Acute Glaucoma

Acute glaucoma, also known as angle-closure or narrow-angle glaucoma, is an obstruction to the outflow of aqueous humor from the posterior to the anterior chamber through the trabecular meshwork, canal of Schlemm, and associated structures. This condition results in an elevation of intraocular pressure and damage to the optic nerve, resulting in a loss of peripheral vision, eye pain, and redness. This type of glaucoma, although not common, may occur as a primary disease or secondary to other conditions and constitutes an ophthalmic emergency. Because of associated presenting symptoms, acute glaucoma may be misdiagnosed or missed entirely.

Etiology: The precise pathophysiology of glaucoma is unknown. In the acute form, pupillary blockage limits the progress of the aqueous humor through the trabecular network. The peripheral iris, which blocks the trabecular meshwork, is displaced forward. In susceptible persons, this may be precipitated by emotional stress, sudden darkness (such as in a theater when the lights go out), or the instillation of mydriatics.

Occurrence: The occurrence of acute glaucoma is less than 100 cases in 100,000. In the African-American and Asian populations, the occurrence is less than 500 in 100,000.

Age: The predominant age range is 55 to 70 years old.

Ethnicity: Acute glaucoma is more common in African-Americans, Asian-Americans, and those of Eskimo ancestry.

Gender: Acute glaucoma occurs more often in women.

Contributing Factors: Contributing factors include an anatomically narrow anterior chamber angle, requiring the use of a special examination technique called gonioscopy to identify. This examination technique is beyond the scope of the primary care practitioner, but the condition can be evaluated during the comprehensive eye examination. Other risk factors include sudden eye trauma, hyperopia, small cornea, shallow anterior chamber, Eskimo ancestry, female gender, family history of glaucoma (first-degree relatives have a 2%–5% risk over a lifetime), cataract, neovascularization, and use of certain antidepressants and other drugs with anticholinergic properties (e.g., atropine, preoperative medications, imipramine, inhaled ipratroprium bromide). Very rarely, sneezing or laser treatment can precipitate the condition.

Signs and Symptoms: The presentation is often dramatic but the diagnosis can be missed because of the associated symptoms. The history reveals severe, unilateral eye pain, blurred vision, lacrimation, reports of seeing colored halos around lights, and a red eye. Headache, nausea, and vomiting frequently accompany visual loss. Symptoms are associated with certain activities and tend to occur at times of emotional stress. Examination reveals circumcorneal conjunctival injection, tearing, and a fixed semidilated pupil that is nonreactive to light. Visual acuity, if evaluated, demonstrates a loss in the affected eye.

Diagnostic Tests: Immediately refer patients for a complete ophthalmic examination, including gonioscopy and tonometry.

Differential Diagnosis: Conjunctivitis, uveitis, corneal trauma or infection, and other types of glaucoma may mimic acute glaucoma.

Treatment: The patient with acute glaucoma needs an immediate consultation with and referral to an ophthalmologist; permanent visual loss occurs within 2–5 days if this condition is untreated. Surgical treatment includes peripheral iridectomy or laser iridotomy. Intraocular pressure must be lowered preoperatively, which may require the use of an osmotic diuretic intravenously and/or orally and miotic eyedrops. As the primary health-care provider, you must communicate to the specialist any medical conditions that need monitoring with the use of these agents. Bilateral treatment is indicated because patients are at risk for developing the same problem in the other eye.

Follow-up: The ophthalmologist treating the patient determines follow-up treatment. Periodic eye examinations are recommended by preventive guidelines.

Sequelae: If treated promptly acute glaucoma is not associated with sequelae. If untreated, permanent visual loss will occur.

Prevention/Prophylaxis: Knowing the risk factors for acute glaucoma, the provider should educate patients having those risk factors (see Education). Periodic eye examinations are recommended for prevention.

Referral: As stated previously, refer the patient immediately upon presentation and evaluation of symptoms.

Education: Teach patients with known risk factors (see Contributing Factors) the importance of having regular eye examinations and of reporting symptoms.

Cataracts

A cataract is an opacification of the lens that interferes with the passage of light through the lens, decreasing visual acuity. The location, size, and density of this opacity influence the degree of visual impairment. Nuclear sclerotic cataracts affect contrast sensitivity, progress slowly, and tend to preserve functional reading vision while frequently causing nearsightedness. In contrast, posterior subcapsular cataracts progress more rapidly and interfere with reading vision.

Etiology: Most cataracts are related to the aging process. The gradual thickening or hardening in the lens is believed to be due to oxidative damage to the lens protein.

Occurrence: The rate of visually significant cataracts in persons under age 50 is 2%–5%. After age 75, 92% of the population have some cataract changes, with 46% experiencing a significant vision loss. Cataracts tend to be bilateral, although the rate of progression varies from one eye to the other.

Age: Although subtle changes in visual acuity related to cataract formation occur as early as age 50, the population over age 75 experiences most of the visually significant cataracts.

Ethnicity: No ethnic groups are significantly more prone to cataracts.

Gender: Cataracts occur equally in men and women.

Contributing Factors: Diabetes mellitus, hypertension, poor nutrition, cigarette smoking, high alcohol intake, trauma to the eye, long-term exposure to ultraviolet B radiation (sunlight), and a strong family history of cataracts are risk factors. Use of certain substances including haloperidol, iron, and glucocorticoids also contributes to cataracts. An association between cataracts and glaucoma and intraocular inflammation also exists.

Signs and Symptoms: The patient with a cataract may initially present with an improvement in near vision requiring a new prescription for corrective lenses. Patients may also experience blurred vision or sensitivity to glare from bright light or from automobile headlights during night driving. Complaints of having difficulty reading and distinguishing contrast sensitivities and of seeing a yellow tint or "washed-out" colors are also common. Some patients may not seek evaluation of their symptoms by a health-care provider owing to denial or fear of loss of independence (driver's license being revoked), whereas other patients seek prompt assessment in the hopes of early intervention. A recent history of falls, accidents, or injury is suspicious. Upon physical examination, visual acuity test results are abnormal for one or both eyes (evaluate both near and distance vision). Examine the eye, using an opaque light for opacification of the lens. The cataract may be visible to the naked eye. The red reflex may be absent or the cataract may appear as a black area.

Diagnostic Tests: No diagnostic testing is required other than that for visual acuity and examination of the eye, unless other visual problems are suspected. Refer the patient to an ophthalmologist for complete evaluation after initial screening.

Differential Diagnosis: Differential diagnosis includes corneal scarring, retinal detachment, comorbid conditions such as macular degeneration, chronic glaucoma, or diabetic retinopathy.

Treatment: Treatment is determined after full evaluation by the ophthalmologist. Ultimately, surgical intervention is required with extraction of the cataract and immediate implantation of a plastic intraocular lens, unless contraindicated by other disease conditions. Collaboration with the ophthalmologist is indicated for patients with severe cardiac, respiratory, or neuromuscular conditions that may prevent the patient from lying still or supine as required during the surgery. Patients receiving anticoagulant therapy should also be managed collaboratively. The degree of the patient's visual impairment and its influence on his or her usual daily functioning determines the timing of the surgery. Initially a conservative treatment plan may include prescription of corrective lenses and periodic reevaluation by the ophthalmologist, coupled with a plan for environmental safety and optimization of the patient's functional abilities within his or her visual limitations. This plan may be developed by other members of the health-care team, family, or both. Preoperative medical clearance is required before surgery. Surgery is performed in an outpatient or short procedure unit, with the patient returning home immediately after discharge.

Follow-up: Immediate postsurgical care includes eye protection and application of topical agents prescribed by the ophthalmologist. The patient should be cautioned to avoid straining, lifting, or bending. A follow-up appointment should be made. The family or health-care team should heighten precautions for environmental safety to help the patient avoid injury. Intensive supervision of mentally compromised patients may be required to prevent them from damaging the operative site. Future follow-up includes a reevaluation of visual acuity, prescribing corrective lenses as indicated, and monitoring the unaffected eye for cataract development.

Sequelae: Possible sequelae to cataract surgery include faulty wound closure with aqueous humor leakage, blindness secondary to choroidal hemorrhage, infection, inflammation, retinal detachment, prolapse of the iris into the corneal wound, and secondary glaucoma.

Prevention/Prophylaxis: The patient should be protected from exposure to ultraviolet B radiation by wearing sunglasses designed for this, and/or by wearing a hat with a wide brim to protect the eyes from the sun. Some authorities encourage the use of antioxidants, but their effectiveness is still unproven.

Referral: After the initial visual screening, refer the patient to an ophthalmologist for complete examination and treatment, including postsurgery follow-up.

Education: Provide the patient with information on age-related visual changes, the importance of protecting the eyes from sunlight with ultraviolet-blocking sunglass lenses, maintaining a nutritionally balanced diet, avoiding high alcohol intake, and having periodic eye examinations every 2 years. Instruct the patient to seek prompt evaluation of any vision changes and reassure him or her that, with proper treatment, cataracts will not result in permanent loss of visual acuity.

Chalazion

A chalazion is a mass on the eyelid caused by an inflammation of a meibomian (oil-secreting) gland of the upper or lower eyelid. Meibomian glands lubricate the lid margins.

Etiology: Blockage in a duct leading to the eyelid surface from the gland or obstruction of a meibomian gland results in inflammation, the formation of a hard mass, and/or infection (usually from staphylococcus).

Occurrence: The development of chalazion is common.

Age: Chalazion can occur at any age.

Ethnicity: No ethnic groups are significantly more prone to chalazion.

Gender: Chalazion occurs equally in men and women.

Contributing Factors: Previously unresolved blepharitis, poor hygiene, immunosuppression, and skin conditions such as acne rosacea or seborrheic dermatitis are all contributing factors to development of chalazion.

Signs and Symptoms: A slow-developing painless hard mass, with inflammation of the meibomian gland and possible involvement of the surrounding tissue, characterizes chalazion. Physical examination with inversion of the eyelid reveals a red elevated mass that may become quite large and press against the eye, causing nystagmus.

Diagnostic Tests
- Visual examination: rules out other problems.
- Culture of drainage: if incision and drainage is done, reveals causative organism.
- Biopsy of recurrent chalazion: rules out malignancy.

Differential Diagnosis: Foreign body, hordeolum, blepharitis, and sebaceous cell carcinoma may mimic chalazion.

Treatment: Sulfacetamide sodium ophthalmic ointment is applied thinly to the lid margin with a cotton-tipped applicator, four times a day for 7 days. Antibiotic eyedrops may be used (to prevent secondary bacterial infection in other parts of the eye). Warm compresses to the area reduce inflammation and hasten healing. Incise and drain if no response to medication and treatment is exhibited.

Follow-up: See patient in 1 week to evaluate treatment.

Sequelae: Complete resolution may take several weeks to months.

Prevention/Prophylaxis: Prevention strategies include advising the patient:

- To perform proper lid hygiene (helps prevent recurrence) by gently scrubbing lids with diluted baby shampoo daily or directly applying baby shampoo with cotton-tipped applicator, and then rinsing.
- To avoid sharing towels or washcloths, to lessen spread of infection.
- To wash hands frequently.
- To apply warm compresses several times a day at the first sign of eyelid irritation or if chalazion starts to return; a clean cloth should be used for each warm compress to eye.

Referral: Refer to or consult with an ophthalmologist if the patient has a visual change, eye pain, or impairment to the eye. Refer the patient to a surgeon if the chalazion does not heal spontaneously in 6 weeks, as surgical removal may be necessary.

Education: Explain to the patient the disease process, signs and symptoms, and treatment (including side effects of medications). Discuss prevention strategies.

Chronic Glaucoma

Chronic open-angle or primary open-angle glaucoma (COAG or POAG, respectively) is an insidious disease characterized by increased intraocular pressure severe enough to damage the optic nerve. Progressive over time with a gradual visual field loss, chronic glaucoma is called the "silent blinder" because it often goes unnoticed until the later stages. Variants occur in which intraocular pressure does not increase, but the optic nerve still becomes damaged. Secondary glaucomas are the result of prior or concurrent ocular disease or trauma; they may have open angles caused by steroid-induced pressure increases.

Etiology: The etiology of chronic glaucoma is unknown but the disease is associated with increased intraocular pressure, optic nerve degeneration, and visual field loss. This condition is believed to result from impaired outflow of aqueous humor through the trabecular network or the canal of Schlemm.

Occurrence: Prevalence of chronic glaucoma increases in persons over age 40, approaching 3%–4% by age 75; 90% of cases are the open-angle type. POAG causes 15%–20% of all blindness in the United States.

Age: Over age 40, the incidence increases, with another increase in incidence between the ages of 60 and 75. Onset is earlier in African-Americans.

Ethnicity: African-Americans are at a higher risk than the general population for developing chronic glaucoma. Glaucoma is the primary cause of blindness in African-Americans.

Gender: Chronic glaucoma occurs equally in men and women.

Contributing Factors: Risk factors include age, a positive family history, and African-American ancestry. Some authorities also consider diabetes mellitus, hypertension, and myopia to be risk factors. Risk factors for secondary open-angle glaucoma include chronic use of topical or oral corticosteroids.

Signs and Symptoms: The disease is asymptomatic in the early stages; by the time symptoms develop, significant neural damage has occurred. Eye health specialists frequently discover COAG during routine eye examinations. Patients may present with a complaint of blurred vision, needing a change in corrective lenses, or occasionally seeing a halo around lights.

On routine vision screening, visual acuity may be normal or unchanged from previous screening; visual fields, however, may be decreased. The skilled examiner may detect changes in the cup-to-disk ratio on funduscopic examination. Because it is often difficult to perform a funduscopic examination on older patients without the benefit of a mydriatic agent, referral for specialized ophthalmologic examination is prudent. The ophthalmologic examination may reveal increased intraocular pressure or signs of optic nerve damage without increased pressure.

Diagnostic Tests: Examination by an eye health professional should include specialized visual field testing. White target lights are presented; nerve fiber bundle defects cause typical changes in the way these lights are seen and not seen. Perform funduscopic examination to scrutinize changes in the normal cup-to-disk ratio (cup is usually one-third the size of the disk). In glaucoma the cup-to-disk ratio increases more than 0.6. Other signs include asymmetry in the size or contour of the cup.

Another diagnostic tool used is tonometry, the measurement of intraocular pressure by using a tool to assess the amount of pressure needed to depress the cornea. The applanation tonometer, which is most commonly used for this purpose, requires the application of a topical anesthetic and the use of the slit lamp. Normal intraocular pressure is between 10 and 21 mmHg. Patients with pressures greater than 21 mmHg but with no visual field defects are considered to have "ocular hypertension," which requires reexamination every 6 months. The use of Schiøtz's tonometer by primary health-care professionals to screen for glaucoma is not recommended. Because this instrument is very sensitive, it tends to overdiagnose when used with older patients.

Gonioscopy, another tool used in visual evaluation for glaucoma, helps to distinguish open-angle from closed-angle glaucoma. A handheld lens is used to visualize the outflow area of the aqueous humor, the iridocorneal angle.

Differential Diagnosis: Differential diagnosis includes severe anemia, cerebral neoplasia, vascular occlusive disease, or past history of hemodynamic crisis.

Treatment: COAG cannot be cured; the goal of treatment is to halt progress of the disease and preserve existing vision by stabilizing the intraocular pressure. Topical eyedrops that reduce aqueous production or encourage outflow are the mainstays of treatment. Ophthalmic beta-blockers are often first-line agents because they are well tolerated and require less frequent dosing than does pilocarpine, another popular treatment: only once or twice daily. These agents are absorbed into the systemic circulation and can precipitate heart failure, heart block, or asthma exacerbation in susceptible patients. Betaxolol 0.25% or 0.5%, a selective beta-blocker, is often prescribed for patients with a history of asthma. This drug, which is less effective than the nonselective beta-blockers, frequently requires the addition of a second agent, epinephrine 0.5% or 1% eyedrops or dipivefrin 0.1% eyedrops twice daily. These sympathomimetics decrease aqueous production and may increase outflow; they may be used alone or in combination with another type of agent.

Parasympathomimetics such as pilocarpine facilitate aqueous outflow by contraction of the ciliary body, which opens the trabecula. Pilocarpine, used in concentrations of 1%–4% and administered three or four times daily, is often prescribed in addition to a beta-blocker or sympathomimetic agent. If topical ophthalmic agents do not effectively lower intraocular pressure, systemic carbonic anhydrase inhibitors are added. These may also be used before surgery to lower the intraocular pressure. Acetazolamide 250 mg, the most common systemic carbonic anhydrase inhibitor, is administered one to four times daily.

If medical therapy is unsuccessful, laser trabeculoplasty or filtration surgery, to improve aqueous outflow, is indicated. The laser treatment is considered for elderly patients who cannot tolerate surgery, although the outcome is not as desirable as with surgery. In either case, medication may still be required after surgery.

Follow-up: Monitor patients for compliance with the treatment regimen. If eyedrops are used, ensure that the patient can instill these or teach a family member or neighbor to do it. Monitor medications for adverse effects; the range and frequency of side effects to glaucoma medications is significant. Ensure that patients have regular ophthalmologic follow-up visits. If visual loss is severe, evaluate environment for safety and risk of falls or injury. If the patient is still a licensed motor vehicle operator, driver's license retesting may be indicated in the interest of public safety.

Sequelae: If initial presentation is monocular, the other eye may become affected. Changes in the patient's overall health may have implications for the treatment plan.

Prevention/Prophylaxis: Educate patients about risk factors and about the need for eye examinations, continued monitoring, and adherence to the prescribed regimen. The latter may be a challenge because, if the disease is detected in the asymptomatic stage, the patient may question the need for regular treatment. Also, the frequency and/or complexity of the medication regimen may influence compliance. African-Americans should have periodic eye examinations every 3–5 years, beginning at age 40. Anyone with a family history of glaucoma should have an annual eye examination, beginning at age 40. Patients with hypertension or diabetes should have regular eye examinations, as recommended by their health-care provider. All patients over age 65 should have annual eye examinations.

Referral: Refer patients initially for ophthalmologic examination and diagnosis. Collaborate on the management plan if the patient has significant medical conditions that affect treatment options, particularly pharmacological. Refer patients for periodic follow-up eye examinations or for treatment of complications if they arise.

Education: Educate the patient about the chronicity and progressive nature of the disease, the need to follow the treatment regimen as prescribed, and the need for regular follow-up eye examinations and reporting of symptoms, if any. Reassure the patient that, although the disease is not curable, it can be managed. Educate patients with known risk factors about the need for eye examinations despite the absence of symptoms.

Epistaxis

Epistaxis is bleeding from the nose.

Etiology: Epistaxis results from a spontaneous rupture of a blood vessel in the nose, usually in the anterior septum. The bleeding may be secondary to local infections, systemic infections, drying of the nasal mucous membrane, trauma, arteriosclerosis, hypertension, or bleeding disorders. Trauma is usually the primary mechanism of disruption of the nasal mucosa.

Occurrence: Most people have at least one episode of minor, nonrecurring epistaxis. Only 10% of the population experiences at least one significant nosebleed. The incidence of epistaxis is higher in winter when heating causes drying and cracking of nasal mucosa. Epistaxis is rare without trauma in patients with hypertension or hemophilia but is characteristic of von Willebrand's disease.

Age: Epistaxis occurs most frequently in children and in elderly persons.

Ethnicity: No ethnic groups are significantly more prone to epistaxis.

Gender: Epistaxis occurs equally in males and females.

Contributing Factors: Local trauma to the anterior portions of the nose (digital, as in picking the nose, and blunt, as in nasal fractures) is usually the cause of epistaxis. Local infections such as vestibulitis, rhinitis, and sinusitis may contribute secondarily to the occurrence of epistaxis. Epistaxis may be an early sign of a more significant systemic illness such as scarlet fever, malaria, or typhoid fever. Bleeding disorders such as aplastic anemia, leukemia, thrombocytopenia, liver disease, hereditary coagulopathies, and Osler-Weber-Rendu syndrome may also contribute to the occurrence of epistaxis.

Signs and Symptoms: Usually no signs or symptoms are associated with epistaxis other than the awareness of blood dripping down the posterior nasopharynx, as well as external bleeding.

Diagnostic Tests: No laboratory studies are indicated for minor and nonrecurring epistaxis. For more substantial or recurrent epistaxis, a complete blood count including platelet count, bleeding time, prothrombin time, and partial thromboplastin time may be useful.

Differential Diagnosis: Trauma, inflammation due to rhinitis or infection, vascular disorders, clotting disorders and blood dyscrasias, intranasal foreign bodies, hereditary telangiectasia, and tumors may be underlying causes of epistaxis.

Treatment: Most episodes of epistaxis are mild and self-limited, resolving spontaneously. Epistaxis may be controlled by pinching the nasal alae together for 5–10 min, keeping the patient in an erect sitting position with head tilted forward to prevent blood from going down the posterior nasopharynx. A small piece of cotton soaked in 1 : 1000 epinephrine or a vasoconstricting nosedrop such as phenylephrine may be placed into the vestibule of the nose and pressed against the bleeding site to promote vasoconstriction. An ice pack can be applied over the nose for additional therapy. The mucous membrane can be anesthetized with 4% lidocaine topically and a silver nitrate stick can be applied to the site of bleeding (Fig. 7–1).

Follow-up: For recurrent episodes, follow-up visits are recommended as needed.

Sequelae: Anemia can be a complication of excessive or frequent bouts of epistaxis.

Prevention/Prophylaxis: Discourage patients from picking, constant rubbing, and excessively forceful blowing of the nose and advise them to increase the humidity in the home, especially in winter months. Use of a petrolatum-based ointment such as zinc oxide or bacitracin applied in the nares may decrease drying of the mucosa.

Referral: Consultation with a physician or eye, ear, nose, and throat (EENT) specialist is indicated for:

Bleeding that is not controlled by 15 min of compression.
Evidence of massive bleeding.
Recurrent bleeding within the first hour.
Second episode of epistaxis within 1 week.
Uncontrolled bleeding from the posterior nasopharynx.

The consulting physician may initiate interventions such as the insertion of Merocel nasal tampons or bismuth subnitrate and iodoform paste to control bleeding. Intractable epistaxis may require transantral arterial ligation or emboliation. The use of the potassium-titanyl-phosphate laser (KTP/532) for photoco-

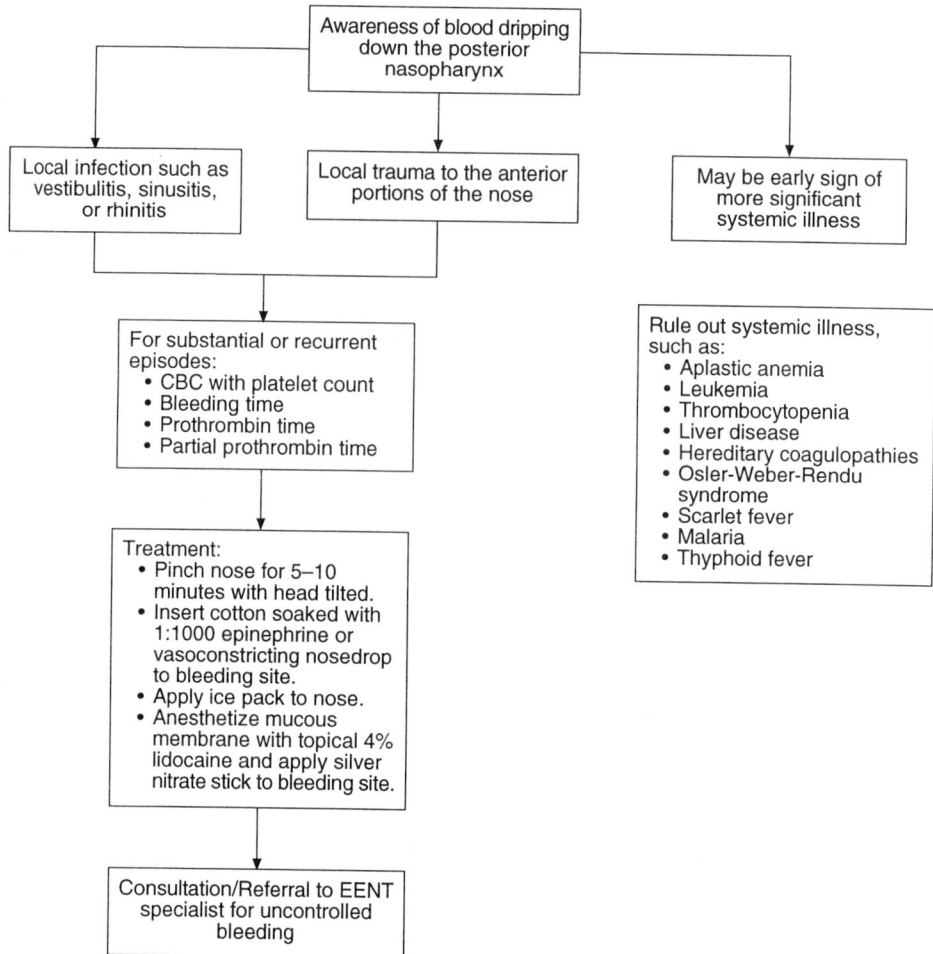

FIGURE 7–1   Epistaxis.

agulation of intranasal telangiectases helps to control epistaxis refractory to traditional surgical therapy.

Education: Discourage picking of the nose and advise patients to increase the humidity in the home, especially in winter months, by means of a humidifier. Petrolatum may be rubbed over the nasal septum twice daily to decrease dryness of mucosa. Teach the patient how to manage simple epistaxis at home and instruct him or her to seek medical attention for excessive (bleeding for more than 1 hr) or recurrent epistaxis.

Hearing Loss

Hearing loss is the decreased ability or complete inability to hear. The loss may involve:

- The external or middle ear: Indicates a mechanical or conductive problem (conductive hearing loss, which is usually reversible).
- The inner ear: Indicates a nerve or sensorineural problem that leads to distortion of sound and misinterpretation of speech (sensorineural hearing loss, which is usually reversible).

Hearing loss may have both conductive and sensorineural components and may be unilateral or bilateral.

Etiology

Sensorineural: This type of hearing loss is caused by a lesion in the organ of Corti or in the central pathways, including the eighth nerve and auditory cortex. Age-related hearing loss (presbycusis) is a form of sensorineural hearing loss that may also be caused by Ménière's disease, tumor, noise damage, genetics, ototoxicity from a variety of medications (such as aminoglycosides, loop diuretics, and antineoplastic agents), syphilis, metabolic disorders such as hypothyroidism, inner ear fistula, and viral syndromes such as mumps.

Conductive: This type of hearing loss is caused by a lesion involving the outer and middle ears to the level of the oval window. This may result from various structural abnormalities, cerumen impaction, perforation of the tympanic membrane, middle ear fluid, damage to the ossicles from trauma or infection, otosclerosis, tympanosclerosis, cholesteatoma, middle ear tumors, temporal bone fractures, injuries related to trauma, and congenital problems.

Occurrence: Prevalence increases after age 40, affecting 25% of all adults age 65–74 and 50% of all adults older than 85.

Age: Sensorineural hearing loss increases with age. Degenerative decline starts at age 20.

Ethnicity: No ethnic groups are significantly more prone to hearing loss.

Gender: Presbycusis is more severe in men than in women; this is attributed to environmental causes.

Contributing Factors: Factors contributing to hearing loss include exposure to loud noises; heredity; ototoxic drugs such as aminoglycoside antibiotics, acetylsalicylic acid (ASA), and quinine; eustachian tube obstruction; chronic middle ear infections; and chronic cerumen impaction. Most cases of sudden unilateral hearing loss in elderly persons are due to thrombotic or embolic obstruction of the internal auditory artery.

Signs and Symptoms: Obtain a complete history of prescription and over-the-counter (OTC) medications. The social and occupational history should include specific questions regarding noise or toxin exposure and any blast injuries. The review of systems should focus on the neurological system, including cranial nerve function such as facial weakness or tingling, loss of taste, or dysphagia.

The patient may complain of difficulty hearing associated with pain, pressure, discomfort, vertigo, and/or loss of balance. Other associated symptoms may include tinnitus, dizziness, blockage, popping, pressure, crackling, trouble hearing distant sounds, or stiffness.

The physical examination includes the otoscopic examination and inspection of the external auditory canal and middle ear. Note any redness, foreign objects, discharge, scaling, lesions, and cerumen. Expect to see minimal cerumen, a pink color, and hairs in the outer third of the ear. The tympanic membrane should have no perforations and be a translucent pearly gray. Changes in the tympanic membrane may be consistent with conductive hearing loss.

Diagnostic Tests

- Audiometry including pure tone and speech testing and impedance (middle ear pressure) testing: detects type and degree hearing loss.
- Weber, Rinne, and/or Schwabach tests: determine conductive or sensorineural hearing loss.
- Computed tomography (CT) scan and/or magnetic resonance imaging (MRI) of the head: detects causes such as tumors (acoustic neuromas, glomus tumor, and cholesteatoma) and traumatic injuries.

Differential Diagnosis: Presbycusis, Ménière's disease, acoustic neuroma, cholesteatoma, and mechanical obstruction may mimic the symptoms of sensorineural or conductive hearing loss.

Treatment: Treat the cause or refer the patient as appropriate. Encouragement, follow-up, and support are very important for the patient with hearing loss.

Conductive Hearing Loss: If hearing loss is caused by cerumen build-up, disimpaction is necessary, using a $1:1$ mixture of H_2O_2 and mineral oil. Place 3 drops in the external ear and wait 1 hr; then lavage with warm saline. If hearing loss caused by infection, treat as appropriate. In the presence of tympanic perforation, ossicle damage, tympanosclerosis, otosclerosis, tumor, or temporal bone injury, refer the patient to a specialist. Stop medications, if indicated, and treat the underlying cause.

Sensorineural Hearing Loss: If hearing loss is sudden and with no apparent cause, high doses of steroids (80 mg/day of prednisone or equivalent) are sometimes used.

If the patient has presbycusis, no specific treatment will reverse the process; therefore, educate and support the patient so that no further damage will occur. Have the patient reduce noise exposure and avoid ototoxic medications. Teach the patient lip-reading when appropriate and instruct the family to speak clearly. Consult a telephone equipment company about the availability of special audio equipment.

Follow-up: See patients as indicated by the cause of the symptom.

Sequelae: Possible complications depend on the cause of the symptom but may include:

- Permanent hearing loss. The patient may need a hearing aid.
- Cerumen removal may damage the external auditory meatus, perforate the tympanic membrane if not done properly, and/or cause otitis media.
- Middle ear problems may progress to chronic ear problems such as perforations and/or cholesteatoma.
- Severe nerve deafness, particularly that associated with tinnitus, may produce severe depression and isolation and occasionally suicide.

Prevention/Prophylaxis: Prevention strategies depend on the cause of the symptom. Advise the patient to use protective devices to guard against occupational or recreational hearing loss, to equalize ear pressure when diving, to chew gum and/or use decongestants in airplanes, to avoid flying or diving if upper respiratory infection (URI) is present, and to avoid ototoxic medications. Teach the patient proper techniques for cerumen removal.

Referral: Refer the patient to or consult with appropriate specialist, as indicated by cause of symptom. Refer patients for audiometry if indicated, especially if no definitive cause for hearing loss is found.

Education: Explain causes of symptoms, measures taken to determine the cause, and symptomatic treatment if any. Advise the patient when to seek medical care. Teach the importance of the use of hearing aids, if indicated, as this can make a significant difference in the patient's quality of life. Advise the patient to contact rehabilitation centers to learn lip-reading skills and/or sign language. Provide support and help the patient resist the temptation to withdraw socially. Educational resource materials are available from the Better Hearing Institute, PO Box 1840, Washington, DC 20013 (800-424-8576) and the National Hearing Aid Helpline, 20361 Middlebelt Rd, Livonia, MD 48152 (800-521-5247).

Oral Cancer

Oral cancer is a potentially malignant tumor of the oral squamous epithelium. The oral cavity includes the lips, floor of the mouth, tongue, buccal mucosa, gingiva, retromolar trigone, and hard palate. The rare tumors of the upper gingiva and hard palate are usually salivary gland adenocarcinomas.

Etiology: Oral cancers are associated with chronic irritation of the squamous epithelial lining of the oral cavity from the ingestion of carcinogenic substances, malnutrition, and systemic illness in susceptible individuals.

Occurrence: Oral cancer accounts for 2%–4% of the malignancies diagnosed annually in the United States. Each year, 36,000 new cases are diagnosed. In recent years, the incidence of lip cancer has declined, whereas the number of tongue cancers has increased.

Age: Oral cancers are usually found in individuals over age 40.

Ethnicity: The incidence of oral cancer is declining among white men but is increasing among African-American men and all women.

Gender: Currently, men are three to four times (depending on the source) more likely than women to develop oral cancer.

Contributing Factors: Tobacco use and heavy alcohol consumption, in isolation or together, are strongly related to the development of oral cancer. Pipe smoking and sun exposure have been implicated in lip cancer. Atrophic glossitis, which is associated with tertiary syphilis, iron deficiency (Plummer-Vinson syndrome), and vitamin deficiencies, predisposes patients to oral cancer. Relationships between oral cancer and Epstein-Barr virus, human papilloma virus, herpes simplex virus, and immunodeficiency states have also been found. No strong association exists between irritation from dentures or teeth and oral cancers.

Signs and Symptoms: Nonhealing, ulcerative lesions on the lip, tongue, or oral mucosa are usually noted first. Leukoplakia, a white patch on the mucosa that cannot be rubbed off, is the most common precancerous lesion. Erythroplasia, a nonpainful, red, velvety lesion, typically on the floor of the mouth, can be carcinoma in situ. Patients may complain that dental appliances are not fitting properly and that they have difficulty chewing. Oral pain and bleeding lesions are usually late signs of malignancy in the oral cavity. Occasionally patients may complain of numbness in the skin around the chin when the lesion involves a nerve. Enlarged submandibular or submental lymph nodes may be found in advanced disease. Unexplained weight loss may be a late symptom.

Diagnostic Tests: All suspicious lesions that have not healed within 2 weeks of occurrence should undergo biopsy and be sent for pathological examination. X-ray films of the mandible and chest may be indicated to assess for metastases or bone erosion. Complete blood count, blood chemistries, and serum ferritin level should be obtained to assess nutritional status. Rapid plasma reagin (RPR) test should be considered for syphilis (Fig. 7–2).

Differential Diagnosis: Nevi, melanotic macule, lesions of Addison's disease, Peutz-Jeghers syndrome, infected hyperkeratosis, candidiasis, syphilitic chancre, keratoacanthoma, lichen planus, frictional keratosis, and hairy leukoplakia may mimic oral cancer.

Treatment: Surgical excision and radiation therapy depends on the size and location of the tumor and on the presence or absence of metastases. Chemother-

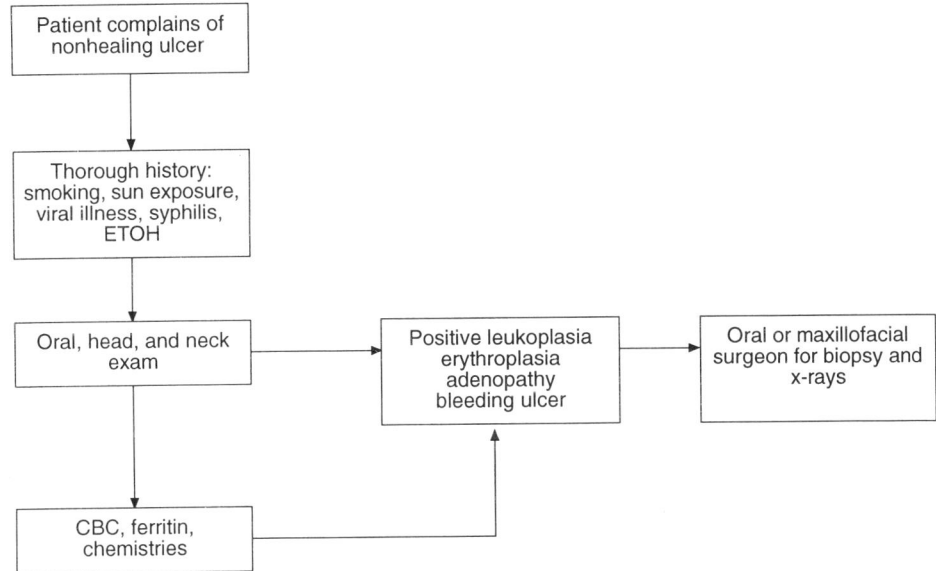

FIGURE 7–2   Oral cancer.

apy is currently not a first-line therapy in oral cancers. Most oral cancers have a cure rate nearly 90% if diagnosed when the size is 3 cm or less and before metastases occurs.

Follow-up: Lifetime surveillance is recommended, as second primary cancers occur in 10%–30% of cases. During the first year, the patient should be seen monthly for focused oral examinations and to assess for reoccurrence of symptoms, in addition to yearly complete physical examinations. Thereafter, follow-up visits should occur every 2 months during the second year, every 3 months during the third year, every 4 months during the fourth year, and then every 6 months. Chest x-ray examinations should be done every 6 months until the fourth year, and yearly thereafter.

Sequelae: Complications of oral cancer include disfigurement and xerostomia from surgery and radiation treatments, malnutrition due to difficulty chewing, infection, second primary cancers, or metastases to lung, regional lymph nodes, or adjacent organs.

Prevention/Prophylaxis: Smoking cessation, treatment for alcoholism, adequate nutrition, and yearly oral examinations can help prevent oral cancer.

Referral: Refer the patient to an oral or maxillofacial surgeon and an oncologist.

Education: Teach patients about the risk factors for developing oral cancer, including smoking and chewing tobacco, alcohol abuse, and poor nutrition. Discuss strategies to help the patient deal with these issues. Advise patients to report any nonhealing oral lesion within 2 weeks of initial occurrence.

Pharyngitis

Pharyngitis is an inflammation of the pharynx.

Etiology: Pharyngitis can be caused by viral infections, bacterial infections, tonsillitis, fungal infections, environmental allergens, and secondary to sinusitis. Most cases of pharyngitis are caused by viruses, including herpangina, hand-foot-and-mouth disease (due to coxsackievirus), and infectious mononucleosis. Treatable bacterial infections are group A streptococcus, *Neisseria gonorrhoeae, Corynebacterium diphtheriae,* groups C and G streptococci, *Haemophilus influenzae, Arcanobacterium haemolyticum, Mycoplasma pneumoniae,* and *Chlamydia pneumoniae.* Noninfectious causes of pharyngitis include pemphigus and systemic lupus erythematosus.

Occurrence: Pharyngitis is one of the most common problems seen in family practice. With an annual cost of treatment of more than $300 million. Viral causes far outnumber bacterial causes of pharyngitis. As many as 20% of healthy people have streptococci in their throats without symptoms, and even among patients with symptomatic pharyngitis, only 50% of those with positive throat cultures demonstrate a serological response to streptococci. Group A streptococcus infections account for 5% of pharyngitis cases.

Age: Pharyngitis can occur at any age but is more common in childhood, adolescence, and young adulthood. Pharyngitis due to group A beta-hemolytic streptococcus is rarely seen in children younger than age 3.

Ethnicity: No prevalence for pharyngitis exists among ethnic groups.

Gender: Pharyngitis occurs equally in males and females.

Contributing Factors: A high risk for or a previous history of rheumatic fever or exposure to someone with streptococcal pharyngitis contribute to the development of pharyngitis.

Signs and Symptoms: Patients with pharyngitis usually complain of a sore throat at rest that often worsens with swallowing. The pharyngeal mucosa may be mildly injected or severely inflamed. Patients with significant viral or streptococcal pharyngitis usually have a purulent exudate of the pharyngeal mucosa, fever greater than 99.5°F, cervical adenopathy, and leukocytosis. Patients with pharyngitis due to herpangina usually have small vesicles or ulcers on the tonsils, pharynx, or posterior buccal mucus, often accompanied by fever, headache, and malaise. Hand-foot-and-mouth disease is usually characterized by sore throat and oral lesions, accompanied by lesions on the hands and feet (patients may also have lesions on arms, legs, and buttocks).

Diagnostic Tests: Differentiating viral from bacterial pharyngitis on the basis of physical examination alone is difficult. Even with careful diagnostic techniques, a precise cause of pharyngitis can be determined in only about 50% of patients. Group A beta-hemolytic streptococcus can be identified by culture or by antigen-detection tests. Because the latter are specific but vary in sensitivity, a positive test result permits early diagnosis and treatment, but a negative test result does not exclude group A streptococcal disease. In these cases, a throat culture is necessary to make a diagnosis. Throat cultures, the "gold standard" for the diagnosis of streptococcal pharyngitis, are done for adults at high risk for or with a previous history of rheumatic fever, for symptomatic patients exposed to someone with streptococcal pharyngitis, and for patients with significant infection. When infectious mononucleosis is suspected, a serology test for heterophil agglutinin and white blood cell count with differential to detect atypical lymphocytes should be done. Pharyngitis, atypical lymphocytosis, and a negative heterophil test result should suggest the possibility of primary cytomegalovirus (CMV) infection or acute human immunodeficiency virus (HIV) infection.

Differential Diagnosis: The differential diagnosis for pharyngitis includes infectious mononucleosis, influenza, stomatitis, rhinitis or sinusitis with postnasal drip, or epiglottitis.

Treatment: Treatment for viral and bacterial pharyngitis includes aspirin for pain and rest. Most cases of pharyngitis are self-limited and do not require antimicrobial therapy. Antibiotic therapy should usually be withheld until and unless culture results are positive for bacteria. Group A beta-hemolytic streptococcus infection should be treated if the culture or antigen detection test result is positive, if the patient is at high risk for development of rheumatic fever, or if the diagnosis is strongly suspected, pending the culture results. Treatment, which is indicated for streptococcal pharyngitis, may be given also for pneumococcal and staphylococcal pharyngitis. Treatment includes penicillin VK 250 mg orally four times a day for 10 days, erythromycin 250 mg orally four times a day for 10 days, or penicillin G benzathine 1.2 million units intramuscularly (IM). Hospitalization and parenteral therapy are indicated when the patient is unable to take oral fluids or if airway obstruction is present.

Follow-up: Recheck the patient in 3–4 days if symptoms do not improve. Patients with streptococcal pharyngitis should have posttreatment throat cultures done only if they are at high risk for rheumatic fever or are still symptomatic.

Sequelae: Complications from pharyngitis include acute rheumatic fever, peritonsillar or retropharyngeal abscesses, life-threatening group A streptococcal infections, cervical lymphadenitis, and acute glomerulonephritis.

Prevention/Prophylaxis: Prophylaxis against streptococcal infection is indicated for the prevention of recurrent rheumatic fever in patients at high risk for contracting streptococcal infection (e.g., children, parents of young children, school teachers, medical and military personnel, patients in crowded living conditions) and those who have had rheumatic fever within the previous 5 years. Prophylaxis can be provided by penicillin G benzathine 1.2 million units IM every 4 weeks, penicillin V 125–250 mg orally twice a day, sulfadiazine 1 g orally every day (for adults with normal renal function and patients with penicillin allergies), or erythromycin 250 mg orally twice a day. Penicillin G benzathine is the drug of choice when medical compliance is an issue.

Referral: A physician should be consulted for patients with cervical adenitis of 3 cm or greater in diameter, peritonsillar or retropharyngeal abscesses, or a prolonged toxic course.

Education: Advise patients to seek medical attention for worsening of pain, dyspnea, drooling, dysphagia, or inability to fully open mouth. Instruct patients to increase oral fluid intake and use hard candy, lozenges, or warm saline gargles to soothe the throat. Patients with streptococcal pharyngitis should not return to school or work until they have been receiving antibiotic therapy for a full 24 hr.

Retinopathy

Retinopathy, noninflammatory disease of the retina, includes hypertensive, diabetic, and circinate retinopathies.

Etiology: The underlying pathology of the retinopathy relates to the underlying etiologic cause. Systemic causes include hypertension (arteriosclerotic), diabetes (diabetic retinopathy), age-related maculare degeneration, blood dyscrasias (thrombocytopenia, severe anemia), sickle-cell disease, toxoplasmosis, and CMV retinitis.

Hypertensive or arteriosclerotic retinopathy is related to the severity of the hypertension. The exact cause of diabetic retinopathy is unknown but directly relates to the duration of diabetes, the patient's age at onset, and glycemic control. Patients with sickle-cell disease are prone to retinopathy as a result of the blockage of small retinal capillaries resulting in neovascularization. Circinate retinopathy (usually bilateral) causes retinal degeneration and is more common among older adults.

Occurrence: Diabetic retinopathy is the leading cause of blindness in the United States. Type 2, or non–insulin-dependent, diabetes mellitus (NIDDM) is common in elderly persons. Diabetic retinopathy develops earlier in older patients, but proliferative retinopathy is less common. Hypertension and age-related macular degeneration are also seen frequently in the elderly.

Age: Elderly patients are prone to various forms of retinopathy. The prevalence of diabetes increases with age (18% between ages 65 and 74).

Ethnicity: Diabetes is most common in Native-Americans. Asian-Americans, African-Americans, and Hispanic-Americans have higher risks of diabetes than whites (1.5–2.0 times higher). Hypertension is also more prevalent among African-Americans.

Gender: Retinopathy occurs equally in men and women.

Contributing Factors: Contributing factors in diabetic retinopathy include age at onset, type of diabetes, duration of disease, poor glycemic control (persistent elevated glycosolated hemoglobin), and early detection of nonproliferative (background) retinopathy. Other factors include poorly controlled hypertension, sickle-cell disease, certain drugs (chloroquine, phenothiazines), and age-related changes (macular degeneration).

Signs and Symptoms: The presenting symptom may be the insidious painless onset of decreased visual acuity. Patients with persistent stage 3 (diastolic readings between 109 and 119 mmHg) or stage 4 (diastolic readings greater than 119 mmHg) hypertension and uncontrolled diabetes (glycosylated hemoglobin [HbA_{1C}] greater than 7%) should be assessed for retinal changes. Visual acuity should be screened in both eyes, using the Snellen chart. Assess pupillary reflex (direct and consensual), extraocular movements, and visual fields by confrontation. A complete funduscopic examination should be done. The funduscopic changes seen in patients with hypertension include arteriolar narrowing, atrioventricular (AV) nicking, flame hemorrhages, and hard and soft exudate. Classic nonproliferative changes in patients with diabetes are microaneurysms and hard and soft exudate. Clinical findings in patients with proliferative retinopathy are cotton wool spots, deep hemorrhages, and neovascularization.

Diagnostic Tests: Measure the patient's blood pressure. Assess for any clinical findings of papilledema in patients with stage 4 (diastolic greater than 119 mmHg) hypertension. Patients with diabetes should have random or fasting serum glucose readings; the desired fasting serum glucose level is 70–110 mg/dL. Glycosylated hemoglobin (HbA_{1C}) levels should be measured every 3–6 months, depending on glycemic control. The range is 4.0%–6.0% of total hemoglobin, with the desired level less than 7%. Patients with known hemoglobin A_1 disease may not yield accurate glycosolated hemoglobin readings.

Differential Diagnosis: In addition to the etiology already reviewed, the differential diagnosis of retinopathy includes glaucoma, cataracts, retinal detachment, CMV retinitis, toxoplasmosis, and retinal vasculitis (related to sarcoidosis).

Treatment: Prevention and early detection is fundamental to preserving vision. Annual ophthalmologic examinations are required. For patients with diabetes, the goal is to optimize glucose control. Patients with hypertension should be treated to control blood pressure (goal is 135/85 mmHg). The parameters and goal of treatment in patients with hypertension and diabetes should be clear and concise. Retinal specialists use a variety of interventions, including laser surgery, to minimize retinal destruction.

Follow-up: Follow-up depends on the findings. A retinal specialist should follow-up patients with retinopathy. Routine monitoring of diabetes and hypertension is required. The staging of retinopathy and the treatment plan require specialty follow-up.

Sequelae: Not all retinopathy is progressive. The condition and its outcome are related to the etiology of the retinopathy.

Prevention/Prophylaxis: Elderly patients should have an annual ophthalmology examination. During routine office visits, perform a fundoscopic examine on the eyes of patients with diabetes and hypertension. Promptly refer the patient to a retinal specialist at the earliest complaint of vision change or alteration in fundi. Patients with diabetes and hypertension should be aware of the goals of treatment and the need to control blood pressure and blood sugar level. Patients should monitor blood glucose and blood pressure at home.

Referral: As stated earlier, all patients with retinopathy should be seen by a retinal specialist. All patients with diabetes and hypertension need to see an ophthalmologist annually. Patients with retinopathy need to be evaluated by a retinal specialist.

Education. Patients should report any alteration in vision. Patients should know the goals of blood pressure and blood sugar control. Educate the patient on the proper use of medications. Finally, patients should understand the importance of follow-up care.

Rhinitis

Rhinitis is an inflammation of the nasal mucosa.

Etiology: Rhinitis may be either allergic or nonallergic. Allergic rhinitis due to the response of the nasal mucosa to airborne allergens in atopic individuals. This response is mediated by immunoglobulin E (IgE). IgE antibodies produced in response to the initial exposure to allergens bind to the nasal mucosa. Reexposure to the allergens causes the release of histamine, leukotrines, and prostaglandins, which results in local vasodilatation and inflammation with increased mucous production. Allergic rhinitis may be seasonal, caused by pollens from trees, flowers, or grasses pollinating in the spring or fall. Perennial allergic rhinitis is often related to environmental exposure to pollutants, animal dander, dust, molds, or cigarette smoke. The subtypes of nonallergic rhinitis include:

- Vasomotor rhinitis, caused by an idiopathic hyperactive nasal mucosa, produces symptoms similar to those of allergic rhinitis. One theory of vasomotor rhinitis proposed that a neurogenic dysfunction causes vascular and glandular hyperactivity of the nasal mucosa.
- Atrophic nonallergic rhinitis is probably due to degeneration and atrophy of nasal membranes and bony structures.
- Primary atopic rhinitis is strongly related to *Klebsiella ozaenae*.
- Rebound rhinitis is due to the overuse of topical nasal decongestants.

Occurrence: Allergic rhinitis occurs in 9%–21% of the population, or more than 20 million people in the United States. Nonallergic rhinitis occurs in 20%–60% of the population.

Age: Allergic rhinitis is most common between ages 10 and 39, declining after age 40. Vasomotor rhinitis is a condition of adulthood and is more common in the elderly. Atrophic rhinitis is associated with aging.

Ethnicity: No prevalence for rhinitis exists among ethnic groups.

Gender: Men and women age 40 and older have roughly the same incidence of rhinitis.

Contributing Factors: Most importantly, allergic rhinitis is usually associated with a strong family history of allergic illnesses, including rhinitis, asthma, and eczema. Exposure to airborne allergens in the environment such as pollution, animal dander, dust mites, molds, or seasonal pollens trigger allergic rhinitis. A variety of factors are thought to contribute to nonallergic rhinitis, including anatomic abnormalities, infections, medications (especially in the elderly), immunodeficiency, tumors of the nasopharynx and paranasal sinuses, Wegener's granulomatosis, pregnancy, hypothyroid disease, and leak of cerebral spinal fluid. Vasomotor rhinitis can be triggered by strong odors or fumes, temperature or barometric pressure changes, and psychological factors.

Signs and Symptoms: Patients with allergic rhinitis complain of rhinorrhea with clear thin nasal discharge, sneezing, obstructed nasal passages, and pruritic eyes, nose, and oropharynx. These individuals usually have a family history of allergies, with symptoms during the spring or fall. Patients with perennial allergic rhinitis have the same symptoms associated with environmental irritants. Physical examination may reveal a pale, boggy nasal mucosa, injected conjunctiva, enlarged turbinates, dark discoloration or bags under the eyes, and mouth breathing. The absence of a pale, boggy nasal mucosa, however, does not necessarily rule out allergic rhinitis.

Postnasal discharge and congestion are common complaints in vasomotor rhinitis, although the complaints associated with allergic rhinitis may also be present. Individuals with atrophic rhinitis often complain of a bad taste along with congestion and thick postnasal discharge. The classic symptoms associated with *Klebsiella ozaenae* rhinitis are crusting of nasal secretions, epistaxis, and foul odor. The physical examination, which should include a thorough check for nasal polyps or septal deviation, reveals pink to red, dry nasal mucosa in nonallergic rhinitis. Diagnosis is usually made from the history and physical examination.

Questions for the patient should include:

- Does the patient associate the symptoms with a season, place, time of day, or activity?
- Is there a family history of allergic diseases?
- Do symptoms seem to occur during times of stress or during weather or temperature changes?
- Does the patient use intranasal drugs such as cocaine?

Symptoms of infection, such as fever, purulent nasal discharge, and tenderness over the sinuses, should be ruled out on examination. Assess for adenopathy, otitis, and wheezes in the lungs, to determine the presence of infection (Fig. 7–3).

Diagnostic Tests: If you suspect allergic rhinitis, perform a nasal smear for eosinophils. An eosinophil count greater than 500 cells/mm^3 is positive for allergy, whereas an elevated neutrophil count in a nasal smear suggests infection. A complete blood count may help to determine if infection is present, but the eosinophil count is not helpful in diagnosing allergic rhinitis. Specialized allergy skin testing may be performed. Radiographic sinus films may be made if infection is suspected.

Differential Diagnosis: Viral or bacterial upper respiratory infection, sinusitis, otitis media, nasal polyps, deviated nasal septum, hypothyroid disease, tumor, and foreign body in the nose may mimic rhinitis.

Treatment: When allergic rhinitis is suspected, environmental control measures can effectively relieve symptoms and avoid the adverse effects of medications. Patients with seasonal allergies should avoid outdoor activities during peak pollen periods, from 11 AM to 3 PM. Windows should be kept closed to decrease pollen levels indoors, and air filters for the home may be helpful.

The two most common causes of perennial allergic rhinitis are dust mites and domestic animals. The patient should wash bedding weekly in hot water, cover mattresses and pillows in plastic, keep pets out of the bedroom, and remove carpeting when possible. Desensitization by immunotherapy, which may cure allergic rhinitis, should be initiated by an allergist after testing.

Pharmacological therapy is directed at control of the symptoms. As first-line therapy, antihistamines are recommended to control rhinorrhea, sneezing, and nasal and eye pruritus. Antihistamines are most effective when taken before symptoms occur, although they can be effective when used intermittently for symptomatic relief. The first-line antihistamines are inexpensive and available over-the-counter but usually cause mild to severe sedation. Diphenhydramine 12.5–25 mg qid, brompheniramine 4–12 mg bid, and chlorpheniramine 4–12 mg bid are the most sedating, but the patient may develop tolerance for this side effect. Clemastine 1.34–2.68 mg bid is the least-sedating first-line antihistamine. The lowest possible dose of these medications should be used in elderly persons to avoid excessive sedation. Because of their anticholinergic effects, these drugs may worsen certain conditions that are common in the elderly patient, such as benign prostatic hypertrophy, bladder neck obstruction, and narrow-angle glaucoma.

Second-generation antihistamines are relatively free of central nervous system (CNS) and anticholinergic side effects, and very effectively relieve allergic rhinitis symptoms. These drugs include loratadine 10 mg qid (or once daily with hepatic impairment), cetirizine 10 mg qid, azatadine 1 mg bid or qid, and fexofenadine 60 mg bid (or once daily with decreased renal function). These

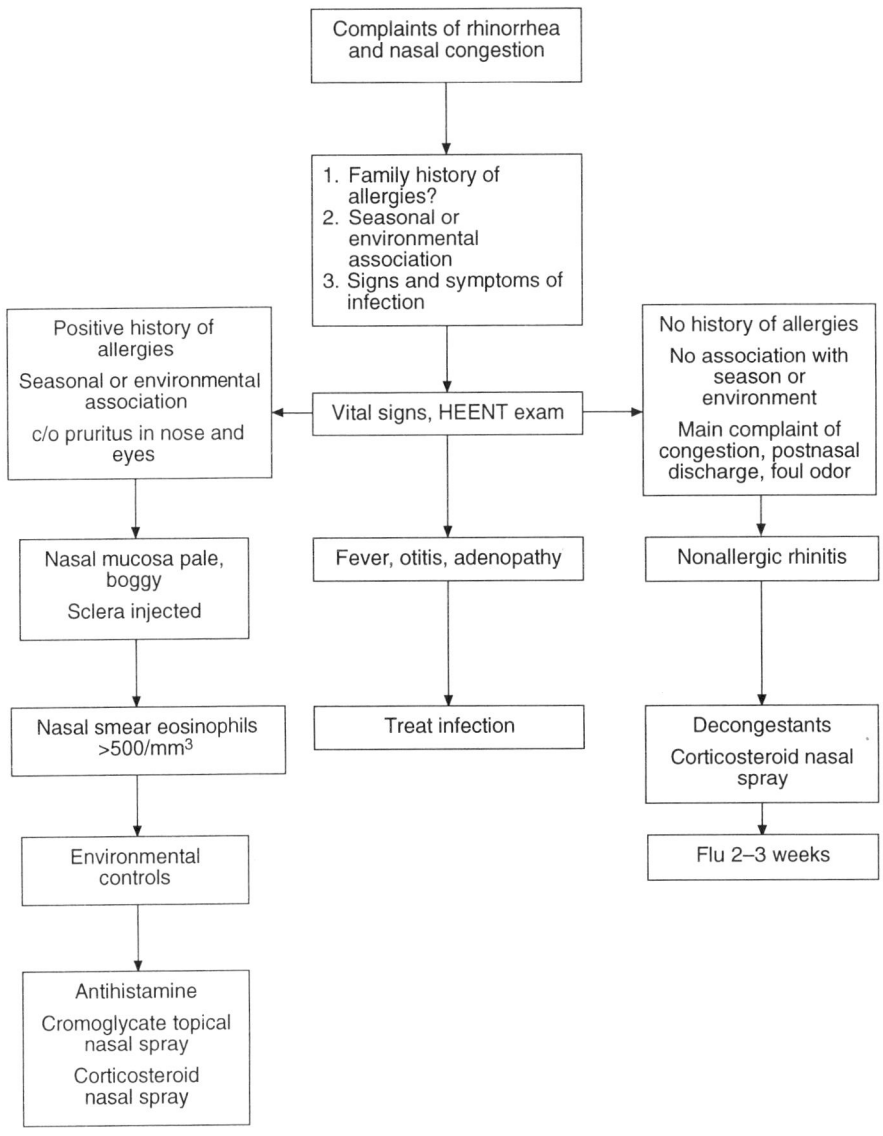

Complaints of rhinorrhea
and nasal congestion

1. Family history of
   allergies?
2. Seasonal or
   environmental
   association
3. Signs and symptoms of
   infection

Positive history of
allergies

Seasonal or environmental
association

c/o pruritus in nose and
eyes

Vital signs, HEENT exam

No history of allergies

No association with
season or
environment

Main complaint of
congestion, postnasal
discharge, foul odor

Nasal mucosa pale,
boggy

Sclera injected

Fever, otitis, adenopathy

Nonallergic rhinitis

Nasal smear eosinophils
>500/mm^3

Treat infection

Decongestants

Corticosteroid nasal
spray

Environmental
controls

Flu 2–3 weeks

Antihistamine

Cromoglycate topical
nasal spray

Corticosteroid
nasal spray

Referral to
allergist/ENT

FIGURE 7–3 Rhinitis.

antihistamines should not be prescribed for patients taking antifungal medications, macrolide antibiotics, tricyclic antidepressants, or class Ia antiarrhythmics, as their interaction with these drugs may cause life-threatening cardiac dysrhythmias. They are also contraindicated for patients with a history of congestive heart failure, coronary artery disease, or liver disease.

Decongestant medications decrease nasal mucosa swelling but have little effect on the other symptoms of rhinitis. Pseudoephedrine and phenylpropanolamine are best used intermittently for only short periods, as they have many CNS side effects. Decongestants are contraindicated in elderly patients with poorly controlled hypertension, coronary artery disease, and a history of cerebral vascular accident. These medications are recommended to decrease severe nasal congestion and enhance the penetration of topical therapies. Topical sodium cromoglycate 4% is effective as needed to control symptoms of allergic rhinitis because of its direct antiinflammatory effect on eosinophils and neutrophils. Topical corticosteroid nasal sprays are effective in most types of rhinitis when used regularly. These sprays are available in once-a-day doses and in aqueous or aerosol preparations to suit patient preferences. Ipratropium bromide nasal spray controls watery rhinorrhea when used two to four times a day. Topical nasal preparations avoid systemic side effects but may cause local irritation and dryness of the nasal mucosa.

Oral corticosteroids are recommended only for severe nasal obstruction such as that caused by rebound rhinitis or nasal polyps. Prednisone 0.5 mg/kg daily for 3–5 days should be effective, and no tapering is necessary. Therapy can be initiated with oral corticosteroids but continued with topical corticosteroids.

Follow-up: Have the patient return in 2–3 weeks to review his or her response to medications and understanding of the principles of care and prevention.

Sequelae: Epistaxis and sinusitis are complications of rhinitis.

Prevention/Prophylaxis: Teach patients with allergic rhinitis to avoid irritants and to try to control environmental risk factors. Discuss the need to take antihistamines or use nasal sprays before exposure to irritants, to prevent symptoms.

Referral: When symptoms persist or worsen, refer the patient to an ear, nose, and throat (ENT) specailist or allergist.

Education: Discuss environmental control with the patient. Avoid the use of OTC nasal sprays for more than 3 consecutive days. Teach the patient about the sedating side effects of antihistamine medications.

BIBLIOGRAPHY

General

Abrams, WB, Beers, MH, and Berkow, R: The Merck Manual of Geriatrics, ed 2. Merck Research Laboratories, Whitehouse Station, NJ, 1995.

Bates, B: A Guide to Physical Examination and History Taking, ed 5. JB Lippincott, Philadelphia, pp 155–196.

Berg, D: Handbook of Primary Care Medicine. JB Lippincott, Philadelphia, 1993, pp 647–658.

Braunwald, E, et al (eds): Harrison's Principles of Internal Medicine, ed 13. McGraw-Hill, New York, 1994.

Carpenito, LJ: Handbook of Nursing Diagnosis, ed 5. JB Lippincott, Philadelphia, 1993.

Collins, RD: Algorithmic Diagnosis of Symptoms and Signs. Igaku-Shoin, New York, 1995.

Dambro, M: Griffith's 5 Minute Clinical Consult. Williams and Wilkins, Baltimore, 1997.

Doenges, ME, Moorhouse, MF, and Geissler, AC: Nursing Care Plans: Guidelines for Individualizing Patient Care, ed 4. FA Davis, Philadelphia, 1997.

Fischbach, F: A Manual of Laboratory Diagnostic Tests, ed 2. JB Lippincott, Philadelphia, 1984.

Gorroll, AH, May, LA, and Mulley, AG: Primary Care Medicine: Office Evaluation and Management of the Adult Patient, ed. 3. JB Lippincott, Philadelphia, 1995.

Hurst, JW (ed): Medicine for the Practicing Physician, ed 4. Appleton and Lange, Norwalk, CT, 1996.

Isselbacher, KJ, et al: Harrison's Principles of Internal Medicine, ed 13. McGraw-Hill, New York, 1994.

Jarvis, C: Physical Examination and Health Assessment. WB Saunders, Philadelphia, 1992, pp 276–307.

Lonergan, ET (ed): Geriatrics. Appleton and Lange, Norwalk, CT, 1996.

Noble, J (ed): Primary Care Medicine, ed 2. CV Mosby, St. Louis, 1996.

Pfenninger, JL, and Fowler, GC: Procedures for Primary Care Physicians. CV Mosby, St. Louis, 1994.

Rakel, R: Manual of Medical Practice. WB Saunders, Philadelphia, 1996.

Rakel, R: Textbook of Family Practice, ed 8. WB Saunders, Philadelphia, 1995.

Schroeder, SA, Krupp, MA, Tierney, LM, and McPhee, SJ: Current Medical Diagnosis and Treatment, ed 28. Norwalk, CT, Appleton and Lange, 1989, pp 101–103.

Schwartz, MH: Textbook of Physical Diagnosis, ed 2. WB Saunders, Philadelphia, 1994.

Seidel, Ball, Dains, and Benedict: Mosby's Guide to Physical Examination, ed 2. Mosby Year Book, St. Louis, 1991, pp 164–263.

Sellers, R: Differential Diagnosis of Common Complaints, ed 3. WB Saunders, Philadelphia, 1996.

Semia, TP, Beizer, JL, and Higbee, MD: Geriatric Dosage Handbook. Lexi-Comp, Cleveland, OH, 1995.

Stanley, JA: Eye. In Lonergan ET (ed): Geriatrics. Appleton and Lange, Stamford, CT, 1996.

Swartz, M: Textbook of Physical Diagnosis, ed 3. WB Saunders, Philadelphia, 1998.

Tierney, LM, McPhee, SJ, and Papadakis, MA (eds): Current Medical Diagnosis and Treatment, ed 36. Appleton and Lang, Stamford, CT, 1997.

Uphold, CR, and Graham, MV: Clinical Guidelines in Adult Health. Barmarrae Books, Gainesville, FL, 1994.

Uphold, C, and Graham, MV: Clinical Guidelines in Family Practice, ed 2. Barmarrae Books, Gainesville, FL, 1994.

US Department of Health and Human Services, Public Health Service: Clinician's Handbook of Preventive Services. Government Printing Office, Washington, DC, 1994.

US Preventive Service Task Force Guide to Clinical Prevention Services, ed 2. Williams and Wilkins, Baltimore, 1996.

Wachtel, R, and Stein, M: The Care of the Ambulatory Patient. CV Mosby, St. Louis, 1996.

Woolf, J, Jones, J, and Lawrence, R (eds): Health Promotion and Disease Prevention in Clinical Practice. Williams and Wilkins, Baltimore, 1996.

Yoshikawa, TT, Cobbs, EL, and Brummel-Smith, K: Practical Ambulatory Geriatrics, ed 2. CV Mosby, St. Louis, 1998.

Acute Glaucoma

Richter, CU: Management of glaucoma. In Gorroll, AH, May, LA, and Mulley, AG (eds): Primary Care Medicine: Office Evaluation of the Adult Patient, ed 3. JB Lippincott, Philadelphia, 1995.

Schachat, AP: Glaucoma. In Barker, LR, Burton, JR, and Zieve, PD (eds). Principles of Ambulatory Medicine, ed 4. Williams and Wilkins, Baltimore, 1995.

Stanley, JA: Eye. In Lonergan, ET (ed): Geriatrics. Appleton and Lange, Stamford, CT, 1996.

Yoshikawa, TT, Cobbs, EL, and Brummel-Smith, K: Practical Ambulatory Geriatrics, ed 2. CV Mosby, St. Louis, 1998.

Cataracts

Steinert, RF: Management of cataracts. In Goroll, AH, May, LA, and Mulley, AG (eds): Primary Care Medicine: Office Evaluation of the Adult Patient, ed 3. JB Lippincott, Philadelphia, 1995.
US Department of Health and Human Services, Public Health Service, Agency for Health Care Policy and Research: Clinical Practice Guideline Number 4: Cataract in Adults: Management of Functional Impairment. AHCPR Publication No 93-0542, Rockville, MD, 1993.

Chronic Glaucoma

Richter, CU: Management of glaucoma. In Goroll, AH, May, LA, and Mulley, AG (eds): Primary Care Medicine: Office Evaluation of the Adult Patient, ed 3. JB Lippincott, Philadelphia, 1995.
Schachat, AP: Glaucoma. In Barker, LR, Burton, JR, and Zieve, PD (eds): Principles of Ambulatory Medicine, ed 4. Williams and Wilkins, Baltimore, 1995.

Epistaxis

Alvi, A, and Joyner-Triplett, N: Acute epistaxis. How to spot the source and stop the flow. Postgrad Med 99:83–90, 94–96, 1996.
Corbridge, RJ, Djazaeri, B, Hellier, WP, and Hadley, J: A prospective randomized controlled trial comparing the use of merocel nasal tampons and BIPP in the control of acute epistaxis. Clin Otolaryngol 20(4):305–307, 1995.
Kotecha, B, et al: Management of epistaxis: A national survey. Ann R Coll Surg Engl 78:444–446, 1996.
Lavy, J: Epistaxis in anticoagulated patients: Educating an at-risk population. Br J Haematol 95:195–197, 1996.
Strong, EB, Bell, DA, Johnson, LP, and Jacobs, JM: Intractable epistaxis: Transantral ligation vs. embolization: Efficacy review and cost analysis. Otolaryngol Head Neck Surg 113(6):674–678, 1995.
Valentino, J: Common EENT symptoms: Epistaxis. In Rakel, R (ed): Saunders Manual of Medical Practice. WB Saunders, Philadelphia, 1996.
Vickery, CL, and Kuhn, FA: Using the KTP/532 laser to control epistaxis in patients with hereditary hemorrhagic telangiectasia. South Med J 89(1):78–80, 1996.
Wilson, WR: Approach to epistaxis. In Gorroll, AG, May, LA, and Mulley, AG (eds): Primary Care Medicine: Office Evaluation of the Adult Patient, ed 3. JB Lippincott, Philadelphia, 1995.

Oral Cancer

Fischer, DS: Follow-up of cancer: A handbook for physicians. Lippincott-Raven, Philadelphia, 1996.
Greenspan, JS: Oral manifestations of disease. In Isselbacher, KJ, et al (eds): Harrison's Principles of Internal Medicine, ed 13. McGraw-Hill, New York, 1994.
Kelly, JP: Screening for oral cancer. In Gorroll, AH, May, LA, and Mulley, AG: Primary Care Medicine: Office Evaluation and Management of the Adult Patient, ed 3. JB Lippincott, Philadelphia, 1995.
Lebovics, RS: Malignant tumors of the head and neck. In Isselbacher, KJ, et al (eds): Harrison's Principles of Internal Medicine, ed 13. McGraw-Hill, New York, 1994.
Parker, RG, Rice, DH, and Casiato, DA: Head and neck cancers. In Casciato, DA, and Lowitz, BB (eds): Manual of Clinical Oncology. Little, Brown, Boston, 1995.
Rubright, WC, et al: Risk factors for advanced stage oral cavity cancer. Arch Otolaryngol Head Neck Surg 122:621, 1996.
Schantz, SP, Harrison, LB, and Hong, WK: Cancer of the head and neck. In DeVita, VT, Hellma, S, and Rosenberg, SA (eds): Cancer: Principles and Practices of Oncology, JB Lippincott, Philadelphia, 1993.
Smith, C, Pindborg, JJ, and Binnie, WH: Oral Cancer: Epidemiology, Etiology, and Pathology. Hemisphere Publishing, New York, 1990.

Pharyngitis

Bronze, MS, and Dale, JB: The reemergence of serious group A streptococcal infections and acute rheumatic fever. Am J Med Sci 311:1, 41–54, 1996.

Burwick, F: Common respiratory symptoms: Sore throat. In Rakel, RE (ed): Saunders Manual of Medical Practice. WB Saunders, Philadelphia, 1996.

Dagnelie, CF, van der Graaf, Y, and De Melker, RA: Do patients with sore throat benefit from penicillin? A randomized double-blind placebo-controlled clinical trial with penicillin V in general practice. Br J Gen Pract 46:589–593, 1996.

Kiselica, D: Group A beta-hemolytic streptococcal pharyngitis: Current clinical concepts. Am Fam Physician 49:1147–1154, 1994.

Little, P, and Williamson, I: Sore throat management in general practice. Fam Pract 13:317–321, 1996.

Middleton, DB: Pharyngitis. Prim Care 23:719–739, 1996.

Schlager, TA, et al: Optical immunoassay for rapid detection of group A beta-hemolytic streptococci. Should culture be replaced? Arch Pediatr Adolesc Med 150:3, 245–248, 1996.

Simon, HB: Approach to the patient with pharyngitis. In Goroll, AH, May, LA, and Mulley, AG (eds): Primary Care Medicine: Office Evaluation of the Adult Patient, ed 3. JB Lippincott, Philadelphia, 1995.

Vukmir, RB: Adult and pediatric pharyngitis. A review. J Emerg Med 10:607–616, 1992.

Retinopathy

Davidson, JK: Clinical Diabetes Mellitus: A Problem-Oriented Approach, ed 2. New York: Thieme Medical Publishers, pp 427–437, 1991.

Rhinitis

Austen, KF: Diseases of immediate type hypersensitivity. In Isselbacher, KJ, et al (eds): Harrison's Principles of Internal Medicine, ed 13. McGraw-Hill, New York, 1994.

Guarderas, JC: Rhinitis and sinusitis: Office management. Mayo Clin Proc 71:882, 1996.

Mygind, N, and Naclerio, RM (eds): Allergic and Non-allergic Rhinitis Clinical Aspects. WB Saunders, Philadelphia, 1993.

Pittman, A, and Fillinghast, J: Allergy and immunology. In Carey, CF, Lee, HH, and Woltje, KF: The Washington Manual of Medical Therapeutics, ed 29. Lippincott-Raven, Philadelphia, 1998.

Self, T, Alloway, RR, and Dempster, JS: Treatment of rhinitis. Am Acad Nurse Pract 8(3):135–143, 1996.

Tan, R, and Corren, J: Optimum treatment of rhinitis in the elderly. Drugs Aging 7:168, 1995.

CHAPTER **8**

CHEST DISORDERS

Cardiac Assessment

Differentiating normal from abnormal cardiac function in an elderly individual can be a challenge because one in two older persons has cardiac disease. More specifically, almost half of all individuals over age 60 have severe coronary artery narrowing with a respective increase in myocardial demand. Of these, fewer than 50% have clinical signs and symptoms of this process. Cardiovascular disease is the most prominent cause of disability in this age group, and the leading cause of death, accounting for about half of all deaths among elderly persons.

CHANGES IN CARDIAC STRUCTURE AND FUNCTION

In an older person the changes in structure and function of the heart depend on the physiologic changes over time, the negative effects of a risky lifestyle, and the specific presence of cardiac disease.

The primary structural change associated with the aging process is the appearance of the barrel chest. Rib cage calcification, intercostal muscle weakening, and kyphoscoliosis all contribute to this finding. The size of the heart remains essentially unchanged, although some increase in left ventricular wall thickness has even been demonstrated in older individuals who do not have cardiovascular disease. Left ventricular hypertrophy is usually due to increased cardiac demand, most likely caused by an increase in peripheral resistance. Peripherally the vessels become atherosclerotic and arteriosclerotic, and the systolic pressure increases with age.

Fat deposits accumulate around the sinoatrial node. The number of pacemaker cells has usually decreased by age 75. Baroreceptors become less sensitive with age, and the response to changes in blood pressure is often blunted.

152

These physiologic changes have little functional impact on the aging heart at rest, but with exercise or stress they render the aging heart less capable of increasing—and sustaining an increase in—cardiac output. The maximal heart rate declines approximately 30% between ages 20 and 80. Cardiac dilatation and increased stroke volume compensate somewhat for the diminished heart rate during exercise.

CLINICAL EXAMINATION FEATURES

Because of the structural changes in the chest wall, the point of maximal impulse (PMI) is often not visible and the apical pulsation is more difficult to feel in the presence of a barrel chest. Although a slight increase in the anteroposterior diameter is considered normal, patients with this increase should be assessed for pathology (e.g., cardiomegaly, overinflated airways).

Auscultation in the geriatric patient frequently reveals changes in normal heart sounds, extra heart sounds, bruits, and murmurs. The S_1 is more easily heard, and splits of the first heart sound are more easily detected because of an ejection sound that occurs when the aortic valve cusp tissue fails to fold into the vessel wall during ejection. A change in the loudness of S_1, accompanied by a slow heart rate, may indicate heart block. The S_2 split on inspiration is narrower or absent because of decreased compliance of the pulmonary vasculature. An opening snap occurs when the mitral or tricuspid valve produces minor vibrations of increased intensity caused by more rapid cusp movement or a resistance to inflow caused by cusp fusion. An audible opening snap is the best physical sign of mitral stenosis but it becomes less obvious in the older adult whose valves are rigid and calcified.

Ventricular filling sounds, best heard with the stethoscope bell, are caused by the halting of the ventricle after ventricular filling. The physiologic S_3, heard most clearly at the apex, disappears by the fourth decade as the ventricle stiffens and filling becomes less rapid. An S_3 in an individual over 50 is usually pathologic and reflects an increased filling rate, usually indicating heart failure or mitral regurgitation. Early diastolic filling is reduced in healthy elderly persons, resulting in an end diastolic volume maintained by an increase in atrial contribution to left ventricular filling. This condition may cause an S_4, which, in the absence of other findings, is considered normal in elderly persons.

The carotid arteries should be assessed routinely for the presence of bruit. Asymptomatic carotid bruit is a risk factor for stroke. Studies demonstrate that a vessel is occluded more than 50% by the time a bruit can be heard. In elderly persons, assess the top level of the internal jugular pulsation when evaluating jugular venous pressure. Do no use the external jugular veins, as they may be sclerosed and appear to be falsely distended or may yield a falsely low pressure reading.

Prolonged extra heart sounds (murmurs), particularly systolic ones, are quite common in elderly individuals. Systolic murmurs, which often indicate aortic valve disease, occur in more than 50% of individuals over age 70. The soft systolic ejection murmur is due to the dilatation and the decrease in compliance of the aorta caused by stiffening of the aortic cusps without obstruction (aortic sclerosis). Loud murmurs, which usually indicate aortic stenosis, are often accompanied by a slow rising carotid pulse and left ventricular hypertrophy. An apical pansystolic or late systolic murmur also occurs frequently in older persons, resulting from floppy valves that become regurgitant over time. The two most common causes of mitral regurgitation are papillary muscle dysfunction (usually due to myocardial infarction) and mitral annular calcification. Diastolic murmurs, which are always pathologic in elderly persons, may be caused by heart block, aortic regurgitation, or mitral stenosis.

In the older adult, additional features of cardiac disease may be seen on physical examination of systems other than the heart. The eye examination might reveal the thick corneal arcus seen with lipid abnormalities or the funduscopic findings of atherosclerosis. The skin may demonstrate xanthomas or cholesterol nodules and changes in skin temperature, indicating a metabolic or peripheral vascular disease causing or contributing to cardiac disease. The presence of edema must be determined. The following lists the clinical cardiac examination features in the geriatric patient:

Structural wall changes common.
S_1 more easily heard.
S_2 split narrower.
S_4 common.
Systolic murmurs common.
Bruits (carotid, abdominal) common.

ASSESSMENT OF RISK FACTORS FOR CORONARY ARTERY DISEASE

Although some risk factors for coronary artery disease can be remedied, others cannot. The two most important risk factors for atherosclerosis that cannot be remedied are advanced age and male gender. The major remediable risk factors are high blood pressure and cholesterol levels and smoking.

Since the 1970s mortality from coronary artery disease has shown a pronounced decline in the United States. Most of this decline has been attributed to changes in lifestyle. The decline in cardiovascular disease has occurred in older as well as younger age groups, suggesting that the effects of risk factor modification persist well into later life.

Blood Pressure

The systolic blood pressure (BP) rises with age; the diastolic pressure remains the same or drops a bit. Established hypertension is a risk factor for cardiovascular disease in the geriatric age group, with systolic elevations posing a greater risk than diastolic elevations. Overall, the risk for both genders of experiencing a cardiovascular event or death is two to three times higher in those with significant hypertension (BP greater than 165/95 mmHg) than in those who are normotensive (BP less than 140/90 mmHg).

Isolated systolic hypertension (ISH) is defined as a systolic pressure greater than 160 mmHg (140–159 is considered borderline) and a diastolic pressure of less than 90 mmHg. Aggressive treatment of ISH has demonstrated a significant reduction in stroke, myocardial infarction, and sudden cardiac death.

Cholesterol

Serum cholesterol levels rise with age, up to age 60; thereafter, these levels begin to drop. The risk of the effects of an elevated cholesterol level persists from middle age to extreme old age, with total cholesterol remaining a significant predictor of new coronary events in both men and women regardless of a history of previous coronary artery disease. Studies show that a drop of 10% in total cholesterol is associated with a reduction of 15%–20% in coronary heart disease over a 2-year period (Swales, Fletcher, and Bulpitt, 1993). Aggressive efforts are often indicated to lower low-density lipoprotein (LDL) levels and raise high-density lipoprotein (HDL) levels for cardiac protection.

Smoking

Smoking is a significant risk factor for coronary heart disease. Studies show that smoking is responsible for about 30% of the annual mortality from coronary artery disease compared with nonsmokers; smokers have a 70% greater annual risk of death from coronary artery disease and more than twice the annual risk of sudden cardiac death (SAM, 1994). These risks seem to be related to the current level of smoking and to be reversible when smoking is discontinued. In several studies, former smokers over age 65 had mortality rates similar to those of nonsmokers, including those who had given up smoking in the previous 1–5 years (LaCroix et al., 1991).

Additional proven or postulated risk factors for cardiovascular disease in the elderly include obesity, lack of exercise, left ventricular hypertrophy, and impaired glucose tolerance.

Elderly individuals are most likely to have a combination of risk factors, which has a cumulative effect on increasing the risk of coronary artery disease. Control of hypertension is clearly the most potentially remediable risk factor. Evidence is compelling for discontinuation of cigarette smoking at any age. More information is needed regarding the effectiveness and feasibility of lowering cholesterol levels, weight reduction, improved exercise plans, and strict control of blood glucose levels, with respect to the incidence of coronary heart disease, particularly in those of most advanced age.

NONINVASIVE CARDIAC STUDIES

Electrocardiogram

The electrocardiogram (ECG) remains the most widely applied diagnostic tool in cardiology. Several aging changes noted in apparently healthy individuals have little prognostic significance:

- Decrease in the prevalence of sinus bradycardia and sinus arrhythmia on the resting ECG.
- Increase in the prevalence and density of supraventricular and ventricular ectopic beats.
- Mild PR interval prolongation.
- Leftward shift of the QRS axis.

Even though the increase in QRS voltage, presence of Q waves and ST-T wave abnormalities have been seen in healthy older adults, these findings, which are also often associated with increased cardiac risk, should cause suspicion.

In general, the criteria for a normal ECG reading do not differ for older individuals. Abmormalities that suggest the presence of heart disease include atrial fibrillation, left bundle branch block, ST-T wave changes, and left ventricular hypertrophy. Studies using an ambulatory 24-hr ECG, which involves a small portable tape recorder, have revealed that the prevalence of arrhythmia increases with age. Studies have consistently demonstrated that ventricular arrhythmias occur frequently, sinus bradycardia is uncommon, and second- and third-degree atrioventricular block is very uncommon in apparently healthy older individuals (Camm, Katritsis, and Ward, 1994). Prognostic inferences from ambulatory ECG readings in elderly persons are weak; in fact, several studies have failed to demonstrate any significant relationship between symptoms, sudden deaths, and ventricular ectopic beats. Most arrhythmias are brief and produce no symptoms, so an inability to find an arrhythmia does not exclude the possibility of a rhythm disturbance. In elderly individuals it is often difficult to establish a direct correlation between symptoms and transient cardiac arrhythmia. A sustained arrhythmia found on ambulatory recording of a patient with central nervous system symptoms may suggest that the symptoms are related to the arrhythmia, so treatment might then be initiated. Because an episodic ECG might not reveal this disturbance, the use of a 24-hr monitoring device is recommended in selected individuals, particularly those who suffer from convulsions, fainting, or falls.

The exercise ECG (exercise stress test) helps in the further diagnosis of an older individual with suspected or known coronary artery disease. Determination of the duration or degree of exercise, the heart rate response, the blood pressure response, ST-segment depression or elevation, and the presence of exercise-induced arrhythmias is the primary target of stress testing. Exercise thallium-201 imaging can be used for risk stratification of the elderly with coronary artery disease. If the patient cannot perform exercise stress testing, a pharmacologic stress can be induced with intravenous (IV) dipyridamole-thallium. Testing using drug-induced stress has yielded a sensitivity and specificity for older individuals with coronary artery disease similar to that for younger individuals.

Echocardiography

Echocardiography involves applying reflected ultrasound waves above audible frequency to the evaluation of the heart. This allows imaging of the internal cardiac structures that are of different densities, such as the myocardium, valves, and cardiac chambers. Both single- and double-dimensional images can be done. Doppler echocardiography can be used to measure the characteristics of blood in the heart. Echocardiography provides detailed information about the cardiac anatomy and physiology, and serial studies can monitor the progression of disease. The studies, which are inexpensive and safe, are particularly well suited to the elderly population. These studies may eliminate the need for the invasive cardiac catheterization in the older adult with valvular disease. Echocardiography is particularly useful in examining diastolic functioning of the ventricles in elderly persons with heart failure who have normal systolic function and do not respond well or even may deteriorate on conventional therapy.

Normal findings of echocardiography in the elderly include calcification of the aortic and mitral valves. Calcification of the mitral ring and dilatation and calcification of the aortic arch may also occur. Common findings include mitral, tricuspid, and aortic regurgitation; mitral leaflet prolapse; increased left ventricular mass; and dilated and tortuous aorta.

The echocardiogram, which is valuable in the examination of valvular disease in the elderly, facilitates the differentiation between aortic valve sclerosis and stenosis. It is also sensitive to the detection of the high-frequency fluttering on the anterior leaflet of the mitral valve caused by aortic regurgitation. In mitral stenosis, valve leaflets are thickened and cusp mobility is reduced; doppler echocardiography can easily detect the presence and etiology of mitral regurgitation. Mitral annular calcification is a common degenerative condition in the elderly; this technnique can demonstrate the severity of the calcification. Infective endocarditis, primarily a clinical diagnosis, frequently presents atypically and asymptomatically in the elderly; the echocardiogram may demonstrate vegetative abscesses or valvular incompetencies. Additional use for echocardiograms may include:

- Follow-up of patients with valve replacements.
- Evaluation for the presence of left ventricular hypertrophy and cardiomyopathies.
- Evaluation for aortic aneurysm, dilatation, or dissection or the presence of pericardial disease.

Transesophageal imaging uses the esophagus as an acoustic window to the heart and the thoracic aorta. Because of the proximity to the heart permitted by this technique, it consistently provides high-quality imaging.

Chest X-Ray Examination

Cardiac findings based on a chest x-ray examination are difficult to interpret because of chest wall deformities. An increase in the cardiothoracic ratio, lengthening of the aorta, aortic tortuosity, and mild dilatation of the aortic knob are common findings that may not indicate cardiovascular disease. Cardiac disease is assessed best in the posteroanterior (PA) view, in which the heart is closer to the film and unmagnified. It is preferable to use an erect rather than a supine PA view. The chest x-ray is useful for assessing chamber enlargement, particularly for assessing the left atrium and the left ventricle. The x-ray examination also helps to identify the findings of pulmonary venous hypertension, dilatation of vessels, interstitial edema, pleural effusion, and valvular thickening and calcification and is useful in follow-up examinations for patients with valve replacements, pacemaker insertions, or both.

INVASIVE CARDIAC STUDIES

Noninvasive methods for evaluation of cardiovascular functioning in the elderly are always preferred to the invasive methods of cardiac catheterization and angiography. In patients with aortic disease, cardiac catheterization is used to measure right heart and pulmonary artery pressures and sometimes to confirm the pressure gradient across the aortic valve, further define the coronary anatomy, assess the quality of obstructed vessels, and estimate the amount of the myocardium supplied by each coronary artery. Because the use of this procedure carries considerable risk it is imperative to plan what information is necessary and then to perform the test as expeditiously as possible. As many elderly patients have borderline renal function, the toxic potential of the radiographic dye must be considered in the risk-benefit analysis.

Arrhythmias

An arrhythmia is a disturbance of cardiac rhythm. Cardiac arrhythmias, which occur in either the presence or absence of underlying heart disease, may be life threatening or be an incidental finding. Arrhythmias may be differentiated by type or mechanism. The most prevalent forms of arrhythmias in a geriatric population are listed here:

1. Sick sinus syndrome: pathologic bradyarrhythmia with an alternating supraventricular tachyarrhythmia (brady-tachy syndrome).
2. Supraventricular tachyarrhythmia: three primary categories.
   - Arrhythmias primarily of atrial origin (i.e., atrial premature beats, ectopic atrial rhythms, multifocal atrial tachycardia, atrial flutter, and atrial fibrillation).

- Arrhythmias arising primarily within the atrioventricular (AV) node (i.e., AV nodal reentrant tachycardia, junctional premature beats, and nonparoxysmal junctional tachycardia).
- Arrhythmias that are partially supraventricular in origin (i.e., preexcitation syndomes).
3. Ventricular arrhythmias: ventricular ectopic beats is the most common variety.

Etiology: Most arrhythmias are thought to be caused by abnormalities either in impulse formation (disordered automaticity) or in impulse conduction (allowing reentry), or by a combination of the two. Increased automaticity is an accentuation of the inherent ability of many cardiac tissues to generate an independent rhythm. Reentry consists of a wave of excitation repeatedly circulating around a fixed anatomic obstacle.

Occurrence: Studies show that asymptomatic older patients with no known structural heart disease have an incidence of up to 40% of sinus arrhythmia, supraventricular or ventricular premature beats, or supraventricular tachycardia.

Age: The prevalence of ventricular arrhythmia increases with age, occurring in 80% of healthy older adults age 60–85. Atrial fibrillation is diagnosed in 4.8% of women and 6.2% of men over age 65 at baseline examination, and its prevalence is strongly associated with advanced age, particularly in women. Although no specific data are available, the incidence of junctional arrhythmias and tachycardias related to the accessory pathway may be lower in elderly individuals because of an age-related reduction in accessory pathway conduction.

Ethnicity: Not available.

Gender: Arrhythmias occur more often in men than in women. (See also "Age.")

Contributing Factors: Preexisting heart disease is a contributing factor to arrhythmias, with structural disease becoming more prevalent with age. Fibrosis or calcification in the vicinity of the AV node causes conduction disturbances. Atrial arrhythmias may be caused by a mechanical obstruction to atrial emptying with subsequent left atrial dilatation, myocardial ischemia, and increased sympathetic activity.

An *age-related factor* associated with tachyarrhythmias is increased left atrial size. This enlargement may contribute to the increase in supraventricular ectopy. Increases in ventricular ectopic beats may be related to left ventricular enlargement. The overload of ionized calcium in the older myocardium may contribute to ectopy. Age-related factors associated with bradyarrhythmias include an age-related decline in the number of pacemaker cells and presence of fat deposits around the sinoatrial (SA) node. HIS bundle cells are replaced with fibrous tissue, and adipose tissue and amyloid are deposited; this is also associated with conduction disturbance.

Systemic diseases (i.e., thyrotoxicosis, infection, hypoxemia, hypercapnea) can cause circulatory disturbances that may provoke an arrhythmia. *Drugs* that can cause an arrhythmia include digitalis and other antiarrhythmics, aminophylline, and alcohol. *Electrolyte disturbances,* particularly hyperkalemia, hypokalemia, hypercalcemia, and hypocalcemia, can precipitate ectopic beats.

Signs and Symptoms: The history, physical examination, and ECG studies represent the cornerstone to evaluation of arrhythmias. Arrhythmias may cause symptoms due to a reduced blood flow or inadequate cardiac pump function. In the history, the patient may describe sensations that accompany abnormal cardiac rhythm such as pounding, racing, or skipped beats. Older adults are less likely to complain of palpitations and more likely to present with manifestations of heart failure or hypoperfusion (i.e., impaired mental function, dizziness, syncope). Along with the history of present illness, previous diagnosis and treatment for arrhythmia and cardiac disease should be elicited.

In the physical examination, concentrate on the cardiac and peripheral vascular systems. Check the pulses for one full minute to determine rate and regularity. Assess normal and extra heart sounds. S_1 intensity may provide information about the relation of atrial to ventricular contraction. The longer the PR interval, the softer the S_1. Note intermittent extra heart sounds (S_3 and S_4). The jugular vein must be assessed. In AV dissociation (when the atria and ventricles contract independently), giant A waves (cannon waves) may be observed. Provoking maneuvers should not be attempted by the advanced practice nurse but may be attempted by a cardiologist. These maneuvers include carotid massage (for atrial arrhythmias only), mild exercise, psychological stress, pharmacologic stress, and electrical programmed stimulation (EPS).

Diagnostic Testing: Diagnostic testing includes a 12-lead ECG done with a rhythm strip, lasting at least 2–3 min. Include exercise testing for those with a clinical history suggesting exercise-induced arrhythmia. An ambulatory 24-hr ECG (Holter monitoring) helps to quantify arrhythmias with reference to symptoms. Event recorders are best suited for documenting less-frequent but more-prolonged bouts of arrhythmias. Patient-activated loop memory devices, which record the ECG prior to the symptomatic event, are most useful. HIS bundle electrograms involve the insertion of a transvenous electrode catheter into the right ventricle, to record depolarizations and the intervals. This method is most useful for distinguishing AV block from an ectopic focus.

In EPS, multipolar catheter electrodes are introduced into the venous or atrial circulation and advanced to various intracardiac positions to monitor the electrical activity or to induce an arrhythmia. EPS is most useful for determining sinus node dysfunction, AV block, intraventricular conduction disturbances, preexcitation syndromes, supraventricular tachycardia, ventricular tachycardia, and unexplained syncope or palpitations. It is used also to monitor cardiac activity in survivors of sudden cardiac death.

Differential Diagnosis: Clarify the diagnosis with precision. Note reversible and precipitating causes of an arrhythmia and coexisting diseases.

Treatment: The incidence of asymptomatic arrhythmias of questionable clinical significance is high. Arrhythmias are never treated in isolation; some are benign and some are not.

The risk of treatment is considerable (Table 8–1). Aggressive therapeutic treatment is indicated when patients are symptomatic and the urgency of therapy depends on the associated hemodynamic disturbance.

Three major factors determine how well a patient tolerates an arrhythmia: heart rate, duration of the arrhythmia, and presence and severity of associated underlying heart disease. Arrhythmias often cannot be controlled unless underlying cardiac problems are discovered and treated. No antiarrhythmic "wonder drug" exists and the bothersome and potentially dangerous side effects necessitate determination of clear indications and use of the utmost caution. Pharmaceutic agent selection is based on the electrophysiology of the rhythm disturbance, the mechanism of action, and the side effects of the drug. Conditions common in the elderly that can affect the choice, dosing, efficacy, and safety of antiarrhythmic therapy include decreased hepatic or renal function, decreased serum albumin levels, and electrolyte abnormalities.

The broad categories of arrhythmia treatment include medications, pacemakers, antitachycardia devices, implantable automatic cardioverter defibrillators, catheter ablative procedure, and specific maneuvers. Vagal maneuvers (carotid massage or the Valsalva maneuver) may terminate or slow AV nodal reentry or AV reentry types. These maneuvers are associated with high risk of emboli dislodgment. The carotid arteries should be assessed for bruit before administering massage. Because of the high mortality associated with antiarrhythmic surgery, this is not recommended in elderly individuals. The specifics of treatment are not detailed in this text because all assessment and management

TABLE 8–1 ARRHYTHMIAS AND SUGGESTED RESPONSES

Arrhythmia	Significance	Treatment
Supraventricular premature complexes, unsustained tachycardias, asymptomatic	Low	Only if symptomatic or caused by concurrent disease
Atrial tachycardias, asymptomatic	Low, if slow and no associated disease	Only if symptomatic or caused by concurrent disease
Ventricular arrhythmias, sustained and symptomatic	High	As beneficial in elderly person as in young persons
Ventricular arrhythmias, asymptomatic	Low	No evidence of effectiveness

From Horowitz, LN, and Lynch, RA: Managing geriatric arrhythmias I: General considerations. Geriatrics 46(3):31, 1991.

must be done in close collaboration with a physician; much of the treatment is initiated by the specialist in the hospital setting.

Follow-up: Because of their low therapeutic ratio, drug dosing and plasma concentrations of the antiarrhythmics are based on therapeutic monitoring. Side effects are significant, including the negative ionotropic effect, which can precipitate heart failure or proarrhythmia in the presence of structural heart disease. Extracardiac side effects can also be significant, including anticholinergic effects, gastrointestinal effects, and neurologic toxicity with some antiarrhythmic agents. Monitor patients after pacemaker insertion with regular follow-up appointments and ECG testing, specifically looking for pacemaker failure, infection, thromboembolism, perforation or dislodgment, and complicating arrhythmias.

Sequelae: Regardless of age, the nature and severity of underlying heart disease are of much greater prognostic significance than the arrhythmia alone. The following rhythm disturbances have been reported to carry a poor prognosis in patients with coronary artery disease: frequent ventricular premature contractions (VPCs) (greater than 10/min), multiform VPCs, ventricular couplets, R-on-T phenomenon, and ventricular tachycardia.

Syncope can occur secondary to asystole. Bradycardia can contribute to complete heart block and to the development of heart failure in patients with associated ventricular dysfunction. Tachycardia can precipitate angina and circulatory arrest in patients with coronary artery disease. Bradyarrhythmias or tachyarrhythmias can cause systemic embolism and stroke. Atrial fibrillation can result in heart failure and a low cardiac output state. The risk of stroke related to atrial fibrillation increases with age.

The Cardiac Arrhythmia Suppression Trial (CAST) demonstrated that patients treated for prognostically significant arrhythmias may have a higher mortality from sudden cardiac death if Class IC (flecainide and encainide) agents are used (Greenberg et al., 1995).

Prevention/Prophylaxis: All patients with atrial fibrillation should be considered for long-term low-intensity warfarin therapy. Aspirin, though less effective in preventing stroke, is an alternative for some patients in whom warfarin is contraindicated. Electrolyte imbalances should be monitored and metabolic disturbances treated. Patients receiving digitalis should be monitored for toxicity.

Referral: All patients with treatable arrhythmias require collaborative management. Clinically significant ventricular arrhythmias or any symptomatic arrhythmia is managed by the specialist in the coronary care unit. A primary care physician may handle many atrial arrhythmias and low-grade ventricular arrhythmias; however, a specialist should be consulted for all clinically significant ventricular arrhythmias, arrhythmias resistant to routine therapy, or arrhythmias whose clinical significance is in doubt.

Education: Carefully instruct all patients receiving antiarrhythmics about the therapeutic effects, side effects, and potentially adverse effects of these medications. Because patients with pacemakers are vulnerable to external electrical fields, they should be instructed to recognize this potential and avoid exposure. Patients with pacemakers must also be aware of signs and symptoms of pacemaker failure.

Congestive Heart Failure

Congestive heart failure (CHF) is a syndrome in which the heart cannot pump an adequate supply of blood, in relation to venous return, to meet the metabolic needs of the tissues.

Etiology: Causes of acute and chronic CHF in elderly individuals are essentially the same as those in the general adult population. Most CHF patients have coronary artery disease, chronic hypertension, or both. Common causes of CHF in elderly persons include coronary artery disease (CAD), ischemic heart disease, aortic stenosis, mitral regurgitation, diastolic dysfunction, metabolic disorders such as diabetes or hyperthyroidism, dysrhythmias, and fluid overload.

Distinction is made between systolic and diastolic dysfunction. Systolic dysfunction relates to the inability of the heart to contract normally and expel sufficient blood, whereas diastolic dysfunction is related to the heart's inability to relax and fill normally.

Occurrence: More than 3 million Americans have heart failure, with an additional 400,000 new cases diagnosed each year. The prevalence of heart failure increases with age from approximately 3% in persons ages 45–64, to 6% in persons age 65–74, and 10% in those age 75 and over. CHF is associated with a very high mortality rate. Mortality for people with New York Heart Association Class IV heart failure at 1 year exceeds 40%.

Age: The average annual incidence for development of the first clinical evidence of heart failure in men and women increases more than fourfold from 45–54 to age 65–74. CHF is the most common diagnosis-related group (DRG) in patients over 65. The number of CHF cases is expected to double in the next 40 years.

Gender: Postmenopausal women have an increased risk of cardiovascular disease, which can lead to CHF.

Ethnicity: Blacks have higher rates of CHF discharges, perhaps from the higher prevalence of hypertension and dilated cardiomyopathy found in this group. No reports have been published on the prevalence of CHF that are generalizable to a racially mixed population of older people.

Contributing Factors: Aging is associated with changes in the heart and vasculature that may cause or exacerbate CHF. Diastolic filling also changes. Other contributing factors for CHF include risk factors for heart disease in general. Independent predictors for CHF include hypertension, diabetes, cigarette smoking, and elevated LDL levels.

Signs and Symptoms: Classic symptoms of CHF include paroxysmal nocturnal dyspnea, orthopnea, dyspnea on exertion, decreased exercise tolerance, fatigue and weakness, dry, hacking cough (especially when lying down), lower extremity swelling, and abdominal discomfort associated with ascites or hepatic engorgement. In elderly persons, the presenting symptoms of CHF may be distorted by comorbid conditions, and dyspnea may not be experienced when the patient's physical activity is limited. Instead of the classic dyspnea seen in younger patients, lethargy or restlessness may prevail. Additionally, the decrease in peripheral perfusion may present as acute confusion, a cerebrovascular accident, uremia, an ischemic or gangrenous extremity, or pulmonary emboli secondary to venous stasis. Finally, the patient may not be able to express symptoms clearly, secondary to preexisting dementia or depression.

Signs of CHF may include elevated jugular venous pressure, positive hepatojugular reflux, extra heart sounds (S_3, S_4), crackles that do not clear with coughing, and peripheral edema in the absence of venous insufficiency.

Diagnostic Tests: Laboratory studies should include a complete blood count, serum electrolytes, creatinine, blood urea nitrogen (BUN), and albumin, as well as liver function tests. Levels of T4 and thyroid-stimulatory hormone (TSH) should be checked on patients over age 65 with heart failure without obvious etiology. Evaluation of CHF should include an electrocardiogram (ECG), which can demonstrate the presence of acute ischemic events, arrhythmias, medication effects, changes from old ECG results, and ventricular hypertrophy. Chest x-ray examination may reveal pulmonary congestion and cardiac enlargement. However, diagnosis of CHF in an elderly patient by chest x-ray examination may be made difficult by the presence of comorbid conditions such as pulmonary parenchymal disease or kyphoscoliosis. Echocardiography can differentiate between systolic and diastolic dysfunction and is useful in evaluation of the heart wall's motion, observation of pericardial effusions, and measurement of the ejection fraction. Echocardiograms are critical to the assessment of valvular lesions. Exercise thallium testing may help demonstrate ischemia. Cardiac catheterization allows for the determination of the severity of myocardial dysfunction and valvular lesions, as well as for the assessment of heart pressures and the presence of coronary artery disease.

Differential Diagnosis: Dyspnea, the primary symptom of heart failure, can be caused by obstructive airway disease, parenchymal lung disease, pulmonary emboli, chest wall or respiratory muscle disease, heart disease, deconditioning, renal failure, anemia, abdominal masses, and anxiety neurosis.

Treatment: Correction of the reversible causative factors is the primary therapy in heart failure. Diuretics are used to reduce volume overload and high ventricular filling pressures in both systolic and diastolic failure. Use caution with diuresis in diastolic dysfunction because overdiuresis may increase symptoms of heart failure. Hydrochlorothiazide (usually 25 mg qd) is useful for patients with mild to moderate CHF without severe renal impairment. Metolazone (2.5–10 mg qd) is a long-acting diuretic. Loop diuretics, such as furosemide (Lasix), are more potent than thiazide diuretics. Elderly patients should be started on 10 mg of Lasix qd initially. The usual maintenance dose is 40 mg qd but can be increased to 160 mg qd if necessary to achieve diuresis. Hospitalized patients with severe volume overload may require doses of intravenous (IV) Lasix as high as 240 mg bid to obtain brisk diuresis. Bumetanide is the least ototoxic diuretic.

Digoxin is indicated for patients with atrial fibrillation or flutter with normal or reduced ejection fractions, or for patients with impaired ejection fractions with sinus rhythm. Loading doses of oral digoxin are not usually necessary for the elderly individual, unless a rapid effect is needed. The pharmacokinetics of digoxin are altered in elderly persons because of their reduced lean body mass and altered creatinine clearance. Patients with reduced renal function should be started on 0.125 mg qd or lower and titrated to an adequate serum digoxin level. Digitalis toxicity may occur at therapeutic serum levels in older adults.

Vasodilators are used in CHF to relieve compensatory vasoconstriction. Intravenous (IV) nitroglycerine is the drug of choice for heart failure in the setting of ischemic heart disease. IV nitroglycerine is started at 5 μg/min with an infusion pump and titrated to effect. All patients with heart failure should be given a trial of angiotensin-converting enzyme (ACE) inhibitors unless the following contraindications are present: renal insufficiency (serum creatinine of 3 or greater), hyperkalemia (higher than 5.5). For patients who develop hypotension (systolic pressure of less than 90 mmHg), decrease the diuretic first, then add the ACE inhibitor if blood pressure stabilizes. Captopril is first given in a test dose of 6.25 mg. If no untoward reactions occur, patients may be given captopril 12.5 mg tid or enalapril 2.5 mg bid, increased slowly if needed. The ELITE study demonstrated that losartan (angiotensin II receptor blocker) may be superior to captopril, through a demonstrated lower mortality rate (Aronow, 1998). Patients that cannot tolerate ACE inhibitors may be managed on hydralazine and isosorbide dinitrate.

Patients with severe or intractable CHF may be treated with beta-adrenergic agonists (dopamine, dobutamine, amrinone, or milrinone).

Diastolic failure is treated primarily with diuretics. Calcium channel blockers and ACE inhibitors are also helpful. Vasodilators cause significant hypotension in diastolic failure.

Patients with CHF and coronary artery disease may be evaluated for revascularization. The goal of coronary artery bypass grafting (CABG) is to prevent further injury to the myocardium or to restore nonfunctional but still viable myocardium. Most studies evaluating the effect of CABG on survival in CHF patients have shown positive results. Predictors of increased risk for perioperative mortality include repeat CABG, emergent CABG, ejection fraction below 20, and age. Risk increases by about 5% annually, after age 60. Percutaneous transluminal coronary angioplasty (PTCA) has not been shown to improve survival.

Indications for valvular surgery in elderly patients include severe valvular lesion and symptoms. Mortality is increased when the patient has severely depressed left ventricular function, inoperable coronary disease, pulmonary hypertension, multiple medical problems, poor functional status, or a poor nutritional state.

Balloon valvuloplasty has been used successfully in patients considered at too high a risk for surgery.

Heart transplantation is not indicated for CHF patients of advanced age, but is considered individually in younger patients.

Mild aerobic exercise increases functional capacity and improves the quality of life for CHF patients. Dietary sodium should be restricted to 2 or 3 g/day. Discourage alcohol. Fluid restriction is not necessary unless there is hyponatremia, but patients with CHF should avoid excessive fluid intake.

Follow-up: Ask the patient about the presence of symptoms of heart failure as noted previously. Determine and document the most strenuous activity that the patient can perform without significant symptoms. Ask general questions related to the patient's quality of life, such as sleep patterns, sexual difficulties, and coping behaviors. Complete review of all medications, including nonprescription medications as necessary. Laboratory work should be done as needed, including electrolyte, creatinine clearance, and digoxin levels when indicated.

Sequelae: The most severe complication of CHF is end-organ disease. Hepatic and renal failure can result from CHF in final stages.

Prevention/Prophylaxis: Reducing cardiac risk factors in elderly persons affects coronary disease as strongly as it does in younger age groups. Encourage risk factor reduction using age-specific guidelines to facilitate changes in lifestyle.

Referral: Warning signs for the need for hospitalization include prolonged weight gain, palpitations, persistent or recurrent dizziness, agitation or cognitive changes, inability to sleep because of paroxysmal nocturnal dyspnea, abdominal pain, and inability to walk.

Education: Education and the use of support groups are very important in patients with CHF because noncompliance provides a major cause of morbidity and unnecessary hospital admissions. Instruct patients and their families about the nature of CHF, necessary medications, dietary restrictions, worsening CHF, and prognosis. Explain typical symptoms of worsening CHF (orthopnea, paroxysmal dyspnea, leg edema, or exercise intolerance) and instruct patients to contact their health-care provider if these should occur. Have the patient contact the health-care provider if daily weight changes by more than 2–4 lb. Practitioners should recommend that CHF patients receive vaccination against influenza and pneumococcal disease. Encourage patients to complete advance directives regarding their health-care preferences.

Hypertension

Hypertension may occur in two forms in elderly persons. Isolated systolic hypertension (ISH) is a systolic blood pressure greater than 140 mmHg and a diastolic pressure less than 90 mmHg. Systolic-diastolic hypertension (SDH) is a systolic pressure greater than 140 mmHg and a diastolic pressure greater than 90 mmHg. Blood pressure is measured twice, separated by 2 min, then averaged. If the first two readings differ by more than 5 mmHg, additional readings should be obtained and averaged.

Etiology: The pathophysiology of both ISH and SDH in the elderly involves loss of vascular tissue elasticity causing an increase in peripheral vascular resistance. Patients with ISH have increased aortic stiffness and high peripheral vascular resistance. Patients with SDH have a decrease in cardiac output and intravascular volume and an increase in peripheral vascular resistance and left ventricular mass. Secondary forms of hypertension may be due to renal parenchymal damage, primary aldosteronism, and pheochromocytoma.

Occurrence: Of adults in the United States, 15%–20% are hypertensive. More than 15 million people over age 65 (more than 60% of the U.S. elderly population) have elevated systolic pressure, with or without elevations in diastolic pressure.

Age: SDH hypertension usually begins in middle age and levels off at about age 55. The prevalence of ISH continues to rise even after age 80.

Ethnicity: The prevalence of systolic and diastolic hypertension is greater in African-Americans (more than 70% of elderly African-Americans) than it is in elderly white or Mexican-Americans.

Gender: In over-65 age group, black women have the highest rate, followed by African-American men, Mexican-American men, white men, Mexican-American women, and white women.

Contributing Factors: A variety of factors contribute to elevations in blood pressure in the elderly. Physiologic age–related changes include reduced myocardial compliance, diminished β-adrenergic sensitivity, blunted baroreceptor reflexes, extracellular fluid volume contraction, decreases in renal functional capacity, and altered activity in the renin-angiotensin system.

Other factors include obesity (particularly intra-abdominal fat); physical inactivity (may raise blood pressure, owing to more constricted peripheral vessels); alcohol (daily consumption of more than two alcoholic drinks having a vasopressor effect); sodium consumption (salt-sensitive response greater in all persons over age 60, in blacks, and in obese individuals). Additional influences include smoking (causing slow repeated rises in blood pressure) and insomnia (causing more sustained elevations in blood pressure, which normally is lowest late in the day and during sleep and highest in early morning hours).

Signs and Symptoms: Usually no symptoms are associated with elevations in blood pressure, unless the hypertension is a malignant or accelerated type or is due to a secondary cause. The history should elicit the duration of the hypertension, previous treatment for hypertension, family history of hypertension, and presence of diabetes or coronary artery disease. Risk factors including smoking, sedentary lifestyle, high intake of sodium and/or fat should be determined. Ask the patient about signs and symptoms of conditions such as stroke, transient ischemic attack, myocardial infarction, angina, and renal disease, which could indicate target-organ damage. All medications (prescribed and over-the-counter [OTC]) should be thoroughly reviewed. Psychosocial history should be examined for potential stressors.

The physical assessment technique for measuring blood pressure includes having the patient be in a basal (resting) state for 5 min prior to measurement and using a relaxed bare arm and the proper size cuff. Measure the blood pressure with the patient lying or sitting; then have the patient stand, wait 2 min, and recheck the blood pressure. The pulse should be checked as well, and if a drop in blood pressure is not followed by a compensatory rise in pulse (increase greater than 10 beats/min), then the patient may have baroreceptor reflex impairment. The initial physical examination should include two or more blood pressure measurements, each separated by 2 min.

The physical examination in the hypertensive patient should also include an assessment for target organ disease such as retinopathy, cardiac enlargement, arrhythmias, murmurs, extra heart sounds, abdominal masses, neck and abdominal bruits, weak or absent peripheral pulses, and edema.

Diagnostic Tests: Measurement of the blood pressure is all that is required; if elevated, three blood pressure readings taken on different occasions should be averaged. Labile or "white coat" hypertension is blood pressure that is elevated when measured in the physician's office in association with a normal 24-hr blood pressure reading (Fig. 8–1).

Diagnostic errors can be avoided in the elderly by checking for pseudohypertension. Blood vessels that have become rigid from arteriosclerosis are difficult to occlude with the sphygmomanometer; this can yield falsely high blood pressure readings. Perform Osler's maneuver by pumping the cuff to higher than the patient's recorded systolic blood pressure; then, if the radial or brachial artery is still palpable pseudohypertension may be present. If pseudohypertension is suspected, the electronic oscillometric device can be used to provide readings that more closely correspond to intra-arterial levels; otherwise, the more invasive intra-arterial measurement may be done.

A postprandial fall in blood pressure is common in elderly persons, with the maximal drop noted 60 min after eating (particularly a high-carbohydrate meal). Postprandial hypotension is thought to be due to increased splanchnic blood flow, which decreases systemic vascular resistance; it may also be due to a rise in plasma insulin levels.

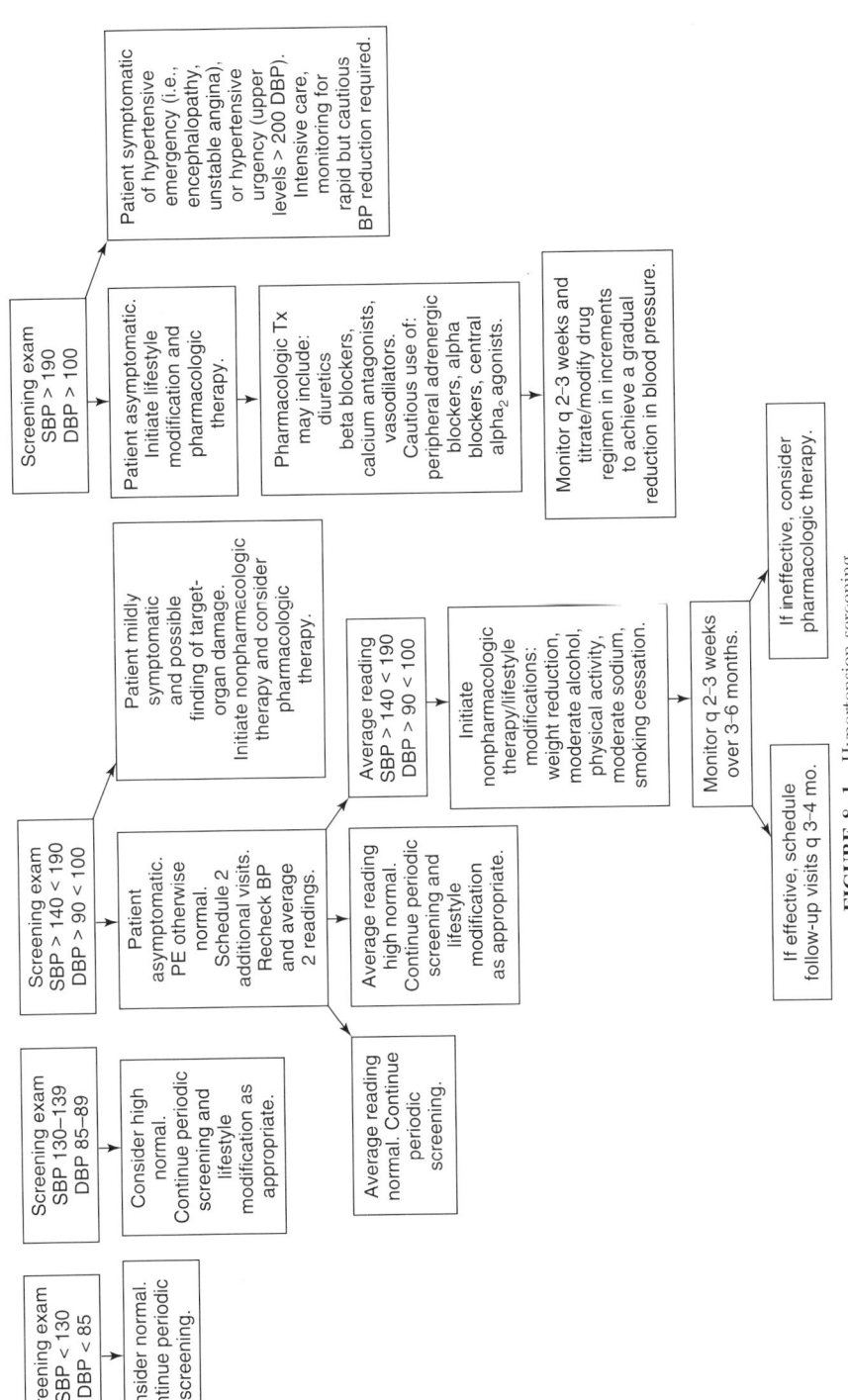

FIGURE 8-1 Hypertension screening.

Screening exam SBP <130 DBP <85
Consider normal. Continue periodic screening.

Screening exam SBP 130–139 DBP 85–89
Consider high normal. Continue periodic screening and lifestyle modification as appropriate.

Screening exam SBP > 140 < 190 DBP > 90 < 100
Patient asymptomatic. PE otherwise normal. Schedule 2 additional visits. Recheck BP and average 2 readings.

Average reading normal. Continue periodic screening.

Average reading high normal. Continue periodic screening and lifestyle modification as appropriate.

Patient mildly symptomatic and possible finding of target-organ damage. Initiate nonpharmacologic therapy and consider pharmacologic therapy.

Average reading SBP > 140 < 190 DBP > 90 < 100
Initiate nonpharmacologic therapy/lifestyle modifications: weight reduction, moderate alcohol, physical activity, moderate sodium, smoking cessation.

Monitor q 2–3 weeks over 3–6 months.

If effective, schedule follow-up visits q 3-4 mo.

If ineffective, consider pharmacologic therapy.

Screening exam SBP >190 DBP > 100
Patient symptomatic of hypertensive emergency (i.e., encephalopathy, unstable angina), or hypertensive urgency (upper levels > 200 DBP). Intensive care, monitoring for rapid but cautious BP reduction required.

Patient asymptomatic. Initiate lifestyle modification and pharmacologic therapy.

Pharmacologic Tx may include: diuretics beta blockers, calcium antagonists, vasodilators. Cautious use of: peripheral adrenergic blockers, alpha blockers, central alpha$_2$ agonists.

Monitor q 2–3 weeks and titrate/modify drug regimen in increments to achieve a gradual reduction in blood pressure.

169

The clinician must avoid an auscultory gap error. In some elderly individuals, a wide gap between the first Korotkoff's sound and subsequent beats is noted. If the cuff is not inflated high enough, the systolic pressure can be underestimated. This can be avoided by palpating the radial pulse and inflating the cuff beyond the disappearance of the palpable pulse.

Other diagnostic work that may be done to examine target organ damage includes urinalysis; 12-lead electrocardiogram; complete blood count; and creatinine, potassium, glucose, sodium, calcium, total lipoprotein, high-density lipoprotein, and triglyceride levels.

Differential Diagnosis: The differential for hypertension includes the determination of the type (isolated systolic, systolic-diastolic, and/or secondary cause). A secondary cause for hypertension is suspected if the onset of systolic-diastolic hypertension occurs after age 55, the hypertension is difficult to treat, or the clinical or laboratory findings suggest a cause.

Treatment: The aim of therapy is to reduce the systolic blood pressure to less than 140 mmHg and the diastolic blood pressure to 90 mmHg or less if tolerated. Lifestyle modifications are the initial mode of therapy unless the systolic blood pressure is greater than 190 mmHg or the diastolic pressure is greater than 100 mmHg, in which case pharmacologic therapy is indicated immediately.

As a lifestyle modification, weight reduction is noteworthy because even small amounts of weight (10 lb) loss in obese persons can lead to significant reductions in blood pressure. This may be due to increased insulin sensitivity when weight is lost. Sodium restriction should be moderate (2.5–5 g sodium/day), because of salt sensitivity in elderly persons. Increased physical activity is encouraged because repetitive aerobic exercise lowers the blood pressure by dampening the sympathetic nervous system. The BP then remains lower for 12 hr as a result of persistent postexercise vasodilatation. Moderate alcohol consumption is advised, to no more than 1 oz/day. Discontinuation of smoking is strongly advised for improvement in cardiovascular health. Other lifestyle changes include increasing potassium intake from fresh fruits and vegetables, relaxing to decrease stress, reducing fat and caffeine intake, and maintaining adequate calcium and magnesium intake.

If after 3–6 months nonpharmacologic therapy has not been effective and the blood pressure remains elevated, then pharmacologic therapy is indicated. Drug therapy may be initiated sooner if the patient has target-organ disease or multiple cardiac risk factors. Blood pressure reduction with pharmacologic therapy should be done in slow increments of drug modifications every 3–4 months unless hypertension is severe.

Diuretics are the initial drug of choice for older adults, as they are the only classification shown to reduce both cerebrovascular and cardiovascular morbidity and mortality. A low-dose diuretic (hydrochlorothiazide 12.5–25 mg/day) is recommended. The relatively few adverse reactions to this low-cost drug may include electrolyte depletion, glucose intolerance, hyperuricemia, and serum lipid elevations. Loop diuretics (Lasix 20 mg or Bumex 0.5 mg initially) may be necessary in elderly persons with creatinine clearance less than 30 mL/min.

Beta-blockers are thought to decrease the blood pressure by decreasing cardiac output interfering with renin and having a central effect. However, findings from recent studies on the role they play in decreasing cardiovascular events are less impressive. Beta-blockers remain the drug of choice, however, for patients with a history of myocardial infarction or angina. Side effects include fatigue, exercise intolerance, worsened insulin sensitivity, glucose intolerance, and increased triglyceride levels. These agents are contraindicated in patients with chronic obstructive pulmonary disease. Beta-blockers in combination with thiazide diuretics may work well for older patients.

Calcium channel blockers, which provide vasodilatation and promote diuresis, are widely used as first-line drug but have not been well studied. The few adverse effects found among older adults include conduction defects, peripheral edema, headache, and constipation.

Other drug classifications are preferred for certain patients. These include ACE inhibitors for those with heart failure. Drugs that exaggerate postural changes in blood pressure or cause cognitive dysfunction should be used with caution.

In the event of an inadequate response or compliance and quality of life issues related to the drug therapy, the drug dose may need to be increased, another drug substituted, or a second agent from another classification added. Once the hypertension has been controlled for 6 months, the dose may need to be stepped down. In some older frailer individuals with poor prognosis and comorbidities, the benefits of drug therapy are too small to outweight the risks involving the quality and quantity of life.

Follow-up: See the patient every 2–4 weeks until antihypertensive therapy stabilizes the blood pressure. After control has been established, a visit may be required every 3–4 months. Electrolyte, serum glucose, and lipid levels need to be monitored in selected patients; orthostatic blood pressure must be measured at each visit. The clinician needs to monitor the J-curve phenomenon. This refers to the point at which mortality increases owing to compromised coronary filling, which appears to occur when the diastolic pressure is reduced to 70–85 mmHg.

Sequelae: Recent national clinical trials show that reductions in blood pressure decrease the rate of cardiovascular and cerebrovascular events, even in individuals over age 80 (JNC VI, 1997). The elevation in systolic blood pressure, which is the single greatest risk factor for coronary artery disease in elderly persons, interacts with other risk factors to compound it. A well-documented relationship exists between blood pressure elevation and stroke, transient ischemic attacks, sudden death, congestive heart failure, aneurysms, and renal failure.

Prevention/Prophylaxis: Compliance with antihypertensive therapy is the best way to reduce blood pressure. Prevention of obesity and avoidance of smoking are important primary prevention strategies.

Referral: In accelerated or malignant hypertension, end-organ damage from hypertension occurs over a brief period of time. Patients with a diastolic pressure greater than 120 mmHg or symptoms indicating a hypertensive emergency (e.g., hypertensive encephalopathy, intracranial hemorrhage, unstable angina, or acute myocardial infarction) need an intensive care setting to monitor urine output and arterial and central venous and pulmonary capillary wedge pressure. Patients with associated conditions including heart failure, high-grade retinopathy, acute cerebrovascular ischemia, and progressive renal insufficiency also require close collaboration with the physician.

Education: Patients need specific information on the disease and management. On each visit the patient should discuss the medication management and demonstrate the ability to comply. Consult a dietician to provide the appropriate nutritional instructions.

Ischemic Heart Disease

Ischemic heart disease (IHD) is the imbalance between the supply and demand for blood flow to the myocardium.

Etiology: The pathophysiology of myocardial ischemia in younger or older adults is related to an imbalance between myoycardial demand and coronary perfusion. This imbalance precipitates ischemia, which is frequently manifested as angina but may instead present silently as an acute event (i.e., sudden death or myocardial infarction).

Pathologic mechanisms that interfere with blood flow (supply) include narrowing of a major coronary artery (usually caused by fixed coronary arteriosclerosis), spasms of the coronary arteries, changes in the normal arterial tone, thrombus formation, or arteritis.

The amount of oxygen required by the myocardium (demand) is determined by the blood pressure, heart rate, left ventricular size and thickness, and the contractility state.

Occurrence: Although IHD is on the decline, it remains the leading cause of death for elderly men and women. Among those over age 70, the prevalence of ischemia presenting as angina is estimated at 22%; however, estimated prevalence based on thallium test results is near 60%. Some studies have estimated the ratio of silent to symptomatic ischemic episodes to be as high as 7:1.

Age: The prevalence increases dramatically with age, peaking in the eighth decade.

Ethnicity: Not available.

Gender: The incidence of IHD is greater in men, peaking in the sixth and seventh decades. In women, IHD increases steadily with age, peaking in the eighth decade.

Contributing Factors: Age-related changes in myocardial and circulatory pathophysiology include reduced left ventricular compliance, amyloid deposits, diastolic dysfunction, increased aortic impedance, and peripheral vascular resistance.

Other factors predictive of risk for IHD include elevations in the systolic blood pressure, plasma glucose, body mass index, and total serum cholesterol.

Signs and Symptoms: The key symptom of IHD is chest pain, but anginal equivalents in elderly individuals may include fatigue or breathlessness. The classic feature of ischemic pain include characterizations of dull, crushing substernal pain associated with dyspnea; diaphoresis; nausea; and sometimes palpatations. Some individuals may describe the feeling as a heaviness or pressure sensation rather than pain.

Chest pain in elderly persons is more likely to be of mild intensity, located elsewhere than in the substernal region, and last a shorter time than in younger individuals. The discomfort is often triggered by physical exertion, lasts a few minutes, and subsides with rest or sublingual nitroglycerine. The discomfort may radiate to the neck, left shoulder, arm, or lower jaw. Precipitants to ischemic episodes include emotional stress, heavy meal consumption, and/or exposure to cold air. The altered pain perception in older adults changes the classic presentation of ischemia, which may lead to misdiagnosis and undertreatment. IHD among elderly individuals is more likely to coexist with other conditions, particularly gastroesophageal reflux disease (GERD); therefore, it may be impossible to differentiate the two conditions.

Stable angina is described as discomfort associated with increased myocardial demand at a stable, constant, and predictable level. Often patients show signs of autonomic dysfunction including elevated heart rate, elevated blood pressure, and diaphoresis. Unstable angina is characterized by angina occurring at rest, variant angina (Prinzmetal's angina), and discomfort patterns that change suddenly with less prediction.

Physical examination findings during an ischemic episode may be nonexistent or may include extra heart sounds, mild hypertension, tachycardia, or tachypnea. A paradoxic split of S_2 may indicate an alteration in left ventricular function associated with ischemic discomfort.

Diagnostic Tests: The ECG must be performed immediately in the patient with ischemic pain. ST-segment depression or elevation or T-wave inversion in the absence of left ventricular hypertrophy strongly support the diagnosis of myocardial ischemia. Q waves may be evidence of an old myocardial infarct. In the evaluation of the chronic stable ischemic patient, exercise ECG testing is the most useful diagnostic test. Exercise thallium scintigraphy demonstrates defects in myocardial perfusion with exercise. Older adults may not be able to exercise to 90% of the predicted maximum heart rate owing to coexisting musculoskeletal or respiratory disease, in which case stress may be induced pharmacologically with dipyridamole or adenosine (Fig. 8–2).

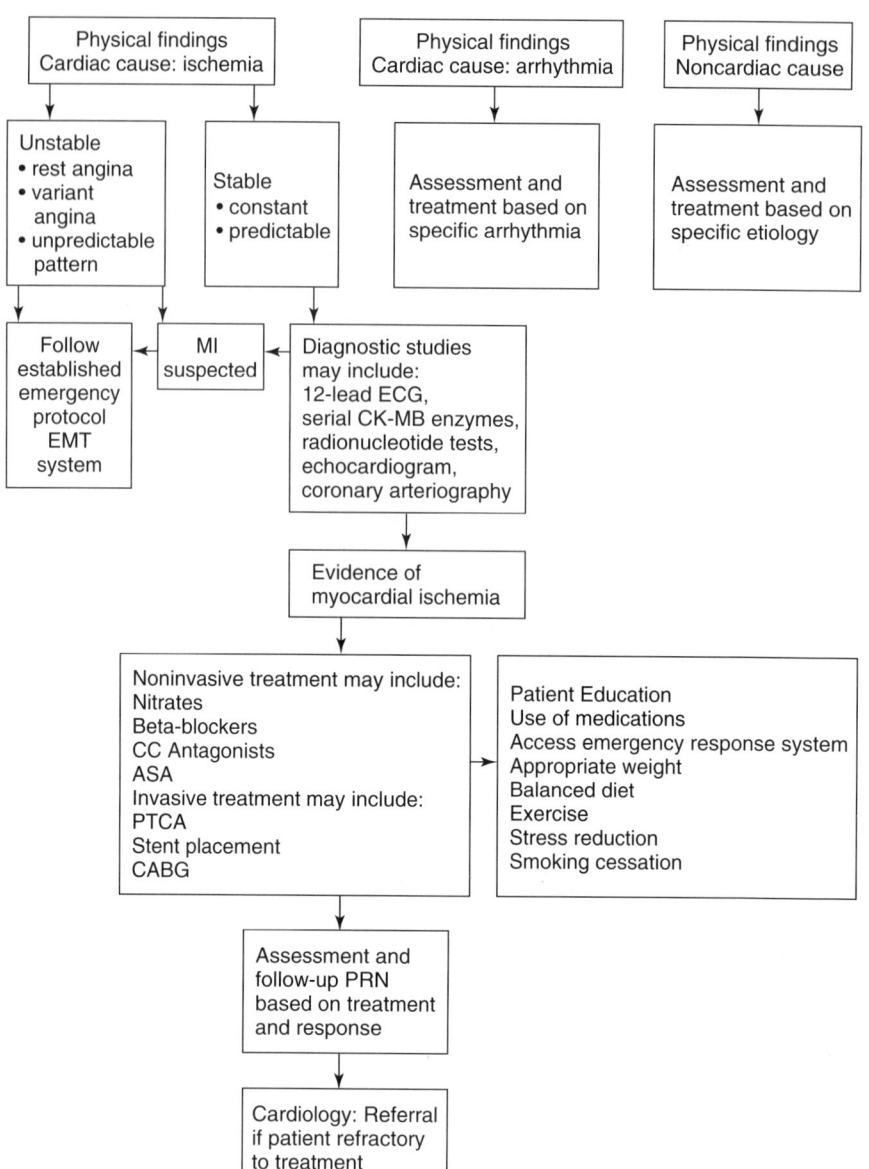

FIGURE 8–2 Suspected ischemic chest discomfort.

Measurement of left ventricular filling pressure (pulmonary capillary wedge pressure) might be done during painful ischemic episodes. Echocardiography performed during dobutamine infusion and then immediately after exercise can diagnose, localize, and assess the severity of ischemia-induced left ventricular dysfunction.

The more invasive technique of cardiac catheterization is performed in those for whom pharmacologic therapy fails: patients who have had myocardial infarction or who have unstable angina. This test may also provide more detail about the coronary arteries in patients for whom angioplasty or coronary artery bypass grafting is being considered. Coronary angiography is also sometimes done to exclude coronary artery disease in patients who are incapacitated by the pain or fear of it.

Differential Diagnosis: Ischemic heart disease must be differentiated from other, superimposed diseases that may increase myocardial oxygen demand and decrease its supply (i.e., anemia, infection, hyperthyroidism, and arrhythmias).

Chest pain from IHD must be differentiated from pleuritic, costochondral, or pericardial pain. This type of pain can also mimick gastrointestinal reflux disease, herpes zoster, and panic disorder.

Treatment: The immediate goal of treatment is to decrease oxygen consumption and increase the blood supply to the myocardium by reducing vascular tone, improving collateral flow, and preventing platelet plugs and thrombosis. The treatment regimens are similar for both symptomatic and asymptomatic elderly persons. The primary drugs used to accomplish this include nitrates, beta-blockers, calcium antagonists, thrombolytics, and aspirin.

Nitrates decrease the preload through venous dilatation and decrease the afterload through arterial dilatation. Nitroglycerine given sublingually 0.3–0.6 mg or used as a lingual spray 0.4 mg often provides relief during the ischemic episode. The anti-ischemic effect is diminished if nitroglycerine is given continuously because tolerance develops rapidly; therefore, intermittent dosing is preferred with a scheduled nitrate-free period. Longer-acting nitrate preparations such as isosorbide dinitrate (10–40 mg qid) exert an antianginal effect for 2–4 hr, and cutaneous application can be effective for 3–5 hr. Because elderly persons are particularly sensitive to vasodilators, they may demonstrate an exaggerated drug response; therefore, smaller doses and careful titration are recommended. Side effects include headache and dizziness.

Beta-blockers decrease myocardial oxygen demand by decreasing the heart rate, blood pressure, and myocardial contractility. Propranolol 10–40 mg qid daily is used to treat elderly persons; longer-acting drugs (e.g., atenolol) can be given once a day. Contraindications to these agents include conduction disturbances, chronic obstructive pulmonary disease, and congestive heart failure. These drugs:

Are lipofilic and last longer in elderly persons.
Frequently cause fatigue and lethargy.

Increase triglyceride levels.

Decrease HDL and cholesterol levels.

Must be tapered (abrupt withdrawal has been associated with exacerbation of angina, precipitation of myocardial infarction, and sudden death).

Calcium antagonists decrease coronary and peripheral vascular resistance and reduce coronary artery spasm. They are generally well tolerated in elderly patients, but significant side effects include peripheral edema and constipation. Using various combinations of the three drugs may yield an additive effect: however, the patient needs to be monitored carefully for adverse effects.

Acetylsalicylic acide (ASA) 75–300 mg affords protective benefit to individuals with angina. ASA is given after an acute myocardial infarction to reduce platelet aggregation. Daily doses of 20 mg ASA are continued for at least 2 years after the infarction, and even indefinitely for many patients. The risk of gastric irritation and gastrointestinal bleeding exists even with low doses of ASA.

Invasive intervention therapy for geriatric patients also includes intravenous thrombolytic therapy in patients with known or suspected acute myocardial infarction (see Myocardial Infarction). Mechanical intervention with percutaneous transluminal coronary angioplasty (PTCA) is used to revascularize elderly patients with acute or chronic manifestations of coronary artery disease. Elderly patients with all forms of angina tolerate well and benefit from PTCA, particularly those with comorbid factors that limit the appropriateness for a surgical procedure (i.e., coronary artery bypass graft [CABG]). A high rate of restenosis occurs after PTCA. Other percutaneous interventions available include lasers, atherectomy devices, stents, and intra-aortic balloon counterpulsation.

The longer-term goals for patients who have end-organ damage from IHD are to relieve symptoms and allow patients to resume their preferred lifestyle. CABG is a revascularization procedure that is very effective in alleviating ischemic symptoms. CABG has an advantage over PTCA in that its results are more durable and revascularization is more complete. The patient most likely to benefit maximally is one with the potential to return to an active lifestyle who can tolerate the 3–4 months of cardiac rehabilitation. Comorbid factors known to effect the outcome negatively include diabetes, cerebral and peripheral vascular disease, a history of recent myocardial infarction, systemic hypertension, renal insufficiency, pulmonary disease, obesity. Elderly women have a considerably higher risk of death and complications from IHD than their male counterparts.

Follow-up: Patients with IHD disease must be monitored for the effectiveness of prescribed drugs and any potential adverse effect. Changes in features of symptoms and disease progression should be determined and CABG readings monitored as indicated.

Sequelae: Silent ischemia has the same prognosis as symptomatic ischemia. Angina is associated with a twofold to threefold increase in the risk of death when ECG abnormalities are also present. ECG abnormalities compatible with ischemia are associated with mortality even in the absence of chest pain.

Complications from coronary artery disease include congestive heart failure, acute myocardial infarction and associated problems, arrhythmias, and sudden death.

Prevention/Prophylaxis: Risk factor modification includes control of systolic hypertension, cholesterol levels, and elimination of smoking. A sedentary lifestyle predisposes an individual to coronary artery disease, particularly in the presence of other risk factors. Physical conditioning tends to lower the blood pressure; those who are physically active have slightly higher plasma HDL levels than those who are sedentary. Other strategies to manage risk include weight control, hypolipidemic therapy if indicated, and perhaps estrogen therapy in the postmenopausal woman. Low-dose aspirin therapy (325 mg every other day) may reduce the risk of myocardial infarction; however, its use is associated with adverse effects. Its risk and benefits must be examined individually in patients.

Referral: Unstable patients with IHD require hospitalization because approximately 20% of these patients suffer myocardial infarction. Collaborate closely with the physician regarding patients who are refractory to treatment.

Education: Advise patients to report changes in the pattern or intensity of angina. All patients should be instructed to call emergency services when experiencing chest pain because the differential diagnosis is difficult to determine without technological equipment.

Myocardial Infarction

Myocardial infarction (MI) is necrosis of heart tissue caused by lack of blood supply. MIs can be transmural or subendocardial (non–Q wave MI).

Etiology: MI generally occurs after the abrupt decrease in coronary blood flow to the myocardium following a thrombotic occlusion of a coronary artery already narrowed by atherosclerosis. In most cases this atherosclerotic plaque ruptures or ulcerates and a mural thrombus forms in the coronary artery.

Occurrence: Coronary disease is the most frequent cause of death in people age 65 and older. Mortality rates from coronary artery disease are decreasing in the general population but remain high in the elderly population. Mortality from MI among patients older than 75 is 32%, compared with 5% in patients younger than 55. More than 50% of in-hospital mortality from MI occurs in patients older than 65, and 80% of patients who die from MI are 65 or older. Elderly persons admitted to the hospital more often have non–Q wave MIs, which are associated with higher postdischarge mortality, theoretically because of the higher incidence of diffuse coronary disease and existing poor myocardial perfusion.

Age: Postmortem studies show that coronary atherosclerosis, which often begins to develop before age 20, is widespread even among asymptomatic adults. Aging itself may be a risk factor for MI in both men and women.

Ethnicity: Not available.

Gender: MI is much more prevalent in men than in women up to age 74, after which the occurrence increases steeply with age in both genders. On average, women develop heart disease 10 years later than men and suffer MIs and sudden death 20 years later than men.

Contributing Factors: Risk factors for heart disease and MI in elderly individuals are essentially the same as in the younger population. Risk factors include hypertension, hyperlipidemia, diabetes, physical inactivity, obesity, and stress. Cigarette smoking is associated with new coronary events for elderly men and women. Postmenopausal women are at increased risk because of the loss of estrogen and its cardioprotective effect.

Aging alters the cardiovascular system in ways that reduce cardiac reserve and efficiency, thus compromising the ability to respond to stress or illness. The cardiovascular system becomes less compliant as diastolic filling of the ventricles declines and afterload increases secondary to increased stiffness in the ascending aorta. This results in moderate hypertrophy of the left ventricle, causing a more precarious balance between myocardial oxygen supply and demand. Other changes in the elderly cardiovascular system include decreased responsiveness to β-adrenergic stimulation, decreased baroreceptor sensitivity, and an increased dependence on a higher end-diastolic volume to maintain cardiac output.

Signs and Symptoms: With advancing age the presentation of acute MI will be less likely to include the classic symptoms of crushing substernal chest pain, nausea, vomiting, and diaphoresis. Rather, a vague ache or discomfort may be present. Elderly persons may not recognize that throat, shoulder, or abdominal pain may be referred cardiac pain. Dyspnea is the second most common symptom of MI in both younger and older populations. For patients 85 and older, syncope, acute confusion, or stroke may be the only presenting symptom. Some elderly patients may present only with faintness, weakness, giddiness, or restlessness.

Upon physical examination, the patient may be anxious and weak and may appear cyanotic. Arrhythmias may be noted on the ECG. The skin may be diaphoretic, cold, and clammy. Thrills, heaves, and an abnormal point of maximum impulse (PMI) may be palpated. Peripheral pulses may be irregular, slow, fast, or thready. Auscultation may reveal an S_3 or S_4, pericardial friction rub, murmurs, or crackles. The physical examination must focus on ruling out diagnoses other than MI (Fig. 8–3).

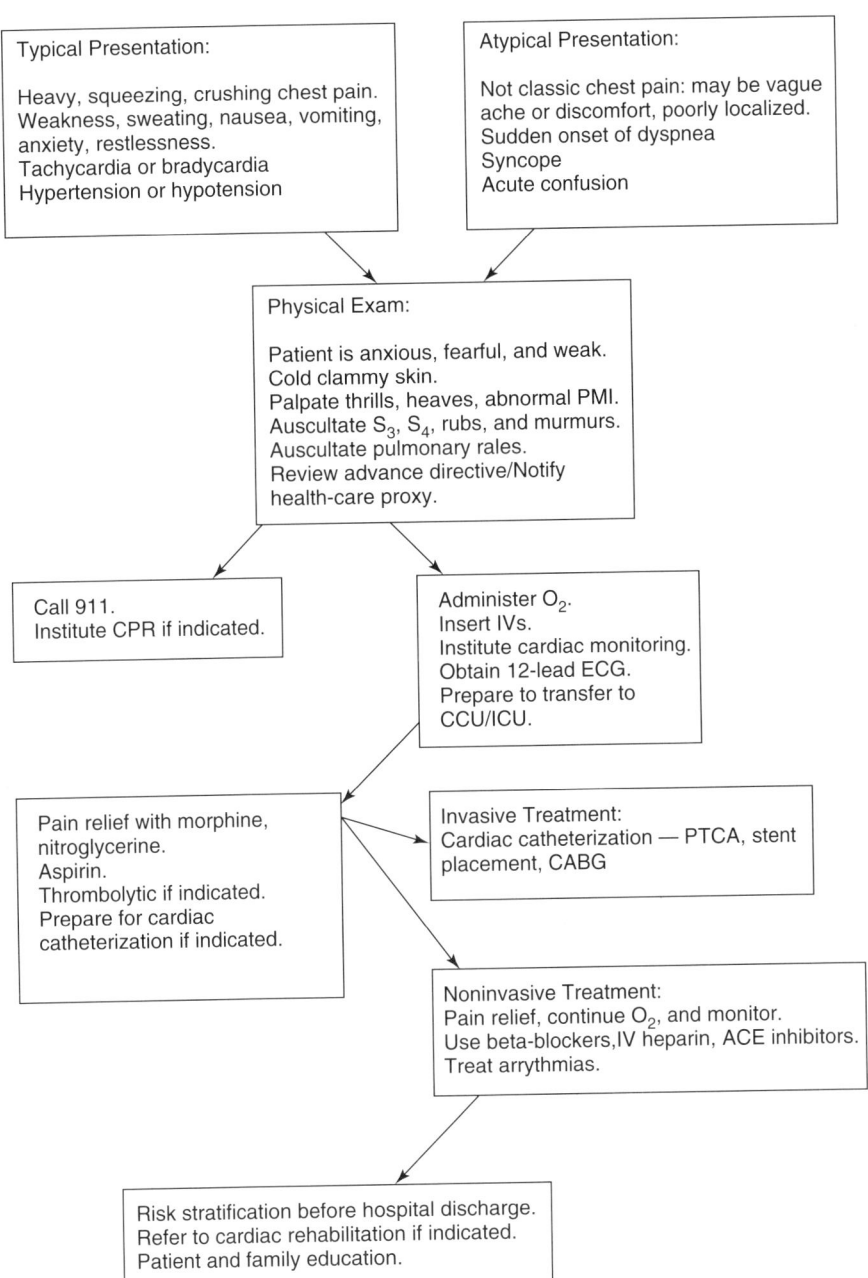

Typical Presentation:

Heavy, squeezing, crushing chest pain.
Weakness, sweating, nausea, vomiting,
anxiety, restlessness.
Tachycardia or bradycardia
Hypertension or hypotension

Atypical Presentation:

Not classic chest pain: may be vague
ache or discomfort, poorly localized.
Sudden onset of dyspnea
Syncope
Acute confusion

Physical Exam:

Patient is anxious, fearful, and weak.
Cold clammy skin.
Palpate thrills, heaves, abnormal PMI.
Auscultate S_3, S_4, rubs, and murmurs.
Auscultate pulmonary rales.
Review advance directive/Notify
health-care proxy.

Call 911.
Institute CPR if indicated.

Administer O_2.
Insert IVs.
Institute cardiac monitoring.
Obtain 12-lead ECG.
Prepare to transfer to
CCU/ICU.

Pain relief with morphine,
nitroglycerine.
Aspirin.
Thrombolytic if indicated.
Prepare for cardiac
catheterization if indicated.

Invasive Treatment:
Cardiac catheterization — PTCA, stent
placement, CABG

Noninvasive Treatment:
Pain relief, continue O_2, and monitor.
Use beta-blockers,IV heparin, ACE inhibitors.
Treat arrythmias.

Risk stratification before hospital discharge.
Refer to cardiac rehabilitation if indicated.
Patient and family education.

FIGURE 8–3 Myocardial infarction.

Diagnostic Tests: Along with a chest x-ray examination, complete blood count, clotting profile, electrolytes, and cardiac enzymes, evaluation for acute MI includes serial ECGs. Changes on the ECG indicative of MI include Q waves and ST-segment elevation in leads facing the infarction. ST-segment depression is sometimes present. With the increased incidence of non–Q wave infarctions, the presence of a single normal ECG does not rule out MI, which is why serial ECGs are necessary. However, ECGs may be nondiagnostic or difficult to interpret in elderly people because of possible abnormalities such as left bundle branch block, left ventricular hypertrophy, and previously unrecognized MIs.

In older adults, the cardiac enzyme profile may be atypical. Creatine kinase (CK), an enzyme found in myocardial cells, is released into the bloodstream when cells are damaged within 3–8 hr after the onset of pain. Because the baseline CK in elderly patients may be significantly lower than normal, even those with MI may not develop CK levels high enough to be interpreted as abnormal, owing to decreased muscle mass. CK-MB, an isoenzyme of CK, may be more sensitive, especially with serial measurements. Troponin is a cardiac-specific marker for acute MI, and elevations usually occur early after myocardial cell injury. Lactate dehydrogenase (LDH) levels are occasionally useful in patients with delayed presentation because this enzyme remains elevated for several days. Other tests for MI include echocardiography, technetium pyro-phosphate, or stress thallium scans.

Differential Diagnosis: The pain from MI can be similar to that of acute pericarditis, pulmonary embolism, acute aortic dissection, or costochondritis. Many conditions can present as cardiac disease in the elderly, including cor pulmonale, pneumonia, esophageal spasm, gastroesophageal reflux disease, hiatal hernia, gallbladder disease, osteoarthritis of the spine, muscle injury, and panic disorder.

Treatment: Many studies have examined pharmacologic and interventional treatments for acute MI, but often these have excluded elderly people. Nitrates, the cornerstone for therapy of ischemic pain, reduce preload and improve coronary perfusion. Chest pain should be treated with sublingual nitroglycerine, repeated three times, 5 min apart, unless the patient is hypotensive. Intravenous (IV) nitrates have been shown to limit infarct size and reduce pain, complications, and mortality. IV nitroglycerine is started at 5 μg/min on an infusion pump and titrated to desired effect. Frequent monitoring is necessary because harmful effects can be seen if the systolic blood pressure drops below 90 mmHg. Morphine sulfate, 2–4 mg every 10 min, up to 20 mg, is also effective for pain relief. Supplemental oxygen should be given if saturation is less than 94%. Aspirin should be given as soon as possible if there is no obvious contraindication. Aspirin 75–160 mg/day should be continued for life after an MI.

Thrombolytic agents, such as tissue-type plasminogen (tPA) and streptokinase (SK), have become the standard treatments for MI. Indications for thrombolysis are based on the existence of chest pain and specific ECG changes that indicate a transmural infarction. Studies show this therapy is frequently omitted for elderly patients. Reasons for this include frequent delay in seeking medical care, atypical presentation of MI, and a higher prevalence of non–Q wave MIs. Fear of hemorrhage following use of thrombolytics must be weighed against the proven gains in survival for all age groups, especially for those presenting early with MI. A variety of studies suggest that SK may be as beneficial as tPA in treating the elderly MI patient. It is considerably less expensive.

Current practice includes IV heparin following tPA. For patients not receiving thrombolytics, low-dose subcutaneous heparin or low-molecular-weight heparin is indicated for prophylaxis of deep venous thrombosis. Elderly patients with large anterior MIs and heart failure, as well as those with documented left ventricular thrombus, should receive full heparin anticoagulation for 3–5 days, followed by 3 months of warfarin.

Beta-blockers, which have been shown to limit infarct size, decrease chest pain, and improve prognosis, are generally well tolerated in patients age 65–75. Some conditions that contraindicate the use of beta-blockers in the elderly include bronchospastic lung disease, marked bradycardia, hypotension, depression, and diabetes. Studies show that beta-blockers are underused in the elderly; age alone should not determine their use. In acute MI, metoprolol or atenolol is given as a 2.5–5 mg IV every 5 min, for a total of 15 mg and 10 mg, respectively.

At about 3 days after an MI, angiotensin-converting enzyme (ACE) inhibitors are recommended for every elderly patient with an ejection fraction less than 40% and no obvious contraindication to their use. Captopril is first given as a test dose of 6.25 mg. If tolerated, captopril 50–100 mg is given daily. Calcium channel blockers have limited use in the MI patient. Prophylactic use of lidocaine does not improve survival, and the altered metabolism in elderly persons may promote toxicity, causing symptoms such as agitation and seizures.

In terms of interventional management of elderly MI patients, direct percutaneous transluminal coronary angioplasty (PTCA) may be a valuable alternative in those for whom thrombolytics are contraindicated. Coronary artery bypass graft (CABG) is preferred for patients with left main stenosis and those with moderately severe left ventricular depression. Emergency PTCA or CABG in elderly patients presenting with cardiogenic shock or heart failure is associated with high morbidity and mortality.

Follow-up: Risk stratification for future cardiac events following stabilization from MI is necessary. Tests to evaluate for ischemia or myocardium at risk include low-level exercise test, IV dipyridamole followed by nuclear perfusion scanning with thallium-201, and dobutamine echocardiography. Left ventricular function can be determined by echocardiography or radionuclide ventriculogram. Routine coronary angiography is not recommended for all MI patients but should be performed on patients with demonstrable ischemia. Patients at high risk for sudden death from arrhythmias should undergo electrophysiologic evaluation.

Sequelae: Increasing age is associated with more complications after MI including heart failure, arrhythmias, pulmonary edema, cardiogenic shock, cardiac rupture, and death.

Prevention/Prophylaxis: Secondary prevention in the elderly MI patient includes use of aspirin, beta-blockers, and ACE inhibitors unless there are absolute contraindications to these agents. Lipid-lowering therapy is also beneficial. Reduction of risk factors is necessary. Cardiac rehabilitation can be as beneficial in older MI patients as in younger ones. Emotional support remains important.

Referral: Suspicion of acute MI should prompt transfer of the patient to an environment equipped with cardiac monitoring and the ability to administer advanced cardiac life support. As hospitalization continues, consultation with a variety of disciplines, such as surgery, social work, and physical therapy, may be necessary.

Education: Individualized teaching following MI for each patient and family should be provided, using age-specific teaching methods. Teach the basic definitions of coronary artery disease, angina, and MI. Patients need information on the healing process following MI, when to return to work or resume normal daily activities, and when to resume sexual relations. Give an exercise prescription. Involve patients and families in a discussion of the psychologic adjustment following MI. Encourage risk factor reduction. Health-care practitioners should work with patients to set goals and design plans. Give the patient information on community resources, such as the American Heart Association or support groups in their area. Smoking cessation should be encouraged.

Medication teaching and review is very important. Health-care providers should be aware of all medications prescribed for the patient. Teach patients about the desired effects and common side effects of their medications. Review what to do if medication cannot be taken or obtained. Discuss interactions with over-the-counter medications.

Teach elderly patients about altered pain perception that can occur with age and with diseases such as diabetes. Teach patients and their families about warning signs such as chest pain or pressure, shortness of breath, indigestion, choking, sweating, dizziness, palpitations, severe weakness, and loss of consciousness. Establish a clear plan for obtaining prompt medical attention.

Valvular Heart Disease

Valvular heart disease (VHD) is damage to a valve or valves of the heart, causing cardiac dysfunction. The most prevalent types of VHD in elderly persons include:
- Aortic stenosis and regurgitation.
- Mitral stenosis.
- Mitral valve prolapse.

Combined stenosis and regurgitation is not uncommon.

- **Aortic stenosis:** an abnormal narrowing of the aortic valve orifice.
- **Aortic regurgitation:** retrograde blood blow through an incompetent aortic valve into the left ventricle during ventricular diastole.
- **Mitral stenosis:** an abnormal narrowing of the mitral valve orifice.
- **Mitral regurgitation:** retrograde blood flow during systole from the left ventricle into the left atrium through an incompetent mitral valve.
- **Mitral valve prolapse:** mitral regurgitation associated with a bulging of one or both mitral valve leaflets into the left atrium during ventricular systole.

Etiology: In the elderly, the predominant causes of valvular heart disease include age-related degenerative calcification, myxomatous degeneration, papillary muscle dysfunction, infective endocarditis, and rheumatic disease. Valvular stenosis usually results in elevated pressures in the chamber upstream from the stenosis. In valvular regurgitation, a portion of the ejected volume of blood leaks back into the upstream cardiac chamber.

Occurrence: Occurrence of VHD varies according to the type of valvular disease; only limited information is available.

Age: Aortic stenosis, the most clinically significant valvular lesion in elderly persons, increases in frequency with age and is found in 5.5% of those over age 75. Isolated aortic regurgitation is rarely seen and is usually accompanied by some degree of mitral valve involvement. Rheumatic heart disease remains the predominant cause of mitral valve disease, which is almost always acquired before age 20 and becomes clinically apparent by the fifth decade. Mitral regurgitation is more common than mitral stenosis in elderly individuals. About 6% of individuals over age 60 have mitral annular calcification that causes mitral regurgitation.

Ethnicity: Not significant.

Gender: Mitral annular calcification (a frequent cause of mitral regurgitation) affects women two to three times more frequently than it affects men. Mitral valve prolapse is more common in elderly men than in elderly women.

Contributing Factors: Age-related fibrotic thickening of valvular tissue or dilatation and calcification of the valve annulus may contribute to and cause hemodynamic abnormalities. Valvular stenosis of rheumatic origin can gradually progress throughout adult life. Other factors that may contribute to or cause valvular disease include metastatic carcinoid tumors; methysergide (used to treat migraines); rheumatoid arthritis (can produce nodules in the leaflets); systemic lupus (can cause small vegetations, thickening, and regurgitation in the leaflets); and radiation therapy.

Signs and Symptoms

Aortic Stenosis: The majority of patients are asymptomatic. For those with symptoms, the prognosis is poor. Chest pain is an early symptom. Presyncope followed by effort syncope occurs in about one-third of patients with symptoms. Exertional dyspnea may herald the development of congestive heart failure.

Physical findings include a characteristic loud, rough systolic ejection murmur in the second right intercostal space at the midclavicular line that is well transmitted into the neck. This murmur, which peaks in intensity in mid to late systole, may be associated with a thrill. S_1 is often soft, and the aortic component of S_2 is soft or absent. An S_4 is common. The pulse pressure is narrow; there is a slow rise in the carotid pulse.

Aortic Regurgitation: In chronic aortic regurgitation, patients are asymptomatic for many years. When the left ventricle can no longer manage the increased stroke volume, patients may experience effort intolerance and dyspnea. Chest pain and palpitations may be present.

The presentation of acute severe regurgitation is different in that left ventricular compensation and stroke volume changes have not yet occurred. The presenting symptoms may include tachycardia and dyspnea due to pulmonary venous congestion.

Physical findings with chronic aortic regurgitation include a wide pulse pressure and possibly bounding pulses. Systolic and diastolic thrills may be present on the precordium. S_1 is normal or soft. S_2 may be physiologically split, but A_2 may be soft or not heard owing to a high-frequency, early diastolic murmur. An atrial gallop and S_3 are often present. An apical diastolic rumble, the Austin Flint murmur, may be heard.

The clinical features of acute aortic regurgitation are dominated by the sudden severe heart failure. The pulse pressure may be narrowed because of elevated left ventricular diastolic pressure. The S_1 is soft, a prominent summated gallop is common, and the diastolic murmur is harsh and shortened by the elevated ventricular filling pressure.

Mitral Stenosis: The symptoms of mitral stenosis, dyspnea on exertion and lethargy resulting from elevated left atrial and pulmonary venous pressures, are generally associated with valve areas of less than 1.5 cm (normal is 4 cm).

The clinical findings include a loud S_1 and an apical diastolic rumble with presystolic accentuation. An opening snap may also be present, but it may be soft or not heard at all because of valve stiffness and calcification.

Mitral Regurgitation: For patients with mitral regurgitation, the main complaints are fatigue and a gradual decrease in exercise tolerance, which appear only when the ventricle begins to fail.

The clinical features vary, depending on the pathologic cause; however, a holosystolic murmur at the apex is a nearly constant feature. If the disease is severe, the apex beat is hyperdynamic and displaced laterally, and an S_3 is usually found.

Mitral Valve Prolapse: Chest pain and palpitations are the most prominent symptoms in elderly as well as young persons, although older patients are more likely to be disabled by the symptoms. Other symptoms that may represent an arrhythmic etiology are dizziness and syncope. Heart failure is a common presentation.

The clinical picture includes a midsystolic click(s) and a late systolic or holosystolic murmur characteristic of mitral regurgitation. In some patients the murmur, click, or both are not appreciated until the patient stands or performs the Valsalva maneuver. An apical S_3-S_4 gallop is usually present at the time of heart failure.

Diagnostic Tests: In aortic stenosis, the ECG is abnormal in most cases, demonstrating QRS or T-wave changes reflecting left ventricular hypertrophy. Chest x-ray examination usually reveals aortic dilatation; dense calcification is generally seen on lateral film. Chest films may show cardiac enlargement when congestive heart failure is advanced. Echocardiography demonstrates thickening and calcification of the aortic valve with decreased mobility of the leaflets. Doppler measurement of intracardiac blood velocity can help determine hemodynamic severity. Cardiac catheterization measurement of the systolic pressure gradient across the aortic valve is the definitive method for assessing aortic stenosis in patients being considered for surgery or when there is a discrepancy between the clinical findings and the diagnostic tests.

In aortic regurgitation, if the process is acute, the ECG findings may be normal. If chronic, a left ventricular hypertrophy and strain is seen. Cardiomegaly found on the chest x-ray examination is demonstrated with left ventricular enlargement. Echocardiography shows left ventricular muscle thickness and early diastolic fluttering of the anterior mitral valve leaflet. Color Doppler imaging can further determine the presence of aortic regurgitation; however, its severity is best determined by the more invasive cardiac catheterization with angiography.

In mitral stenosis, P waves may suggest left atrial enlargement and (in the elderly) the ECG more commonly reveals atrial fibrillation. Chest x-ray examination nearly always reveals left atrial enlargement. Echocardiography with Doppler flow studies is diagnostic of thickening of the mitral leaflet, reduced motion, and parallel movement of anterior and posterior leaflets in diastole; the flow study also assesses the severity of the stenosis. Cardiac catheterization is sometimes performed in those with an uncertain degree of stenosis after noninvasive studies and in those being considered for surgery.

In mitral regurgitation, the ECG shows left atrial enlargement or atrial fibrillation, and the chest x-ray examination shows left ventricular dilatation; in nonrheumatic forms of mitral regurgitation these are less distinctive. Echocardiography delineates overall ventricular function and Doppler studies show the jet and severity of the regurgitation. Transesophageal echocardiography is a more precise way of visualizing the regurgitant jet.

In mitral valve prolapse, the ECG may show left ventricular enlargement and atrial hypertrophy, and atrial fibrillation is a frequent finding in the elderly. The chest x-ray examination will display pulmonary congestion with moderate cardiac enlargement.

Differential Diagnosis: The diagnosis of VHD in elderly persons is sometimes overlooked because the early symptoms are vague and nonspecific. Murmurs in older adults are common and frequently determined to be functional or insignificant. The barrel chest of an older individual may obscure a murmur; in fact, with an increased anteroposterior diameter, a left ventricular hypertrophy may not be detected.

Murmurs have been associated with conditions other than valvular disease (i.e., hypertension, anemia, thyroid disease) so this differential must be considered.

Patients with established valvular heart disease need to have a specific determination of the etiologies of valvular involvement.

Treatment

Aortic Stenosis: Symptoms of aortic stenosis (angina, heart failure, syncope) are associated with substantial valvular obstruction and a risk of sudden death; therefore, medical therapy is associated with poor prognosis. Aortic valve replacement (AVR) is associated with a higher mortality (5%–15%) in elderly persons than in younger individuals. Factors associated with greater operative risk include emergency surgery, left ventricular dysfunction, significant coronary disease, cachexia, additional valve replacement, or concomitant CABG. The proper selection of the type of valve is important in elderly patients. The bioprosthetic valves are advantageous in that their use obviates the need for systemic anticoagulation (which is associated with substantial morbidity and mortality in the elderly). The disadvantage of this valve type is that the tissue degrades, and 30%–40% of patients will require reoperation in 10 years. The mechanical valves are more durable and have better hemodynamic profiles, but these require lifelong anticoagulation therapy.

Aortic balloon valvuloplasty (ABV) is an alternative treatment method; however, as it is associated with rapid restenosis and significant residual outflow obstruction, it is reserved as a palliative procedure for the symptomatic patient who is not a surgical candidate or as a bridge to surgery.

Aortic Regurgitation: Acute aortic regurgitation always warrants surgery. Chronic aortic regurgitation requires medical treatment of the early signs of heart failure with digitalis, diuretics, and vasodilators. Because no ideal aortic valve prosthesis exists, valve replacement for aortic insufficiency is considered only for the severely symptomatic chronic patient who is unresponsive to medical therapy.

Mitral Stenosis: Therapies for the symptomatic patient with mitral stenosis include medical therapy, commissurotomy, and mitral valve replacement. The patient with symptoms of mild heart failure is managed with diuretics and salt restriction. Because atrial fibrillation occurs in most patients with moderate to severe stenosis, anticoagulation is often indicated. Because of the high risk associated with anticoagulation in the elderly patient, however, a less aggressive approach to therapy may be taken. Digitalis, beta-blockers, or calcium channel blockers may be used to control rate.

When the patient has severe symptoms of mitral stenosis, valve replacement or commissurotomy is indicated. Recently, percutaneous balloon mitral valvuloplasty has been used as a nonsurgical alternative. Contraindications for this procedure include concomitant mitral regurgitation and left atrial thrombus.

Mitral Regurgitation: Medical management of mitral regurgitation includes use of digitalis, diuretics, and vasodilators to reduce the symptoms of heart failure and reduce the regurgitant volume. Mitral valve surgery is considered in the symptomatic patient with progressive disease before signs of irreversible left ventricular dysfunction are present. The mortality associated with mitral valve replacement is 10%–15% but may be as high as 50% in the higher-risk patient (i.e., in the presence of severe left ventricular dysfunction, concomitant coronary artery disease requiring revascularization, multivalve surgical procedures, emergency surgery, or advanced age).

Mitral valve repair is associated with a lower operative mortality than mitral valve replacement, and might be preferred in some individuals. When mitral annular calcification is the etiology, medical therapy is prudent because the operative risk is substantially higher in patients with this disease process. Acute mitral regurgitation from papillary muscle rupture or chordal rupture requires patient stabilization followed by surgery, which still carries a very high mortality.

Mitral Valve Prolapse: Medical management may stabilize the patient; anticoagulation to prevent emboli is warranted. Mitral valve surgery is needed in patients with progressive ventricular dilatation.

Follow-up: For patients treated medically for valvular disease, close follow-up to monitor the effectiveness of treatment, adverse effects of medication, and progressiveness of the disease process is indicated. Diuretics, digitalis, and anticoagulation therapy all require meticulous attention. Surgically treated patients are monitored for valve function, fluid balance, and anticoagulation.

Sequelae: Valve replacement risks include thrombus formation, infection, or rupture at the attachment points to the valve ring. Infective endocarditis, which may occur with artificial valves, has a high risk of mortality and requires reoperation. There is a high prevalence of gallstones in patients with prosthetic valves, thought to be due to low-grade intravascular hemolysis.

In patients who are not surgical candidates, the symptoms of heart failure are progressive and disabling. Even in surgical patients, the symptoms of heart failure may recur or persist.

Prevention/Prophylaxis: In patients with prosthetic valves, the risk of thrombo-embolism decreases with an individualized antithrombolitic regimen. The specific therapy is determined based on the comorbid state and the patient's overall status.

Consider prophylactic antibiotic therapy in all patients with valvular disease, especially those with valve replacement, rheumatic heart disease, aortic regurgitation, or mitral valve prolapse with significant mitral regurgitation murmurs.

Referral: All patients with symptoms of progressive valvular disease must be managed collaboratively with the physician. Many will require further collaboration with a cardiologist. The Practice Guidelines for Cardiothoracic Surgery Concerning Valvular Heart Disease include the indication for surgery. In general, these include symptoms that cannot be controlled with medical therapy or indications of a threat to survival (i.e., angina, dyspnea, effort syncope or progressive impairment of ventricular contractility, and infective endocarditis).

Education: Elderly persons constitute 40%–60% of all cases of endocarditis. Instruct all at-risk patients in the importance of good dental care and antibiotic prophylaxis.

Instruct all patients with valve disease requiring medication therapy to report lack of therapeutic effect or any adverse effects of these drugs. Teach the patient to be aware of drug-food interactions (e.g., green leafy vegetables and anticoagulants). Teach the patient with disabling heart failure about energy-conserving measures. Patients with hemodynamically significant valvular heart disease should generally avoid participation in competitive sports.

Assessment of the Respiratory System

In order to assess the respiratory system accurately in the older adult, the nurse practitioner must be familiar with changes in tissue and in the musculoskeletal and respiratory systems that are caused by aging.

The aging process is characterized by a loss of elasticity and flexibility in collagen and elastin tissue components; this impedes the normal expiratory recoil of the lung. The concurrent decrease in body water composition dries mucous membranes and interferes with the protective functions of the upper airway in expelling foreign material. Loss of elastin also affects the alveoli and the basement membrane of the capillary wall where gas exchange occurs. A thickening occurs in both areas, which limits the amount of diffusion. Musculoskeletal changes, including calcification of costal cartilage and weakening of inspiratory muscles, result in a relaxation of the skeletal contours and an increased anteroposterior diameter, causing a barrel chest, although not as pronounced as that found in patients with chronic obstructive pulmonary disease (COPD). An exaggeration of the thoracic curvature may also occur, with some tracheal displacement. Expiratory muscles must work harder because expiration is no longer a passive act, resulting in use of accessory muscles. The residual capacity of the lungs is increased and inspiratory reserve capacity lessened. Air tends to fill the apices and not the bases. Because of decreased muscular strength, the cough reflex is not as forceful or effective. All of these changes occur gradually and are hardly noticeable unless a physiologic challenge or stress arises. Even in such an event, exertional dyspnea may be the only observed change in the healthy older adult. Healthy lifestyle behaviors also serve to mitigate these age-related changes.

Healthy older adults or those with stable, chronic problems are unlikely to seek care unless there is a change in functional capabilities related to breathing, such as decreased exercise tolerance, shortness of breath with exertion, or easy fatiguability. In frail elderly persons, an increase in respirations, sweating, or anorexia may be the only indication of a respiratory problem. History questions should address the symptom using the OLDCART or PQRST symptom analysis format; these are discussed in Chapter 17. Is there a prior history of the problem or of any respiratory problem? Does the patient use tobacco or has he or she used it in the past? Is there a history of occupational exposures or lung problems? Has the possibility of tuberculosis been eliminated? Is the patient a silent aspirator? Any changes in medications, including the use of OTC, herbal and homeopathic remedies should be addressed. Is there a cough, sputum production, or hemoptysis? Is the patient wheezing? If there is pain, have cardiac or musculoskeletal causes been ruled out? If there is dyspnea, is it related to activity or does it occur at rest or when lying down? How many pillows are used? Specific questions about changes in endurance, stair-climbing, or activities of daily living (ADLs) are necessary to quantify the extent of the problem. Does the problem interfere with eating? Has there been a 10-lb weight loss or gain in the past 6 months? Has the patient received the influenza vaccine and pneumococcal vaccine? Is human immunodeficiency virus (HIV) a consideration?

Physical assessment of the respiratory system begins with general observation of the patient: rate and ease of respirations at rest, conversational ability (limited by breathing problems), use of accessory muscles, posture, color, pursed lips, circumoral or nailbed cyanosis, and capillary refill. The chest and upper back should be exposed for full inspection and examination. Are both sides symmetric, with equal respiratory effort and diaphragmatic movement? Is there any evidence of kyphosis, lordosis, or scoliosis? Rapid respiratory rates are common with pneumonia, fever, or COPD.

Palpation of the posterior chest to confirm equal chest expansion is done by placing the thumbs on the chest wall near the vertebrae at T9–10 and spreading the hands. A small fold of skin should be between the thumbs. When the patient takes a deep breath per your instruction, the thumbs should move apart symmetrically. If pneumonia or consolidation is suspected, palpating for tactile fremitus may be helpful. Using the ball of the hand (metacarpophalageal area of the palm)

TABLE 8–2   NORMAL BREATH SOUNDS

Sound Characteristics	Auscultation Sites
Vesicular: soft, low pitch, inspiration greater than expiration	Peripheral lung fields
Bronchial: loud, high pitch, inspiration less than expiration	Trachea, larynx
Bronchovesicular: moderate, inspiration equal to expiration	Main bronchi; upper sternum; upper back between scapulae

or the ulnar side of the hand, feel the vibrations in a side-to-side pattern while the patient says, "ninety-nine." The vibrations should feel the same on either side and be stronger in the upper areas. Increased fremitus occurs with marked consolidation, such as lobar pneumonia. Percussion of the posterior chest for resonance and symmetry is the next step, again using a side-to-side approach. Dullness is indicative of increased density as found with pneumonia, tumor growth, or pleural effusion. Hyperresonance is found with air trapping in emphysema or with pneumothorax. Auscultation of posterior breath sounds for symmetry, presence or absence of adventitious sounds, and air movement is done with the patient seated, with his or her arms resting on the knees to retract the scapulae. The patient is instructed to take a deep breath through the mouth, with the mouth open, inhaling and exhaling. Decreased breath sounds are common with emphysema, pleurisy, or pleural effusion. Wheezing is commonly heard with asthma or acute bronchitis, although it may also be part of the "background" of chronic bronchitis or asthmatic COPD. Crackles are heard with congestive heart failure (CHF), pulmonary edema, or pneumonia; basilar crackles that clear with coughing or deep breathing are not pathologic. Normal breath sounds are shown in Table 8–2. Older patients become lightheaded with deep breathing and may need this part of the examination to be spaced out over time. If pneumonia is suspected, vocal fremitus techniques such as bronchophony, egophony, or whispered pectoriloquy may be indicated. Examination of the anterior chest follows the same sequence. The right middle lobe is auscultated anterolaterally.

Chronic Bronchitis

Chronic bronchitis is a daily chronic cough with increased sputum production lasting for at least three consecutive months in at least two consecutive years. The cough is usually worse on wakening.

Etiology: Chronic bronchitis is caused by inflammation and hypertrophy of the bronchial and bronchiolar walls. Hyperplasia and hypertrophy of goblet cells in smaller airways and of mucous glands around cartilaginous airways contribute to mechanical obstruction.

Occurrence: At high risk are those with a long history of cigarette smoking. Chronic obstructive pulmonary disease (COPD) affects more than 14 million people in the United States.

Age: Chronic bronchitis is most common among those in their sixth or seventh decade of life.

Ethnicity: Not significant.

Gender: Chronic bronchitis more common in men than in women.

Contributing Factors: Frequent exposure to tobacco smoke either by direct or second-hand smoke inhalation, industrial gases or fumes, dust particles, aerosol sprays, dander, frequent respiratory infections, and repeated allergic responses all contribute to the development of chronic bronchitis.

Signs and Symptoms: The patient may experience changes in appetite or activity tolerance. Symptoms may include chronic cough with copious sputum, wheezing, recurrent respiratory infections, fatigue, and dyspnea on exertion. Signs may include neck vein distention during expiration in absence of heart failure, increased anteroposterior diameter of thorax, rhonchi and wheezes, prolonged expiration, hyperresonance on percussion, decreased heart and breath sounds, tachypnea, ruddy skin color, and clubbing of nailbeds (Fig. 8–4).

Diagnostic Tests

- Chest x-ray examination: Hyperinflation of lungs and enlarged heart.
- Pulmonary function tests: Increased residual volume, decreased vital capacity and forced expiratory volume in 1 sec (FEV_1), with forced expiratory flow (FEF) 25–75% most diagnostic of chronic bronchitis.
- Electrocardiogram (ECG): Atrial arrhythmia; peaked P waves in leads II, III, and aVF, with occasional right ventricular hypertrophy.
- Laboratory studies: Complete blood count (CBC), normal; arterial blood gases (ABGs), decreased Pao_2 and HCO_3 (early stage); decreased Pao_2, increased $Paco_2$ and HCO_3, normal or decreased pH (advanced stage). Sputum should be cultured if infection is suspected (most common organisms are *Streptococcus pneumoniae* and *Haemophilus influenzae*).

Differential Diagnosis: Carcinoma of the lung, asthma, interstitial lung disease, congestive heart failure, pneumonitis, bronchiectasis, chronic rhinitis, chronic sinusitis, diseases of the external auditory canal, pharyngitis, and extrinsic compression lesions should be considered when diagnosing chronic bronchitis.

Treatment: Treatment is individualized to the patient's condition with the focus on recognition and treatment of complications. Symptomatic relief and support through pulmonary rehabilitation is recommended. These patients are com-

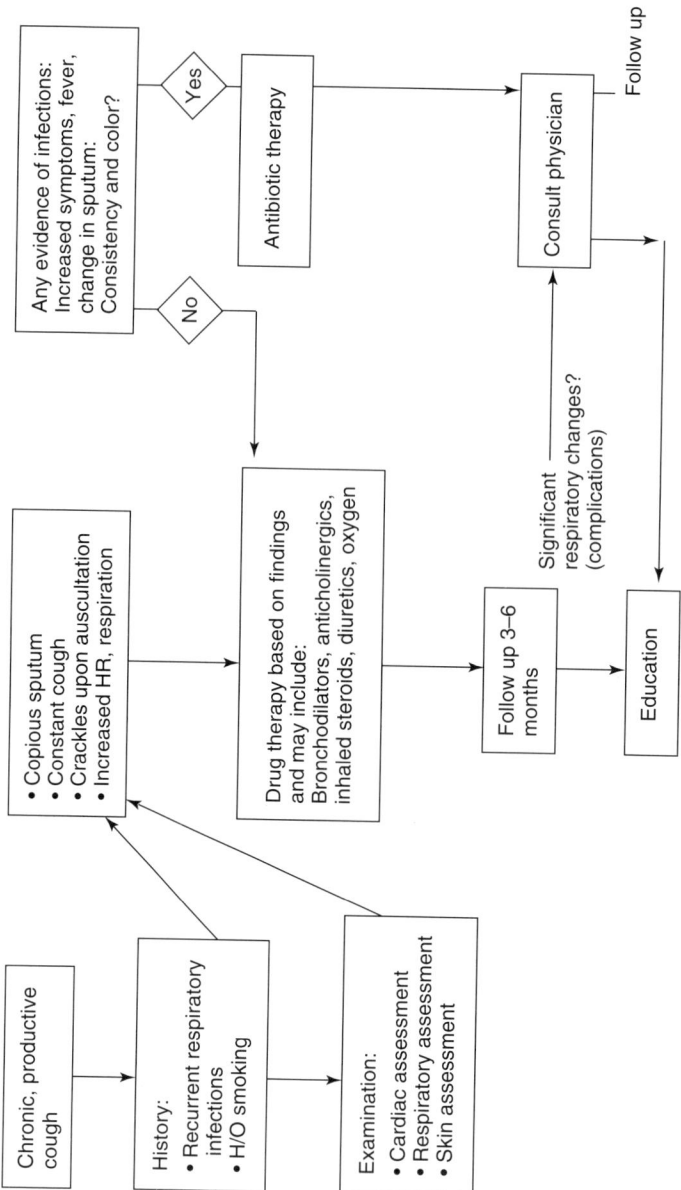

FIGURE 8–4 Chronic bronchitis.

monly taking multiple medications simultaneously (e.g., bronchodilators, steroids, diuretics, and oxygen). Usually, β_2 selective agonists and anticholinergic agents are used, allowing longer therapeutic duration without many side effects (metaproterenol metered-dose inhaler [MDI] 2 puffs q 4–6 hr or 10–20 mg PO tid, or albuterol MDI 2 puffs q 4–6 hr or 2–4 mg PO tid, or theophylline 100–300 mg PO (10–12 mg/kg) bid, or ipratropium bromide MDI 2 puffs qid). The use of a spacing chamber can improve the delivery of a metered dose. For inflammatory flare-ups or if the bronchodilator is ineffective, a steroid may be added to the regimen. An inhaled steroid (beclomethasone dipropionate 2 puffs qid) for 7–10 days may be helpful. If this is ineffective, oral prednisone 5–10 mg PO qid is commonly used. In severe cases, an aerosol bronchodilator q 4 hr for several days is administered. Infections may be treated with trimethoprim-sulfamethoxazole DS bid, amoxicillin 250–500 mg tid, or erythromycin 250 mg qid for 10 days. Oxygen therapy should be initiated for a Pao_2 of 55 at rest.

Follow-up: The degree of dyspnea reflects the effectiveness of treatment. Follow-up visits should be scheduled for 3–6 months, and as needed. Monitor for signs and symptoms of complications. Further evaluation is individualized to the assessment findings.

Sequelae: Monitor for bronchopulmonary infections, bronchial pneumonia, cor pulmonale, pulmonary hypertension, polycythemia pulmonary embolism, spontaneous pneumothorax, and progression to emphysema.

Prevention/Prophylaxis: Prophylactic measures include annual influenza vaccine; pneumococcal vaccination (once in a lifetime); avoidance of crowds, especially during cold and flu seasons; and avoidance of extreme variations. A home humidifier may be helpful in thinning secretions. Postural drainage three to four times a day may also aid in mobilizing secretions. Smoking cessation and the avoidance of second-hand smoke is essential in the prevention of chronic bronchitis.

Referral: Refer to a physician or specialist if complications occur with no response to treatment.

Education: Compliance to the treatment regimen is facilitated through the patient's knowledge of the respiratory system, the disease process, precipitating factors of the disease, drug education, proper use of inhalers, and signs and symptoms of complications. Maintenance of hydration allows for clearance of low-viscosity mucus. For patients in a poor nutritional state, the use of liquid oral supplements is recommended. Advise patients to reduce alcohol consumption because alcohol depresses the respiratory drive. Encourage aerobic exercise as tolerated. Patients should be cautioned about using OTC medications such as cough suppressants, narcotics, sleeping pills, antihistamines, and oxygen therapy. Participation in a pulmonary rehabilitation program and support group should also be encouraged.

Chronic Obstructive Pulmonary Disease

Chronic obstructive pulmonary disease (COPD) is characterized by progressive obstruction of airflow, which becomes irreversible. COPD may take the form of emphysema, chronic bronchitis, unremitting asthma, or (usually) a combination of these. Airway hyperreactivity may also be present. Although most patients with COPD have a combination mixture of the aforementioned entities, usually one predominates.

Etiology: *Emphysema* is characterized by obstruction to airflow caused by abnormal airspace enlargement distal to terminal bronchioles. No fibrosis occurs, but the walls of the airspaces are destroyed, possibly because of oxidative changes from protease-antiprotease imbalance. Air becomes trapped, hindering effective O_2 and CO_2 exchange.

The clinical diagnosis of *chronic bronchitis* is based on certain symptom criteria. A chronic, productive cough, typically worse on awakening and lasting for three consecutive months in two sequential years, is considered diagnostic after other causes of mucous hypersecretion have been ruled out. Inflammation in the lining of the airways results in hyperplasia of goblet cells, edema and inflammation of mucosa, and hypertrophy of mucous glands.

Unremitting *asthma* is a chronic inflammatory airway disorder with hyperactivity of the airway. In older patients, asthma tends to become less reversible, at which point it becomes a chronic obstructive disease.

Smoking is a prominent factor in the development of almost all types of COPD.

Occurrence: Prevalence of COPD in elderly persons has been steadily increasing since 1971; an estimated 17 million diagnosed patients exist in the United States, with almost as many in the asymptomatic to early symptomatic period. It is the fifth major cause of death.

Age: Because of the natural history of the disease (including a 20- to 40-year preclinical period of damage), the elderly population is most affected. The incidence for all forms of COPD is 130 in 1000 for patients over age 60. The mortality rate, 200 in 100,000 for age 65–70 years, jumps to 450 in 100,000 for the 75 and above age group.

Ethnicity: Mortality from COPD is higher among whites than among non-whites.

Gender: More men than women are diagnosed with COPD.

Contributing Factors: *Smoking* is the primary cause of COPD. Early age at starting, total pack-years, and current smoking practice contribute to COPD mortality. Other contributing factors for COPD include

Air pollution.

Occupational exposures.

Severe viral pneumonia at a young age.

Passive smoking.

Alcohol consumption.

Airway hyperactivity.

Possibly viral infection.

Rarely, a genetic component due to α_1-antitrypsin deficiency.

Changes in the weather cause exacerbation of symptoms; environmental allergens and biochemical mediators also play a role in asthmatic COPD.

Signs and Symptoms: Symptoms of *emphysema* include mild exertional dyspnea progressing to difficulty breathing at rest, barrel chest, diminished breath sounds, occasional wheezing, occasional respiratory infections, infrequent cough or sputum production, use of accessory muscles for respiration, weight loss. Symptoms of *chronic bronchitis* include frequent productive cough, especially in the morning; frequent infections; wheezing; decreased breath sounds; and cyanosis. *Asthma* symptoms include periodic dyspnea; wheezing; decreased breath sounds; cough, especially at night; cyanosis; and nocturnal and seasonal exacerbation of symptoms.

Because the older COPD patient usually has a combination of more than one type of COPD, symptoms often vary.

A careful history regarding onset and timing of symptoms, changes in activity and exercise patterns, smoking, and occupational background helps to establish diagnosis. Physical examination will not reveal early stages of COPD but does help in establishing a baseline and uncovering comorbidities. Initially, the patient may present frequently with sinus or respiratory infections. As the disease progresses, changes in the respiratory pattern (such as prolonged expiration, pursed-lip breathing, and use of accessory muscles of respiration) can be seen. Weight loss is frequently seen in the later stages of emphysema, when the patient becomes dyspneic while trying to eat. Right-sided heart failure and cor pulmonale seen in the later stages may present as jugular venous distention, hepatomegaly, or peripheral edema. The patient's color may appear ruddy or dusky, depending on oxygenation. In the early to middle stages, chest auscultation may reveal longer expirations, with wheezing on forced expiration. Later, as the chest hyperinflates, breath sounds become distant and percussion is hyperresonant. Wheezes can sometimes be heard (most frequently with chronic bronchitis); the presence of crackles suggests possible pulmonary edema or pneumonia. The chest takes on a barrel-like appearance. Hyperinflation restricts diaphragmatic movement. As the cardiovascular system attempts to compensate, tachycardia or a gallop rhythm commonly occurs.

Diagnostic Tests: Perform spirometry to establish a baseline on every patient over age 40 who smokes. FEV_1 less than 80% after adjustment for height, age, gender, and race indicates compromised air flow. Reduction in FVC may be due to air trapping from obstructive disease or to restrictive lung disease; total lung capacity (TLC) differentiates the two (Table 8–3, Table 8–4). Patients

TABLE 8–3   NORMAL PERCENT OF PREDICTED FOR SPIROMETRY

FEV₁ Percent (FEV₁/FVC)		FVC Percent of Predicted	
>70%	Normal	>80%	Normal
61–69%	Mild obstructive lung disease	66–79%	Mild restrictive
45–60%	Moderate obstructive lung disease	50–65%	Moderate restrictive
<45%	Severe obstructive lung disease	<50%	Severe restrictive

Reduction in FVC may be due to air trapping from obstructive disease or to restrictive lung disease; TLC differentiates the two.

receiving bronchodilator therapy should be told not to use this medication on the day of spirometry testing until after the test is over (Fig. 8–5).

Bronchodilator Response: To rule out asthma in a patient with respiratory symptoms suggestive of COPD who is not using a bronchodilator, obtain a baseline FEV₁ and then give a trial of an inhaled or nebulized β-agonist. Measure the FEV₁ again. An increase of 200 mL, or 15%, is clinically significant, indicating some reversibility of damage. An increase of greater than 20% suggests an asthmatic component to the COPD.

A complete blood count (CBC) helps to measure the degree of secondary polycythemia (advanced COPD with hypoxemia), detecting the presence of infection by an increased white blood cell (WBC) count, or, if eosinophilia is present, considering an allergic or asthmatic component. Chest x-ray examination in those having advanced COPD with emphysema may reveal hyperinflation, bullae or blebs, and a flat hemidiaphragm. In chronic bronchitis, increased markings suggest "dirty lungs," and cardiomegaly may be present. A chest x-ray may be indicated also when pneumonia is suspected, or to rule out other pulmonary problems. Unless you suspect hypoxemia or hypercapnia, evaluation of arterial blood gases (ABGs) is not necessary. Pulse oximetry, frequently used to determine oxygen saturation, is readily available, noninvasive, and a reliable guide to monitoring oxygen therapy. If cardiac involvement is severe, an ECG in advanced COPD may demonstrate evidence of right-axis deviation, sinus

TABLE 8–4   PERCENT OF PREDICTED FOR TLC*

>80%	Normal	All lung volumes are decreased in restrictive disease.
66–79%	Mild restrictive	
50–65%	Moderate restrictive	
<50%	Severe restrictive	

*TLC is normal or increased in COPD; residual volume is increased. FEV₁/FVC ratio is reduced.

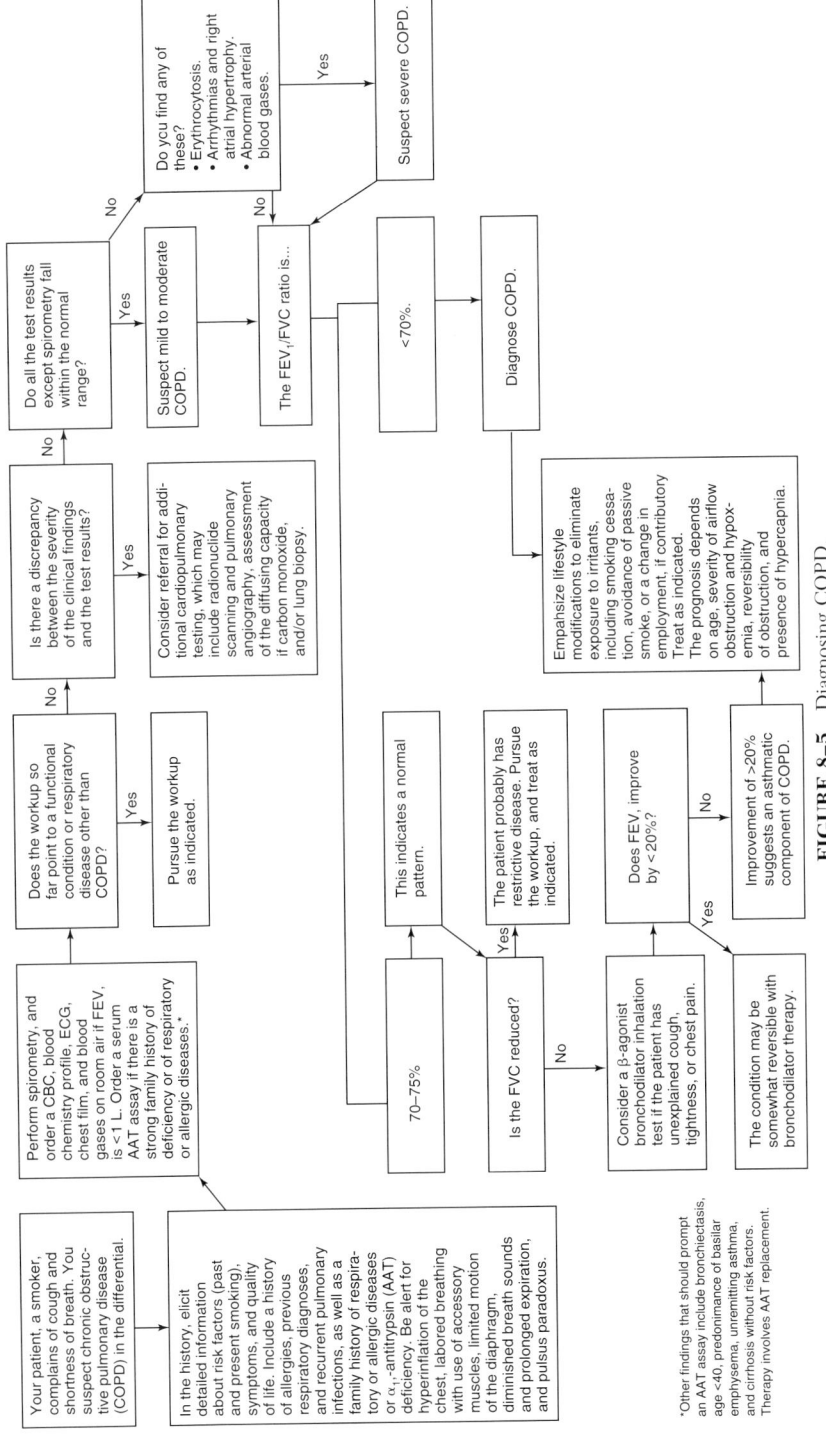

Your patient, a smoker, complains of cough and shortness of breath. You suspect chronic obstructive pulmonary disease (COPD) in the differential.

In the history, elicit detailed information about risk factors (past and present smoking), symptoms, and quality of life. Include a history of allergies, previous respiratory diagnoses, and recurrent pulmonary infections, as well as a family history of respiratory or allergic diseases or α_{1}-antitrypsin (AAT) deficiency. Be alert for hyperinflation of the chest, labored breathing with use of accessory muscles, limited motion of the diaphragm, diminished breath sounds and prolonged expiration, and pulsus paradoxus.

Perform spirometry, and order a CBC, blood chemistry profile, ECG, chest film, and blood gases on room air if FEV_1 is < 1 L. Order a serum AAT assay if there is a strong family history of deficiency or of respiratory or allergic diseases.*

Does the workup so far point to a functional condition or respiratory disease other than COPD?

No → Is there a discrepancy between the severity of the clinical findings and the test results?

Yes → Pursue the workup as indicated.

No → Do all the test results except spirometry fall within the normal range?

Yes → Consider referral for additional cardiopulmonary testing, which may include radionuclide scanning and pulmonary angiography, assessment of the diffusing capacity of carbon monoxide, and/or lung biopsy.

Yes → Suspect mild to moderate COPD.

No → Do you find any of these?
• Erythrocytosis.
• Arrhythmias and right atrial hypertrophy.
• Abnormal arterial blood gases.

Yes → Suspect severe COPD.

No → The FEV_1/FVC ratio is...

70–75% → This indicates a normal pattern.

<70%. → Diagnose COPD.

Is the FVC reduced?

Yes → The patient probably has restrictive disease. Pursue the workup, and treat as indicated.

No → Consider a β-agonist bronchodilator inhalation test if the patient has unexplained cough, tightness, or chest pain.

Does FEV_1 improve by <20%?

Yes → The condition may be somewhat reversible with bronchodilator therapy.

No → Improvement of >20% suggests an asthmatic component of COPD.

Emphasize lifestyle modifications to eliminate exposure to irritants, including smoking cessation, avoidance of passive smoke, or a change in employment, if contributory. Treat as indicated. The prognosis depends on age, severity of airflow obstruction and hypoxemia, reversibility of obstruction, and presence of hypercapnia.

FIGURE 8–5 Diagnosing COPD.

*Other findings that should prompt an AAT assay include bronchiectasis, age <40, predominance of basilar emphysema, unremitting asthma, and cirrhosis without risk factors. Therapy involves AAT replacement.

tachycardia, and pulmonary hypertension with the presence of ongoing S waves in the lateral precordial leads.

Differential Diagnosis Differential diagnosis includes lung cancer, bronchiectasis, acute bronchitis, occupational lung disease, and acute viral infection.

Treatment: Individualize treatment goals according to the stage of disease, comorbidities, and patient goals. Use collaborative management with a physician specializing in respiratory problems. Smoking cessation is a primary goal of treatment. If the patient is ready to quit, Zyban (bupropion [Wellbutrin]) sustained-release, 150 mg PO daily for 3 days, then twice a day for 7–12 weeks, can be prescribed, after you establish its compatibility with the other medications the patient may be taking. Follow-up phone calls weekly for the first few weeks may help maintain the patient's motivation. Adequate hydration is important. Treat infections early and aggressively to prevent complications or further loss of lung function. The patient should receive yearly influenza vaccine unless contraindications exist. Pneumococcal vaccine should also be given once, with the option to repeat in 5 or 6 years, if the individual's condition permits, an option that is recommended for high-risk patients. Whether or not to repeat the pneumococcal vaccine is a clinical decision.

The use of antibiotic prophylaxis in acute exacerbations of COPD is a matter of controversy. Most authorities agree that low-level antibiotic therapy benefits the patient when fever, purulent sputum, or other symptoms of a bacterial infection exist. The practice of prescribing for COPD patients prophylactic antibiotics during the winter to prevent infection is not recommended. When choosing a suitable agent, keep in mind that typical respiratory organisms include *Streptococcus pneumoniae, Haemophilus influenzae,* and *Moraxella catarrhalis.* Amoxicillin 250 mg, tab 1 PO tid; ampicillin 250 mg, tab 1 PO qid; Ceclor 250 mg, tab 1 PO tid; doxycycline 100 mg, tab 1 PO bid; and Bactrim DS (trimethoprim-sulfamethoxazole [TMP/SMZ]), tab 1 PO bid are all usually effective when prescribed for 7–10 days. The patient or caregiver should be instructed to call if symptoms worsen after 3 days of antibiotic therapy. Consult with a pulmonary or internal medicine specialist if the patient does not improve. For most COPD patients, inhaled anticholinergics and bronchodilators are the mainstay of therapy. This is problematic if the patient cannot learn how to administer a metered-dose inhaler (MDI). Older patients should use a spacer chamber. An alternate approach, requiring more time and usually someone other than the patient to set up, is medication delivery via nebulizer. This can be administered with an oral mouthpiece or a mask; mininebulizers are available for home or long-term care settings. For patients with nonasthmatic COPD, the use of an ipratropium (Atrovent) MDI can be instituted; the usual dosage is 2–4 puffs qid. Ipratropium is also available as nebulizer therapy. It is *not* effective in treating acute bronchospasm; patients should be instructed about this and advised to use their β-agonist inhaler for acute problems or to seek urgent care. Anticholinergics should be used cautiously in patients with narrow-angle glaucoma, prostatic hypertrophy, or bladder neck obstruction, and they are contraindicated in patients who are allergic to atropine. Because of the route of administration (inhalation), side effects are minimal. Combivent, a combination of ipratropium and albuterol in an MDI, is also available. The usual dosage is 1–2 puffs up to four times daily. Beta-agonist MDI therapy is most effective in treating patients with asthmatic COPD, but it is also used to treat those with nonasthmatic COPD. β-agonist MDI is a powerful bronchodilator that usually provides a measure of relief upon administration. This drug is given either as needed, in patients with less severe disease, or on a regular administration basis for moderate to severe COPD. The most commonly used agent is albuterol (Proventil, Ventolin) MDI, 1–2 puffs q 4–6 hr; albuterol is also available for nebulizer.

Other frequently prescribed inhaled bronchodilators are

Metaproterenol sulfate (Alupent, Metaprel) MDI, 2 puffs q 4 hr, also available in nebulizer or oral form.
Pirbutrol acetate (Maxair) MDI, 2 puffs q 4–6 hr.
Salmeterol xinafoate (Serevent) MDI, 2 puffs bid (q 12 hr).
Terbutaline sulfate (Brethaire) MDI, 2 puffs q 4–6 hr.

The effects of beta-agonists are antagonized by beta-blockers. Beta-agonists are sympathomimetic agents that cause transient tachycardia, nervousness, and elevation in blood pressure. Use beta-agonists cautiously with cardiovascular disease, and note that concurrent therapy with xanthines (e.g., theophylline) or other sympathomimetics (often found in OTC decongestants or cold remedies) will exaggerate side effects.

The decision to institute treatment with an inhaled beta-agonist is a clinical one, based on trial use and effect. In the past, reports were published of sudden death associated with administration of beta-agonists; further investigation revealed that the medication was being used inappropriately (too frequently) in most cases. Patients should be instructed to seek care if their breathing changes or it does not respond to the prescribed medication regimen.

The use of methylxanthines such as theophylline and aminophylline has decreased significantly. They are now considered third- or fourth-line agents, to be used when inhaled bronchodilators and/or anticholinergic agents do not control symptoms well. Dosage is individualized, with the timed-release forms being preferred. Significant side effects occur, including increased nervousness or agitation, increased heart rate, and gastrointestinal (GI) effects. Also, many drug interactions are associated with the methylxanthines. These drugs are contraindicated in patients taking H2 blockers, fluoroquinolones, or macrolide antibiotics.

Frequent drug level measurements are required to monitor for methylxanthine toxicity; subtherapeutic drug levels, especially in older patients, are not usually adjusted because of lack of monitoring. Doses should be reduced in the presence of hepatic or cardiac disease or a history of seizures.

Oral corticosteroids and sometimes inhaled steroids are prescribed for patients with COPD that is refractory to treatment or for those experiencing an exacerbation. Collaborate with a pulmonary disease specialist regarding the management of these patients. The use of steroids should never be taken lightly. In the older patient with COPD, many things need to be considered. If the patient has a history of cor pulmonale, average doses of oral steroids can cause fluid retention and precipitate an episode of right-sided heart failure. Prednisone 20 mg PO daily may be sufficient to control symptoms. Short courses of oral steroids are preferred to a maintenance course whenever possible.

Patients with asthmatic COPD may use inhaled corticosteroids instead of oral corticosteroids or after tapering off the use of oral corticosteroids. Because of the potential of these drugs to mask infection, careful monitoring is required. Instruct patients to rinse their mouth and equipment after using the inhaler, to prevent oral candidiasis. Commonly used inhaled steroids include beclomethasone dipropionate (Beclovent, Vanceril); flunisolide (AeroBid, AeroBid-M); triamcinolone acetonide (Azmacort). Dosage for all three of these drugs is 2 puffs qid, then reduced to 2 puffs bid. Another inhaled steroid is fluticasone propionate (Flovent), available in three dosage strengths: 40 μg, 110 μg, and 220 μg/puff. Dosage for each is 2 puffs bid.

If the patient has cor pulmonale from pulmonary hypertension, low-level loop diuretic therapy helps to control fluid build-up. Monitor these patients for hypokalemia.

Use the foregoing information as a guideline. You are responsible for reviewing the medication regimen, including drug action, side effects, interactions, dosing, and contraindications before initiating a new medication or making changes to an existing medication regimen. In addition to medication management, quality of life and functionality are important issues to consider when treating patients with COPD. Every patient should have an advanced directive. Reconditioning for stable patients with moderate COPD can improve function and alleviate anxiety. A program of flexibility and aerobic training three to five times weekly is helpful.

Realistic goals should be established and endurance built up gradually. In addition to physical exercise, instruction in anxiety management, breathing and relaxation exercises, including pursed lip and abdominal breathing, may help to enhance O_2 and CO_2 exchange and relieve dyspnea. For the patient with severe COPD, maintaining comfort and any element of functionality is helpful. When dyspnea is unrelieved by medications and interferes with functionality, low-level oxygen therapy may be instituted, either temporarily during and after an acute exacerbation or on a long-term basis. Medicare criteria must be met for long-term therapy to be reimbursable. Type of oxygen delivery is determined by the duration and activity level of the patient. Liquid systems or small canisters of compressed gas permit mobility outside of the home.

Nutrition is a treatment concern for many older patients with COPD. The exertion of breathing burns extra calories and tires these patients so much that they cannot eat. Medications may also contribute to anorexia. Small, frequent feedings with easily chewed and digested foods are recommended. Supplementation with a liquid nutritional preparation may help. Consultation with a nutritionist may also be indicated.

Several surgical options including lung volume reduction therapy, lung resections, transplants, and laser bullectomy are available in selected circumstances. Consultation with a pulmonary specialist is advised, with possibility of referral to a thoracic surgeon.

If the patient is at home, supportive services such as home care nurse, physical therapy, and home health aide may be instituted after an acute exacerbation of COPD. End-stage COPD patients may be candidates for hospice care, if this is in accord with their wishes. In any case, a large part of the treatment for any COPD patient is support and understanding.

Follow-up: A newly diagnosed patient should be seen frequently until an optimal treatment plan is in place and disease education has been completed. For stable patients who are maintaining their usual activities of daily living (ADLs), routine reassessment every 3–6 months is advisable, with instructions to the patient or caregiver to schedule an interim visit if there is a change in status, increased symptoms, or an infection. For stable patients with other significant comorbidities, visits every 3 months are advisable.

Patients who are unstable or have had an acute exacerbation will need more frequent follow-up visits initially. Collaborative management with these patients is strongly advised; during the immediate postacute period, a pulmonary specialist should manage the patient.

Sequelae: COPD can lead to infections, particularly respiratory (pneumonia, recurrent bronchitis, viral infections), cor pulmonale, pulmonary hypertension, malnutrition, acute or chronic respiratory failure, steroid-induced myopathy or Cushing's syndrome, bullous lung disease, polycythemia, and sleep-related hypoxemia. Depression is frequently associated with COPD.

Prevention/Prophylaxis: COPD is almost 100% preventable by avoidance of smoking.

Referral: Collaborative management is advised in all but stable, moderately ill patients. Refer patients to a pulmonary specialist during instability, for hospital and post-acute care and for determination of the need for oxygen therapy. Refer patients to a surgeon if the option of surgery is deemed appropriate. Refer patients to physical therapy for reconditioning; occupational therapy may also be helpful in teaching breathing techniques and energy-conserving measures. Postacute COPD patients dwelling in the community should be referred for home care. Also, refer all patients to community resources and support groups.

Education: Teach the patient, family, and/or caregivers about the disease process and its management, the role of smoking in causing the disease, the possibility of reversibility in the early/moderate stage with smoking cessation, medications, oxygen therapy precautions, and the need to seek care early if infection develops, dyspnea increases, or a change in cognitive status occurs. Advise patients of the need for regular follow-up visits, even if no symptoms are present.

Lung Cancer

Lung cancer is a malignant neoplasm of the parenchyma of the lung. Most (82%) of lung neoplasms are non–small cell lung cancer (NSCLC), which includes squamous cell carcinoma, adenocarcinoma, and large cell carcinoma. Small cell lung cancer (SCLC) accounts for 18% of lung malignancies and includes the histologic subtypes oat cell, polygonal cell, lymphatic, and spindle cell.

Etiology: Research has shown conclusively that more than 85% of lung cancer cases are associated with tobacco smoking. The inhalation of other carcinogens, usually through occupational exposure, account for most other cases of lung cancer. Patients with preexisting diseases that involve the lungs, such as chronic obstructive pulmonary disease (COPD), prior lung cancers, and sarcoidosis are at increased risk for developing lung cancer. Radiation exposure may cause lung cancer. Some research suggests that there may be a genetic predisposition to carcinoma of the lung.

Occurrence: Lung cancer is the most common cause of cancer-associated deaths in the United States. Annually, more than 170,000 new cases are diagnosed, and more than 157,000 individuals die from lung cancer.

Age: Lung cancer can occur at any age but there is a dramatic increase in new diagnosis after age 40.

Ethnicity: Not significant.

Gender: The male-to-female ratio is 4:3, although the incidence of the disease is growing faster for women than for men. In 1995 in the United States, there were approximately 96,000 new cases for men, compared with 73,900 for women.

Contributing Factors: The cumulative dose or pack-years for cigarette smoking is directly related to the risk of developing lung cancr. The more cigarettes smoked per day and the longer the individual has smoked, the higher the risk of developing lung cancer. The risk of lung cancer is 30 times higher in smokers than in nonsmokers. Cigar and pipe smokers, as well as passive smokers, have double the risk. The risks of developing lung cancer steadily decline for people who quit smoking and approach that of a nonsmoker after 15 years of abstinence. Individuals who have smoked for more than 20 years will probably always have a slightly increased risk of developing the disease, even after 15 years as a nonsmoker.

Asbestos exposure alone increases the risk of developing pulmonary carcinoma but when combined with smoking the risk increases to 90 times that of a nonsmoker. Other inhaled agents implicated in the development of the disease are radon, arsenic, nickel, chromates, halo ethers, alkylating compounds, and polycyclic aromatic hydrocarbons. Air pollution is also thought to contribute to the development of lung cancer.

Signs and Symptoms: Unfortunately, signs and symptoms of lung cancer are usually present only after the disease has progressed beyond the early stages. Routine screening for the disease with chest x-ray examination is not recommended because it is neither specific nor sensitive. Symptoms suggestive of lung cancer include smoking, a new or changing cough, hoarseness, hemoptysis, anorexia, cachexia, unexplained weight loss, dyspnea, hypoxia, wheezing, unresolving pneumonia, and chest wall pain. Patients may initially present with symptoms related to extrathoracic disease including tracheal obstruction, esophageal obstruction with dysphagia, laryngeal nerve paralysis, phrenic nerve paralysis with elevated hemidiaphragm, sympathetic nerve paralysis or Horner's syndrome, pleural effusion due to lymphatic obstruction, Pancoast's syndrome involving the eighth cervical and first and second thoracic nerves, or superior vena cava syndrome from vascular obstruction.

Patients with pericardial and cardiac extension of tumor may have symptoms of arrhythmia, tamponade, or failure. The presenting illness in patients with lung cancer may be paraneoplastic syndromes including hypercalcemia, hypophosphatemia, hyponatremia with syndrome of inappropriate antidiuretic hormone, and hypercoaguable states. Occasionally, skeletal-connective syndromes, clubbing, and osteoarthropathy are initial symptoms of lung cancer.

Diagnostic Tests: After a history and physical examination suggestive of disease, a chest x-ray examination and sputum for cytology are indicated for further screening. Complete blood count and chemistries are performed to assess for paraneoplastic syndromes. Definitive diagnosis of lung cancer is established by tissue pathology and histology. Computerized tomography scans are ordered by specialists for staging of the disease (Fig. 8–6).

Differential Diagnosis: Tuberculosis, infectious granuloma, pneumonia, empyema, bronchiectasis, abscess, sarcoidosis, pneumonitis, and asbestosis can all mimick lung cancer.

Treatment: Surgical resection and radiation therapy are indicated for NSCLC. Chemotherapy for NSCLC is usually palliative. Chemotherapy and radiation are the treatments of choice in SCLC. Combination chemotherapy used to treat SCLC includes cyclophosphamide, adriamycin, and vincristine or VP-16.

Follow-up: Patients should be seen for follow-up every 2 months following treatment for lung cancer. Every visit will include a chest x-ray examination. During years 2–5 follow-up should be every 3 months with a chest x-ray examination. Yearly examinations are advised thereafter.

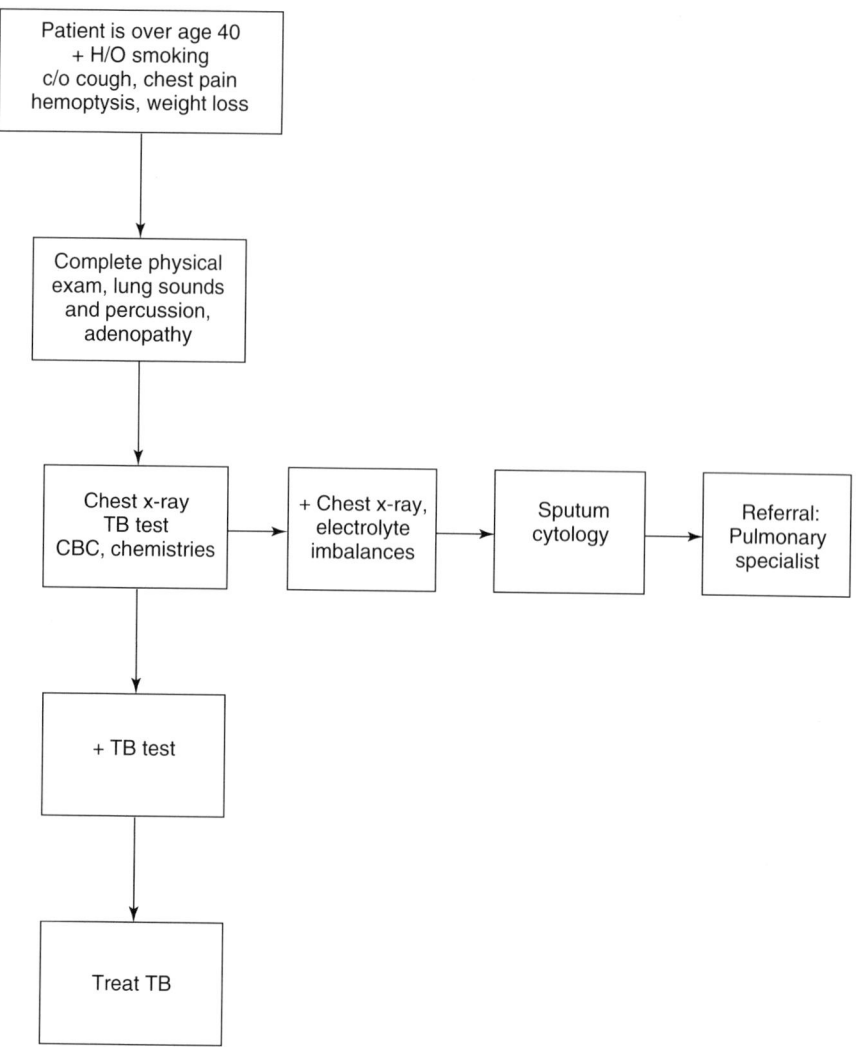

FIGURE 8–6   Lung cancer.

Sequelae: Disability and death are the chief sequelae of lung cancer. The 5-year survival rate is 13% for NSCLC and less than 10% for SCLC.

Prevention/Prophylaxis: Prevention of lung cancer should focus on smoking cessation.

Ask about and record the tobacco use status of every patient, advise patients who smoke to quit, and offer smoking cessation treatment at every office visit.

Referral: Upon suspecting lung cancer, refer the patient to a pulmonary specialist and possibly a cardiothoracic surgeon and an oncologist.

Education: Many smoking cessation programs are available. Examples include the American Academy of Family Physicians Stop Smoking Kit (800-227-2237), various pamphlets from the American Cancer Society (800-227-2345), and A Healthy Beginning Counseling Kit from the American Lung Association (800-315-8700).

The primary health-care provider can assess the smoker's motivation to quit and offer motivational intervention based on the "4 Rs:"

Risks: Review acute, long-term, and environmental risks with the patient. Encourage the patient to identify risks that are most important to him or her.
Rewards: Help the patient to identify potential benefits of quitting.
Repetition: Reinforce risks and rewards identified by the patient on a regular basis.
Relapse prevention: Communicate caring, concern, and encouragement.

Let the patient talk about feelings related to quitting smoking. Provide education about the process of smoking cessation. Guide the patient in the use of nicotine replacement therapies such as gum or a patch. Provide information about support groups and community programs available to help with smoking cessation.

Pneumonia

Pneumonia, an acute lower respiratory tract infection of the lung parenchyma, can be bacterial or viral. Bacterial pneumonia is the most common type in older adults. Pneumonia is also classified as community acquired or nosocomial (acquired from a hospital or nursing home).

Etiology: The most common cause of community-acquired pneumonia is *Streptococcus pneumoniae*, followed by *Staphylococcus aureus, Haemophilus influenzae,* and other gram-negative and anaerobic bacteria. In patients with COPD, *S. pneumoniae, H. influenzae, Moraxella catarrhalis,* and *Legionella* species predominate. Aspiration pneumonia is most often caused by anaerobes and *S. pneumoniae.* Nosocomial infections in the older patient are caused by a variety of organisms including *Klebsiella pneumoniae, S. pneumoniae, Staph. aureus, H. influenzae, Pseudomonas aeruginosa, Escherichia coli,* anaerobes, *Legionella,* or *Chlamydia* species. It is often the norm to have a mixture of organisms.

Occurrence: The annual incidence of community-based pneumonia is 1200 in 100,000 and of nosocomial, 800 in 100,000.

Age: Pneumonia is the most common cause of death caused by infectious disease in older patients. Elderly persons are at 5–10 times the risk of younger adults for dying of pneumonia. Up to 60% of cases occur in patients age 65 or older.

Ethnicity: Not significant.

Gender: More men than women are diagnosed with pneumonia.

Contributing Factors: Comorbidities, influenza, chronic pulmonary conditions, smoking, alcoholism, malnutrition, colonization of the oropharynx by gram-negative bacteria, institutional setting, decline in immune function, hospitalization, use of sedating medications, and diminished cough reflex may contribute to development of pneumonia. Swallowing problems from esophageal or neurologic conditions or the presence of a feeding tube can lead to aspiration pneumonia. Risk factors for pneumonia-related death include age over 65, comorbid disease (e.g., diabetes, renal insufficiency, congestive heart failure [CHF]), fever more than 101°F, immunosuppressed state and/or pneumonia caused by *S. aureus*, gram-negative rods, aspiration, and/or airway obstruction.

Signs and Symptoms: Typical symptoms include fever, chills, cough, and rusty or thick sputum, with associated gastrointestinal (GI) upset or anorexia, malaise, and diaphoresis. These characteristic symptoms are frequently absent, particularly in the frail elderly, leading to a lag time before diagnosis. In the older patient, mental status changes (i.e., confusion), new onset or increased frequency of falls, increased respiratory rate, hypotension, anorexia, a marked functional decline, and new onset of urinary incontinence are typical symptoms. Caregivers or family members may report that the patient is not his or her usual self. Physical examination of the chest reveals crackles that do not clear with cough or deep breathing. Increased respiratory rate (greater than 24 breaths/min) is typical. If the patient is not able to deep breathe adequately, crackles may be absent. Dullness to percussion, egophony, and bronchial breath sounds may be present. A fever of 100°F, with tachycardia, may be present. Signs of dehydration may also occur. The patient may appear anxious, restless, or withdrawn. Concurrent symptoms of CHF may appear.

Diagnostic Tests: A complete blood count (CBC) should be done to assess hemodynamic status and leukocytosis or leukopenia. A hemoglobin of less than 9.0 is associated with increased morbidity related to the pneumonia. An elevation of the white blood cells (WBCs) to greater than 15,000 suggests an active immune response; increased mortality is associated with a leukopenic response of less than 5000. Normal WBCs with a shift to the left can also be seen. Blood cultures are also recommended because of the possibility of bacteremia. If fluid-electrolyte imbalance is a consideration, a chemistry panel consisting of blood urea nitrogen (BUN), creatinine, and electrolytes is indicated. This information can be used to establish the creatinine clearance before prescribing drug therapy. If liver function is questionable, testing should be done to establish a baseline prior to prescribing. A chest x-ray should be done. The presence of an infiltrate is confirmatory for pneumonia; incidental findings may include CHF or COPD changes. The presence of hilar adenopathy with peripheral infiltrate, cavitation in the upper lobe, and/or miliary infiltrate suggests tuberculosis. Because chest x-ray findings lag behind the clinical picture, in the absence of positive evidence, treatment should be based on the clinical presentation. A sputum specimen for Gram stain and/or culture is helpful, if it can be obtained without causing major trauma to the patient. Sputum for acid-fast bacilli (AFB) should be obtained if tuberculosis is suspected. Dermal skin testing with purified protein derivative (PPD) is indicated; a positive response in older patients is an indurated area greater than 10 mm after 48–72 hr. (See Tuberculosis, for more information and confounding variables.) If the patient is a known positive reactor, retesting should not be done.

In patients with comorbidities affecting oxygenation, pulse oximetry is indicated to evaluate O_2 saturation and need for oxygen therapy. If the patient is hospitalized, arterial blood gases (ABG) may be drawn.

Differential Diagnosis: Differential diagnosis includes other causes of pulmonary infection including influenza or parainfluenza, adenoviruses, fungal agents, toxoplasma, tuberculosis, pulmonary embolism with infarction, vasculitis of the pulmonary bed, and pneumothorax.

Treatment: A critical element in treatment is the choice of setting. For community-dwelling older patients, the presence of a responsible caregiver and a supportive home environment is necessary. Temporary measures to increase support and monitor status of response may be introduced by ordering home health services. If the patient fails to recover or deteriorates despite these interventions, hospitalization should be contemplated. Failure to drink fluids or signs of hemodynamic instability are definitive criteria for hospitalization.

For older patients in the long-term care setting, familiarity with the setting is important in making a decision about where to treat the patient. If oxygen therapy and parenteral administration of fluids and medications are available by nursing staff or through a contractual arrangement covered by health insurance, then the patient should be maintained in that setting. The health and safety of other patients in the facility must also be considered. Objective criteria for hospital admission include:

- Acute medical problem necessitating hospitalization regardless of pneumonia diagnosis.
- Severe electrolyte or hematologic abnormalities.
- Significant abnormalities in vital signs (heart rate greater than 140 beats/min; systolic blood pressure less than 90 mmHg; respirations greater than 30 breaths/min).
- Altered mental status.
- Hypoxemia on room air (Pao_2 less than 60 mmHg).

Antimicrobial treatment is usually empirical and is directed at eradicating the most frequently occurring agents in the patient's setting. If diagnostic testing yields a definite organism, treatment is directed toward its elimination. Empiric therapy for community-acquired pneumonia includes second-generation cephalosporins such as cefaclor (Ceclor) 250 mg PO tid, cefprozil (Cefzil) 500 mg PO bid, or cefuroxime (Ceftin) 125–500 mg PO bid; duration of therapy is 10 days. Loracarbef (Lorabid), a cephalosporin-type beta-lactam antibiotic, 400 mg PO bid for 14 days or amoxicillin clavulanate (Augmentin), an aminopenicillin and beta-lactamase inhibitor, 875 mg PO bid for 10 days may be given. Augmentin is contraindicated in the presence of penicillin allergy; additionally, a cross-sensitivity to cephalosporins exists in some penicillin-allergic patients, so caution must be used. Sulfamethoxazole with trimethoprim DS (Bactrim/Septra; TMP/SMX) is effective against gram-negative *H. influenzae* but may not eradicate the gram-positive coccal organisms; dosage is 1 tablet bid for 10 days. The use of this agent is contraindicated in patients allergic to sulfate. Erythromycin 500 mg PO qid or clarithromycin (Biaxin) 250–500 mg PO bid, for 10 days, are both macrolide antibiotics, effective as alternatives in penicillin- or sulfa-allergic patients. Erythromycin has significant GI effects that interfere with compliance. The macrolides are also effective in *Legionella*-type infections; because of the severity and potential mortality associated with these infections, hospitalization is usually indicated.

For patients in long-term care settings, ceftriaxone (Rocephin), a third-generation cephalosporin, has been used successfully, because of its gram-negative and gram-positive activity. It can be given intramuscularly, 2 g initially, followed by 1 g intramuscularly (IM) q 12 hr. Injection is painful; the drug can be diluted with 1% lidocaine (without epinephrine) and given in two injections at separate sites. After a 7-day course, the patient can be switched to an oral second-generation cephalosporin and treatment continued for another 7–14 days.

Levofloxacin (Levaquin), a quinolone antibiotic, is also available for treatment of both community-acquired and long-term care resident cases of pneumonia. Dosage is 500 mg daily, orally or by intravenous (IV) infusion, for 7–14 days.

This information is intended as a guideline; each provider is responsible for reviewing the medication regimen, including action, side effects, interactions, dosing, and contraindications, before initiating a new medication or making changes to existing medication regimens.

In addition to antimicrobial treatment measures, supportive and restorative measures are necessary for optimal recovery. Oxygen therapy based on determinations of ABGs or pulse oximetry during the acute phase is one such entity. Nutritional supplementation may also be indicated. Physical therapy measures for strengthening and ambulation may be initiated during the acute recovery period and continued during convalescence or replaced by restorative nursing measures.

Follow-up: Follow-up depends on comorbidities and response to prescribed treatment regimen. Independent community-dwelling older adults or caregivers should be instructed to call if symptoms worsen, if no response occurs after 3–5 days of treatment, or if symptoms recur. A follow-up visit after completion of treatment, to assess response and further interventions, is helpful. Patient teaching regarding self-care and increasing functional status can be given at this time, with further visits depending on individual status. Follow-up chest x-ray examination, if indicated, should be delayed for at least 6 weeks because resolution will take 6–12 weeks to occur. Frail elderly persons in a long-term care setting will need more frequent and prolonged monitoring after an acute episode of pneumonia.

Sequelae: The older patient with comorbidities is especially prone to complications, including severe deconditioning and decline in ADL level. If nutrition is poor, coexisting lung disease is present, or both, the patient may never return to baseline. Adult respiratory distress syndrome (ARDS) or multiple organ dysfunction syndrome (MODS) may also occur, resulting in significant morbidity and mortality. Superinfections, recurrence, or opportunistic infections may occur in susceptible patients.

Prevention/Prophylaxis: Older patients should have an annual influenza vaccination. If unable to take the influenza vaccine and living in a long-term care setting, the patient may receive amatadine or rimantadine prophylaxis during the peak influenza period. The pneumococcal vaccine is administered once in patients age 65 or older. Antibiotics should be prescribed prudently. Teach patients with comorbidities to avoid contact with persons having known respiratory infections.

Referral: Refer patients with comorbidities to infectious disease, internal medicine, or pulmonary specialists for inpatient management and initial follow-up. Manage patients in long-term care settings collaboratively, until a return to baseline is achieved. Refer patients to a dietician for nutritional guidance and to physical therapy (PT) for reconditioning, strengthening, and increasing level of activities of daily living (ADLs). Refer patients to home care services (nursing, PT, home health aide) as needed for in-home support.

Education: Teach groups of older adults (especially those with comorbidities) about preventive measures. Educate patient and caregivers in management, including the importance of nutrition and hydration and deep breathing exercises.

Pulmonary Embolism

Pulmonary embolism (PE) is the occlusion of one or more pulmonary vessels by a traveling thrombus originating from a distant site. Although a blood clot is the most common embolism, fat, air, bone marrow, tumor cells, amniotic fluid, and foreign material can also occlude the pulmonary vasculature.

Etiology: Pulmonary embolism is usually caused by a dislodged thrombus from one of the veins of the legs or pelvis (deep vein thrombosis [DVT]).

Occurrence: Between 600,000 and 700,000 cases diagnosed each year, with 100,000–200,000 deaths annually.

Age: The incidence of pulmonary embolism tends to increase with age.

Ethnicity: Not significant.

Gender: The incidence of pulmonary embolism is equal for men and women.

Contributing Factors: Virchow's triad of stasis or prolonged immobility, hyper-coagulation, and venous trauma (endothelial injury with inflammation of the vessel lining) represent risk factors for PE. Stasis may be occupational or medical (e.g., congestive heart failure [CHF]; postsurgical paralysis, chronic illness or debilitation, tumor compression). Venous trauma damaging the deep veins of the legs; orthopedic procedures from arthroscopy to hip, knees, or pelvic repair; or trauma from falls, burns, or crush injuries may contribute to thrombus formation and lead to PE. Hypercoagulation is associated with connective tissue diseases, malignant tumors, and stroke. A genetic factor involving inactivated protein C occurring in about 5% of the population also predisposes these individuals to hypercoagulation. Other risk factors include use of estrogen, advanced age, and obesity. Additionally, a past history of DVT or PE is associated with recurrence.

Signs and Symptoms: Signs and symptoms of PE tend to be nonspecific, so the diagnosis is frequently missed. This is particularly problematic with older pa-tients who tend to have diminished response or atypical presentations. Dyspnea (acute onset), anxiety or apprehension, pleuritic chest pain, cough, tachypnea, and accentuation of the pulmonic component of S_2 are frequently present and may be accompanied by diaphoresis, syncope, tachycardia, S_3 gallop, hypoxemia, and/or hemoptysis. Physical examination usually reveals tachypnea. Auscultation of the lungs may be normal or may demonstrate localized wheezing, consolida-tion, or friction rub. Jugular venous distention and atrial arrhythmia may be present. Examination of the legs, especially of the iliofemoral and popliteal areas, may reveal signs of DVT; the arms, abdomen, and pelvic areas should also be examined for pain, erythema, or palpable vein cords. Although DVT occurs in the calf area of the leg as well, these thrombotic areas account for less than 5% of pulmonary emboli.

Diagnostic Tests: Arterial blood gases (ABGs) may show normal Pao_2 in up to 40% of patients with PE because of hyperventilation. Chest x-ray findings may be abnormal but nonspecific; small, unilateral pleural effusions are seen in up to 50% of patients with PE. Electrocardiogram (ECG) helps rule out cardiac problems such as myocardial infarction and pericarditis. The ventilation-perfusion ($\dot{V}/\dot{Q}$) ratio scan is the most commonly employed diagnostic test for PE; normal results rule out clinically significant PE. Recent research has shed doubt on the ability of the $\dot{V}/\dot{Q}$ scan to diagnose PE accurately in the absence of a high index of suspicion. Pulmonary angiography, the most definitive study for PE, is invasive and very expensive; therefore, it is used primarily when results of a $\dot{V}/\dot{Q}$ scan or lower extremity study are inconclusive and the patient is unstable. Currently, newer forms of computed tomography (CT) scanning are being tested for PE diagnosis, as is magnetic resonance angiography (MRA) (Fig. 8–7).

Differential Diagnosis: Differential diagnosis includes pneumonia, myocardial infarction, pericarditis, CHF, pleural effusion, panic attacks, hyperventilation syndrome, pneumothorax, esophageal rupture, gastritis, gastric or duodenal ulcer, gastroesophageal reflux disease (GERD), and asthma.

Treatment: Anticoagulation using intravenous (IV) heparin with conversion to oral warfarin (Coumadin) is the cornerstone of treatment. Anticoagulation decreases PE-associated mortality from approximately 30% to 8%. Heparin therapy is guided by partial thromboplastin time (PTT) determinations q 6 hr after heparin dose until the therapeutic range is achieved (1.5 to 2 times the normal range of 30–45 sec). PTT is then checked once daily and the warfarin therapy is initiated at 5–10 mg PO daily. Prothrombin time (PT) is measured to maintain the patient with an international normalized ratio (INR) in the therapeutic range of two to three times control levels. Heparin therapy is continued for approximately 5 days after beginning the warfarin to ensure adequate anticoagulation. Warfarin is used for long-term maintenance of 3–6 months, with measurements of the INR three times during the initial week of therapy, tapering to twice weekly for 2 weeks, then once weekly or every other week. Dosage is adjusted based on these results. If the patient is not a candidate for anticoagulation, placement of a vena cava filter is effective to block emboli before they reach the lungs. Selected patients may be candidates for thrombolytic therapy immediately after PE.

Follow-up: Follow-up visits are on an individualized basis. Anticoagulation is usually continued for a minimum of 3 months after the PE. Further therapy is based on risk factors for PE, potential for recurrence, and risks associated with anticoagulation. Close monitoring for control of anticoagulation is essential.

Sequelae: Unrecognized PE can be fatal; many are diagnosed at autopsy. Other complications include alveolar collapse, atelectasis, and pulmonary infarction. The condition tends to recur. Complications from anticoagulation include uncontrolled bleeding and hematoma.

Prevention/Prophylaxis: Patients should avoid controllable risk factors for PE. Encourage frequent ambulation, use of antiembolic stocking, safety precautions to avoid injury to lower extremities, evaluation of possible hypercoagulation pathology, and prophylactic anticoagulation following orthopedic surgery for high-risk patients. Prolonged sitting should be avoided.

Referral: Refer patients to internal medicine or emergency medicine for emergent evaluation and initial treatment plan. Once stable, patients can be managed on warfarin with INR testing in their usual place of residence. Patients may also be candidates for low molecular weight heparin treatment, which is currently investigational for PE but approved for DVT.

Your patient is apprehensive and has chest pain, dyspnea, tachypnea, and cough. You detect increased intensity of the pulmonic portion of the second heart sound and identify one or more risk factors for lower-extremity deep vein thrombosis (DVT).* You suspect pulmonary embolism (PE).†

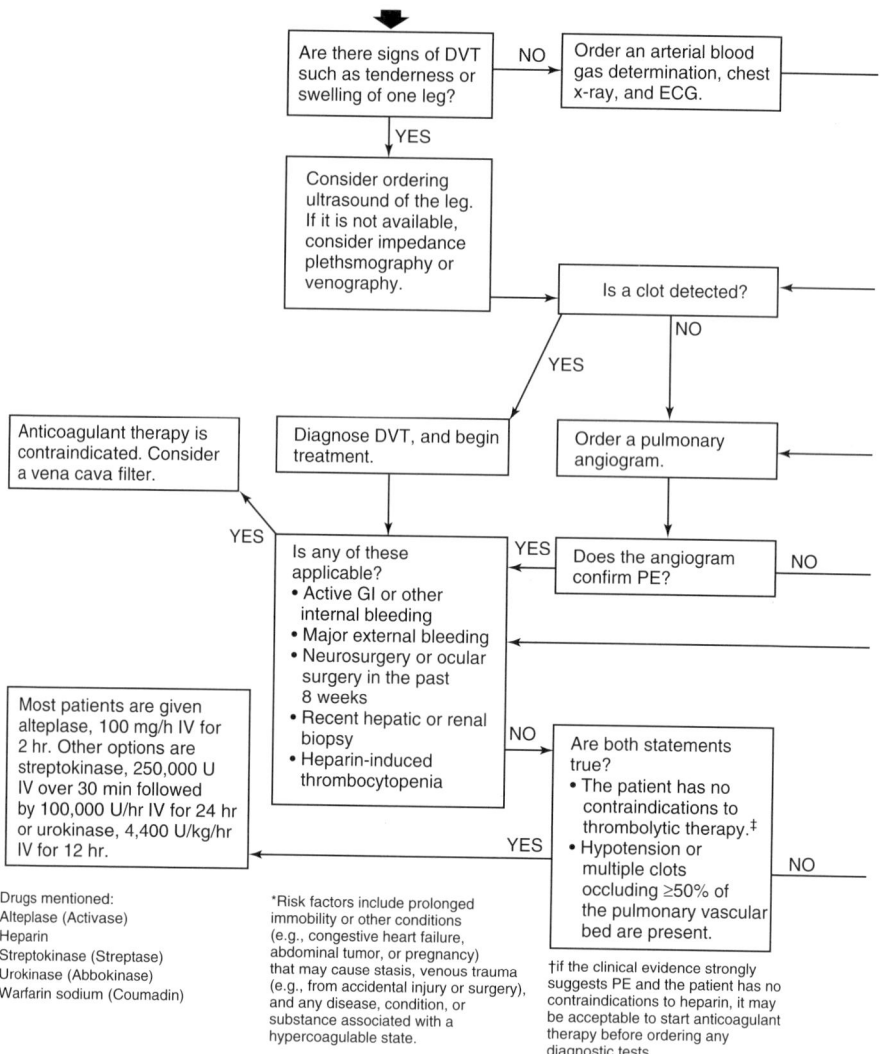

Drugs mentioned:
Alteplase (Activase)
Heparin
Streptokinase (Streptase)
Urokinase (Abbokinase)
Warfarin sodium (Coumadin)

*Risk factors include prolonged immobility or other conditions (e.g., congestive heart failure, abdominal tumor, or pregnancy) that may cause stasis, venous trauma (e.g., from accidental injury or surgery), and any disease, condition, or substance associated with a hypercoagulable state.

†if the clinical evidence strongly suggests PE and the patient has no contraindications to heparin, it may be acceptable to start anticoagulant therapy before ordering any diagnostic tests.

FIGURE 8–7 Initial management of pulmonary embolism.

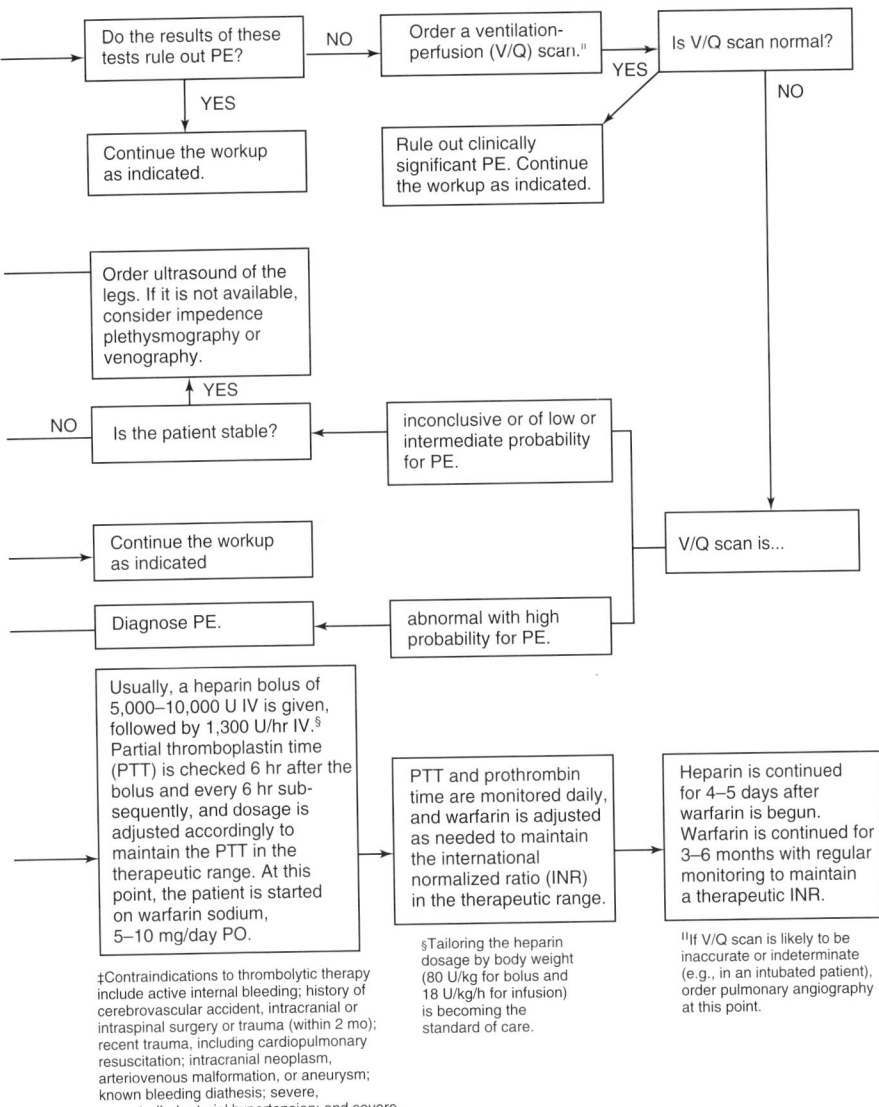

FIGURE 8–7 Continued

Education: Teach the patient, family, or caregiver about risk factors and preventive measures, disease pathology, monitoring for signs of recurrence, and need for compliance with anticoagulation therapy. Instruct the patient to use a soft toothbrush and an electric razor, and to report bleeding gums, hemoptysis, and any blood in stool or urine. Advise patients to avoid aspirin, to consult with their health-care provider prior to taking any over-the-counter (OTC) medications, and to take precautions to avoid bumping or bruising themselves.

Pulmonary Tuberculosis

Tuberculosis (TB), a chronic necrotizing infection caused by a slow-growing acid-fast bacillus (AFB), *Mycobacterium tuberculosis*. TB is the most common infectious disease among humans. The primary site for most cases of TB is the lungs; extrapulmonary TB, which can affect any organ or tissue, is more common among individuals infected with the human immunodeficiency virus (HIV).

Etiology: The infection spreads by inhalation of airborne particles or droplets produced by persons with active pulmonary or laryngeal tuberculosis during coughing, sneezing, singing, and other expiratory efforts. The development of infection after exposure depends on the exposed person's ability to mount an effective immune response on the cellular level. In the initial 2–4 weeks before cellular immunity response occurs, direct pulmonary infection may develop, or lymphohematogenous circulation may lead to miliary, meningeal, or TB adenitis. When T cells recognize the specific antigen, they become sensitized, engaging the macrophages in destroying or containing the tubercle bacilli. This leads to healing, with no residual or calcified lymph nodes in the pulmonary or tracheobronchial areas. This latent stage is typical of 90%–95% of infected persons, leaving them at lifelong risk for reactivation. Tuberculin skin testing documents exposure at this point.

Occurrence: TB occurs worldwide. An estimated 10 million in the United States are infected with TB, with 3 million deaths annually. More than 20,000 new cases occur each year; 90% of these are a reactivation of previous infection (recrudescent, postprimary), and 10% are new infections.

Age: Immunosuppressed patients of any age are more commonly affected. Children and adolescents are more likely to have primary disease; adults and elderly persons are more likely to have recrudescent disease.

Ethnicity: Persons born in geographic areas where TB is more prevalent, including Asia, Africa, and Latin America, are at higher risk. Native Americans are at higher risk because of environmental factors (crowding, poor health, poor nutrition).

Gender: Occurs in men more frequently than in women.

Contributing Factors: Contributing factors include

- A compromised immune system (especially from HIV infection) or prolonged corticosteroid or other immunosuppressive therapy.
- Close contact with an individual with active TB (household contacts, sharing a common ventilation system).
- Substance abuse.
- Malnutrition.
- Residence in a long-term care facility.
- Homelessness.
- Medically underserved, low-income aggregates, including African-American, Latin-American, and Native American.
- Correctional system inmates.
- Coexistence of chronic medical conditions such as diabetes mellitus; silicosis; lymphoma, leukemia, and other malignancies; chronic renal failure; history of gastrectomy; and body weight 10% below ideal.

Signs and Symptoms: Typical presentation includes cough, hemoptysis, weight loss, anorexia, adenopathy, fever, night sweats, decreased activity level, and pleuritic pain. In the average population, the onset is gradual and may go undetected for some time. In the older patient, these findings are not usually present, or they are so subtle and so intermingled with other chronic illness symptoms as to be undistinguishable. Weight loss, unexplained fever, or anorexia may be the only symptoms. Typical simulations include pneumonia, bronchitis, or CHF with pleural effusion. Extrapulmonary TB may manifest with symptoms typical to the site involved (e.g., urinary incontinence or frequency and urgency for bladder TB). Physical examination may be unrevealing: nonspecific signs such as fever or weight loss may be the only findings. In some persons, a positive tuberculin test reaction is the only manifestation. Chest examination may demonstrate crackles that do not clear with cough in advanced apical disease. If pleural effusion is present, percussion in the area may be dull. In the presence of large cavities, amphoric breath sounds may be present on auscultation.

Diagnostic Tests: The standard intradermal test to screen for exposure to TB or detect an active case of TB is the Mantoux test, with intermediate purified protein derivative (PPD) 5 units. The test is very technique specific; if administered too deeply, without producing the required bleb, it is invalid and must be repeated at another site. Interpretation of the result is also subject to error; the area of induration or hardness, not erythema, must be measured with a millimeter ruler 48–72 hr after the agent is administered. The results demonstrate the ability of the person tested to mount a delayed type hypersensitivity (DTH) response to prior infection. Appropriate measurement parameters for reactive and nonreactive results are as follows:

- *Induration of 0 mm:* Nonreactive: seen in patients with anergy or no infection; presence of active TB still possible (close contacts of persons with recently diagnosed TB should be retested in 8–12 weeks).

- *Induration of 5 mm:* Reactive: seen in patients with known or suspected HIV infection; in close contacts of a patient with active TB; in intravenous (IV) drug abusers of unknown HIV status; and in those with chest x-ray findings suspicious of prior TB.
- *Induration of 10 mm:* Reactive: seen in residents of long-term care facilities (nursing homes, prisons); foreign-born persons; children under age 4; HIV-negative IV drug abusers; low-income, medically underserved groups; health-care workers in settings where patients with TB are likely to be found; high-risk racial and ethnic groups; those with medical problems placing them at increased risk of active TB.
- *Induration of 15 mm:* Reactive: seen in good health, with no known TB risk factors.

When reporting or recording results, specify reactive or nonreactive and the millimeter measurement for induration. Many older patients have an impaired DTH response to the tuberculin testing. For this reason, "boosting" is recommended if the initial test results in an induration of less than 10 mm, to avoid false-negatives. Within 7–10 days after the initial test is read, a second test is administered; the result of the second test is considered the authentic result. Immunosuppressed individuals who cannot mount a response to the PPD may be given an anergy panel (*Candida, Trichophyton,* and mumps).

Use of steroids may cause a false-negative skin test result; recent vaccination with bacille Calmette-Guérin (BCG) can cause a false-positive result. For specific details regarding protocol in these and other atypical cases, consult Centers for Disease Control (CDC) or State Health Department guidelines.

Diagnosis of pulmonary TB is based on positive bacteriologic cultures, including sputum for AFB yielding positive results on staining and growing *M. tuberculosis* on culture. Cultures may take 4–6 weeks, so treatment is begun once an assumption of active disease is made. Drug sensitivities should be ascertained with cultures to identify strains resistant to typical first-line agents. Early morning sputa are optimal; it may be necessary to collect induced specimens.

Chest x-ray in reactivated disease may show nodular or patchy infiltrates in the apical or upper lobe areas posteriorly and inferiorly; apical lordotic views are helpful. Cavitary nodules are also frequently seen. In primary disease, nonspecific infiltrates in any areas or the presence of pleural effusion may be visualized; if concurrent hilar adenopathy is present, TB is a prime consideration.

When extrapulmonary foci are suspected, special testing of the involved organ systems is conducted.

Because most TB in elderly persons represents a reactivation of an old lesion, drug resistance is less likely than with newly acquired infection.

Differential Diagnosis: Pneumonia, lymphoma, fungal infections, CHF, pleural effusion, and lung cancer can mimic TB.

Treatment: Prior to treatment, obtain baseline values for liver function, bilirubin, CBC blood urea nitrogen (BUN), creatinine, and serum uric acid. For newly diagnosed, active TB, initial treatment consists of combined therapy using four first-line drugs: isoniazid (INH), rifampin (RIF), pyrazinamide (PZA), and ethambutol (EMB), until culture results are complete. Several treatment options are available. The most commonly used is presented here (for further information, consult with the CDC).

Daily for 2 months:	INH 5 mg/kg (300 mg max)
	RIF 10 mg/kg (600 mg max)
	PZA 15–30 mg/kg (2 g max)
	EMB 15–25 mg/kg (1 g max)
Then daily for 4 months:	INH and RIF (see preceding dosage schedule)

In lieu of daily therapy for 4 months, the same agents (INH, RIF) can be used as follows:

INH 15 mg/kg (900 mg max) two or three times weekly by directly observed therapy (DOT).

RIF 10 mg/kg (600 mg max) two or three times weekly by DOT.

For HIV-positive individuals, length of treatment is 12 months. The basis for treatment is

Availability of two drugs to which the bacterium is susceptible.

Prolonged treatment is needed.

Compliance is key to successful control of disease.

Follow-up: Patients being treated for active pulmonary TB should have sputum for AFB smear and culture performed monthly until a negative culture is obtained. If cultures are not negative after 3 months, reevaluate treatment. Follow-up cultures at 6 and 12 months are advisable to detect late relapse. Chest x-ray examination should be done at 2–3 months and at therapy termination to evaluate response. Periodic liver enzymes are necessary, especially if the patient is taking INH, to monitor for effects on hepatotoxicity. For the frail elderly adult in a long-term care setting, more frequent monitoring for adverse effects of treatment including anorexia, polyneuropathy, or development of medication-induced hepatitis is warranted. DOT is the norm in these settings, so compliance is less of a concern. Refer community-dwelling elderly persons to the local or state health department for follow-up, monitoring of medication compliance and side effects, patient and family education, and testing of close contacts. Tuberculosis is a reportable disease.

Many agencies charged with monitoring and control have outreach services such as home visits. Emphasize to patients that compliance is critical to successful control. If no follow-up visitation is available through the monitoring agency, see the patient for monthly follow-up visits in the office.

Sequelae: Possible complications include development of drug-resistant organisms, particularly if a patient is noncompliant with the prescribed treatment.

Secondary infection of cavitary lesions and development of treatment-associated hepatitis or polyneuropathy are possible. If treatment is ineffective, spread of disease to other close contacts can occur.

Prevention/Prophylaxis: For older patients residing in long-term care settings, PPD testing before admission to the facility is required unless there is documented evidence of a positive test result in the past. If the initial test result is nonreactive (less than 10 mm induration after 48–72 hr), a second test should be performed within 2 weeks to evaluate for the booster phenomenon. Anergy testing can be performed if indicated. Annual retesting is recommended. Patients with a positive PPD reaction, including booster, need a chest x-ray to evaluate for active disease. Staff are required to have tuberculin skin testing at initial employment and annually.

The decision to institute chemoprophylaxis is a clinical judgment, based on a comparison of individual factors with the risk of developing TB versus the risk of INH toxicity. Recommendations for preventive therapy are as follows:

- Household members and other close contacts of patient with active TB.
- Recent PPD converter.
- Prior history of untreated TB.
- Reactive skin test and abnormal chest x-ray film consistent with inactive, old TB lesions.
- Reactive skin test, age under 35 years.
- Reactive skin test and risk factor for activation of TB such as silicosis, diabetes mellitus, HIV, end stage renal disease, malnutrition, and prolonged immunosuppressive or corticosteroid therapy.
- Chemoprophylaxis drug is INH 300 mg PO daily for 6 months in an otherwise healthy person. In immunosuppressed individuals with abnormal but stable chest x-ray findings, duration of therapy is 9 months, except for HIV-positive individuals, for whom duration is 12 months.

Referral: Patients may be referred to a government-associated community agency such as the health department or to an infectious disease or pulmonary specialist for initial evaluation and management recommendations. Refer patients with concurrent positive HIV status or confirmed acquired immunodeficiency syndrome (AIDS) to specialized treatment services or collaborate in management with specialists in this area. Refer patients with severe anorexia or malnutrition to a dietician.

Education: Teach patient, caregivers, close contacts, and paraprofessional providers about the nature of the disease, its mode of transmission, screening and control measures, and follow-up required. Teach the patient or caregiver about medications, drug actions and possible side effects, length of treatment, and need for compliance.

Restrictive Lung Disease

Restrictive lung disease refers to a heterogenous group of disorders that share a common abnormal ventilatory function. Restricted breathing is characterized by small tidal volume and rapid rate. The hallmark of restrictive pattern is a decrease in lung volumes, principally total lung capacity (TLC) and vital capacity (VC).

Etiology: Restrictive lung diseases, which have a variety of etiologies, are divided into subgroups based on the location of the pathology:

Restrictive/parenchymal/interstitial: In addition to a decrease in TLC and VC, residual volume (RV) is also decreased. Forced expiratory flow rates are maintained.

- Sarcoidosis.
- Idiopathic pulmonary fibrosis.
- Pneumoconiosis.
- Occupational lung disease.
- Drug/radiation-induced interstitial lung disease.

Restrictive/extraparenchymal: Abnormalities can be predominantly in inspiration or in both inspiration and expiration.

- Neuromuscular.
  - Diaphragmatic weakness/paralysis.
  - Myasthenia gravis.°
  - Muscular dystrophies.°
  - Cervical spine injuries.°
  - Guillain-Barré syndrome.°
- Chest wall.
  - Kyphoscoliosis.
  - Obesity.
  - Ankylosing spondylitis.°

° Limitations may be both inspiratory and expiratory.

Occurrence: The incidence of restrictive lung disease is undeterminable because several distinct entities are involved. Occupational lung diseases are common in farmers and in those who work with silica asbestos, beryllium, or cotton.

Age: Occupationally induced disease is seen predominantly in the older population; other restrictive lung diseases may occur at any age.

Ethnicity: Not significant.

Gender: The incidence is higher in men than women, for occupational types of restrictive lung disease.

Contributing Factors: Risk factors vary with etiology, including exposure to occupational dust, abnormalities in skeletal structure, and autoimmune disorders.

Signs and Symptoms: Patients have a gradual onset of dyspnea, initially occurring only with exertion, and progressing dyspnea at rest. The breathing pattern is rapid and shallow. A nonproductive cough may also be present. A careful history may disclose prior occupational risk factors. Use of tobacco should also be ascertained; it is not uncommon for patients to have a mixed pattern of obstructive and restrictive disease. Physical findings may reveal skeletal abnormalities such as kyphoscoliosis, limiting lung expansion. The initial presentation of breathing problems often occurs after an acute respiratory viral infection.

Physical assessment of the lung may be initially unremarkable. With progression of the disease, you will typically hear inspiratory crackles (Velcro) at the bases. You may see cyanosis and clubbing of fingers and toes. In the end stages, signs of right-sided heart failure, including cor pulmonale, appear.

Diagnostic Tests: Pulmonary function testing (PFT) is valuable in distinguishing obstructive from restrictive disease, and in characterizing the type of restrictive (extraparenchymal or parenchymal) disease (Table 8–5). The FEV_1/FVC ratio is normal. Other changes were identified earlier (see Etiology).

Interstitial lung diseases share some common findings on chest radiographs including the appearance of increased interstitial markers. Typical descriptive terms for x-ray findings include honeycomb pattern, miliary pattern, ground-glass pattern, and nodular appearance. High-resolution CT scan can detect early interstitial disease with a normal chest x-ray film, determine the extent of the disease, and offer a guide for bronchoscopy with biopsy and broncheolar lavage. In the late stages, arterial blood gases (ABGs) help to identify the degree of hypoxemia and CO_2 retention.

Differential Diagnosis: Infectious or neoplastic diseases, chronic obstructive pulmonary disease (COPD), and congestive heart failure (CHF) can mimic restrictive lung disease.

Treatment: Therapy depends on the cause of disease and the disease progression. Smoking cessation should be pursued aggressively if this is an issue. Occupational exposures should be avoided. Corticosteroid therapy with prednisone 1 mg/kg per day initially is indicated for most interstitial diseases, tapering after 8–12 weeks to maintenance. If corticosteroid treatment is ineffective, cytotoxic agents including azathioprine (Imuran) and cyclophosphamide (Cytoxan) have been tried. In the end stage, administer supplemental O_2 for supportive care. Lung transplantation may be considered in selected cases.

TABLE 8–5 RESTRICTIVE VERSUS OBSTRUCTIVE PFT

	FVC%	FEV₁%	FEV₁/FVC
Restrictive	↓	↓	N
Obstructive	↓ or N	↓	↓

Follow-up: Follow-up visits are scheduled as indicated by symptoms and comorbidities. Periodic chest x-ray films or PETs may help to chart course and to evaluate response to treatment.

Sequelae: Use of corticosteroids or immunosuppressives may result in increased risk of infection. Pulmonary hypertension and right-sided heart failure may occur. Restrictive lung diseases are chronic.

Prevention/Prophylaxis: Give patients the pneumococcal pneumonia and influenza vaccine. Advise patients to avoid known exposures, tobacco use, and persons with acute, infectious upper respiratory illness.

Referrals: Initially refer patients to pulmonary specialist for bronchoscopy, and consider collaborative management. If immunosuppressives are used, refer the patient for initial recommendations and periodic reevaluation.

Education: Teach the patient about chronic disease management, regular self-care habits, and early intervention in acute illness.

Upper Respiratory Tract Infection

An upper respiratory tract infection (URI), also known as the common cold, is usually caused by a virus and results in inflammation of the nasal passages. Most URIs are self-limiting and accompanied only by minor somatic complaints.

Etiology: URIs are usually caused by a virus such as rhinovirus; influenza A, B, and C viruses; parainfluenza viruses; respiratory syncytial viruses; coronaviruses; adenoviruses; and enteric cytopathogenic human orphan (ECHO) viruses. Additionally, *Mycobacterium avium* and *Pneumocystis carinii* have been found in older patients who are not immunosuppressed. In 40% of cases, no agent can be identified. The usual mode of transmission is hand-to-hand from contaminated nasal secretions. The incubation period is 1–3 days, with the usual URI lasting 6–10 days.

Occurrence: URIs are the most common cause of short-term disability in the United States, occurring in 31 in 100 people per year.

Age: URIs occur more frequently in children than in adults.

Ethnicity: Native Americans and Eskimos are at higher risk than other ethnic groups and may suffer more frequent complications of colds.

Gender: URIs occur equally in men and women.

Contributing Factors: Risk factors for developing URIs include exposure to infected individuals, contact between nose or conjunctiva and contaminated fingers. Older persons with diabetes get more frequent URIs than the general population.

Signs and Symptoms: Most common signs and symptoms include nasal obstruction and stuffiness (80%–100% of patients), sneezing (50%–70%), and scratchy throat (50%). Other signs and symptoms include cough (40%), hoarseness (30%), malaise (20%–25%), headache (25%), and fever above 100°F (less than 1%). Physical examination may reveal mucopurulent nasal drainage, nasopharyngeal mucosal swelling, and lymphadenopathy. (Pharyngeal exudates are unusual in viral infections and more common in bacterial infections.)

Diagnostic Tests

Laboratory: Complete blood count (CBC) if symptoms persist for more than 10 days or the patient has a fever above 100°F. Nasal smear for eosinophils is indicated if allergic rhinitis is suspected. Throat cultures are needed if streptococcal pharyngitis is suspected. Monospot test may be performed to rule out mononucleosis.

Procedures: Skin testing may be performed in patients with rhinitis when the diagnosis is not clear.

Differential Diagnosis: Symptoms of influenza, chronic rhinitis, sinusitis, Epstein-Barr virus, mumps, and rubeola mimic those of URIs. The use of medications such as nasal sprays (when use is continuous), antihypertensives, hormones, psychotropic drugs, aspirin, and nonsteroid anti-inflammatory drugs (NSAIDs) can cause symptoms similar to those of URIs.

Treatment: URIs are usually managed on an outpatient basis.

Physical: URIs are treated with rest, increased fluid intake, and symptom relief measures such as humidified air.

Pharmacologic: Over-the-counter (OTC) medications may be taken for pain, fever, congestion, or cough relief. Topical nasal and oral decongestants are available, with topical decongestants preferred owing to fewer systemic side effects. The nasal decongestant of choice is oxymetazoline; the oral decongestant of choice is pseudoephedrine. When a cough is nonproductive or prevents normal rest and activities, it may be treated with a cough suppressant that contains dextromethorphan or codeine. Rinsing with mouthwashes, sucking on lozenges or hard candy, gargling with warm saline, and using products with local anesthetics such as benzocaine or phenol may provide subjective relief of sore throat pain. The use of antihistamines, vitamin C (ascorbic acid), and expectorants is controversial.

Follow-up: See the patient if symptoms last longer than 6–10 days or if the patient develops fever associated with systemic symptoms, difficulty breathing, or purulent nasal drainage.

Sequelae: Possible complications include lower respiratory tract infection, sinusitis, and aggravation of asthma symptoms.

Prevention/Prophylaxis: Advise the patient to perform frequent proper handwashing, avoid touching the face, and avoid contact with infected people.

Pneumococcal and influenza vaccinations are recommended for all older adults.

Referral: Usually neither referral nor consultation is necessary if the patient has an uncomplicated URI.

Education: Explain the disease process, signs and symptoms, and treatment (including side effects of medications). Discuss prevention strategies and when to contact a health-care provider.

BIBLIOGRAPHY

Cardiac Assessment

Brecker, SJD, and Oldershaw, PJ: Chapter 6: Echocardiography. In Martin, A, and Camm, AJ (eds): Geriatric Cardiology: Principles and Practice. John Wiley and Sons, New York, 1994.

Camm, AJ, Katritsis, D, and Ward, DE: Chapter 7: Clinical electrocardiography and electrophysiology in the elderly. In Martin, A, and Camm, AJ (eds): Geriatric Cardiology: Principles and Practice. John Wiley and Sons, New York, 1994.

Constant, J: Chapter 4: Clinical findings in the elderly heart patient. In Messerli, FH (ed): Cardiovascular Disease in the Elderly, ed 3. Kluwer Academic Publishers, Boston, 1993.

Fleg, JL: Chapter 3: Electrocardiographic findings in older persons without clinical heart disease. In Tresch, DD, and Aronow, WS (eds): Cardiovascular Disease in the Elderly Patient. Marcel Dekker, New York, 1994.

Fleg, JL, Gerstenblith, G, and Lakatta, EG: Chapter 3: Pathophysiology of the aging heart and circulation. In Messerli, FH (ed): Cardiovascular Disease in the Elderly, ed 3. Kluwer Academic Publishers, Boston, 1993.

Gardin, JM: Chapter 4: Echocardiographic measurements in elderly patients without clinical heart disease. In Tresch, DD, and Aronow, WS (eds): Cardiovascular Disease in the Elderly Patient. Marcel Dekker, New York, 1994.

Kannel, W: Range of serum cholesterol values in the population developing coronary artery disease. Am J Cardiol 76:69c–77c, 1995.

LaCroix, AZ, et al: Smoking and mortality among older men and women in three communities. N Engl J Med 324:1619–1625, 1991.

Lakatta, EG: Changes in cardiovascular function with aging. Eur Heart J 11(Suppl C):22–29, 1990.

Leatham, A: Chapter 5: Clinical examination. In Martin, A, and Camm, AJ (eds): Geriatric Cardiology: Principles and Practice. John Wiley and Sons, New York, 1994.

Lowenthal, D: Geriatric Cardiology. In Cardiovascular Clinics 22:2. FA Davis, Philadelphia, 1992.

Schulman, SP: Chapter 1: Normal aging changes of the cardiovascular system. In Tresch, DD, and Aronow WS (eds): Cardiovascular Disease in the Elderly Patient. Marcel Dekker, New York, 1994.

Scientific American Medicine: Coronary artery disease. In Rubenstein, E, and Federman, DD (eds): Scientific American Medicine, 1978–1998. Scientific American Medicine, Inc, New York, 1994.

SHEP Cooperative Research Group: Prevention of stroke by antihypertensive drug treatment in older persons with isolated systolic hypertension. JAMA 265:3255–3264, 1991.

Swales, JD, Fletcher, AE, and Bulpitt, CJ: Chapter 2: Epidemiology. In Messerli, FH (ed): Cardiovascular Disease in the Elderly, ed 3. Kluwer Academic Publishers, Boston, 1993.

Tresch, DD, and Aronow, WS: Chapter 11: Recognition and diagnosis of coronary artery disease in the elderly. In Tresch, DD, and Aronow, WS (eds): Cardiovascular Disease in the Elderly Patient. Marcel Dekker, New York, 1994.

Wilson, AG: Chapter 9: The chest radiograph. In Martin, A, and Camm, AJ (eds): Geriatric Cardiology: Principles and Practice. John Wiley and Sons, New York, 1994.

Arrhythmias

Aronow, WS: Treatment of ventricular arrhythmias in older adults. J Am Geriatr Soc 43:688, 1995.

Arrhythmias and conduction disorders. In Abrams, WB, Beers, MH, and Berkow, R (eds): The Merck Manual of Geriatrics, ed 2. Merck Research Laboratories, Whitehouse Station, NJ, 1995.

Chung, M, and Klein, A: Atrial fibrillation. In Rubenstein, E, and Federman, DD (eds): Scientific American Medicine, 1978–1998. Scientific American Medicine, Inc, New York, 1997.

Furberg, CT, et al: Prevalence of atrial fibrillation in elderly subjects (The Cardiovascular Health Study). Am J Cardiol 74:236, 1994.

Greenberg, HM, et al: Interactions of ischeaemia and encinide/flecainide treatment: A proposed mechanism for the increased mortality in CAST I. British Heart Journal 74(6):631–635, 1995.

Horowitz, LN, and Lynch, RA: Managing geriatric arrhythmias I: General considerations. Geriatrics 46(3):31, 1991.

Lynch, RA, and Horowitz, LN: Managing geriatric arrhythmias II: Drug selection and use. Geriatrics 46(4):41, 1991.

Langberg, JJ, and LeLurgio, DB: Ventricular arrhythmias. In Rubenstein, E, and Federman, DD (eds): Scientific American Medicine, 1978–1998. Scientific American Medicine, Inc, New York, 1997.

Murgatroyd, FD, Bashir, Y, and Camm, AJ: Chapter 20: Cardiac arrhythmias in the elderly. In Camm, AJ, and Martin, A: Geriatric Cardiology: Principles and Practices. John Wiley and Sons, New York, 1994.

Ravikishore, AG, and Camm, AJ: Chapter 4: Dangerous and treatable cardiac arrhythmias in elderly people. In Sinclair, AJ, and Woodhouse, KW (eds): Acute Medical Illness in Old Age. Chapman and Hall, London, 1995.

Rippe, JM, and Albert, JS: Chapter 3: Arrhythmias. In: Manual of Cardiovascular Diagnosis and Therapy. Little, Brown, Boston, 1985.

Spratt, KA, Michelson, EL, and Dreifus, LS: Chapter 8: Disturbances in cardiac rhythm. In Messerli, FH (ed): Cardiovascular Disease in the Elderly, ed 3. Kluwer Academic Publishers, Boston, 1993.

Tchou, PJ, and Trohman, RG: Supraventricular tachycardia. In Rubenstein, E, and Federman, DD (eds): Scientific American Medicine, 1978–1998. Scientific American Medicine, Inc, New York, 1997.

Congestive Heart Failure

Aronow, WS: The ELITE study. Drugs and Aging 12(6):423–428, 1998.

Braunwald, E: Heart failure. In Harrison's Principles of Internal Medicine, ed 13. McGraw-Hill, New York, 1994.

Cannon, L, and Marshall, J: Cardiac disease in the elderly population. Clin Geriatr Med 9:3, 1993.

Dracup, K, Dunba, S, and Baker, D: Rethinking heart failure. AJN 95:7, 1995.

Dec, GW, and Hutler, AM: Congestive heart failure. In Rubenstein, E, and Federman, DD (eds): Scientific American Medicine, 1978–1998. Scientific American Medicine, Inc, New York, 1997.

Guerra-Garcia, H, Taffet, G, and Luchi, R: Congestive heart failure: Treatment modifications in the elderly. Consultant 34:4, 1994.

Heart Failure: Evaluation and Care of Patients with Left-Ventricular Systolic Dysfunction. AHCPR Clinical Practice Guideline, Agency on Health Care Policy and Research, US Dept. of Health & Human Services, Rockville, MD, 1994.

Luchi, R, Taffet, G, and Teasdale, T: Congestive heart failure in the elderly. J Am Geriatr Soc 39:8, 1991.

Massie, B, and Wolfe, C: Heart failure. In Messerli, F (ed): Cardiovascular Disease in the Elderly, ed 3. Kluwer Academic Publishers, Boston, 1993.

Rich, MW: Epidemiology, pathophysiology and etiology of congestive heart failure in older adults. J Am Geriatr Soc 45:968–974, 1997.

Hypertension

Gifford, R: Managing hypertension in the elderly: Dispelling the myths. Cleve Clin J Med 62:29, 1995.

Joint National Committee: The sixth report of the Joint National Committee on Detection, Evaluation, and Treatment of High Blood Pressure. Arch Intern Med 157:2413–2446, 1997.

Kaplan, N: Hypertension in the elderly. Annu Rev Med 45:27–35, 1995.

Kaplan, N: Southwestern Internal Medicine Conference: The promises and perils of treating the elderly hypertensive. Am J Med Sci 305(3):183, 1993.

Kochar, M: Hypertension in elderly patients. Postgrad Med 91(4):393, 1992.

National High Blood Pressure Education Program Working Group: National High Blood Pressure Working Group report on hypertension in the elderly. Hypertension 23:275, 1994.

Oparil, S, and Calhoun, DA: High blood pressure. In Rubenstein, E, and Federman, DD (eds): Scientific American Medicine, 1978–1998. Scientific American Medicine, Inc, New York, 1997.

Rippe, JM, and Alpert, JS: Chapter 11: Hypertension. In Manual of Cardiovascular Diagnosis and Therapy. Little, Brown, Boston, 1985.

Weinburger, M: Hypertension in the elderly. Hospital Practice 103 (May 15):103–120, 1992.

Ischemic Heart Disease

Elder, A, and Fox, K: Chapter 17: Ischaemic heart disease in the elderly. In Martin, A, and Camm, AJ: Geriatric Cardiology: Principles and Practice. John Wiley and Sons, New York, 1994.

Fazar, E, Lazar, J, and Frishman, W: Angina pectoris and silent ischemia in the elderly: A management update. Geriatrics 47(7):24, 1992.

Frishman, W: Treatment of myocardial ischemia and myocardial infarction in the elderly. South Med J 86(10):S29, 1993.

Howell, J, and Hedges, J: Differential diagnosis of chest discomfort and general approach to myocardial ischemia decision making. Am J Emerg Med 9(6):571, 1991.

Hutler, AM: Ischemic heart disease: Angina pectoris. In Rubenstein, E, and Federman, DD (eds): Scientific American Medicine, 1978–1998. Scientific American Medicine, Inc, New York, 1997.

Limacher, M: Chapter 6: Clinical features of coronary heart disease in the elderly. In Lowenthal, D (ed): Cardiovascular Clinics 22(2):63–71, FA Davis, Philadelphia, 1992.

Pepine, C, and Pepine, A: Chapter 13: Intervention therapy for coronary artery disease in the elderly. In Lowenthal, D (ed): Cardiovascular Clinics 22(2):175, FA Davis, Philadelphia, 1992.

Salley, R, and Robinson, C: Ischemic heart disease in the elderly: The role of coronary angioplasty and coronary artery bypass grafting. South Med J 86(10):S15, 1993.

Segal, B: Managing angina in the elderly: An update. Geriatrics 44(1):55, 1989.

Myocardial Infarction

Cannon, L, and Marshall, J: Cardiac disease in the elderly population. Clin Geriatr Med 9:3, 1993.

Carnevali, D, and Patrick, M: Nursing Management for the Elderly, ed 3. JB Lippincott, Philadelphia, 1993.

Devlin, W, et al: Comparison of outcomes in patients with myocardial infarction aged >75 years with that in younger patients. Am J Cardiol 75(8):573–576, 1995.

Fulmer, T, and Walker, M (eds): Critical Care Nursing of the Elderly. Springer, New York, 1991.

Herlitz, J, et al: Optimal treatment after acute myocardial infarction in the elderly. Drugs Aging 6:3, 1995.

Pasternak, RC, and Braumwald, E: Acute myocardial infarction. In Isselbacker, KJ, et al (eds): Harrison's Principles of Internal Medicine, ed 13. McGraw-Hill, New York, 1994.

Sinclair, D: Myocardial infarction: Considerations for geriatric patients. Can Fam Physician 40:1172–1177, 1994.

Sokolyk, S, and Tresch, D: Treatment of myocardial infarction in elderly patients. Compr Ther 20:10, 1994.

Suarez, G, et al: Prediction on admission of in-hospital mortality in patients older than 70 years with acute myocardial infarction. Chest 108:1, 1995.

Thompson, L, Wood, C, and Wallhagen, M: Geriatric acute myocardial infarction: A challenge to recognition, prompt diagnosis, and appropriate care. Critical Care Nursing Clinics of North America 4:2, 1992.

Tresch, DD: Management of the older patient with acute myocardial infarction. J Am Geriatr Soc 46:1157–1162, 1998.

Valvular Disease

Booth, DC, and Demaria, AN: Chapter 11: Valvular heart disease in the elderly. In Messerli, FH (ed): Cardiovascular Disease in the Elderly, ed 3. Kluwer Academic Publishers, Boston, 1993.

Valvular heart disease. In Abrams, WB, Beers, MH, and Berkow, R (eds): The Merck Manual of Geriatrics, ed 2. Merck Research Laboratories, Whitehouse Station, NJ, 1995.

Currie, PJ: Valvular heart disease: A correctable cause of congestive heart failure. Postgrad Med 89:123, 1991.

Griffin, BP: Valvular heart disease. In Rubenstein, E, and Federman, DD (eds): Scientific American Medicine, 1978–1998. Scientific American, Inc, New York, 1998.

Kaiser, G: Practice guidelines in cardiothoracic surgery. Ann Thorac Surg 59:1264, 1995.

Marzo, KP, and Herling, IM: Chapter 9: Valvular disease in the elderly. In Fran, KL, and Brest, AN (eds): Cardiovascular Clinics 23:175, FA Davis, Philadelphia, 1993.

McEwan, JR, and Oakley, CM: Chapter 18: Valve disease in the elderly. In Martin, A, and Camm, AJ (eds): Geriatric Cardiology: Principles and Practices. John Wiley and Sons, New York, 1994.

Tresch, DD: Atypical presentations of cardiovascular disorders in the elderly. Geriatrics 42(10):31, 1987.

Respiratory Assessment

Abrams, WB, Beers, MH, and Berkow, R: The Merck Manual of Geriatrics, ed 2, Merck Research Laboratories, Whitehouse Station, NJ, 1995.

Bates, B, Bickley, LS, and Hoekelman, RA: A Guide to Physical Examination and History Taking, ed 6. JB Lippincott, Philadelphia, 1995.

Ebersole, P, and Hess, P: Toward Healthy Aging, ed 4. CV Mosby, St Louis, 1994.

Eliopoulos, C: Health Assessment of the Older Adult, ed 2. Addison-Wesley Nursing, Redwood City, CA, 1990.

Jarvis CA: Physical Examination and Health Assessment, ed 2. WB Saunders, Philadelphia, 1996.

Mezey, MD, Rauckhorst, LH, and Stakes, SA: Health Assessment of the Older Individual, ed 2. Springer, New York, 1993.

Chronic Bronchitis

Bornbrand, L, Hoole, AJ, and Pickard, CG: Manual of Clinical Problems in Adult Ambulatory Care, ed 2. Little, Brown, Boston, 1992.

Cole, RB, and Mackey, AD: Essentials of Respiratory Disease, ed 3. Churchill Livingstone, New York, 1990.

Heath, JM: Outpatient management of chronic bronchitis in the elderly. Am Fam Physician 48:841, 1993.

Hodgkin, JE, Kigin, CM, Nett, LM, and Tiep, BL: Your role in COPD in home care. Patient Care 26:147, 1992.

Hofford, JM: Metered dose inhaler therapy for asthma, bronchitis, and emphysema. J Fam Pract 34:485, 1992.

Hoole, AJ, et al: Patient Care Guidelines for Nurse Practitioners, ed 4. JB Lippincott, Philadelphia, 1995.

Reichel, W: Care of the Elderly: Clinical Aspects of Aging, ed 4. Williams & Wilkins, Baltimore, 1995.

Rosen, MJ: Treatment of exacerbation of COPD. Am Fam Physician 45:693, 1992.

Staab, A, and Lyles, M: Manual of Geriatric Nursing. Scott, Foresman, Glenview, IL, 1990.

COPD

Celli, BR, Cosentino, A, Fiel, S, and Petty, TL: The challenge of COPD: Step by step through the workup. Patient Care 31(2):21–52, 1997.

Celli, BR, et al: The challenge of COPD: Therapeutic strategies that work. Patient Care 31(5):101–118, 1997.

Celli, BR, et al: The challenge of COPD: Managing the special problems of chronic lung disease. Patient Care 31(7):87–98, 1997.

Chernecky, CC, and Bergey, BJ: Laboratory Tests and Diagnostic Procedures, ed 2. WB Saunders, Philadelphia, 1997.

Dambro, M: Griffith's 5 Minute Clinical Consult. Williams & Wilkins, Baltimore, 1997.

King, TE, and Newman, K: The aging lung, chronic obstructive pulmonary disease, asthma, and pulmonary rehabilitation. In Jahnigen, DW, and Schrier, RW: Geriatric Medicine, ed 2. Blackwell Scientific, Cambridge, MA, 1997.

Stauffer, JL: Disorders of the airways. In Tierney, LM, McPhee, SJ, and Papadakis, MA (eds): Current Medical Diagnosis and Treatment, ed 36. Appleton & Lange, Norwalk, CT, 1997.

Zopey, L, and Williams, AJ: Chronic obstructive pulmonary disease and asthma. In Yoshikawa, TT, Cobbs, EL, and Brummel-Smith, K: Practical Ambulatory Geriatrics, ed 2. CV Mosby, St Louis, 1998.

Lung Cancer

Fischer, DS: Follow-up of Cancer: A Handbook for Physicians. Lippincott-Raven, Philadelphia, 1996.

Ginsberg, RJ, Kris, MG, and Armstrong, JG: Non-small cell lung cancer. In DeVita, VT, Hellman, S, and Rosenberg, SA (eds): Cancer: Principles and Practices of Oncology. JB Lippincott, Philadelphia, 1993.

Gorroll, AH, May, LA, and Mulley, AG: Primary Care Medicine: Office Evaluation and Management of the Adult Patient, ed 3. JB Lippincott, Philadelphia, 1995.

Ihde, DC, Pass, HI, and Glatstein, EJ: Small cell lung cancer. In DeVita, VT, Hellman, S, and Rosenberg, SA (eds): Cancer: Principles and Practices of Oncology. JB Lippincott, Philadelphia, 1993.

Minna, JD: Neoplasms of the lung. In Isselbacher, KJ, et al (eds): Harrison's Principles of Internal Medicine, ed 13. McGraw-Hill, New York, 1994.

Tabbarah, HJ, Lowitz, BB, and Livingston, RB: Lung cancer. In Casciato, DA, and Lowitz, BB (eds): Manual of Clinical Oncology. Little, Brown, Boston, 1995.

Uphold, CR, and Graham, MV: Clinical Guidelines in Adult Health. Baramarrae Books, Gainesville, FL, 1994.

US Department of Health and Human Services. Smoking cessation: Information for specialists. Oncol Nurs Forum 23:1475, 1996.

Wolpaw, DR: Early detection in lung cancer: Case finding and screening. Med Clin North Am 80:63, 1996.

Pneumonia

American Thoracic Society: Guidelines for the initial management of adults with community acquired pneumonia: Diagnosis, assessment of severity, and initial antimicrobial therapy. Am Rev Resp Dis 148:1418–1426, 1993.

Chernecky, CC, and Bergey, BJ: Laboratory Tests and Diagnostic Procedures, ed 2. WB Saunders, Philadelphia, 1997.

Dambro, MR: Griffith's 5 Minute Clinical Consult. Williams & Wilkins, Baltimore, 1997.

Fitzgerald, MA. Pharmacologic update: Management of pneumonia in elderly people. J Am Acad Nurse Pract 8(5):237–241.

King, TE: Lung disorders in the elderly. In Jahnigen, DW, and Schrier, RW: Geriatric Medicine, ed 2. Blackwell Scientific, Cambridge, MA, 1997.

Mick, D: Pneumonia in elders. Geriatr Nurs 18(3):99–102.

Reddy, U, and Thadepalli, H: Respiratory infections. In Yoshikawa, TT, Cobbs, EL, and Brummel-Smith, K: Practical Ambulatory Geriatrics, ed 2. CV Mosby, St Louis, 1998.

Stauffer, JL: Disorders of the airways. In Tierney, LM, McPhee, SJ, and Papadakis, MA (eds): Current Medical Diagnosis and Treatment, ed 36. Appleton & Lange, Norwalk, CT, 1997.

Pulmonary Embolism

Abrams, WB, Beers, MH, and Berkow, R: The Merck Manual of Geriatrics, ed 2. Merck Research Laboratories, Whitehouse Station, NJ, 1995.

Dambro, MR: Griffith's 5 Minute Clinical Consult. Williams & Wilkins, Baltimore, 1997.

Dietzen, DL: Pulmonary embolus. In Rakel, RE: Saunders Manual of Medical Practice. WB Saunders, Philadelphia, 1996.

Dobbin, KR: Low molecular weight heparins: The future of thromboembolic therapy. Nurse Pract 23(3):98–107, 1998.

Hampson, NB, Panacek, EA, and Tapson, VF: Pulmonary embolism: Common, elusive, and deadly. Patient Care 31(13):75–88, 1997.

Pulmonary TB

Dambro, MR: Griffith's 5 Minute Clinical Consult. Williams & Wilkins, Baltimore, 1997.

Gonzalez-Rothi, RJ: Resurgent TB: Stopping the spread. Patient Care 31(9):97–118, 1997.

King, TE: Lung disorders in the elderly. In Jahnigen, DW, and Schrier, RW: Geriatric Medicine, ed 2. Blackwell Scientific, Cambridge, MA, 1997.

Morbidity and Mortality Weekly Report: Guidelines for preventing the transmission of Mycobacterium tuberculosis in health-care facilities. MMWR 43(RR-13):59–68, 1994.

Pettit, J: Question and answer: Tuberculosis in the elderly. Journal of the American Academy of Nurse Practitioners 8(3):131–134, 1996.

Stauffer, JL: Pulmonary tuberculosis. In Tierney, LM, McPhee, SJ, and Papadakis, MA (eds): Current Medical Diagnosis and Treatment, ed 36. Appleton & Lange, Norwalk, CT, 1997.

Warner, L: Infectious disease. In Lonergan, ET (ed): Geriatrics. Appleton & Lange, Stamford, CT, 1996.

Restrictive Lung Disease

Addison, TE: Pulmonary disease. In Lonergan, ET (ed): Geriatrics. Appleton & Lang, Stamford, CT, 1996.

Black, JM, and Matassarin-Jacobs, E: Luckmann and Sorensen's Medical-Surgical Nursing, ed 4. WB Saunders, Philadelphia, 1993.

Dambro, MR: Griffith's 5 Minute Clinical Consult. Williams & Wilkins, Baltimore, 1997.

Reynolds, HY: Interstitial lung diseases. In Isselbacher, KJ, et al (eds): Harrison's Principles of Internal Medicine, ed 13. McGraw-Hill, New York, 1994.

Speizer, FE: Environmental lung diseases. In Isselbacher, KJ, et al (eds): Harrison's Principles of Internal Medicine, ed 13. McGraw-Hill, New York, 1994.

Weinberger, SE, and Drazen, JM: Disturbances of respiratory function. In Isselbacher, KJ, et al (eds): Harrison's Principles of Internal Medicine, ed 13. McGraw-Hill, New York, 1994.

Zaman, MK: Interstitial lung disease. In Rakel, RE: Saunders Manual of Medical Practice. WB Saunders, Philadelphia, 1996.

Upper Respiratory Infection

Dambro, M: Griffith's 5 Minute Clinical Consult. Williams & Wilkins, Baltimore, 1997.

Goroll, A, May, L, and Mulley, A: Primary Care Medicine. Lippincott-Raven, Philadelphia, 1995.

Greene, H: Medical Decision Making. CV Mosby, St Louis, 1993.

Greenberger, N, and Hinthorn, D: History Taking and Physical Examination. CV Mosby, St Louis, 1993.

Hurst, JW (eds): Medicine for the Practicing Physician, ed 4. Appleton & Lange, Norwalk, CT, 1996.

Noble, J (ed): Primary Care Medicine, ed 2. CV Mosby, St Louis, 1996.

Pfenninger, JL, and Fowler, GC: Procedures for Primary Care Physicians. CV Mosby, St Louis, 1994.

Rakel, R: Manual of Medical Practice. WB Saunders, Philadelphia, 1996.

Rakel, R: Textbook of Family Practice, ed 8. WB Saunders, Philadelphia, 1995.

Sellers, R: Differential Diagnosis of Common Complaints, ed 3. WB Saunders, Philadelphia, 1996.

Swartz, M: Textbook of Physical Diagnosis. WB Saunders, Philadelphia, 1994.

Tierney, LM, McPhee, SJ, and Papadakis, MA: Current Medical Diagnosis and Treatment, ed 35. Appleton & Lange, Norwalk, CT, 1996.

Uphold, C, and Graham, MV: Clinical Guidelines in Family Practice, ed 2. Barmarrae Books, Gainesville, FL, 1994.

US Preventive Service Task Force: Guide to Clinical Prevention Services, ed 2. Williams & Wilkins, Baltimore, 1996.

Wachtel, R, and Stein, M: The Care of the Ambulatory Patient. CV Mosby, St Louis, 1996.

Woolf, J, Jones, J, and Lawrence, R (eds): Health Promotion and Disease Prevention in Clinical Practice. Williams & Wilkins, Baltimore, 1996.

CHAPTER **9**

PERIPHERAL

VASCULAR DISORDERS

Vascular problems represent one of the few areas of assessment in which diagnosis may be made on the basis of careful history taking and thorough physical examination. The extremities are easy to examine; careful inspection, auscultation, and palpation can detect even subtle changes in an affected extremity. The temperature of the examination room should be comfortable for the patient, to minimize vasoconstriction. Cigarette smoking by the patient can also affect findings.

Inspection of the entire body surface may reveal systemic manifestations of disease such as diabetes, hypertension, or hyperlipidemia. Examination of the ocular fundi may reveal emboli of the retinal vessels or arcus, which are seen in patients with atherosclerosis or abnormal lipid metabolism. Xanthomas may also suggest lipid metabolism abnormalities.

Inspection of the legs should involve comparison of both legs, noting skin color, hair distribution, venous pattern, size (swelling or muscle atrophy), and any skin lesions or ulcers. The toes (and spaces between the toes) should be inspected for hair distribution and any cracks in the skin or signs of tinea. Thick-ridged nails occur with arterial insufficiency. Other involvement of the skin may be manifested by petechial lesions that imply microemboli of platelet thrombi, cholesterol, and atherosclerotic debris. Unilateral swelling of the leg indicates a local acute problem. Brown discoloration occurs with chronic venous stasis.

The dorsum of the hand is used to test temperature of the legs. Both legs are compared at symmetric areas. A foot or leg that feels cool unilaterally indicates an arterial deficit.

A positive Homan's sign occurs in about 35% of cases of deep vein thrombosis, but also occurs with superficial phlebitis and with injury to the Achille's tendon and gastrocnemius muscle. For this test, flex the patient's knee and press the calf muscle forward against the tibia, or sharply dorsiflex the foot against the calf.

230

Peripheral arterial pulses should be graded on the four-point scale:

0 Absent pulse.
1 Severe impairment.
2 Moderate impairment.
3 Slight impairment.
4 Normal pulses.

If finding the popliteal pulse proves difficult, turn the patient prone and lift his or her lower leg while bending it slightly. The pulse may be felt just lateral to the medial tendon. A normal popliteal pulse is often not palpable.

The abdominal aorta can be palpated easily, except in obese patients. Pulsations can be felt by exerting deep pressure with the fingertips over the periumbilical area while the patient is lying with the feet drawn up and the thighs slightly parted.

Pretibial edema is assessed by depressing the skin over the tibia for 5 sec before releasing. Grading is on a 1 to 4 scale, ranging from mild to severe indentation of the skin.

Auscultation over the large arteries should follow palpation. The carotid, subclavian, iliac, and femoral arteries, as well as the abdominal aorta, should be auscultated also. Applying too much pressure with the stethoscope may produce bruits over normal arteries.

After completion of the traditional physical examination, estimation of the blood flow to the patient's lower limb is required. Buerger's postural test is easily performed. It is based on the fact that about 60 to 75 mmHg of systolic pressure is needed to keep a supine patient's foot warm when it is raised 60–75 degrees for 1–2 min. In this position the patient flexes and extends the ankles and toes to the point of fatigue while the examiner supports the legs, keeping the patient's knees straight. When arterial flow is defective, the feet become pale and veins on the dorsum of the foot empty. Then the feet are lowered as the patient sits up, and the examiner notes how long it takes for reactive rubor or venous filling to develop. Color should return within 10 sec.

In addition, the legs should be tested for strength and sensation. Motor and sensory loss occurs with severe arterial deficits, especially in patients with diabetes.

Abdominal Aortic Aneurysm

A true abdominal aortic aneurysm (AAA), a localized dilatation of the abdominal aortic wall by more than 3 cm, is the most common type of arterial aneurysm. The abdominal aorta passes from the aortic hiatus of the diaphragm into the abdomen, descending ventrally to the vertebral column and ending at the fourth lumbar vertebra where it divides into the two common iliac arteries.

Etiology: Most AAAs are a complication of atherosclerosis. Other, less frequent causes are trauma, infection, syphilis, cystic medial necrosis, inflammation, and

Marfan's syndrome. The vast majority of AAAs are infrarenal; only about 5% infringe on visceral vessels, most commonly the renal arteries.

Occurrence: The incidence of AAA has been estimated at 10 to 20 in 1000 population. It is estimated that 28,000 new patients are diagnosed with AAA each year.

Age: In persons older than age 50 the prevalence of AAA is 3%. Aneurysms developing in patients over age 65 are almost always arteriosclerotic in origin. An estimated 1 in 250 people over age 50 dies because of rupture of an AAA.

Ethnicity: Although no dominant ethnic group is represented, a hereditary basis for the disease is suggested.

Gender: Men are affected by aneurysmal disease 10 times more often than women.

Contributing Factors: In patients with known peripheral vascular disease, the prevalence of AAA has been reported to be nearly 10%. Other factors associated with AAA include history of hypertension, family history of aneurysm, and clinical evidence of atherosclerotic complications in other vessels. Risk factors for atherosclerosis include hypercholesterolemia, diabetes, smoking, and hypertension.

Signs and Symptoms: Most patients with AAAs are asymptomatic except in the presence of bleeding, dissection, rupture, or impending rupture. Symptoms may include mild to severe abdominal, flank, and/or lower back pain. The patient may complain of a "second heart" sensation in the abdomen after feeling a pulsatile epigastric mass. More than 50% of AAAs are asymptomatic when discovered by routine physical examination. About 50% of AAAs are associated with a bruit. Most AAAs are palpable in the periumbilical area, often slightly left of the midline. Because one-quarter to one-third of patients with AAA also have significant arterial occlusive disease, a systematic evaluation should be performed (Fig. 9–1).

Diagnostic Tests: Abdominal ultrasound is virtually 100% accurate, providing precise information on the aneurysm's size, shape, and location. Ultrasound is also recommended by some practitioners as a screening test for obese elderly individuals, especially those with risk factors for aneurysm. About 70%–90% of patients with syphilitic aneurysms test positive serologically for syphilis. Anteroposterior (AP) and cross-table lateral abdominal radiograms document AAAs in 70%–80% of patients because the aneurysm wall is frequently calcified. Computed tomography (CT) and magnetic resonance imaging (MRI) are more expensive and should be used only in special situations, such as a suspected leak in an otherwise stable patient, or to confirm the extent of visceral artery involvement or inflammatory changes.

Differential Diagnosis: Because various agents can produce aortic aneurysms, it is important to search for syphilis, hypertension, and associated valvular or congenital heart disease. An ectatic abdominal aorta without aneurysm may also

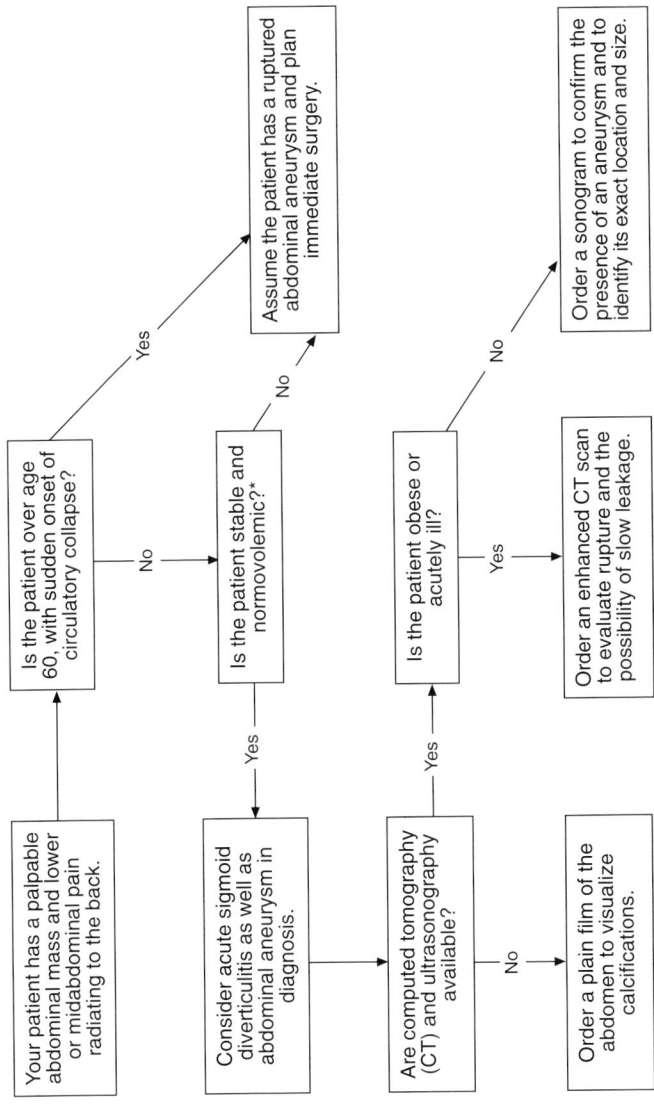

FIGURE 9-1 Suspected abdominal aortic aneurysm.

*Don't rely on the absence of peripheral pulses to confirm ruptured aneurysm.
They disappear only when the patient has become extremely hypovolemic.

be palpable and may be confused with an AAA. Other acute causes of abdominal pain may mimic rupture of an AAA, and cholelithiasis must be excluded.

Treatment: The risk of rupture in patients with aneurysms greater than 6 cm in transverse diameter is so great that almost all such individuals must be referred for possible surgical repair. Elective repair of aneurysms less than 4 cm in elderly people is slightly more controversial. Generally, a 4-cm aneurysm is predicted to grow to 6 cm in 4 years.

Recent studies demonstrate a slowing of the expansion of large aneurysms (greater than 5 cm) with the use of beta-blockers (Gadowski, Pilcher, & Ricci). Contraindications to the use of beta-blockers include congestive heart failure and diabetes mellitus in patients taking medications (either insulin or oral agents). If no contraindications to a cardioselective beta-blocker exist, atenolol at 25 mg daily may be used. Because many patients with AAA also have peripheral vascular disease, labetolol may be appropriate. This drug should be avoided, however, in patients susceptible to bronchospasm.

All patients with AAAs should be kept normotensive (with systolic blood pressure less than or equal to 120 mmHg, if possible) through medication. Patients with AAA who smoke should stop immediately, as growth rates for AAA may be higher in patients who continue to smoke.

Surgical repair of AAA prolongs life, and elective repair has an operative mortality rate of less than 3%. However, even the worst operative mortality rate (13%, for patients with heart disease) is better than that found after nonsurgical management.

Follow-up: Patients with small aneurysms (less than 4 cm) can be followed with serial examination and ultrasound every 3–6 months. Any size symptomatic AAAs or asymptomatic AAAs greater than 5 cm in diameter should be excised, with mandatory surgical referral.

Sequelae: The most likely complication of AAA is rupture. Infrequent complications are thrombi to the lower extremities and infection of the aneurysm, with *Salmonella* being the most common causative organism.

Prevention/Prophylaxis: Because AAAs are most often due to atherosclerosis, the same preventive measures are applicable in peripheral vascular disease and AAA. Patients with aortitis or AAA caused by syphilis should be treated with 2.4 million units of benzathine penicillin intramuscularly (IM) each week for 3 weeks, 500 mg of tetracycline PO qid for 30 days, or 500 mg of erythromycin PO qid for 30 days.

Referral: Physician referral for all symptomatic AAA patients is essential. Physician consultation after initial diagnosis of asymptomatic AAA is recommended.

Education: Patients and their families should be taught the importance of follow-up, how to manage hypertension and other risk factors, and to recognize symptoms that should be reported to the physician immediately. The risks of operative versus nonoperative treatment should be explained to the patient and family.

Peripheral Vascular Disease

Peripheral vascular disease (PVD) refers to a disease or process that limits blood flow to the extremities and vital organs other than the heart. These processes may involve the arterial, venous, or lymphatic systems, but are most often due to enlarging atherosclerotic plaques in the distal aorta or in major bifurcations or areas of angulation in the iliac, femoral, and popliteal arteries.

Etiology: Atherosclerotic plaques may be fatty streaks, fibrous plaques, or complicated lesions. Fatty streaks are early lesions that occur in the intima of arteries. Fibrous plaques, areas of intimal thickening, are the most frequently occurring type of lesion. Complicated plaques, calcified fibrous plaques with potential for necrosis and thrombosis, are most often associated with symptoms.

Occurrence: In general, PVD is present in 10% of the elderly population. Persons with diabetes, either non–insulin-dependent diabetes mellitus (NIDDM) or insulin-dependent diabetes mellitus (IDDM), account for 30%–50% of patients undergoing surgery for PVD and for 60%–70% of surgeries involving vascular reconstruction below the popliteal artery.

Age: PVD is rare in nondiabetic persons before the fifth decade. The 65- to 74-year-old group is associated with the highest rate of newly symptomatic PVD.

Gender: Before age 50, the ratio of male-to-female risk is 2 : 1. After age 65, the risk ratio is closer to 1 : 1.

Ethnicity: Recently published data from the Atherosclerosis Risk in Communities (ARIC) study show that blacks have higher levels of coagulation proteins, which is thought to be a risk factor for atherosclerosis.

Contributing Factors: Smoking is the chief risk factor contributing to PVD. Patients who do not quit smoking after developing arterial occlusion have a 10-fold greater incidence of limb amputation. Significant risk factors also include obesity, hyperlipidemia, hypertension, diabetes mellitus, and family history of PVD. Less often, disorders that affect blood viscosity, such as polycythemia, are risk factors. Early hysterectomy or ovariectomy is a risk factor in women.

Signs and Symptoms: PVD has three general patterns of presentation. The most common presentation of lower limb atherosclerosis is a patient age 65–75 with a calf that aches or burns, usually during walking (indicating femoropopliteal disease). Persistent pain must be differentiated from intermittent pain, known as intermittent claudication, which has come to mean discomfort associated with exertion. However, in patients over age 70, the classic symptom of claudication (pain occurring in the calf, hip, or buttock area that is relieved by rest) may be absent. Older adults may instead describe numbness, coldness, and pain in the foot at rest. Foot pain at rest indicates that blood flow is 10% of normal. Individuals with this symptom often are not ambulatory owing to advanced age or disability and do not have pain until basal tissue requirements are not met.

Physical examination confirms the diagnosis of PVD. Absent or markedly decreased peripheral pulses are the cardinal sign. The posterior tibialis pulse is always present in healthy individuals, whereas the dorsalis pedis pulse may be absent in approximately 5% of the healthy population. Patent arteries tend to have more prominent pulses with aging.

Another cluster of presenting symptoms may commonly be found in 40- to 60-year-old men presenting with a history of smoking and hyperlipidemia. These symptoms include weakness and aching of the pelvic muscles and thighs with exercise (aortoiliac disease). These patients may complain of decreased ability to maintain an erection and probably have a family history of vascular disease. Examination reveals a decrease in muscle mass and tone in the lower extremities, bruits over the distal aorta and iliac arteries, and decreased femoral pulses.

The third type of clinical presentation is of a man or woman who has had diabetes mellitus with poor control for several years. The patient's chief complaint is of aching pain in the anterior tibial muscles and the foot, particularly the metatarsal arch, while walking. If rest pain is present, it must be distinguished from peripheral neuropathy, which tends to be more bilateral. Physical examination shows absent dorsalis pedis and anterior tibialis pulses, but more proximal pulses may be palpable. The foot and ankle show trophic changes such as fragile skin with rubor, absent toe hair, nail thickening, muscle wasting, and nonhealing ulcers. In these cases, the occlusive lesions are found in the distal tibial and peroneal arteries.

Other findings include blanching of the foot during elevation, poor capillary refill after skin compression, and temperature differences between the affected foot and the unaffected foot. The feet should be elevated above heart level for at least 20 sec to determine whether pallor develops. When the foot is moved to the dependent position, pallor that lasts for more than 30 sec or rubor that develops after 20 sec indicates less than 10% of normal blood flow capacity.

Diagnostic Tests: The ankle/brachial index can be measured using a blood pressure cuff and a handheld Doppler. The ankle component is determined by detecting the initial flow through the dorsalis pedis artery as the ankle blood pressure cuff is deflated. The systolic pressures at the forearm and the ankle are compared. The ratio should be 1 or greater. In the active elderly person with claudication, the ratio is less than 1 but greater than 0.5. In patients with rest symptoms, the ratio is less than 0.5. The sensitivity of the ankle/brachial index improves by taking measurement during exercise; in a patient with significant disease, the ratio during exercise is less than that at rest. Vascular duplex scanning can provide useful data about the location and severity of lower limb arterial disease. Because arteriography is invasive, this technique is used for initial diagnosis only if the severity of symptoms forces a consideration of vascular surgery.

Differential Diagnosis: Acute arterial insufficiency may result when an embolus from the left atrium, ventricle, or aorta lodges in the peripheral circulation. Patients with pain from arteritis demonstrate one or more of the following: increased erythrocyte sedimentation rate, fever, lethargy or weight loss, or rash. Pain from osteoarthritis of the lower back can be distinguished by history and physical examination. Thromboangiitis obliterans (Buerger's disease) is found almost solely in men under age 35 who smoke heavily. With this condition, the upper extremities are often involved, along with the legs. In Raynaud's phenomenon, the hands and tips of the ears and nose, as well as the feet, may be involved. Patients with Raynaud's phenomenon tend to have cool hands and feet, even in a warm environment. The appearance of Raynaud's phenomenon after age 40 is almost always an indicator of internal disease. Refer to Fig. 9–2.

Treatment: Management of PVD should begin by helping patients to reduce risk factors early in life. Once PVD is recognized, the goal is to prevent complications. The feet must be protected, inspected daily, and toenails trimmed carefully. Bunions, corns, and calluses should be cared for by a qualified professional and any infection, including dermatophytosis, treated promptly. All forms of tobacco use should cease immediately. Obese patients should lose weight.

Walking at least 30–60 min daily develops collateral circulation and improves symptoms. Cycling and swimming are acceptable alternatives for patients with musculoskeletal problems. All patients who are able to should walk to the point of calf discomfort daily.

Vasodilators and anticoagulants are of no benefit in atherosclerotic disease. Pentoxifylline (Trental) is still unproven by placebo-controlled study, but recent studies suggest that exercise tolerance improved in elderly patients given pentoxifylline 400 mg tid (with meals). Nondiabetic patients may respond better to this drug than diabetic patients. Individual patients must weigh their improvement against the expense and bother of taking a medication three times daily indefinitely. If no improvement has occurred at the end of an 8-week trial of this dosage of pentoxifylline, the drug may be discontinued. A new drug, clopidogrel (Plavix), is indicated for use in atherosclerotic peripheral arterial disease (PAD). It is also an inhibitor of platelet aggregation. The dosage is 75 mg PO qd. The CAPRIE study demonstrated a relative risk reduction of 23.8% when the use of clopidogrel was compared with the use of aspirin in patients with PAD. Events defined in this study were either nonfatal (ischemic stroke, myocardial infarction [MI], intracranial hemorrhage, amputation, or vascular death) or fatal (events in the previous category as well as death from nonvascular events).

Follow-up: Monthly follow-ups are recommended to evaluate patient response to pharmacologic and nonpharmacologic therapy.

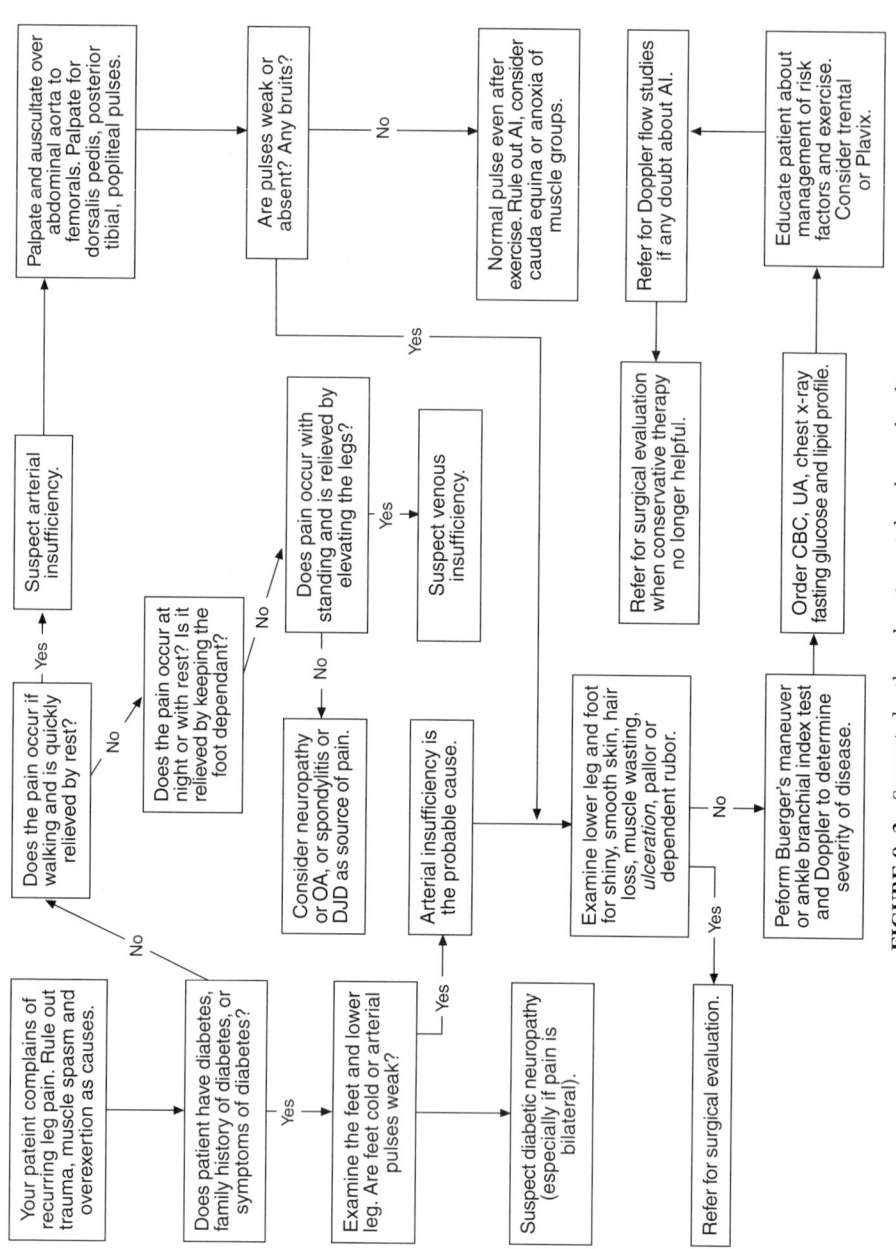

FIGURE 9–2 Suspected arthrosclerotic peripheral vascular disease.

Sequelae: Approximately one-third of patients with atherosclerosis experience worsening of their symptoms, requiring revascularization. Patients with pain at rest or gangrene are at high risk for amputation if revascularization is not undertaken.

Prevention/Prophylaxis: Preventing PVD before the initial onset of symptoms is accomplished by controlling the modifiable risk factors discussed earlier. Once a patient is diagnosed with PVD, the goal is to delay the progression of symptoms by changing lifestyle, risk factors, and using pharmacologic therapy, including lipid-lowering agents, to modify other risk factors. Patients should be taught prophylactic measures to protect the skin of the feet and toes.

Referral: Indications for referral for surgery include claudication that is intolerable to the patient, ischemic rest pain, impending gangrene, and nonhealing ulceration.

Education: Most areas of education are discussed as a part of treatment, as PVD management focuses on prevention and teaching. Patients should be taught to report promptly any change in symptoms, especially nonhealing ulcers.

BIBLIOGRAPHY

Assessment

Jarvis, C: Physical Examination and Health Assessment. WB Saunders, Philadelphia, 1992.
Woods, B: Clinical evaluation of the peripheral vasculature. Cardiol Clin 9:413, 1991.

Abdominal Aortic Aneurysm

Ahronheim, J: Handbook of Prescribing Medications for Geriatric Patients. Little, Brown, Toronto, 1992.
Carpenito, L: Nursing Diagnosis: An Application to Clinical Practice, ed 3. JB Lippincott, New York, 1989.
Friedman, S: Peripheral vascular diseases. In Abrams, W, and Berkow, R (eds): The Merck Manual of Geriatrics. Merck Sharp & Dohme Research Laboratories, Rahway, NJ, 1990.
Gadowski, G, Pilcher, D, and Ricci, M: Abdominal aortic aneurysm expansion rate: Effect of size and beta adrenergic blockade. J Vasc Surg 19:727, 1994.
Ham, R, and Sloane, P: Primary Care Geriatrics: A Case-Based Approach. Mosby Year Book, Baltimore, 1992.
Jones, C: Peripheral vascular disease and arterial aneurysms. In Barker, L, Burton, J, Zieve, P (eds): Principles of Ambulatory Medicine, ed 4. Williams & Wilkins, Baltimore, 1995, pp 1298–1310.
MacSweeney, S, et al: Smoking and the growth of small abdominal aortic aneurysms. Lancet 344:651, 1994.
Meadors, F: Outpatient surveillance of abdominal aortic aneurysms. J Ark Med Soc 91:85–87, 1994.
Sung, J, et al: Racial differences in mortality from cardiovascular disease in Atlanta, 1979–1985. J Natl Med Assoc 84:259, 1992.
Upton, C, and Graham, M: Clinical Guidelines in Adult Health. Barmarrae Books, Gainesville, FL, 1993.
Woods, B: Clinical evaluation of the peripheral vasculature. Cardiol Clin 9:413, 427, 1991.
Yoshikawa, T, Cobbs, E, and Brummel-Smith, K: Ambulatory geriatric care. CV Mosby, Boston, 1993.

Peripheral Vascular Disease

Ahronheim, J: Handbook of Prescribing Medications for Geriatric Patients. Little, Brown, Toronto, 1992.

CAPRIE Steering Committee: A randomised, blinded trial of clopidogrel versus aspirin in patients at risk of ischaemic events (CAPRIE). Lancet 348(9038):1329–1339, 1996.

Carpenito, L: Nursing Diagnosis: An Application to Clinical Practice, ed 3. JB Lippincott, New York, 1989.

Friedman, S: Peripheral vascular diseases. In Abrams, W, and Berkow, R (eds): The Merck Manual of Geriatrics. Merck Sharp & Dohme Research Laboratories, Rahway, NJ, 1990.

Ham, R, and Sloane, P: Primary Care Geriatrics: A Case-Based Approach. Mosby Year Book, Baltimore, 1992.

Jones, C: Peripheral vascular disease and arterial aneurysms. In Barker, L, Burton, J, Zieve, P, (eds): Principles of Ambulatory Medicine, ed 4. Williams & Wilkins, Baltimore, 1995, pp 1298–1310.

Sung, J, et al: Racial differences in mortality from cardiovascular disease in Atlanta, 1979–1985. Natl Med Assoc 84:259, 1992.

Upton, C, and Graham, M: Clinical Guidelines in Adult Health. Barmarrae Books, Gainesville, FL, 1993.

Woods, B: Clinical evaluation of the peripheral vasculature. Cardiol Clin 9:413, 427, 1991.

Yoshikawa, T, Cobbs, E, and Brummel-Smith, K: Ambulatory Geriatric Care. CV Mosby, Boston, 1993.

CHAPTER **10**

ABDOMINAL

DISORDERS

Accurate history taking of abdominal complaints is essential for completing an assessment of the older adult. The physical examination is often unremarkable, and laboratory findings may not provide diagnostic information because the presentation of illness in the older adult is usually subdued. Explore with the patient any episodes of anorexia, dyspepsia, dysphagia, heartburn, nausea, regurgitation, vomiting, diarrhea, tenesmus, or constipation. Determine the sequence of events that triggered each symptom. Inquire about precipitating factors such as a meal, position of the body, use of caffeine or alcohol, and smoking. Were any other symptoms presented that can be clustered to form a differential diagnosis? It is important to discern from patients what therapeutic measures they have initiated to alleviate the symptoms. Determine if the treatment is a previously prescribed regimen, an over-the-counter (OTC) medication, or a home remedy. Explore with the patient when the last time a fecal occult test was performed and if a sigmoidoscopy examination was ever performed.

The physical examination of the abdomen begins with inspection. The practitioner can consider the abdomen to be divided into four quadrants, visualizing an imaginary vertical line from the sternum to the pubis passing through the umbilicus, and a horizontal line drawn through the umbilicus. Carefully examine for scars, lesions, dilated veins, or other marks. Determine if the abdomen is concave or protuberant. Is an umbilical or abdominal wall hernia present? Is a lift noticeable?

Auscultation follows inspection of the abdomen. Using the diaphragm, place the stethoscope lightly against the skin. Listen for bowel sounds, vascular bruits, and rubs. Bowel sounds are produced by peristalsis. A murmur heard in the abdomen may be an aortic aneurysm. A constant systolic-diastolic bruit may occur

241

when the patient has an arteriovenous fistula in the renal vessels. Other sites to auscultate for bruits during the abdominal examination include the iliac arteries and the femoral arteries. When auscultating bowel sounds, take the time to listen for presence of bowel sounds. Generally, people who are hungry have active bowel sounds, whereas those who have just ingested a meal may have quiet bowel sounds. Bowel sounds described as high pitched, rumbling, or tinkling are known as borborygmi. A rushing sound is associated with bowel obstruction. If bowel sounds are absent, listen for 5 minutes; suspect peritonitis, mesenteric thrombosis, or advanced intestinal obstruction when bowel sounds are absent. Listen for a loud succussion splash over the abdomen of a patient in whom you suspect a gastric obstruction or dilatation.

Part of a focused assessment of the abdomen would include testing of the gag reflex, which may be weakened in an older adult; an absent gag reflex is abnormal. Perform light palpation to discern abdominal masses, enlarged organs, and areas of tenderness. Using the palm and extended fingers of the right hand, press about 1 cm deep. If a patient has complained of abdominal pain, always paplate in a quadrant away from the identified location. Once you discover the tender area, maintain pressure over this area to determine the consistency of the pain. If the pain diminishes despite the applied pressure to the area, inflammation is unlikely. If you suspect intraabdominal tenderness, proceed to deep palpation. Check for referred rebound tenderness by applying pressure with the tips of the fingers to a site distant from the area of questionable tenderness, then quickly removing them from the abdomen. If tenderness is elicited remote from the area palpated after release of pressure, consider peritoneal irritation. A mass detected in the lower abdomen upon palpation warrants further rectal and/or pelvic examination. Rectal examination includes determining presence or absence of stool, checking for presence of hemorrhoids, and sphincter tone and guaiac testing. Ask the patient to strain down gently as if having a bowel movement to relax the anal sphincter.

Percussion of the abdomen is performed to determine the density of tissue of the abdominal organs by the sound emitted when tapped. It is normal to hear tympanic sounds over the stomach, whereas dullness is expected over a distended bladder. Dullness noted over other areas of the abdomen is a deviation from the norm. Definitive percussion is used to ascertain the size and shape of the liver and spleen. Because the liver decreases in size starting at about age 50, the normal range of liver size in an older person would be 6–12 cm.

Acute Renal Failure

Acute renal failure (ARF) is a rapid reduction of renal function, associated with azotemia, with or without oliguria. Classification of ARF falls into three categories:

Prerenal, stemming from poor renal perfusion.

Postrenal, caused by obstruction.

Intrinsic, caused by injury to the kidney (e.g., from glomerulonephritis or tubular necrosis).

Etiology: ARF occurs when the amount of blood flow to the kidneys is decreased or the renal tubules are damaged from a toxin or ischemia, resulting in an abrupt decline in renal function. Intravascular volume depletion, prolonged ischemic damage to the kidney, and any obstruction to the flow in urine can cause ARF. This reduction in the glomerular filtration rate (GFR) is evidenced by a rise in the plasma creatinine level.

Occurrence: An estimated 5% of patients admitted to the hospital develop ARF; this percentage increases with the acuity of the patient and the length of hospitalization.

Age: ARF can occur in patients of all ages. Considering the high percentage of hospitalized older adults who experience congestive heart failure, sepsis, or surgical procedures with associated volume depletion, development of ARF is possible in all critically ill or older surgical patients. The incidence of mortality increases with age.

Ethnicity: No known prevalence exists among ethnic groups.

Gender: ARF occurs equally in men and women.

Contributing Factors: Heatstroke, dehydration, vomiting, diarrhea, congestive heart failure, cirrhosis, and early sepsis are precursors to prerenal ARF. Surgical patients are susceptible to ARF because of volume depletion. Intrinsic cases of congestive heart failure result from patient exposure to nephrotoxic drugs (angiotensin-converting enzyme [ACE] inhibitors, certain nonsteroid anti-inflammatory drugs [NSAIDs], aminoglycoside therapy), tubular necrosis, interstitial nephritis, and chronic disease such as polyarteritis or systemic lupus erythematosus. Obstructions caused by bladder, pelvic, or retroperitoneal tumors, calculi, and prostatism, and a neurogenic bladder may contribute to postrenal ARF.

Signs and Symptoms: The signs and symptoms of acute renal failure depend on the disease category of ARF. A thorough history is important to discern all causes of ARF; multiple causes may be identified in an individual patient. The patient may complain of anorexia, headache, fatigue, vomiting, diarrhea, muscle cramps, somnolence, weakness, back pain, foul-smelling concentrated urine, oliguria, or xerostomia. Delirium and dehydration may be the first indications of ARF in a frail older adult. All causes of altered renal perfusion, trauma, infection, and obstruction should be explored. Physical examination may reveal ecchymosis, hypertension, petechiae, crackles, rash, tachycardia, and tachypnea. Examine for signs of volume depletion and infection. Palpate the kidneys for tenderness and the bladder for enlargement. Rectal and vaginal examinations are done when obstruction is suspected.

Diagnostic Tests: Urinalysis is examined for sediment, osmolarity, and urine sodium and creatinine levels. In prerenal and postrenal ARF, the sediment is usually normal, but sometimes hyaline casts are present. Tubular epithelial cells, cellular casts, and debris are common findings in acute tubular necrosis. In prerenal disease, the blood urea nitrogen (BUN)–plasma creatinine clearance ratio is usually greater than $20:1$, whereas in acute tubular necrosis the ratio is less than $15:1$. Laboratory findings in ARF consist of hyponatremia, hyperkalemia, hypocalcemia, azotemia, and decreased creatinine clearance. Table 10–1 depicts the use of indices to distinguish prerenal azotemia from intrinsic azotemia. Renal ultrasonography or computed tomography (CT) should detect a normal-sized or slightly enlarged kidney in ARF.

Differential Diagnosis: Determining the reasons for ARF delineates the differential diagnosis. Glomerulonephritis, systemic vasculitis, urinary tract obstruction, and pyelonephritis need to be considered when diagnosing ARF.

Treatment: Patients with ARF require hospitalization and often intensive care. Treatment measures are aimed at reversing correctable causes of ARF. For patients with intrinsic ARF, therapy is directed toward complications such as hyponatremia, hyperkalemia, medication dosage, anemia, or metabolic acidosis. Hemodialysis, peritoneal dialysis, and hemofiltration may be considered by the nephrologist in severe cases. For patients with elevated serum phosphorus levels, give oral phosphate-binding agents such as aluminum-containing or calcium carbonate antacids to maintain the serum phosphorus level at less than

TABLE 10–1   URINE DIAGNOSTIC INDICES IN SEPARATION OF PRERENAL FROM INTRINSIC FACTOR RENAL AZOTEMIA

Diagnostic Index	Prerenal Azotemia	Intrinsic Renal Azotemia
Fractional excretion of sodium (%)° $\dfrac{U_{NA}P_{Cr}}{P_{NA}U_{Cr}} \times 100$	<1	>1
Urine sodium concentration (mmol/L)	<10	>20
Urine creatinine to plasma creatinine ratio	>40	<20
Urine urea nitrogen to plasma urea nitrogen ratio	>8	<3
Urine specific gravity	>1.018	<1.012
Urine osmolality (mmol/kg H_2O)	>500	<250
Plasma BUN/creatinine ratio (mg/dL)	>20	$<10–15$
Renal failure index° $\dfrac{U_{NA}}{U_{Cr}/P_{Cr}} \times 100$	<1	>1
Urinary sediment	Hyaline casts	Muddy brown granular casts

°Most sensitive indices.

5.5 mg/dL. Order a low-protein diet with 0.5 g/kg of body weight per day of protein to prevent a rise in the BUN level. Use urinary catheters cautiously in older adults because a high prevalence of infection is associated with catheterization.

Follow-up: Management of the patient recovering from ARF depends on the initial cause(s) of the kidney dysfunction, if the reversible cause was corrected, and if any sequelae occurred. Dietary management may require interdisciplinary consultation to include physician specialists, nutritionist, nursing staff, patient and family members. For patients who recover from a reversible cause of ARF, monitor serum creatinine level every 3 months until renal function stabilizes.

Sequelae: Volume overload resulting in pulmonary edema, hypertensive crisis, hyperkalemia, anemia, infections, cardiac disease, hemorrhage to include upper gastrointestinal bleeding, and death are possible complications of acute renal failure.

Prevention/Prophylaxis: ARF can be avoided in some instances when nephrotoxic medications are indicated for medical therapy. Monitor renal function, adjust medication dosages accordingly, and try alternative medications if the potential exists for developing ARF. For surgical patients, ARF can often be prevented if you monitor fluid balance, blood volume, and blood pressure.

Referral: All patients with ARF require hospitalization. Referral to a specialist is recommended; these patients often have concomitant problems that a specialist would manage in the acute care setting. Postrenal ARF may require collaboration with a nephrologist, urologist, and radiologist.

Education: For the reversible causes of ARF, teach patients to avoid dehydration and excessive heat, to avoid taking any OTC medications before contacting their provider, and, if applicable to their case, to recognize the signs and symptoms of congestive heart failure.

Bladder Cancer

Ninety percent of bladder cancers are transitional urothelial cell cancer, 8% are squamous cell cancer, and the remainder are adenocarcinoma. In bladder cancer, the posterior and lateral walls of the bladder are involved more frequently than the superior wall. Bladder cancer can be categorized as superficial, invasive, and metastatic.

- Superficial, or early, bladder cancer occurs when the lesion is located on the surface of the mucosa or when the tumor penetrates the mucosa and submucosa only.
- Invasive bladder cancer develops when lesions pervade the bladder muscularis or the perivesical fat.

- Metastatic bladder cancer is characterized by lymph node, visceral, or bone tissue.

Etiology: Occupational exposure to aniline dye, leather processing, paint, rubber, and possibly tobacco tars, because of suspected chemical carcinogens, have been linked to the development of bladder cancer. Squamous cell bladder cancer has been linked to chronic infection with *Schistosoma haematobium*.

Occurrence: More than 50,000 new cases of bladder cancer are diagnosed in the United States yearly.

Age: The average age of onset is in the late 60s.

Ethnicity: *S. haematobium* infection is prevalent in Africa and the Middle East. The incidence of bladder cancer increases among people from the industrialized areas of the northeastern United States because of their higher exposure to carcinogens.

Gender: Bladder cancer is 2.5 times more common in men than in women.

Contributing Factors: History of smoking increases the risk of bladder cancer. Pelvic irradiation, certain drugs (e.g., cyclophosphamide), and abnormal tryptophan metabolism contribute to the development of bladder cancer. Excessive coffee consumption, use of some artificial sweeteners (e.g., sodium saccharin and sodium cyclamate), and overuse of phenacetin-containing analgesics have been suggested risk factors. Exfoliation of cancer cells by cystoscopy, brushing, or transurethral biopsy or resection may spread bladder cancer cells to other sites within the bladder that may be irritated from instrumentation.

Signs and Symptoms: Hematuria, pyuria, burning, and frequency are very common in the presentation of bladder cancer. Symptoms of advanced cancer may include pelvic or flank pain and lower extremity edema due to lymphatic or a venous blockage. The clinician should palpate and percuss for evidence of any kidney enlargement and perform a prostate examination on men and pelvic examination on women. Additionally, the examination should be directed toward searching for possible sites of metastasis in the lungs, liver, bone, and lymph nodes.

Diagnostic Tests: Initial workup for bladder cancer should include a complete blood count (CBC) with differential, which may show a microcytic anemia and/or an infection, a renal function test to determine possible renal parenchymal disease, and urinalysis. A urinalysis result of greater than 5 RBCs per high-power field warrants a referral to a urologist for a cystoscopy with biopsy and a bimanual examination while under general anesthesia. Intravenous pyelography may be ordered to rule out ureteral obstruction with hydronephrosis. Abdominal and pelvic CT scans determine lymphadenopathy. A chest x-ray examination rules out any metastasis to the lungs. Staging of probable disease is based on clinical findings.

Differential Diagnosis: Rule out nephrolithiasis, urinary tract infection, benign prostatic hypertrophy, and other genitourinary cancers such as prostate or renal carcinoma.

Treatment: Management of bladder cancer depends on the stage of the disease. Initially surgical intervention to remove the bladder tumors is warranted. For patients with multiple recurrent superficial bladder cancer, collaboration with an oncologist for chemotherapy may be requested by the urologist following surgery. Intravesical administration of agents such as thiotepa 30–60 mL in 100 mL of sterile water or saline is injected via a catheter into the empty bladder. Advanced disease generally requires surgery, radiation, and chemotherapy with combination agents. The patients' age and health status at the time of diagnosis must be considered in the management of bladder cancer.

Follow-up: Patients with superficial low-grade bladder cancer require a cysto-scopy at designated intervals, although the value of repeated testing has been questioned. The need for supplemental nutritional support, pain management, prevention of complications such as skin breakdown, and an advanced directive should be discussed during future follow-up care.

Sequelae: Metastasis to other parts of the body can occur. Survival of the untreated patient may be less than 2 years.

Prevention/Prophylaxis: Encourage patients who smoke to discontinue tobacco use and decrease exposure to harmful chemicals.

Referral: Refer patients with clinically significant hematuria to a urologist. An oncologist may also be involved in the patient's management of the disease. Patient and family support is important at this time; information pertaining to hospice services should be provided.

Education: Older adults with bladder cancer may need to be educated about palliative support measures when the disease becomes terminal.

Bowel Obstruction

A bowel obstruction is an intestinal blockage classified as a mechanical obstruction or as an adynamic ileus, acute or chronic, simple or strangulated. Bowel obstruc-tions occur both in the small intestine and the colon.

Etiology: A mechancial bowel obstruction results when there is a complete or partial blockage of the lumen of the bowel by a lesion. A simple mechanical obstruction occurs without insult to the vascular or neurological system. Strangu-lation of the bowel in older adults happens when there is a twisting of the bowel, resulting in ischemia of the bowel wall. The bowel may become edematous and infarcted, leading to perforation and gangrene. An adynamic ileus may result from metabolic disturbances such as hypokalemia or when injury or illness causes reduced blood supply to the bowel.

Occurrence: An estimated 20% of all hospital admissions for an acute abdominal condition is for suspected bowel obstruction.

Age: Bowel obstruction from all causes except intussusception is more prevalent in older adults.

Ethnicity: No prevalence is known among ethnic groups.

Gender: Bowel obstruction occurs equally in men and women.

Contributing Factors: Patients with recent history of surgery, vertebral fractures, lower lobe pneumonia, fractured ribs, severe trauma, hypokalemia, and myocardial infarctions are at the risk for developing an adynamic ileus. A mechanical bowel obstruction can be caused by neoplasms, hernias, inflammatory disease, diverticulitis, mesenteric ischemia, stricture formation, volvulus, gallstones, and fecal impactions. Patients with a history of abdominal surgery may develop adhesions that can cause a small bowel obstruction.

Signs and Symptoms: Clinical presentation of bowel obstruction depends on the site and the cause of the obstruction. In adynamic ileus, patients may report hiccups, vomiting, and abdominal distention with cramping. Pain is usually continuous rather than colicky. Obstipation may or may not occur. Fever may be present. Auscultation generally reveals absent or minimum peristalsis. Diffuse minimal abdominal tenderness may be elicited. Presentation of a mechanical small bowel obstruction would include abdominal cramps located in the epigastrium or around the umbilicus, with associated pain that can be more severe the higher the obstruction. Profuse vomiting occurs early with a small bowel obstruction. The vomitus may first consist of mucus and bile in a high small bowel obstruction. With a lower ileal obstruction, the vomitus becomes feculent. Diarrhea may occur in partial small bowel obstruction. Obstipation exists with complete obstruction. The patient may have a low-grade fever. Inspect the abdomen for evidence of surgical scars and external hernias. Borborygmi may be heard on auscultation; however, late in the presentation of a strangulated bowel, peristalsis may be minimal or absent. Abdominal distention is found; the abdomen may not be tender, in the case of a strangulated bowel. With mechanical obstruction of the large bowel, symptoms are similar to a small bowel obstruction, but appear more gradually. The patient complains of persistent constipation leading to abdominal distention. Vomiting may be absent, if the ileocecal valve is functioning. Physical examination reveals loud borborygmi, no abdominal tenderness, and an empty rectal vault. Patients with a strangulating bowel may exhibit signs of shock late in the presentation of the obstruction.

Diagnostic Tests: White blood cells (WBCs) may be slightly elevated to 15,000/mm^3; a shift to the left may occur without an elevation of the WBCs in the older adult. Hematocrit may be elevated in the dehydrated patient. A urinalysis may reveal an increase in specific gravity owing to the excess fluid loss. Serum electrolyte are ordered to determine degree of dehydration and plan for intravenous (IV) fluid replacement. A rise in the BUN could indicate blood in the intestine and/or dehydration. The serum amylase level may be moderately elevated. Positive test result for occult blood in the stool suggests bowel strangulation or carcinoma of the bowel. Chest x-ray and supine and upright plain abdominal films determine presence of air-fluid levels, external hernias, or marked dilatation of the bowel. If possible, the chest x-ray examination should be obtained after the nasogastric tube has been inserted. Colonoscopy is performed to determine the site of the obstruction. Barium enema is also diagnostic for bowel obstruction. Oral barium is contraindicated in patients with a suspected colonic obstruction because a hardened mass of the barium can form above the obstruction.

Differential Diagnosis: Acute appendicitis, cholecystitis, pancreatitis, and diverticulitis must be considered in the diagnosis of bowel obstruction.

Treatment: Initial treatment of a bowel obstruction consists of hospitalization for nasogastric suctioning, urinary catheter to monitor output, and fluid and electrolyte replacement with IV fluids. Prophylactic IV antibiotics may be ordered by the surgeon. For an acute mechancial obstruction, surgery is indicated to correct the underlying cause (e.g., repair a hernia, lyse adhesions, correct a volvulus, or remove a gallstone or high fecal impaction). For patients with adynamic ileus, nasogastric suctioning and IV fluids may be all that is necessary to relieve the obstruction; for other patients with an ileus, colonoscopic decompression may be required. Terminally ill patients with bowel obstruction should receive palliative care, including pain relief and IV hydration.

Follow-up: Postoperative care of the patient with a surgically corrected bowel obstruction includes monitoring for return of bowel function, maintaining fluid and electrolyte balance with IV alimentation, and observing for signs of sepsis. After discharge from the hospital, the patient should return within 2 weeks for surveillance. Patients being treated nonsurgically should also be monitored accordingly; observe for signs of recurrence of the bowel obstruction. If an ileus persists longer than 1 week, an underlying mechanical obstruction should be ruled out and a laparotomy may be necessary.

Sequelae: Following correction of a bowel obstruction, slow return of bowel function is an early complication. The possibility of ensuing bowel obstructions and sepsis needs to be monitored in all patients. For those patients who are not surgical candidates, complications such as perforation and peritonitis should be considered.

Prevention/Prophylaxis: Caregivers must understand the importance of avoiding fecal impactions in patients at risk for this condition.

Referral: Recommend a surgical consultation for patients with susceptible bowel obstruction.

Education: Inform older adults with diagnosed untreated internal and external hernias of the possible complication of bowel obstruction.

Cholecystitis

Cholecystitis, an acute or chronic inflammation of the gallbladder, results from an obstruction of the cystic duct.

Etiology: The pathologic origin of gallstones is unknown. Cholecystitis occurs when the cystic duct becomes obstructed, usually by a gallstone, except in cases involving trauma, recent surgery, or sepsis.

Occurrence: Approximately 10% of the United States population of adults age 40 and older have gallstones; 90% of cases of cholecystitis are associated with gallstones.

Age: Common presentation is in the fifth and sixth decades.

Ethnicity: A high prevalence for cholecystitis exists in older Native Americans and whites; the disease is less prevalent in African-Americans. The prevalence of gallbladder disease is highest in the Pima Indians of Arizona.

Gender: Twice as many women as men have cholecystitis.

Contributing Factors: Obesity is a known predisposing factor to cholecystitis. Diabetes, ileal disease, pancreatic insufficiency, and hyperlipidemia predispose patients to gallstone development. The consumption of a large, fatty meal may result in cholecystitis. Gallstone formation may be attributed to use of exogenous estrogens prescribed for postmenopausal hormone replacement and clofibrate used to treat hyperlipidemia. Gallbladder stasis, a precursor to gallstone formation, occurs with extended treatment of total parenteral nutrition.

Signs and Symptoms. One type of presentation of acute cholecystitis includes nausea, vomiting, malaise, fever (which may be low-grade), and abdominal pain that radiates around the sides to the back as in biliary colic; another type is associated with an acute change in mental status as the only outward sign. Physical examination may reveal right upper quadrant subcostal tenderness and pain upon inspiration (Murphy's sign). In a patient who has reported symptoms for a number of days, rebound tenderness may suggest perforation. Abdominal tenderness, however, may be absent.

Diagnostic Tests: A CBC with differential shows WBCs of 12,000–15,000 with peripheral leukocytosis, although WBCs may not be elevated in older adults. Serum amylase generally is increased, even without evident pancreatitis. Serum bilirubin and alkaline phosphatase levels may also be elevated if biliary obstruction has occurred.

In chronic cholecystitis, however, the laboratory values may be normal. Real-time ultrasonography, the diagnostic procedure of choice for both chronic and acute cholecystitis, shows gallstones, thickening of the gallbladder wall, and, if the common bile duct is obstructed, dilatation of the biliary tract.

Differential Diagnosis: Older adults with a perforated peptic ulcer, appendicitis, liver abscess, diverticulitis, hepatitis, acute pyelonephritis, gastrointestinal carcinoma, and acute pancreatitis have symptoms similar to those of cholecystitis.

Treatment: Patients with acute cholecystitis require hospitalization. Nasogastric suctioning, IV fluids with electrolytes, and intramuscular analgesics for severe pain are ordered. In older adults with suspected infection, IV antibiotics should be given adjusting the dosage for creatinine clearance. Effective single-agent antibiotics such as ampicillin, cephalosporins, ureidopenicillins are recommended, except in cases of extremely debilitated patients. Those with signs of gram-negative sepsis may require combination antibiotic treatment. Surgical intervention should be considered once the patient stabilizes. When surgery is contraindicated in patients with acute calculous cholecystitis, treatment with urodexycholic acid may be considered if an adequate functioning gallbladder is present and gallstones are determined to be composed of cholesterol.

Follow-up: Postoperative management includes monitoring for impending infection, adverse drug reactions and interactions, and changes in functional and mental status. For the frail older adult who is not a surgical candidate, observation for complications is critical. Ultrasound of the gallbladder at 6-month intervals is recommended. For older women still prone to cholelithiasis after surgery, dosages of estrogen preparation may need to be reduced if applicable.

Sequelae: Complications of acute cholecystitis may result from severe inflammation with necrosis to the gallbladder; abscess formation and localized perforation may occur. The mortality rate for persons with perforation is moderately high (about 30%).

Prevention/Prophylaxis: The importance of resting and avoiding risk factors following acute cholecystitis or an exacerbation of chronic cholecystitis needs to be emphasized.

Referral: A surgical consultation is necessary if acute cholecystitis is suspected. A gastroenterologist should be consulted for the frail older adult who is not a surgical candidate.

Education: Encourage patients with chronic cholecystitis and those for whom surgery is contraindicated to report early signs and symptoms of an acute attack, to prevent complications.

Chronic Renal Failure

Chronic renal failure (CRF) can result from any long-term cause of renal dysfunction. In older adults, renal disease is often secondary to other age-related conditions. CRF is characterized by a decrease in the glomerular filtration rate.

Etiology: Chronic renal failure involves progressive, irreversible damage to both kidneys. There are many causes of CRF, including diabetic nephropathy, hypertensive disease, glomerulonephritis, and cystic kidney disease. In a small number of cases (about 6%), the etiology is unknown.

Occurrence: Chronic renal failure is diagnosed in more than 40,000 patients per year in the United States.

Age: Chronic renal failure can occur at any age; the incidence increases with age.

Ethnicity: End-stage renal failure (ESRF) is more prevalent in blacks than in whites.

Gender: The overall incidence of ESRF is higher in men than in women; certain causes of ESRF are more common in women, however, such as type II diabetes, scleroderma, and systemic lupus erythematus.

Contributing Factors: Identified risks factors for chronic renal failure include age, race, sex, and family history of disease. Patients with chronic glomerulonephritis, diabetes, hypertensive and atherosclerotic vascular disease, multiple myeloma, amyloidosis, and Wegener's granulomatosis are susceptible to CRF.

Signs and Symptoms: An older adult may complain of anorexia, fatigue, nocturia, and weakness in the early stages of CRF. As the disease progresses, the patient usually reports nausea, vomiting, stomatitis, an unpleasant or metallic taste in the mouth, muscle cramps and twitches, and depression. Physical examination may reveal hypertension and peripheral neuropathies with sensory and motor deficits. In late-stage disease, confusion, breathlessness, and intractable hiccups are observed. Xerosis with pruritus occurs; the skin turns a yellow-brown. Uremic frost is formed from crystallized urea during the later stages of renal failure.

Diagnostic Tests: In diagnostic testing for CRF, look for impaired renal function, significant proteinuria, and urinary sediment. Increased BUN and a decline in urea clearance occurs in CRF. The rise in serum creatinine parallels the rise in BUN, with the BUN level 10 times that of the serum creatinine. Plasma sodium concentrations may be normal or slightly reduced. Patients are usually acidotic, with the CO_2 level between 15 and 20 mmol/L. Subnormal levels of serum calcium and phosphorus are common in CRF. The urinalysis report may show proteinuria and urinary sediment, which may contain broad waxy casts. Findings of the CBC with indices usually shows a normochromic-normocytic anemia of moderate severity. Ultrasound of the kidneys should be performed in all patients with CRF, to determine kidney size and presence of urinary tract obstruction.

Differential Diagnosis: Consider urinary tract obstruction, vasculitis, and kidney infection when establishing the diagnosis of CRF.

Treatment: Underlying factors that contribute to CRF (e.g., heart failure, nephrotoxins, hypercalcemia, infection) must be treated specifically. When uremia develops, dietary protein restriction in the older adult is often unnecessary because the average daily intake is often under 65 g of protein and 4–5 g of salt. Water restriction is unnecessary unless the patient is in congestive heart failure, has uncontrolled hypertension, or has experienced oliguria. A multivitamin should be included as part of the daily regimen. For patients with hypertension, ACE inhibitors are the treatment of choice; captopril 25 mg tid is recommended. Renal function needs to be monitored with drug therapy. If iron-deficiency anemia is detected, give oral ferrous sulfate 325 mg/day. Patients with hypokalemia require potassium supplementation; monitor potassium-blood levels to determine dosage. Consultation with a nephrologist is necessary to determine the need for dialysis and/or hospitalization.

Follow-up: Once the patient is stabilized, monitor CBC, blood chemistries, urine, and blood pressure. Beginning biweekly, review with the patient diet, fluid intake, and medication usage (including OTC drugs). Dosages of any renally excreted medications that the patient must take should be reduced.

Sequelae: Anemia and pruritus are common complications of CRF. Congestive heart failure also may result from CRF. Patients with pruritus and xerosis should use skin moisturizers; antihistamines are contraindicated because of their sedative effect and potential for central nervous system (CNS) adverse reactions. For untreated patients with a creatinine level of greater than 10, uremia occurs and death is imminent within 3–5 months.

Prevention/Prophylaxis: The use of NSAIDs in the elderly with known history of renal failure should be avoided unless absolutely required.

Referral: When the patient begins to show evidence of deterioration despite supportive treatment, refer him or her to a nephrologist. At this time, discuss the options for vascular and/or peritoneal access for dialysis. For the patient who is not a candidate for aggressive treatment, provide information about local hospice services to the patient and the family.

Education: Inform patients of the importance of obtaining consent from their health-care provider before taking any OTC medications. During hot weather, instruct patients to avoid any strenuous activities and to increase their fluid intake to avoid dehydration and hyperthermia.

Cirrhosis of the Liver

Cirrhosis occurs when there is chronic insult to the liver, resulting in fibrous and nodular regeneration of the existing hepatocytes.

Etiology: Chronic alcoholism is the most common cause of cirrhosis in the United States. The cause of primary biliary cirrhosis, a chronic inflammatory disease of the liver in which the intrahepatic bile duct is destroyed, is unknown.

Occurrence: A prevalent disease in older adults, cirrhosis of the liver accounts for more than 25,000 deaths annually in the general population.

Age: Cirrhosis, which has an increase in onset in older adults is one of the top 10 leading causes of death for patients 55 to 74. Onset of primary biliary cirrhosis is usually before age 65.

Ethnicity: No known prevalence exists among groups.

Gender: Cirrhosis of the liver is equally prevalent in men and women with chronic alcoholism.

Contributing Factors: Chronic alcohol consumption, combined with a poor nutritional intake, contributes to cirrhosis.

Signs and Symptoms: Patients report anorexia, fatigue, pruritus, jaundice, and easy bruising of the skin. AUDIT, which stands for the *Alcohol Use Disorders Identification Test*, is an assessment tool specifically for patients with alcoholism. It allows the practitioner to explore the patient's history of chronic alcohol use and the status of functional impairment. Physical examination may reveal evidence of xanthomata, palmar erythema, spider angiomas, clubbing of fingers, and in men decreased body hair, gynecomastia, and testicular atrophy. Palpation of the liver may reveal a firm, nodular liver.

Diagnostic Tests: CBC with indices may reveal a macrocytic anemia caused by nutritional deficiencies of vitamin B_{12} and folic acid. A decreased serum albumin level and prolonged prothrombin time occur in cirrhosis. The serum aspartate aminotransferase (AST) level is elevated; the alanine aminotransferase (ALT) level is usually above normal but not the degree of the AST. A percutaneous liver biopsy can establish the diagnosis of cirrhosis.

Differential Diagnosis: Liver cancer and alcoholic hepatitis need to be considered in the differential diagnosis of cirrhosis; both conditions, however, can occur concomitantly with alcoholic cirrhosis.

Treatment: Cessation of all alcohol intake is imperative. Nutritional support includes at least 1 g protein per kg of body weight and 2000–3000 kcal/day, unless contraindicated by the presence of hepatic encephalopathy or coma. Multiple vitamin supplements should be prescribed.

Follow-up: Surveillance of the older adult with cirrhosis depends on the stability of the patient and the presence of complications. Stable older adults should have repeat liver function tests 6 months to 1 year following initial diagnosis. Unstable patients may need to be monitored monthly. Complications of cirrhosis, listed in the next section, require additional medical therapy. On return visits observation and testing for changes in mental status and depression may be indicated.

Sequelae: Complications from cirrhosis include ascites, portal hypertension, variceal bleeding, renal failure, or encephalopathy. Alcoholic hepatitis may occur with cirrhosis.

Prevention/Prophylaxis: Cessation of alcohol consumption is critical to the prognosis of cirrhosis.

Referral: A gastroenterologist should be consulted when:

- Varices are suspected.
- Variceal bleeding occurs.
- An esophagogastroduodenscopy is performed.
- Managing complications.

Education: Instruct patients to eliminate all alcohol consumption. Recommend an alcohol treatment program and provide the telephone number for the nearest chapter of Alcoholics Anonymous. An additional organization that may be beneficial to the alcoholic patient is: Secular Rational Recovery Systems (530-621-4374). Patients should be requested not to self-medicate with over-the-counter medications.

Colorectal Cancer

Adenocarcinomas are the most common type of cancer of the large intestine; less common are carcinoid tumors, squamous cell carcinoma, and melanoma. Many colorectal cancers develop from adenomatous polyps of the colon and rectum, which occurs most frequently in the sigmoid and rectum. The invasion of cancer of the colon and rectum occurs by direct extension through the bowel wall, hematogenous metastases, perineural extension, metastases to the region lymph nodes, and intraluminal metastases.

Etiology: The etiology of colorectal cancer is unknown, but the high-calorie, high-fat Western diet has been implicated in its development.

Occurrence: Colorectal cancer is the second most common malignancy in the United States, and it is associated with 50% mortality rate.

Age: The incidence of colorectal cancer increases with age; 90% of the cases of colorectal cancer occur in people age 50 and older.

Ethnicity: Seventh-Day Adventists and Mormons, because of their dietary habits and overall lifestyle, tend to have a lower rate of colorectal cancer than the general population.

Gender: Colorectal cancer occurs equally in men and women. Women who have had a cholecystectomy may be at greater risk for this type of cancer.

Contributing Factors: A family history of colorectal cancer, multiple polyps, and a long history of ulcerative colitis have been linked to the development of colorectal cancer. Patients with a family or personal history of gynecologic cancer and patients diagnosed with Barrett's esophagus have an increased risk of developing colorectal cancer. Reported history of a ureterosigmoidostomy and prior infection from *Streptococcus bovis* have also been implicated. A lower incidence of colorectal cancer has been found in vegetarian populations and in those with a high fiber intake. A regular dietary intake of low-fat and high-fiber foods appears to be protective against colorectal carcinoma.

Signs and Symptoms: A new onset of constipation or diarrhea may suggest colorectal cancer. Associated abdominal pain, bloating, and vomiting may also occur. The patient with rectal cancer may have the sensation of incomplete evacuation. Low back pain or leg pain may also be reported. The patient who has been having intestinal bleeding may experience a change in mental status and weakness from anemia. An abdominal or rectal mass may be palpated. A benign polyp tends to feel soft and pliable, whereas a cancerous mass is generally hard and irregular. An anoscopy may reveal a polyp(s) or frank bleeding.

Diagnostic Tests: A colonoscopy with a biopsy that extends to the cecum is recommended for the diagnosis of colon cancer. A second choice is a barium enema with air contrast studies, preceded by a flexible sigmoidoscopy, although with this technique a biopsy is unattainable. An irregular filling defect found by the barium enema suggests an adenocarcinoma. Additional testing should include a CBC to evaluate for anemia. Consider the possibility of metastasis in older adults with colorectal cancer. Elevated serum albumin and alkaline phosphatase levels imply liver metastases. A chest x-ray examination is ordered to detect pulmonary metastases. Measuring the preoperative carcinoembryonic antigen (CEA) level, which is related to the stage of the cancer, can be used to predict the prognosis of the surgical intervention. CEA levels greater than 5.0 ng/mL are associated with a poor prognosis. Measuring the CEA level before surgery is useful as baseline data in the long-term evaluation of colorectal cancer. Patients who are heavy smokers and/or have history of alcoholic liver disease may have increased levels of CEA. Staging of colorectal cancer is determined after surgery from the pathology reports.

Differential Diagnosis: An inflammatory mass in the colon caused by diverticulitis should be considered in the differential diagnosis; however, a history of weight loss combined with blood in the stool and a mass in the colon generally indicates an adenocarcinoma. Other neoplasms such as prostatic carcinoma and sarcoma need to be ruled out.

Treatment: The extent of treatment for colorectal cancer depends on how invasive the cancer is in the colon and surrounding sites and the condition of the patient at the time of diagnosis. Patients should be referred to a surgeon for consideration of a radical resection; presence of metastatic disease does not necessarily rule out surgery. The use of chemotherapeutic agent fluorouracil combined with levamisole is an effective adjuvant therapy after a surgical resection of stage III colorectal cancer, even in older adults.

Follow-up: After curative surgery the following are essential:

- Close monitoring for symptoms of fatigue, weight loss, and change in bowel habits.

- Physical examination especially of the chest and abdomen.
- CBC to rule out anemia.
- Liver function tests and chest x-ray examination to detect indications of metastatic disease.

A colonoscopy should be ordered, yearly unless a new polyp is present, in which case every 6 months. Given the high recurrence rate of colorectal cancer, patients who have had a resection of the colon should have a colonoscopy 3–6 months after the surgery to detect cancerous lesions at the site of the anastomosis and new developments in other sections of the colon. CEA levels should be evaluated every 6 months for the first 2 years after the operation; decreasing levels indicate tumor regression. Initial follow-up after radical resection for patients with a temporary or permanent colostomy should include counseling, a review of ostomy care, and community resource information. Determine the patient's nutritional status, current weight, and possible need for nutritional supplements.

Sequelae: Complications of colorectal cancer include obstruction and perforation. A postresection recurrence of colorectal cancer is common. Bowel adhesions and fibrosis may also occur. The lungs and bone are two sites known for metastasis following colorectal cancer.

Prevention/Prophylaxis: The American Cancer Society recommends that beginning at age 50 all asymptomatic individuals with no risk factors should have an annual fecal occult blood test. A sigmoidoscopy for men and women over age 65 is recommended every 3–5 years. Prolonged prophylactic use of aspirin may reduce the risk of colon cancer.

Referral: A gastroenterologist should be consulted for colonoscopy with biopsy of the lesion. A surgical consultation should be initiated after diagnosis, for consideration of radical resection. If adjuvant chemotherapy is indicated, an oncologist is also consulted. Depending on the outcome of the surgery, consultation with an endostomal therapist may be necessary. The patient and the family should be given information about local hospice services, as needed.

Education: Teach older adults about the importance of routine surveillance for rectal bleeding.

Cystitis

Cystitis is an infection of the wall of the bladder, resulting from an ascending infection from the urethra in 95% of cases. Bacteriuria is the main clinical manifestation of cystitis.

Etiology: The susceptibility to urinary tract infections increases in old age because the host defenses of the body, needed to prevent phagocytose bacteria from coming in contact with the bladder mucosa, are diminished or impaired.

Occurrence: Cysttis is prevalent in older adults, with a 10%–30% rate of infection.

Age: The incidence of cystitis increases with age, especially for men and all institutionalized older adults.

Ethnicity: No known prevalence exists among ethnic groups.

Gender: Cystitis is more prevalent in older women than in older men; the incidence of cystitis increases with age in older men, related to benign prostatic hypertrophy and prostatitis.

Contributing Factors: Predisposing factors to the development of cystitis include indwelling catheters, functional disability, incontinence, cognitive impairment, diabetes, ureteral obstruction, uterine or bladder prolapse, estrogen deficiencies, and a history of vesicoureteral reflux.

Signs and Symptoms: Mental confusion, anorexia, malaise, and incontinence may be the first symptoms of cystitis in an older patient, especially for patients with indwelling catheters or a neurogenic bladder. Patients may report urgency, frequency, and dysuria. Gross hematuria is more common in younger women than in older adults with cystitis. Question patients about their sexual history, to include use of spermicide. Physical examination may reveal fever, tachypnea, and tachycardia. Superpubic tenderness may be elicited upon palpation. Percussion for CVA tenderness may be positive with reported flank pain. Vaginal examination in women should rule out discharge or erythema. In men, the prostate gland should be examined very gently to assess for enlargement, bogginess, and tenderness (Fig. 10–1).

Diagnostic Tests: A dipstick urinanalysis for nitrate and luekocyte esterase (LE) shows a positive LE and positive nitrate with a gram-negative organism. A microscopic urinalysis in symptomatic bacteriuria shows pyuria and bacteria. Pyuria with more than 10 WBCs usually indicates cystitis in 95% of cases. Clinical bacteriuria in women with symptomatic dysuria is defined as greater than 10^2 colony-forming units (CFU)/mL with pyuria of a single or predominant uropathogen grown on the culture. In dysuric men, growths of greater than 10^3 CFU/mL or more of a single or predominant uropathogen is considered clinically diagnostic. If more than one organism is identified, the culture may be contaminated and should be repeated. Identification and susceptibility testing on a urine culture from an indwelling catheter may reveal one or two predominant organisms at 10^4 CFU/mL or more. In asymptomatic women, 10^5 CFU/mL or higher indicates bacteriuria. Organisms causing urinary tract infections are usually aerobes such as *Escherichia coli, Klebsiella, Enterobacter,* staphylococci, *Pseudomonas,* and *Proteus.* Gram's stain of unspun urine detecting one or more bacteria per oil-immersion field is associated with a colony count of more than 10^5/mL.

Differential Diagnosis: Urethritis, prostatitis, pyelonephritis, and vaginitis are considered in the workup for cystitis.

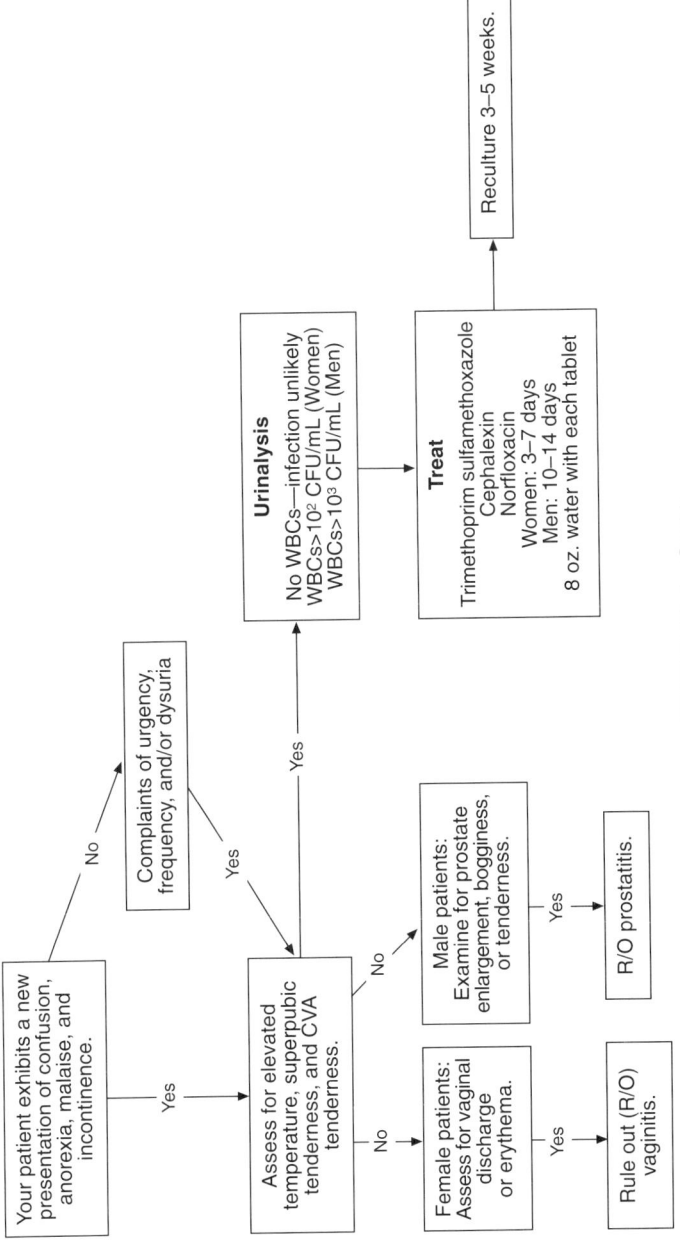

FIGURE 10–1 Cystitis.

Treatment: Older women with symptomatic uncomplicated bacteriuria should be treated with oral trimethoprim sulfamethoxazole 160 mg/800 mg every 12 hr, cephalexin 250–500 mg every 6 hr, or norfloxacin 400 mg every 12 hr, for 3–7 days. Older men with uncomplicated cystitis require medication for 10–14 days. Longer treatments, for 4–6 weeks, may be necessary to sterilize the urinary tract in older men following an infection. Monitor reneal function before dosing medications, however.

Follow-up: Repeat culturing 3–5 weeks after completion of the medication regimen. Relapse occurs when the same organism is found in the culture specimen shortly after cessation of treatment. Reinfection, a reintroduction of the organism from the fecal reservoir, occurs in 10%–25% of all cases of cystitis. Change in treatment is warranted if the organisms are resistant to the original treatment.

Sequelae: Untreated symptomatic cystitis can lead to pyelonephritis, sepsis, shock, and death.

Prevention/Prophylaxis: Prophylactic use of antibiotics by patients with indwelling catheters is not recommended. For older adults who require frequent instrumentation of the lower genitourinary tract or who have frequent cystitis, give trimethoprim/sulfamethoxazole 80 mg/400 mg, ½–1 tablet nightly.

Referral: In complicated cystitis that has progressed to pyelonephritis or urosepsis, consultation with a specialist is recommended for hospitalization.

Education: Inform all patients receiving antimicrobial therapy for cystitis of the necessity of drinking at least 8 oz of water with each tablet. Encourage patients with recurrent cystitis to drink cranberry juice as part of their daily routine.

Diverticulitis

Diverticulitis is an inflammatory condition that involves perforation of one or more colonic diverticula, which are herniations of the mucosa through the muscularis of the colon. It usually occurs in the sigmoid or descending colon. Inflammation of the diverticulum begins at the apex when the narrow opening of the lumen is exposed to fecal residue.

Etiology: Diverticula are common in older adults. Age-related changes in the elastic matrix of the colon and the resulting sluggish fecal mass are thought to cause increased intraluminal pressure of the colon. Diverticular disease is rare in societies that consume high-fiber diets. It is thought that a low-fiber diet produces less bulky stool and increased intracolonic pressure. Diverticulitis, is thought to develop when one or more diverticula are perforated. Because this perforation is usually a localized process, free intraperitoneal air or diffuse peritoneal signs are usually not evident; their presence would indicate a more severe case and the possible need for surgical consultation.

Occurrence: An estimated 65% of older adults will develop diverticulosis by age 85. Only about 5% of the population with diverticulosis will go on to develop diverticulitis, which is usually most severe in older adults.

Age: Diverticulitis is most commonly found in older adults.

Ethnicity: This condition is found almost exclusively in westernized countries or populations that have begun to consume a refined Western diet.

Gender: Diverticulitis occurs equally in men and women.

Contributing Factors: Chronic constipation and the need to strain to defecate contribute to diverticulitis. Chronic use of NSAIDs increases the incidence of diverticulitis.

Signs and Symptoms: Clinical presentation of diverticulitis in an older adult may be suppressed despite the presence of severe disease. Mental confusion may be the first overt indication of diverticulitis in an older adult with known diverticular disease. History of left lower quadrant pain and fever may be present; associated complaints of nausea and vomiting suggest obstruction. Constipation or diarrhea, abdominal cramping without the abdominal pain, and fever may also occur. Joint pain may be reported. Bowel sounds may be normal in mild disease; however, bowel sounds become hypoactive until there is an obstruction, when a tinkling sound may be heard. Localized tenderness is usually present in the left lower quadrant. Rebound tenderness and guarding are signs of peritonitis. A mass palpated in the left lower quadrant may indicate an abscess. Occult rectal bleeding occurs in about 25% of patients with diverticulitis. Tenderness may be elicited during the rectal examination.

Diagnostic Tests: Complete blood count with differential shows a low hemoglobin, indicative of bleeding; the WBC count may show a shift to the left. Erythrocyte sedimentation rate (ESR) is elevated to greater than 30 mm/hr. The urinalysis often shows increased WBCs and hematuria. Supine and upright abdominal x-ray films can detect air-fluid levels—signs of bowel obstruction or free air showing ruptured diverticulum. An ultrasound of the abdomen is ordered to rule out the possibility of an ovarian cyst. A CT scan is the recommended method for determining abscesses. Sigmoidoscopy, colonoscopy, and barium enema are usually avoided during acute diverticulitis because these tests may cause further perforation or leakage of bowel contents. These tests may be performed several weeks after the resolution of the acute episode.

Differential Diagnosis: The differential diagnosis for diverticulitis includes inflammatory bowel disease, ischemic colitis, vascular ectasia, carcinoma of the colon, urologic disorders, and gynecologic carcinomas or abscesses.

Treatment: For mild cases, rest, clear liquids, and oral antibiotics such as amoxicillin and clavulanate potassium 250–500 mg tid or ciprofloxacin hydrochloride 250–500 mg are recommended every 12 hr, and metronidazole 250–500 mg tid can be tried at home for 7–10 days if follow-up occurs within 72 hr. Hospitalization should be considered for older adults, with diverticulitis, owing to the uncertainty of the severity of the disease because of possibly subdued presentation. Acute treatment for hospitalized patients should consist of bed rest, restriction of any fluids by mouth, nasogastric suction if nausea, vomiting, or other indication of obstruction is present, and IV fluids and electrolytes. Various antibiotic regimens are used for treatment of diverticulitis. Because of the need for adequate coverage of bowel flora, commonly used agents include ampicillin/sulbactam sodium 1 g IV every 6 hr or ciprofloxacin 250–500 mg IV bid with metronidazole 250–500 mg IV tid for the treatment of severe diverticulitis. Pay special attention to the patient's renal function and creatinine clearance level.

Follow-up: Older adults with mild cases treated at home with prescribed therapy should expect improvement by the third day. Hospitalized patients require daily monitoring for persistent signs and symptoms of diverticulitis, laboratory values, and response to treatment. Surgical consultation may be necessary if the patient does not respond to treatment and continues to have elevated WBCs, fever, rebound tenderness, pain, and tachycardia.

Sequelae: Complications include bowel perforation, peritonitis, abscess, fistula, hemorrhage, and bowel obstruction.

Prevention/Prophylaxis: Recognition of early signs and symptoms of diverticulitis helps prevent severe cases.

Referral: Severe episodes of diverticulitis require consultation with a gastroenterologist for hospitalization. Repeated episodes may require surgical consultation for an elective sigmoid resection.

Education: Provide information on a high-fiber diet and/or fiber supplementation. Teach patients to increase their fluid intake unless otherwise cautioned, especially when taking fiber supplements.

Esophagitis

Esophagitis is an inflammation of the lining of the esophagus.

Etiology: Patients may develop esophagitis if they:
- Ingest medications improperly.
- Ingest caustic chemicals.
- Have chronic conditions such as scleroderma.
- Are exposed to local radiation treatments.

A bacterial, viral, or fungal infection can cause esophagitis. *Candida albicans* is the most common fungal infection. The herpes simplex I virus can also cause esophagitis. Bacterial esophagitis is rare but can coincide with a fungal or viral infection, making it difficult to diagnose. In gastroesophageal reflux disease, esophagitis is a common complication.

Occurrence: The exact incidence of esophagitis is unknown.

Age: Esophagitis can occur at all ages.

Ethnicity: No known prevalence exists among ethnic groups.

Gender: Esophagitis occurs equally in men and women.

Contributing Factors: In older adults, normal aging changes such as decreased gastric motility and delayed gastric emptying can contribute to the development of esophagitis. Immunosuppressed patients are susceptible to viral, bacterial, and fungal infections. Swallowing certain medications such as aspirin, tetracycline, ferrous sulfate, NSAIDs, and potassium chloride without sufficient fluids and not remaining upright for at least 5 minutes after the medication is taken can cause esophagitis. Substances that lower the esophageal sphincter (coffee, peppermint, alcohol, spicy foods, citric fruits, nifedipine, verapamil, and progesterone) can contribute to esophagitis.

Signs and Symptoms: A history of dysphagia and pain upon swallowing is common. Associated pyrosis, regurgitation, coughing, wheezing, and progressive hoarseness may occur. A fever may be present in patients with an infectious process. Patients should be questioned about medication usage, smoking, intake of substances that lower the esophageal sphincter, sleeping habits, and use of any tight or restrictive clothing. Physical examination usually produces no positive findings. Oral thrush may be found in patients with *Candida albicans.* Palpate for any upper abdominal masses or tendernes. Perform a rectal examination to detect any frank bleeding (Fig. 10–2).

Diagnostic Tests: If suspicion was aroused on the physical examination stool should be checked using the guaiac test to determine if there has been any intestinal bleeding. Laboratory studies are not required when pyrosis is relieved by antacids, position change, or both. For older adults who complain of persistent dysphagia, or dynophagia with or without fever, a barium shallow and/or an endoscopy (with brush and biopsy if stuctural mucosal damage is suspected) is ordered.

Differential Diagnosis: Esophageal stricture, esophageal carcinoma, cholecystitis, and peptic ulcer disease may mimic this disorder.

Treatment: For infectious esophagitis, temporary symptomatic relief can be obtained with sucralfate slurry 1 g/10 mL PO qid. Viscous lidocaine (2%) 15 mL PO every 4 hr as needed to swish and swallow can be used also for short-term temporary relief, unless contraindicated by potential drug interactions or history of cardiac or hepatic disease. For mild cases of *Candida albicans* infection, nystatin oral suspension 400,000–600,000 units qid spaced evenly over 24 hr is prescribed. For more serious cases, such as in patients with AIDS, ketoconazole 200–400 mg PO qid is given. Ketoconazole should not be given at the same time as antacids or H2 blockers. For severe cases of herpes simplex virus–induced esophagitis, IV acyclovir may be given, adjusting the dosage for the patient's weight and creatinine clearance. Esophagitis from radiation can

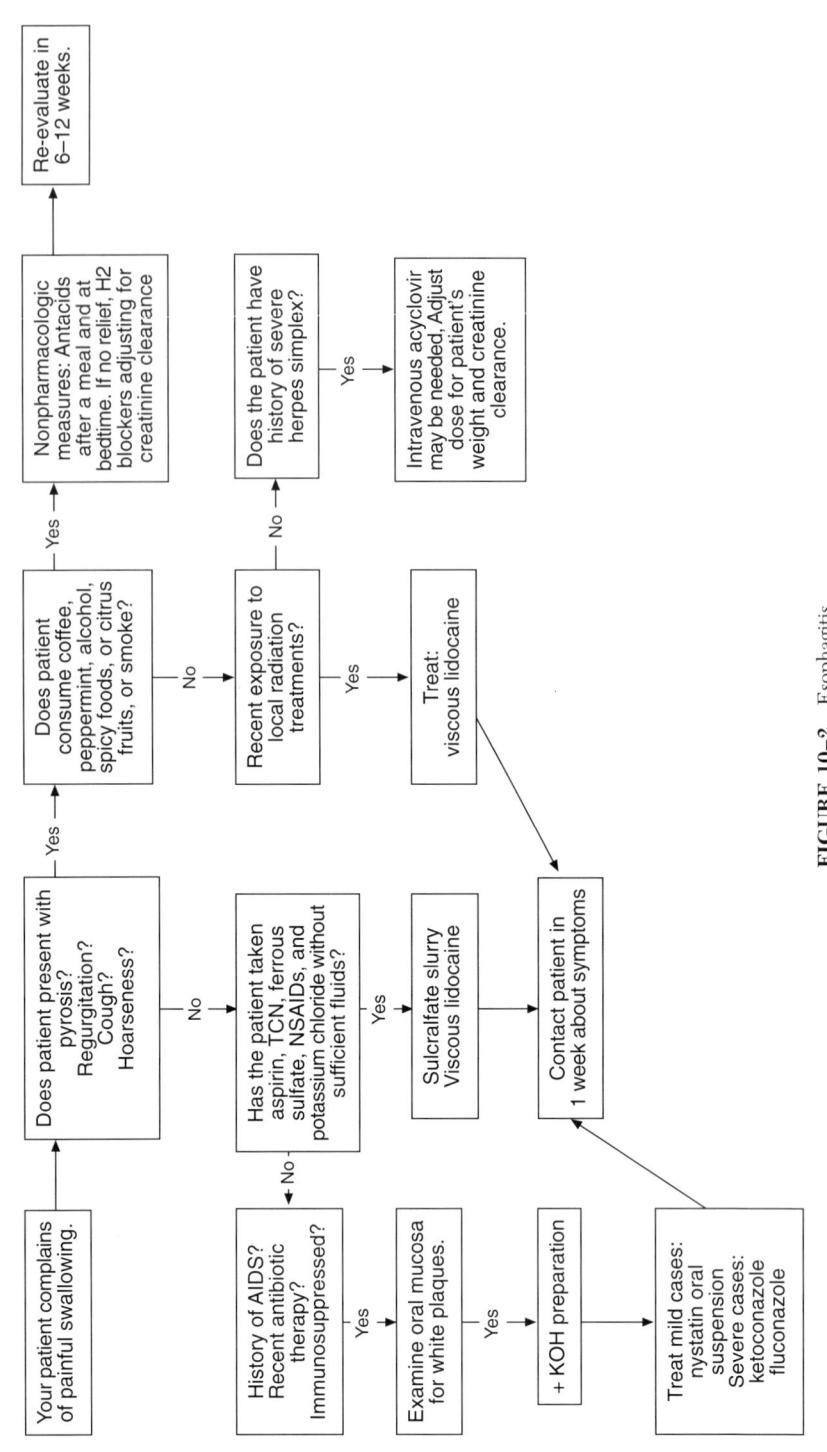

FIGURE 10–2 Esophagitis.

be treated with viscous lidocaine. For esophageal reflux, nonpharmacologic therapy should be initiated, with the use of antacids after meals and at bedtime. Oral H2 blockers such as ranitidine 150 mg PO bid, famotidine 20 mg bid, and nizatidine 150 mg bid, adjusting the dosage for the creatinine clearance. In cases of erosive esophagitis caused by reflux, omeprazole 20 mg once a day for 4–8 weeks is given. Alternatively, patients may be given lansoprazole 30 mg qid before eating for up to 8 weeks, followed by reevaluation.

Follow-up: Patients should report progress at least 1 week after treatment. Repeat endoscopy at 6–12 weeks if the patient is still symptomatic but compliant. Yearly endoscopy is recommended thereafter for patients with severe cases of esophagitis.

Sequelae: Ulceration and bleeding, if reflux esophagitis is present, can occur following esophagitis; Barrett's esophagus with possible adenocarcinoma may be a long-term complication.

Prevention/Prophylaxis: Because of the high recurrence rate of esophagitis, patients should be instructed to follow all nonpharmacologic measures unless otherwise instructed. H2 blockers may be prescribed for an extended time.

Referral: A gastroenterologist should be consulted for the endoscopy and for patients with severe or nonresponsive esophagitis.

Education: Patients with reflux esophagitis should be instructed to raise the head of the bed 4–6 inches with shock blocks. Factors that increase abdominal pressure, such as wearing tight restrictive clothing should be avoided. The patient should avoid smoking and ingestion of fatty foods, coffee, chocolate, peppermints, citric juices, alcohol, and large quantities of fluids with meals. If an H2 blocker is prescribed, the second dose of the medication should be taken with or immediately after the evening meal.

Gastritis

Gastritis is an inflammation of the mucosal lining of the stomach.

Etiology: Gastritis represents a group of disorders characterized by inflammation of the stomach lining; each disorder, however, has distinct clinical attributes, pathogeneses, and histological features. Gastritis may be caused by:

- Infectious agents such as *Helicobacter pylori* or streptococci.
- Autoimmune reactions.
- Food or drug allergies.
- Parasitic disease.
- Physiologic stressors.
- Normal aging changes.
- Prior gastric surgery.

Gastritis is divided first into erosive and nonerosive; a possible inflammatory process within each group may then be categorized as acute or chronic.

Occurrence: Exact incidence of gastritis is unknown.

Age: Although gastritis occurs in all ages, it is a common occurrence in older adults.

Ethnicity: No known prevalence exists among ethnic groups.

Gender: Gastritis occurs equally in men and women.

Contributing Factors: Many factors can precipitate the development of gastritis. Acute gastritis can be caused by physiological stressors, hypovolemic shock, aspirin, NSAIDs, alcohol, radiation, gastric lymphoma, Crohn's disease, and *H. pylori* and other bacterial and viral infections. Chronic gastritis can develop because of gastric atrophy, *H. pylori* infection, bile and pancreatic secretions, and pernicious anemia. Most patients who have had a previous gastrectomy will develop gastritis.

Signs and Symptoms: Anorexia, nausea (with or without vomiting), and epigastric distress aggravated by eating are common with gastritis. Physical examination may be unremarkable in cases of chronic gastritis. Palpate for abdominal masses and liver tenderness. Perform a rectal examination to test for occult blood. Any unaccounted weight loss should be noted. Gastrointestinal (GI) bleeding may be exhibited by "coffee-ground" vomitus, melena, hematochezia, or the passing of bright red blood in a nasogastric tube. Any patient suspected of GI bleeding should be examined for changes in mental status, coolness of the extremities, and pallor of the nailbeds, mucus membranes, and conjunctivae. Assessment should include watching for any changes in cardiac output such as decreasing blood pressure and increased heart rate (Fig. 10–3).

Diagnostic Tests

Complete blood count with indices to detect blood loss and anemia.
Stool guaiac tested.
Gastroscopy with a biopsy, the definitive diagnostic test for gastritis.

Differential Diagnosis: Consider peptic ulcer disease and gastric carcinomas in the differential diagnosis of gastritis.

Treatment: Patients with acute gastritis should avoid offensive agents such as alcohol, NSAIDs, and aspirin. H2 blockers such as famotidine, ranitidine, or nizatidine can be given for 6–8 weeks. An oral dose of ranitidine 300 mg or nizatidine 300 mg daily at bedtime can be ordered. Decrease the dosage of the H2 blockers however, depending on the creatinine clearance. If the creatinine clearance is less than 50 mL/min, reduce the dosage for ranitidine to 150 mg qid. If the creatinine clearance is 20–50 mL/min, the dose for nizatidine should be 150 mg daily. If the creatinine clearance is less than 20 mL/min, give nizatidine 150 mg every other day. Acute hemorrhagic gastritis requires hospitalization for intravenous fluids, nasogastric aspiration, transfusion of blood products as necessary, and monitoring of vital signs. Chronic gastritis from *H. pylori*

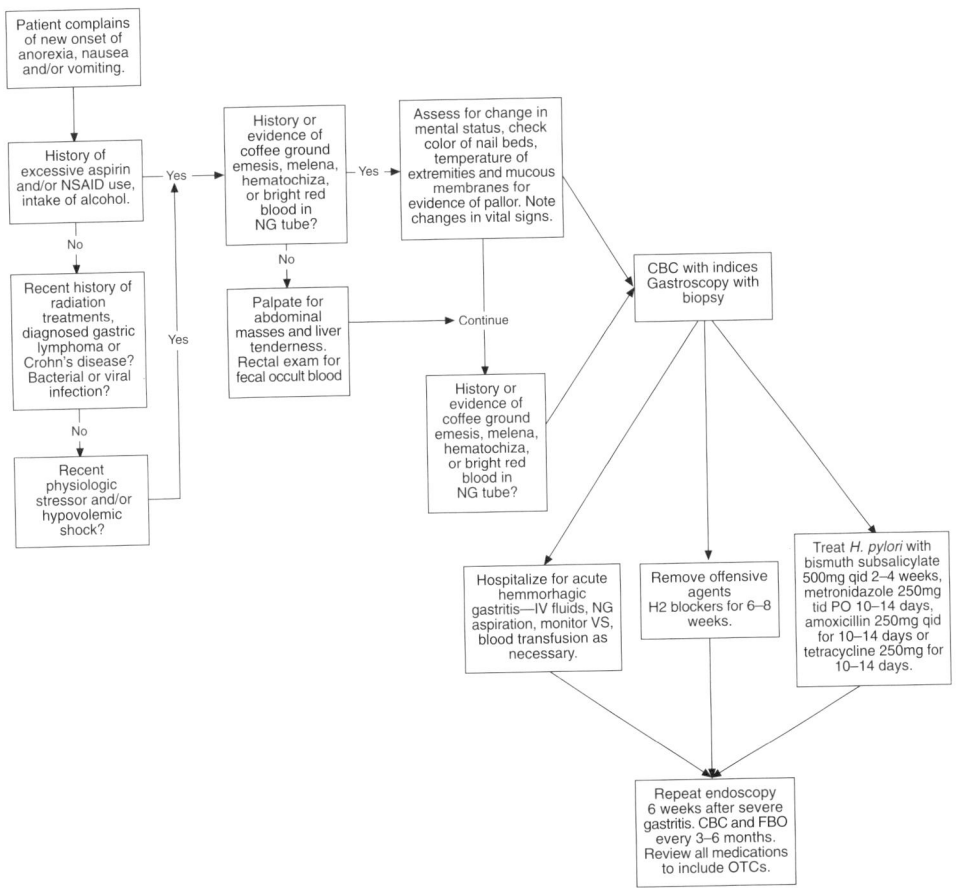

FIGURE 10–3   Gastritis.

can be treated with bismuth subsalicylate 500 mg qid for 2–4 weeks, metronidazole 250 mg PO for 10–14 days, amoxicillin 250 mg qid for 10–14 days, or tetracycline 250 mg qid PO for 10–14 days. The absorption of tetracycline can be decreased if the bismuth is taken at the same time. Diarrhea is a common drug side effect.

Follow-up: A repeat endoscopy is advised after 6 weeks for those patients who had severe gastritis or who continue to have symptoms despite treatment. Obtain a blood count and check stool for occult blood at subsequent office visits every 3–6 months following the diagnosis of gastritis. At each follow-up appointment, review all drugs, including over-the-counter medications.

Sequelae: Acute hemorrhagic gastritis has a high mortality rate in older adults. Patients with untreated chronic gastritis associated with pernicious anemia develop neurological complications.

Prevention/Prophylaxis: Alternative anti-inflamatory or nonnarcotic analgesics should be considered in the treatment of pain or inflammation in older adults with a history of gastritis. Critically ill older adults need to be monitored for signs and symptoms of hypovolemic shock due to acute gastric bleeding.

Referral: Older patients with acute hemorrhagic gastritis require hospitalization, probably with admission to the intensive care unit. Consultation with a gastroenterologist for endoscopy and management of complicated cases of gastritis is recommended.

Education: Advise patients to report any black tarlike stools or frank bleeding to the practitioner immediately. All alcohol product use should be discontinued.

Gastroenteritis

Gastroenteritis is an infectious response of the gastrointestinal tract to various microorganisms that can be viral, bacterial, or parasitic in origin.

Etiology: Gastroenteritis is caused by exposure to:

Viruses such as Norwalk virus, Norwalk-like virus, and Astrovirus.

Bacteria such as *Salmonella, Campylobacter, Shigella, Escherichia coli,* and *Vibrio cholerae.*

Parasites such as *Giardia lamblia.*

Occurrence: Exact incidence of infectious gastroenteritis is unknown because of under-reporting of symptoms. Approximately 30%–40% of gastroenteritis diarrhea in the United States is thought to be viral in origin, with more than 55% of the adult population exposed to a common enteric calci virus.

Age: Gastroenteritis occurs at all ages, but its incidence and the mortality rate from infectious diarrhea are higher in older adults. Epidemic cases of gastroenteritis occur in nursing home populations.

Ethnicity: No known prevalence exists among ethnic groups.

Gender: Gastroenteritis is equally prevalent in both sexes, although diarrhea is more common in women.

Contributing Factors: Specific to the older adult population, age-related factors such as decreased motility, mucosal atrophy, and decreased gastric acidity inhibit natural defense mechanisms against infectious agents. The use of H2 blockers, antacids, anticholinergic drugs, and narcotics increases the potential for developing gastroenteritis. Gastroenteritis can also be caused by emotional stress, viral or bacterial infection, food intolerance, and organic (shellfish, certain mushrooms) or inorganic poisons (sodium nitrate). Travel to another country with a change in surroundings or to an area of poor sanitation standards and facilities can contribute to the development of gastroenteritis. Nursing home populations are susceptible to epidemics because of contact with health-care workers who may not use proper hand-washing techniques. Fecal-to-oral contact has been identified as a mode of transmission of organisms.

Signs and Symptoms: History of possible fecal-to-oral contact, exposure to other patients with gastroenteritis, and ingestion of certain food products such as mayonnaise, custards, fried rice, vegetables, beef, or poultry should be explored. Travel to a foreign country or region that may have contaminated water should be recorded, as should any previous history of diarrhea and related symptoms and the duration of the current episode. A sudden onset of diarrhea, abdominal pain with distension, flatulence, and vomiting may be reported. Associated anorexia, headache, fatigue, dizziness, and myalgias are also symptoms of gastro-enteritis. Fever may or may not occur in the older adult; mental confusion may result from dehydration. The stool's color, odor, amount, and frequency should be described and the presence of any blood or mucus in the stool discerned. Patients' use of prescription drugs, OTC medications, and home remedies needs to be included in the history.

In the physical examination the skin is checked for signs of rashes or dehy-dration and the lymph nodes are assessed for any lymphadenopathy. Abdominal examination may reveal distension, hyperactive bowel sounds, and tenderness. Perform a rectal examination to note any bleeding and color of the stool and to check for an impaction.

Diagnostic Tests: CBC with differential should be ordered. WBC shift to the left may suggest an infection and a decreased hemoglobin value indicates anemia from probable blood loss. Serum electrolyte evaluation shows an increased sodium level in dehydrated patients and decreased potassium resulting from the diarrhea. Elevated serum creatinine and BUN levels also occur in dehydra-tion. Stool samples for blood, ova and parasite, leukocytes, and bacteria are ordered to try to identify the microorganism. A stool culture positive for blood is found in bacterial infections as well as in inflammatory processes; the culture and sensitivity report may show *Salmonella, Campylobacter, Shigella,* and *V. cholerae.* Consider sigmoidoscopy for patients with bloody diarrhea.

Differential Diagnosis: Consider the possibility of fecal impaction, fecal inconti-nence, colorectal cancers, adverse reaction to medications, diverticulitis, mal-absorption, and pseudomembranous colitis if the patient has recently been prescribed an antibiotic.

Treatment: Lost fluids and electrolytes must be replaced. Clear liquids and specially formulated rehydration liquids such as Gatorade should be given as tolerated. Clear broths and crackers may be added to the diet when diarrhea has ceased. Patients should avoid caffeine, dairy products, alcohol, fruits, bran, vegetables, and red meats. Solid foods should be added gradually, starting with rice or potatoes. When the patient no longer has loose stools, foods such as applesauce and bananas and skinless chicken can be added. Physical activity should be limited, to avoid unnecessary exertion. Care should be taken to prevent any skin excoriation or pressure sores. Patients with infectious diarrhea should avoid antidiarrheal medications. Antibiotic therapy is specific to the bacterial or parasitic organisms identified from the stool culture. *Campylobacter* infection is treated with erythromycin 250 mg qid for 5 days or, in the event of sensitivity to erythromycin, ciprofloxacin 500 mg bid for 7 days, adjusting the dose for renal function. *G. lamblia* infection is treated with metronidazole 250 mg tid for 5–10 days. Severe cases of travelers' diarrhea (enterotoxigenic *E. coli*) can be treated with trimethoprim/sulfamethoxazole, 160/800 mg (double strength) PO bid for 5 days or ciprofloxacin 500 mg bid for 3 days.

Follow-up: Contact outpatients 4 days after the onset of symptoms to decide progress. Request nursing home staff to provide a verbal report of the patient's condition on the third or fourth day; note any further outbreak of gastroenteritis. For older adults with chronic diarrhea or other persistent gastrointestinal symptoms, refer to a gastroenterologist.

Sequelae: Dehydration, anemia, and hypovolemic shock could occur in untreated cases of severe infectious diarrhea.

Prevention/Prophylaxis: Older adults with travel plans to foreign destinations should be urged to avoid contaminated water. Avoid ice cubes and brushing teeth with nonbottled water. Discard any foods that contain dairy or egg products that have not been refrigerated for an extended time or exposed to very warm temperatures. Raw or undercooked meat and seafood should be avoided.

Referral: Prefer to a specialist when symptoms persist beyond 4 days, when severe dehydration develops, or when the patient has bloody stools.

Education: Gastroenteritis, although generally self-limiting, can be debilitating. Infections with some microorganisms such as *G. lamblia* can become chronic and result in lactose intolerance, which is common in older adults. Any new case of diarrhea not resolved in 3–4 days requires provider intervention. Use of OTC antiperistaltic agents such as loperamide is contraindicated in infectious diarrhea.

Hernia

A hernia is the protrusion of tissue through a weakened section in the abdominal wall. Abdominal wall hernias usually occur at the groin (inguinal) and umbilicus. Hernias are classified by their severity as reducible, incarcerated, or strangulated.

- A reducible hernia moves easily through the anatomic defect.
- An incarcerated hernia does not return to a normal position automatically or when manipulated externally.
- A strangulated hernia results when an incarcerated hernia develops edema with ischemia to the entrapped bowel.

In addition to these classifications, inguinal hernias may be either direct or indirect. A direct inguinal hernia passes through the posterior inguinal wall, whereas an indirect or congenital inguinal hernia enters in through the internal abdominal inguinal ring along the spermatic cord through the inguinal passage, to exit out the external inguinal ring.

Etiology: Hernia development has been linked to recurrent Valsalva maneuvers and dysfunctional connective tissue resulting from malnutrition or chronic steroid use. In older women, a history of multiple pregnancies and relaxation of the pelvic musculature, combined with loss of extraperitoneal fat, are considered etiologic factors in the development of an obturator hernia.

Occurrence: More than 500,000 herniorrhaphies are performed annually in the United States.

Age: The incidence of femoral hernias in women increases with age. The incidence of male indirect (congenital) hernias decreases with age but that of direct inguinal hernias increases.

Ethnicity: No known prevalence exists among ethnic groups.

Gender: Indirect inguinal hernias are 8 to 10 times more common in men than in women, yet the indirect inguinal hernia is the most common type of hernia in women. Women are three to five times more likely than men to develop a femoral hernia. The obturator hernia is a rare condition that occurs in women only.

Contributing Factors: A chronic cough, ascites, abdominal surgery, and symptomatic prostatism can contribute to development of a hernia because of the associated risk factor of increased intra-abdominal or intrathoracic pressure. Chronic straining for bowel movements, straining to urinate, and lifting heavy objects may be precursors to hernia formation. Hernias also may form at the site of a surgical incision or a large scar.

Signs and Symptoms: Hernias may be asymptomatic, only to be discovered as part of a routine physical examination. A reducible hernia presents as a nontender mass that becomes more pronounced after a Valsalva maneuver. An incarcerated hernia, also a nontender soft mass, is found in the abdominal, femoral, or inguinal area and remains even after gentle manipulation. Patients with strangulated abdominal hernia usually have a tender mass with associated fever, nausea, and vomiting. Physical examination reveals decreased flatus, high-pitched or tinkling bowel sounds, abdominal distension, and tenderness of the mass. No attempt should be made to reduce a strangulated hernia.

Diagnostic Tests: In an uncomplicated asymptomatic hernia, laboratory and diagnostic tests are unwarranted. If there is questionable strangulation from a prolonged incarcerated hernia, laboratory studies for complications may reveal leukocytosis, elevated serum amylase, and guaiac-positive stool. Abdominal series are done postoperatively to look for signs of perforation (free air) or obstruction of the bowel (multiple air-fluid levels).

Differential Diagnosis: An inguinal hernia must be differentiated from a hydrocele or hematocele. Femoral lymphadenopathy, femoral artery aneurysm, and psoas abscess must be ruled out in diagnosis of a femoral hernia. Other causes of a groin mass include an undescended testicle and muscle strain.

Treatment: Surgical repair of strangulated inguinal, umbilical, and femoral hernias is recommended immediately unless the patient is a poor surgical risk. These patients need to be hospitalized, receive intravenous solutions, and remain NPO. Small direct inguinal hernias and painless indirect inguinal hernias do not need immediate attention; however, surgery is generally recommended within 1 week of diagnosis. Patients who are not surgical candidates can be fitted for a truss and monitored for signs of prolonged incarceration. Patients with a small direct, nonpainful hernia should be observed for reduction of the hernia when the patient is supine.

Follow-up: For patients with reducible hernias, observation of the hernia during subsequent physical examination is recommended. Patients suspected of having an incarcerated hernia should be followed up within the week to determine if they are experiencing any tenderness of the mass and if they have been seen by a general surgeon. For the postoperative patient who has had a herniorrhaphy, assess for wound healing and reoccurrence of the hernia.

Sequelae: An untreated inguinal, umbilical, or femoral hernia may become incarcerated and strangulated, with subsequent intestinal gangrene.

Prevention/Prophylaxis: Cessation of cigarette smoking is recommended, to reduce intrathoracic pressure from chronic coughing. Encourage the use of fiber, fluids, and stool softeners for patients who strain with defecation. Patients should avoid lifting heavy objects without proper support.

Referral: Refer the patient to a general surgeon when a hernia is detected. A strangulated hernia requires immediate attention.

Education: Inform the patient with a reducible hernia of the potential complications of an untreated hernia. Teach patients to avoid straining to defecate or urinate. Encourage smoking cessation to reduce the probability of a chronic cough. Instruct the patients on proper techniques for lifting heavy objects.

Irritable Bowel Syndrome

Irritable bowel syndrome (IBS) is a chronic gastrointestinal disorder characterized by persistent abdominal pain and distressed defecation. The two major classifications of IBS are:

- The *spastic colon*, in which bowel movements are variable, alternating between periods of diarrhea and constipation.
- Painless diarrhea, occurring immediately after a meal or upon rising.

Etiology: No anatomic or biochemical cause of IBS is known. This syndrome is a functional disorder of intestinal motility and altered visceral sensation, leading to constipation and/or diarrhea. Stressful and emotional life events often precede or coexist with the presentation of IBS.

Occurrence: A common presentation for patient referral, IBS accounts for almost 50% of all referrals to a gastroenterologist.

Age: Fifty percent of the cases of IBS are diagnosed before age 35. Because most cases of IBS present by age 50, this syndrome is often a chronic condition in older adults.

Ethnicity: This disorder has a higher prevalence among whites than among other ethnic groups.

Gender: Prevalence of irritable bowel syndrome is twice as great in women as in men.

Contributing Factors: Stressful psychosocial situations may hasten an exacerbation of IBS. Certain food products such as fructose, sorbitol, and lactose have been known to alter bowel motor function.

Signs and Symptoms: A thorough dietary history is essential to establish a differential diagnosis of IBS, thereby ruling out the possibility of food intolerance. Explore the patient's psychosocial history to determine the relationships between stressful events and exacerbation of IBS. Determine the onset of symptoms, including the time of day that the pain and gastrointestinal disturbances usually occur. Report of postprandial abdominal pain suggests biliary tract disease, pancreatitis, or peptic ulcer disease. Patients often report loose and frequent stools or alternating constipation and diarrhea. Abdominal pain may be described as colicky. Pain is often relieved by defecation. Abdominal distention, mucus in the stool, and the sensation of incomplete evacuation are other presenting symptoms. Patients often complain of associated symptoms such as fatigue, flatulence, headache, backache, and dyspepsia.

The physical examination is usually unremarkable. Abdominal tenderness may be elicited, especially in the left lower quadrant, but is not very pronounced. Presence of an abdominal mass, lymphadenopathy, hepatosplenomegaly, or ascites in a patient with IBS would prompt further investigation. A routine digital rectal examination generally reveals a tender rectum that is either empty or full of hard firm feces. A pelvic examination in women is recommended to rule out the presence of an ovarian neoplasm.

Diagnostic Tests: When ordering diagnostic tests in older adults, determine the length of time since the last evaluation and the nature of the current symptoms. In general, a CBC and erythrocyte sedimentation rate will rule out anemia and inflammation. If diarrhea is the presenting symptom, stool culture and examination for occult blood, ova and parasites, and bacteria are recommended. For older adults with a new onset of IBS, a sigmoidoscopy with air insufflation and a barium enema with contrast should exclude other gastrointestinal disorders. Sigmoidoscopy usually reveals normal mucosa except for a mild hyperemic bowel in patients with IBS. Introduction of air in the bowel often triggers abdominal pain and bowel spasms. Patients with documented involuntary weight loss of 5% or greater within a 6-month period or with signs of obstruction should have an abdominal CT scan and a small bowel series. Patients with persistent constipation should be evaluated for hypothyroidism. If the presenting symptoms are bloating and abdominal distension with cramping and diarrhea, a trial of 3 weeks of a lactose-free diet is recommended to rule out lactose intolerance.

Differential Diagnosis: Food intolerance, diverticular disease, parasitic diseases, biliary tract disease, colonic polyps, neoplasms, and pancreatic disease should be considered. With older adults, abuse of cathartics needs to be evaluated.

Treatment: Psyllium preparations taken with two glasses of water and high-fiber food products are recommended. Patients who have been on a low-fiber diet should gradually start with 1 Tbs of bran, daily, building up to at least 3 Tbs/day. For patients who choose bulk-forming products, a total of 15–25 g/day is necessary to achieve results. Caution patients with diabetes about using any products that have a high sugar content. Foods that may exacerbate IBS should be avoided (e.g., caffeinated beverages, alcohol, sorbitol-containing candies or gums, citrus fruits for those with fructose intolerance, and milk products for those who have known lactose intolerance). Antispasmodics are not recommended for treatment of IBS in older adults because of the anticholinergic side effects of these medications. If diarrhea is severe, loperamide 2 mg every 4–8 hr can be taken.

Follow-up: With chronic IBS patients, a positive relationship between provider and patient is mutually beneficial. Dietary intervention and stress-reduction techniques should be reviewed and evaluated. In patients with newly diagnosed IBS, evaluation of persistent symptoms is necessary, as IBS is a diagnosis of exclusion.

Sequelae: Older adults with a chronic history of IBS may suffer from concomitant illness such as diverticulosis. Therefore, complications may develop because of other pathological processes mistaken for IBS symptoms. Patients with uncontrollable diarrhea are at risk for dehydration because of fluid and electrolyte loss. Fecal impaction may result from chronic constipation, especially in an immobile, cognitively impaired older patient.

Prevention/Prophylaxis: The patient should use stress-reduction techniques during emotional situations. Patients should avoid all food products that are known to irritate their bowels. Patients with known food intolerance must read nutrition labels and be informed of the inactive contents of medications, which may contain irritating substances.

Referral: Refer patients to a gastroenterologist for sigmoidoscopy. Refer again if patients exhibit persistent abdominal pain or uncontrollable diarrhea despite compliance with treatment and if signs of gastrointestinal bleeding are present. Patients may benefit from sessions of psychotherapy, biofeedback, or hypnosis.

Education: Inform patients that because the increase of dietary fiber could aggravate their IBS symptoms, they should increase gradually to the recommended dose. It may take 3–4 weeks to reach a therapeutic level sufficient to produce results. Inform patients with chronic IBS that, although the disease itself does not lead to a more serious illness, any change in symptoms should be reported to the practitioner.

Liver Cancer

The liver is the most common organ in the body for metastasis from other cancers. Common sites of primary tumors that metastasize to the liver are the lungs, colon, pancreas, stomach, breast, and gallbladder. Hepatocellular cancer is associated with cirrhosis of the liver.

Etiology: The hepatic filtration of arterial and portal venous blood is a major reason for the high prevalence of metastases from primary cancerous sites in the body to the liver. Metastases may also result from an extension from an abdominal tumor or through the lymphatic system. Malignant tumors of the liver are primarily adenocarcinomas.

Occurrence: Primary liver cancer, rare in the United States, accounts for about 2% of all cancers. A malignant lesion is 20 times more likely to be from a metastatic source than from a primary lesion.

Age: Most common onset of disease is in the sixth and seventh decades.

Ethnicity: Primary liver cancer is prevalent in people from Africa and Asia because of the widespread occurrence of hepatitis B and hepatitis C virus.

Gender: Liver cancer is more prevalent in men than in women.

Contributing Factors: The incidence of liver cancer increases for patients who have a history of cirrhosis of the liver and hepatitis B virus. Exposure to certain chemicals such as vinyl chloride and arsenic have been associated with the development of liver cancer.

Signs and Symptoms: Complaints of weakness, weight loss, sweating, and anorexia may be reported. Physical examination reveals cachexia. Auscultation may reveal a bruit over the tumor and tenderness of the liver. A mass may be palpable.

Diagnostic Tests

- The hematocrit may be normal or elevated owing to the overproduction of erythropoeitin by the tumor.
- Leukocytosis may be present.
- Serum alkaline phosphatase may be elevated.

- ALT, AST, and bilirubin are usually elevated.
- Elevated serum α-fetoprotein, not normally present in adults, is found at levels greater than 500 g/L in patients with primary hepatocellular carcinomas.
- When the primary site of the malignancy is the gastrointestinal tract, breast, or lungs, elevated levels of CEA may be found.
- Ultrasound is used to screen for tumors and can detect tumors greater than 3 cm.

Differential Diagnosis: Cirrhosis and chronic hepatitis B or C infection are associated with symptoms similar to those of primary liver cancer. Patients with metastatic malignancy of the liver often present initially with the symptoms of the primary site.

Treatment: The treatment is palliative at best. A surgical resection of the liver is beneficial only if the patient has a resectable tumor; even so, the survival rate remains low. Intrahepatic chemotherapeutic agents such as fluorouracil and floxuridine may alter the growth of the tumor, but the prognosis remains the same. Older patients with known renal function impairment may require a reduced dosage of these agents, compared with a younger population.

Follow-up: Patients and family members should be given the opportunity to explore adjunctive methods of pain relief and relaxation. Following the diagnosis of liver cancer, the focus should be on holistic palliative care, including the intervention of a hospice and services provided by the American Cancer Society.

Sequelae: The prognosis is poor since the tumor grows rapidly and often metastasizes to the lungs or bones. The survival rate for patients is only 4–6 months.

Prevention/Prophylaxis: Hepatitis vaccine is recommended for high-risk patients. Avoidance of chemical exposure, as part of occupational safety, is suggested. Annual ultrasound screening for patients with chronic hepatitis B should be considered as a preventive measure for liver cancer.

Referral: Refer the patient to an oncologist when the diagnosis of liver cancer is suspected. Local hospice care services should be contacted for care for the patient and family.

Education: Although no further medical treatment is aimed at reversal of the disease, the patient needs to know that you will collaborate with the hospice nurses to provide for the patient's comfort throughout the disease process.

Nephrolithiasis

In the western hemisphere the basis of most nephrolithiasis, or kidney stones, is calcium salts, uric acid, cystine, and struvite. Calculi range in size from microscopic to several centimeters in diameter.

Etiology: Kidney stones develop from the supersaturation of urine with stone-forming salts that occurs either by overexcretion of salt or underexcretion of urine. Some preformed nuclei form to create a calculus. Abnormal crystal growth inhibitors are formed as well, because of hypocitraturia or magnesium deficiency. Approximately 70% of diagnosed kidney stones contain calcium; 20%–25% are struvite stones resulting from urinary tract infections; 5% are uric acid calculi; and 2% contain cystine.

Occurrence: An estimated 500,000 cases of kidney stones are diagnosed in the United States yearly.

Age: The average age of onset of a kidney stone is in the third decade. The incidence of kidney stones for women peaks again at about age 55.

Ethnicity: The incidence of kidney stones in whites is three to four times greater than in African-Americans.

Gender: Men are more likely than women to form calcium stones; struvite stones, however, are more common in women because of the higher incidence of urinary tract infections. Cystine stone formation occurs equally in men and women.

Contributing Factors: A dietary intake of certain food substances that augment the formation of kidney stones include dairy products, chocolate, and green leafy vegetables (calcium oxalate stones), eggs, fish, poultry, peanuts, and wheat (cystine stones). Certain medications such as furosemide, nitrofurantoin, probenecid, silicates, theophylline, and vitamins C and D in a small percentage of cases can contribute to the development of nephrolithiasis. A history of hyperparathyroidism, sarcoidosis, Cushing's syndrome, Paget's disease, and immobilization may contribute to the development of calcium phosphate stones. Chronic urinary tract infections may be precursors to struvite stone formation. Fifty percent of patients with gout are predisposed to uric acid stone formation, resulting from prior history and/or family histories of kidney stones.

Signs and Symptoms: Patients may have abrupt, severe, colicky pain in either flank or pain that originates in the flank and radiates to the groin. Pain spreading downward suggests movement of the stone along the ureter. Associated nausea and vomiting may occur. Hematuria may be reported.

Physical examination may reveal local abdominal and costovertebral tenderness. Men complaining of groin pain should receive a testicular examination to rule out testicular torsion. Women with pain radiating to their labia should have a pelvic examination to rule out possible ovarian cysts or tumors. A cursory physical examination for evidence of systemic diseases such as sarcoidosis or cancer should be conducted (Fig. 10–4).

Diagnostic Tests: For patients who have not yet passed a stone, urine collection for recovery of stones or gravel should be ordered. A urinalysis of freshly voided urine may detect crystalluria. An abnormally high or low urine pH may suggest stone formation. A urine specimen should be sent for culture and sensitivity testing to detect the possibility of underlying infection. A CBC with differential

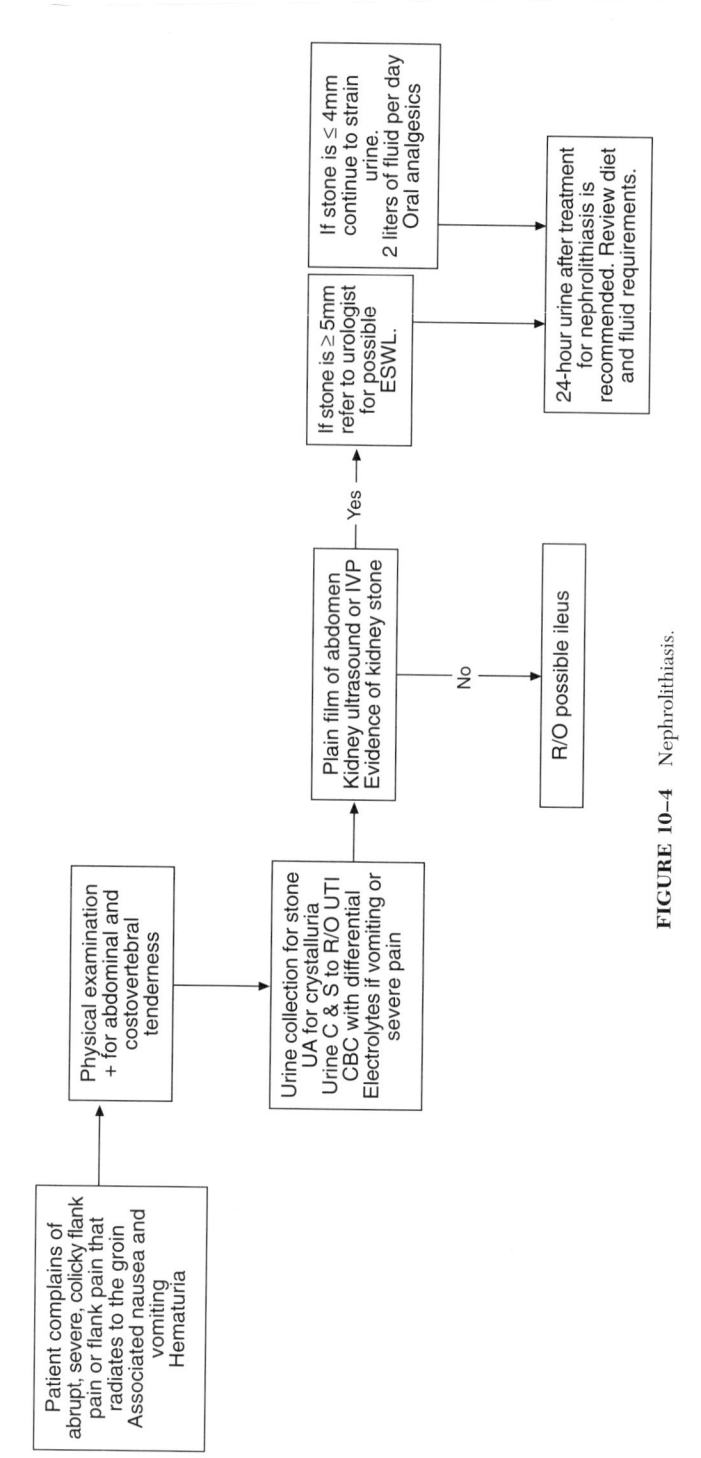

FIGURE 10-4 Nephrolithiasis.

should be ordered to determine the presence of leukocytosis indicative of a concurrent infection. An electrolyte panel should be ordered for patients who have been vomiting or have experienced severe pain, to detect CO_2 levels to rule out associated respiratory alkalosis (low CO_2) or metabolic acidosis (high CO_2). A plain radiographic film of the abdomen can help find the stone and rule out possible ileus. An intravenous pyelogram (IVP) helps detect size, shape, and exact location of the suspected obstruction. For patients who are unable to tolerate an IVP, an ultrasound of the kidneys provides information on probable hydronephrosis.

Differential Diagnosis: Papillary necrosis, hydronephrosis, ileus, diverticulitis, appendicitis, bowel obstruction, mesenteric ischemia, ovarian cyst, and testicular torsion are considered potential sources for localized abdominal pain that may mimic symptoms of nephrolithiasis.

Treatment: Size and location of the stone, coupled with the length of time since the onset of symptoms, directs treatment. Stones 4 mm or smaller usually pass on their own, stones 4–5 mm have a 50% chance of passing without intervention. A stone larger than 5 mm requires immediate referral to a urologist for possible extracorporeal shock-wave lithotripsy (ESWL). Unless contraindicated, intravenous fluids of normal saline can be administered at a rate of 125–150 mL/hr, to help flush out the stone. Instruct patients not in distress and without obstruction to drink 2 L of fluid daily and strain the urine until a stone has passed. Oral analgesics can be prescribed: 1 tablet acetaminophen 300 mg and codeine phosphate 30 mg (this is Tylenol #3) or 1 or 2 tablets acetaminophen 300 mg and codeine phosphate 15 mg (this is Tylenol #2) every 4 hr, without exceeding 4 g acetaminophen a day or 2.5–5 mg hydrocodone component with acetaminophen every 4–6 hr. An adequate fluid intake should continue throughout the day as part of therapy.

Follow-up: A 24-hr urine collection 6 months after treatment for nephrolithiasis is recommended. At this time, also review with the patient the need for compliance with dietary restriction and fluid requirements.

Sequelae: Immediate complications of unresolved kidney stones include obstruction and urinary tract infection. A high incidence of recurrence of kidney stone formation exists; metabolic causes of kidney stones need to be ruled out when dietary measures are unsuccessful.

Prevention/Prophylaxis: An adequate fluid intake daily is essential. To prevent recurrent stones, review a patient's dietary habits to discern if there are any excessive food products that may be factors in kidney stone formation (calcium, purine, protein).

Referral: Refer the patient to a urologist when:

- Obstruction is detected.
- The stone is greater than 5 mm.
- The stone has not passed within 24–48 hr of the onset of pain.

- The patient has complicated diagnostic reports.
- The patient needs complex management.

Education: Inform all patients with nephrolithiasis that there is a high probability of a second occurrence of a kidney stone. Advise the patient, if possible, to strain urine with the provided strainer when experiencing symptoms of kidney obstruction. A daily fluid intake of 10 large glasses of liquid per day is recommended. Explain to patients that fluid intake needs to be increased when urine appears dark yellow. Provide information about any food restrictions that may be deemed necessary to prevent specific stone formation.

Peptic Ulcer Disease

Peptic ulcer disease involves ulcerations of the mucous membrane of the esophagus, stomach, or duodenum. The disease is classified according to the nature and anatomic location of the lesion. Peptic ulcers usually originate near mucosal transition zones in areas exposed to acid, pepsin, bile, and pancreatic enzymes. Gastric ulcers are generally found along the lesser curvature of the stomach between antral and acid-screening mucosa occurring anywhere in the stomach, from the cardia to the pylorus. Duodenal ulcers develop in the duodenal bulb or in the immediate postbulbar area.

Etiology: The etiology of peptic ulcer disease is best characterized as an imbalance between the noxious agents to which the gastrointestinal mucosa is exposed (primarily HCl and pepsin) and the protective factors (mucus production, bicarbonate secretion) that the mucosa uses to resist destruction from such noxious agents. An increase in destructive influences (e.g., with NSAID use) can destroy the mucosa, leading to the development of an ulcer.

Occurrence: Approximately 25 million Americans have experienced peptic ulcer disease.

Age: The predominant age range for gastric ulcers is age 55–65, with rare occurrences before the age of 40. Duodenal ulcers can occur in adults age 25–75. Middle-aged men (age 45–64) and women over age 55 have the highest incidence of peptic duodenal disease.

Ethnicity: Prevalence of peptic ulcer disease is higher in African-Americans and Hispanics than in whites.

Gender: Gastric ulcers are more prevalent in older women than in older men because of the increased use of NSAIDs. The occurrence of duodenal ulcers is twice as common in men than in women.

Contributing Factors: Use of aspirin and other NSAIDs, because of their ability to inhibit prostaglandin synthesis, and smoking are important risk factors. Drinking alcohol can cause gastritis. The use of caffeine and stressful life situations also contribute to the development of peptic ulcer disease. *Helicobacter pylori* infection is a factor in more than 90% of duodenal ulcers and 80% of gastric ulcers.

Signs and Symptoms: Patients with gastric ulcers have a history of dyspepsia, epigastric pain, and/or right upper quadrant pain that radiates to the back following the ingestion of a meal. Patients with duodenal ulcer have pain 1–3 hours after a meal, whereas those with gastric ulcers have pain immediately upon eating. Nocturnal pain may occur. In the older adult definitive symptoms may be absent. Vomiting and anorexia may be reported instead of epigastric pain.

Physical examination of a patient with peptic ulcer disease may be normal. Palpation may reveal upper abdominal tenderness and guarding. Rigidity of the abdomen and absence of bowel sounds may suggest perforation. Patients with chronic duodenal ulcer disease may exhibit signs of dehydration if nausea and vomiting accompany the other symptoms. In patients with suspected gastrointestinal bleeding, signs of shock may be detected. Guaiac stool testing should be done.

Diagnostic Tests: In the diagnostic breath test to detect the presence of *H. pylori*, patients are given ^{13}C- or ^{14}C-labeled urea to drink. The marked carbon is absorbed and is measured as CO_2 in the patient's expired breath. Hemoglobin and hematocrit values are obtained to detect blood loss. Endoscopic gastroduodenoscopy with a biopsy for the detection of peptic ulcer, malignancy, and *H. pylori* remains the "gold standard" in diagnostic testing for this disease.

Differential Diagnosis: Pain associated with angina, gastric carcinoma, gastroesophageal reflux, gallbladder disease, Zollinger-Ellison disease, nonulcer dyspepsia, and irritable bowel syndrome are all probable candidates for the differential diagnosis.

Treatment: The FDA-approved treatment options for *H. pylori*–induced peptic ulcers include:

Omeprazole 20–40 mg qd and clarithromycin 500 mg tid for 2 weeks, then omeprazole 20 mg for 2 weeks.

OR

Ranitidine bismuth citrate (RBC) 400 mg bid and clarithromycin 500 tid for 2 weeks, then RBC 400 mg bid for 2 weeks.

OR

Bismuth subsalicylate 525 mg qid and metronidazole 250 mg qid and 500 mg tetracycline qd for 2 weeks, and an oral dose of ranitidine 300 mg or nizatidine 300 mg daily for 4 weeks.

OR

Lansoprazole 30 mg bid, amoxicillin 1 g bid, and clarithromycin 500 mg bid for 14 days.

The dosage of the H2 blockers may be reduced, depending on creatinine clearance, as follows:

If the creatinine clearance is less than 50 mL/min, the dosage for ranitidine is reduced to 150 mg qid.

If the creatinine clearance is 20–50 mL/min, the dosage for nizatidine is 150 mg daily.

If the creatinine clearance is less than 20 mL/min, nizatidine 150 mg should be given every other day *or* lansoprazole 30 mg bid, amoxicillin 1 g bid, and clarithromycin 500 mg bid should be given for 14 days.

Encourage patients to complete the therapeutic regimen despite the cessation of pain. NSAID-induced peptic ulcers can be treated with H2 blockers.

Follow-up: If a gastric ulcer was detected on endoscopy and the patient continues to have symptoms after 8 weeks of treatment, then referral for endoscopic examination with a biopsy is indicated. Periodic stool guaiac testing and blood counts can detect bleeding.

Sequelae: Complications originating from peptic ulcer disease in the older adult include gastric bleeding, perforation, and gastric outlet obstruction.

Prevention/Prophylaxis: Signs and symptoms of impending recurrence of peptic ulcer disease, including epigastric pain, anorexia, and weight loss, should be identified early. Guaiac stool testing should be performed for all patients taking NSAIDs. Misoprostol 200 g tid has been approved as prophylaxis against NSAID-induced gastric ulcers.

Referral: Refer the patient to a gastroenterologist for initial endoscopy. Refer again if epigastric pain and dyspepsia persist despite treatment and if signs of gastrointestinal bleeding are present.

Education: Avoidance of aspirin and other NSAIDs and tobacco is essential. Reduction of stressful events, coffee (including decaffeinated forms) and other caffeine products, and alcohol is recommended. Caution patients about taking over-the-counter medication preparations without professional advice. The Centers for Disease Control (CDC) has established a *H. pylori* information hot line for physicians and patients at (888-MYULCER).

Gastric Cancer

Gastric cancer is generally classified as early or advanced carcinoma. Gastric cancer usually begins in the distal portion of the stomach and spreads via the lymph or circulatory system.

Etiology: The etiology of gastric cancer is unknown; however, several dietary risk factors are associated with the incidence of stomach cancer. Adenocarcinoma accounts for 95% of all gastric malignancies. Early gastric cancers are generally confined to the mucosa or submucosa; advanced gastric carcinomas penetrate the muscularis propria with lymph node involvement.

Occurrence: More than 20,000 new cases of gastric carcinomas are diagnosed each year in the United States, 90% of which are adenocarcinomas.

Age: The average age at onset of gastric cancer is 55.

Ethnicity: A high incidence of gastric cancer has been found in Native-Americans, African-Americans, Asians, Hispanics, and Scandinavians.

Gender: Gastric cancer is predominantly found in men.

Contributing Factors: Prolonged ingestion of food products that are high in salt and nitrates have an association with gastric cancer because of the presence of bacteria in the stomach, *Helicobacter pylori* being one identified bacteria. Gastric ulcers and adenomatous polyps are known precursors to gastric cancer. Patients with a history of atrophic gastritis resulting from pernicious anemia who have had a partial gastrectomy are at risk for developing gastric cancer.

Signs and Symptoms: Early detection of gastric cancer is often difficult because of the absence of clinical presentation. In more advanced disease, patients may have a vague sensation of fullness following a meal relieved by belching, nausea, with or without anorexia (often to meat), dyspepsia, nonspecific complaints of abdominal pain of varying intensities, and constipation. Weight loss and pallor, if the patient is anemic, may be the only signs noted during physical examination. A palpable mass in the abdomen may be felt in an advanced carcinoma.

Diagnostic Tests: Testing should include:
- CBC with indices to determine presence of anemia.
- Stool testing for occult blood to detect bleeding in the intestinal tract.
- Endoscopy with a biopsy.
- Cytological examination.

Differential Diagnosis: Chronic gastritis, irritable bowel syndrome, and gastric ulcers present with symptoms similar to those of stomach cancer.

Treatment: A partial or complete gastric resection with adjacent lymph nodes is the treatment of choice for gastric cancer. Extensive cancer or metastases negate the need for surgery. Chemotherapeutic agents (most commonly, 5-fluorouracil) have been used alone or in combination with other treatments.

Follow-up: For the patient who has had a gastric resection, continued surveillance every few months is necessary to check for weight loss, bleeding, and obstruction. Laboratory evaluation of CBC, routine liver tests, and measurement of serum CEAs should occur at 3- to 6-month intervals for the first year after surgery. An annual endoscopy is recommended for the next 5 years.

Sequelae: Malnutrition, hemorrhage, obstruction, possibly evasive cancer, and metastases are complications from gastric cancer.

Prevention/Prophylaxis: Patients should eliminate the use of food products that contain nitrates and are highly salted.

Referral: A gastroenterologist should be consulted for the endoscopy and complicated management problems, including annual follow-up endoscopy.

Education: After partial and complete gastrectomy, teach patients about the importance of adequate nutrition. Consuming six small meals a day may be necessary instead of the usual three. Supplementation with vitamins, especially vitamin B_{12}, and minerals such as calcium and iron should be prescribed. Patients may prefer taking nutritional supplements in place of one or more of the meals each day.

BIBLIOGRAPHY

Assessment

DeGowin, R: DeGowin and DeGowin's Bedside Diagnostic Examination. McGraw-Hill, New York, 1987.

Lueckennotte, A: Pocket Guide to Gerontologic Assessment, ed 2. CV Mosby, St. Louis, 1994.

Mezey, M, Rauckhorst, LH, and Stokes, SA: Health Assessment of the Older Individual, ed 2. Springer Publishing, New York, 1993.

Willms, JL, Schneiderman, HS, and Algranti, PS: Physical Diagnosis: Bedside Evaluation of Diagnosis and Function. Williams & Wilkins, Baltimore, 1994.

Acute Renal Failure

Abrams, W, Beers, MH, and Berkow, R: The Merck Manual of Geriatrics, ed 2. Merck Research Laboratories, Whitehouse Station, NJ, 1995.

Brenner, BM, and Lazarus, JM (eds): Acute Renal Failure, ed 3. Churchill-Livingstone, New York, 1993.

Brady, HR, and Breener, B: Acute renal failure. In Isselbacher, KJ, et al (eds): Harrison's Principles of Internal Medicine, ed 13. McGraw-Hill, New York, 1994.

Jennette, JC, and Falk, RJ: Diagnosis and management of glomerulonephritis and basculitis presenting as acute renal failure. Med Clin North Am 74:893, 1990.

Taptich, B, Iyer, P, and Bernocchi-Losey, D: Nursing diagnosis and care planning, ed 2. WB Saunders, Philadelphia, 1994.

Bladder Cancer

Boring, CC, et al: Cancer statistics, 1994. CA 44:7, 1994.

de Kernion, JB, Lowitz BB, and Casciato, DA: Urinary Tract Cancers. Manual of Clinical Oncology.

Lum, BL, and Tori, FM: Adjuvant intravesicular pharmacotherapy for superficial bladder cancer. J Natl Cancer Inst 83:682, 1991.

Raghaven, D, et al: Biology and management of bladder cancer. N Engl J Med 322:1129, 1990.

Bowel Obstruction

Abrams, W, Beers, MH, and Berkow, R: The Merck Manual of Geriatrics, ed 2. Merck Research Laboratories, Whitehouse Station, NJ, 1995.

Silen, W: Acute intestinal obstruction. In Isselbacher, KJ, et al (eds): Harrison's Principles of Internal Medicine, ed 13. McGraw-Hill, New York, 1994.

Taptich, B, Iyer, P, and Bernocchi-Losey, D. Nursing Diagnosis and Care Planning, ed 2. WB Saunders, Philadelphia, 1994.

Tang, E: Bowel obstruction in cancer patients. Arch Surg 130:832, 1995.

Trott, AT, Trunkey, DD, and Wilson, SR: Acute abdominal pain: A guide to crisis management. Patient Care, 1995.

Cholecytitis

Dawes, LG, and Nahrwold, DL: Acute cholecystitis: Update on diagnosis and treatment. J Crit Illness 7:1409, 1992.

Goroll, AH: Management of diverticular disease. In Goroll, AH, May, LA, and Mulley, AG (eds): Primary Care Medicine: Office Evaluation of the Adult Patient, ed 3. JB Lippincott, Philadelphia, 1995.

Greenberger, N, and Isselbacher, KJ: In Isselbacher, KJ, et al (eds): Harrison's Principles of Internal Medicine, ed 13. McGraw-Hill, New York, 1994.

Johnston, DE, and Kaplan, MM: Pathogenesis and treatment of gallstones. N Engl J Med 328:412, 1993.

Quigley, EM, et al: Hepatobiliary complications of total parenteral nutrition. Gastroenterology 104:286, 1993.

Ransohoff, D, Gracie, WA, and Schmitter, JP: Clinical guideline: Guidelines for treatment of gallstones. Ann Intern Med 119:620, 1993.

Pastides, H, et al: A case-control study of the relationship between smoking, diet, and gallbaldder disease. Arch Intern Med 150:1409, 1990

Taptich, B, Iyer, P, and Bernocchi-Losey, D: Nursing diagnosis and care planning, ed 2. WB Saunders, Philadelphia, 1994.

Chronic Renal Failure

Abrams, W, Beers, MH, and Berkow, R: The Merck Manual of Geriatrics, ed 2. Merck Research Laboratories, Whitehouse Station, NJ, 1995.

Lewis, EJ, et al: The effect of angiotensin-converting-enzyme inhibition on diabetic nephropathy. N Engl J Med 329:1456, 1993.

Ravid, M, et al: Long-term stabilizing effect of angiotensin-converting enzyme inhibition on plasma creatinine and on proteinuria in normotensive type II diabetic patients. Ann Intern Med 118:577, 1993.

Taptich, B, Iyer, P, and Bernocchi-Losey, D: Nursing Diagnosis and Care Planning, ed 2. WB Saunders, Philadelphia, 1994.

Whelton, A, Stout, RL, Spilman, PS, and Klassen, DK: Renal effects of ibuprofen, piroxicam and sulindac in patients with asymptomatic renal failure: A prospective, randomized, crossover comparison. Ann Intern Med 112:568, 112.

Zeller, K, et al: Effect of restricting dietary protein on the progression of renal failure patients with insulin-dependent diabetes mellitus. 324:78, 1991.

Cirrhosis of the Liver

Babor, TF, Ramon de la Fuente, and Saunders, J: AUDIT: The alcohol use disorders identification test: Guidelines for use in primary health care, document No. WHO/MNH/DT/89.4. Geneva, World Health Organization. Deaths and hospitalizations from chronic liver disease and cirrhosis—United States, 1980–1989. JAMA 269:569, 1993.

Kettl, P: Detecting problem drinkers in your practice. Patient Care 27, 1995.

Koff, RS: Liver. In Noble, J (ed): Textbook of Primary Care Medicine. CV Mosby, St. Louis, 1996.

Colorectal Cancer

American Cancer Society: 1994 Cancer Facts & Figures. American Cancer Society, Atlanta, 1994.

Fleisher, DE, et al: Detection and surveillance of colorectal cancer. JAMA 261:580, 1989.

Giovannucci, E, et al: Aspirin and the risk of colorectal cancer in women. N Engl J Med 333:609, 1995.

Goroll, AH: Management of gastrointestinal cancers. In Goroll, AH, May, LA, and Mulley, AG (eds): Primary Care Medicine: Office Evaluation of the Adult Patient, ed 3. JB Lippincott, Philadelphia, 1995.

Miller, AD, and Sonnenberg, A: Protection by endoscopy against death from colorectal cancer. Arch Intern Med 155:1741, 1995.

Moertel, CG, et al: Fluorouracil plus levamisole as effective adjuvant therapy after resection of stage III colon carcinoma: A final report. Ann Inter Med 122:321–326, 1995.

Otte, D: Nursing management of the patient with colon and rectal cancer. Semin Oncol Nurs 4:285, 1988.

Schwesinger, MD: Colorectal cancer. In Griffith, HW, Dambro, MR (eds): The Five Minute Consultant. Lea and Febiger, Philadelphia.

Cystitis

Abrams, W, Beers, MH, and Berkow, R: The Merck Manual of Geriatrics, ed 2, Merck Research Laboratories, Whitehouse Station, NJ, 1995.

Avorn, J, et al: Reduction of bacteriuria and pyuria after ingestion of cranberry juice. JAMA 271:751, 1994.

Fang, LS: Approach to dysuria and urinary tract infections in women. In Goroll, AH, May, LA, and Mulley, AG (eds): Primary Care Medicine: Office Evaluation of the Adult Patient, ed 3. JB Lippincott, Philadelphia, 1995.

Fihn, SD: Urinary tract infection. Consultant 32:43, 1992.

Raz, R, and Stamm, WE: A controlled trial of intravaginal estriol in postmenopausal women with recurrent urinary tract infections. N Engl J Med 329:753, 1993.

Stamm, WE, and Hooten, TM: Management of urinary tract infections in adults. N Engl J Med 329:1328, 1993.

Taptich, B, Iyer, P, and Bernocchi-Losey, D: Nursing diagnosis and care planning, ed 2. WB Saunders, Philadelphia, 1994.

Tunkel, AR, and Kaye, D: Urinary tract infections. In Hazzard, WR, et al (eds): Principles of Geriatric Medicine and Gerontology, ed 3. McGraw-Hill, New York, 1994.

Diverticulitis

Guthrie J, Hines C, and Howell D: Don't overtreat diverticular disease. Patient Care 27:12, 1993.

Klein, S, et al: Extraintestinal manifestations in patients with diverticulitis. Ann Intern Med 108:700, 1988.

Goroll, AH: Management of diverticular disease. In Goroll, AH, May, LA, and Mulley, AG (eds): Primary Care Medicine: Office Evaluation of the Adult Patient, ed 3. JB Lippincott, Philadelphia, 1995.

Taptich, B, Iyer, P, and Bernocchi-Losey, D: Nursing Diagnosis and Care Planning, ed 2. WB Saunders, Philadelphia, 1994.

Cheskin, LJ, and Schuster, MM: Colonic disorders. In Hazzard, W, et al (eds): Principles of Geriatric Medicine, ed 3. McGraw-Hill, New York, 1994.

Elfrink, RJ, and Miedema, BW: Colonic diverticula: When complications require surgery and when they don't. Part 3. Postgrad Med 92:97, 1992.

Esophagitis

Amendola, MA, and Spera, TD: Doxycycline-induced esophagitis. JAMA 253:1009, 1985.

Castell DO: Chest pain of undetermined origin: Overview of pathophysiology. Am J Med 92(5a):2S, 1992.

Cohen, S: Pathogenesis of gastrointestinal reflux disease. Ann Intern Med 117:1051, 1992.

Kikendall, JW: Caustic ingestion injuries. Gastrointestinal Clinics of North America 20:847, 1991.

McBane, RD, and Gross, JB, Jr: Herpes esophagitis: Clinical syndrome, endoscopic appearance, and diagnosis in 23 patients. Gastrointest Endosc 37:600, 1991.

Ritcher, JM: Approach to the patient with heartburn and reflux. In Goroll, AG, May, LA, and Mulley, AG (eds): Primary Care Medicine: Office Evaluation of the Adult Patient, ed 3. JB Lippincott, Philadelphia, 1995.

Robinson, M, et al: A comparison of lansoprazole and ranitidine in the treatment of erosive esophagitis. Aliment Pharmacol Ther 9:25, 1995.

Taptich, B, Iyer, P, and Bernocchi-Losey, D: Nursing diagnosis and Care Planning, ed 2. WB Saunders, Philadelphia 1994.

Gastritis

Beam, E: *Helicobacter pylori* and peptic ulcer disease: Understanding this latest pathogen. Clin Rev 5:51, 1995.

Carpenter, H, and Talley, N: Gastroscopy is incomplete without biopsy: Clinical relevance of distinguishing gastropathy from gastritis. Gastroenterology 108:917, 1995.

Clearfield, H: *Helicobacter pylori:* Aggressor or innocent bystander? Med Clin North Am 75:815, 1991.

Fennerty, MB, and Higbee, M: Drug therapy of gastrointestinal disease. In Bressler, R, and Katz, M (eds): Geriatric Pharmacology. McGraw-Hill, New York, 1993.

Gastroenteritis

Barlett, JG: Antibiotic-associated diarrhea. Practical Gastroenterol 16:10, 1992.

Bennish, ML, Salam, MA, and Khan, WA: Treatment of shigellosis. Compression of one or two doses ciprofloxacin with standard 5-day therapy: A randomized, blinded trial. Ann Intern Med 117:727, 1992.

Bennett, RG: Diarrhea among residents of long-term care facilities. Infection control and hospital epidemiology. 14:397, 1993.

Eastaugh, JA: Food poisoning: Bugs and drugs. Hospital Medicine 53, 1993.

Gianella, RA: Enteric infections. Gastroenterology 104:1589, 1993.

Jacobs, R: General problems in infectious diseases. In Tierney, LM, McPhee, SJ, Papadakis, MA, and Schroeder, SA (eds): Current Medical Diagnosis and Treatment. Appleton and Lange, Norwalk, CT, 1993.

Pegues, DA, and Woernle, CH: An outbreak of acute nonbacterial gastroenteritis on a nursing home. 14:87, 1993.

Hernia

Arregui, ME, et al: Laparoscopic inguinal herniorrhaphy—techniques and controversies. Surg Clin North Am 73:513, 1993.

Abrams, W, Beers, MH, and Berkow, R: The Merck Manual of Geriatrics, ed 2. Merck Research Laboratories, Whitehouse Station, NJ, 1995.

Margolies, M: Approach to the patient with an external hernia. In Goroll, AH, May, LA, and Mulley, AG (eds): Primary Care Medicine: Office Evaluation of the Adult Patient, ed 3. JB Lippincott, Philadelphia, 1995.

Monson, JR: Education and debate: Minimally invasive surgery: Advanced techniques in abdominal surgery. Br Med J 307:1346, 1993.

Irritable Bowel

Abrams, W, Beers, MH, and Berkow, R: The Merck Manual of Geriatrics, ed 2. Merck Research Laboratories, Whitehouse Station, NJ, 1995.

Camilleri, M, and Prather, CM: The irritable bowel syndrome: Mechanisms and a practical guide to management. Ann Intern Med 116:1001, 1992.

Lynn, RB, and Friedman, LS: Irritable bowel syndrome. N Engl J Med 329:1940, 1993.

Nanda, R, et al: Food intolerance and irritable bowel syndrome. Gut 30:1099, 1989.

Owens, D, Nelson, D, and Talley, N: The irritable bowel syndrome: Long-term prognosis and the physician-patient interaction. Ann Intern Med 122:107, 1995.

Schuster, MM: Diagnostic evaluation of the irritable bowel syndrome. Gastoenterol Clin North Am 20:269, 1991.

Talley, NJ, O'Keefe, EA, Zinmeister, AR, and Melton, LJ: Prevalence of gastrointestinal symptoms in the elderly: A population-based study. Gastroenterology 102:895, 1992.

Liver Cancer

Drug Information for the Health Care Professional. United States Pharmacopeial Convention, 1995.
Isselbacher, KJ, and Dienstag, JL: Tumors of the liver: In Isselbacher, KJ, et al (eds): Harrison's Principles of Internal Medicine, ed 13. McGraw-Hill, New York, 1994.
O'Mary, SS: Liver cancer: Primary and metastatic disease. Semin Oncol Nurs 4:265, 1988.
Smith, CS, and Paauw, DS: Hepatocellular carcinoma: Identifying and screening populations at increased risk. Postgrad Med 94:71, 1993.
Tsukuma, H, et al: Risk factors for hepatocellular carcinoma among patients with chronic liver disease. N Engl J Med 328:1797, 1993.

Nephrolithiasis

Coe, FL, and Favus, MJ: Nephrolithiasis. In Isselbacher, KJ, et al (eds): Harrison's Principles of Internal Medicine, ed 13. McGraw-Hill, New York, 1994.
Kupin, W, Preminger, G, Segura, J, and Smith, A: A treatment plan for urinary stones. Patient Care 29:22, 1995.
La Porte, J, and Baum, N: Kidney stones. Postgrad Med 87:219, 1990.
Mutgi, A, Williams, JW, and Nettleman, M: Renal colic: Utility of the plain abdominal roentgenogram. Arch Intern Med 151:1589, 1991.
Wilson, D: Clinical and laboratory evaluation of renal stone patients. Endocrinol Metab Clin North Am 19:773, 1990.

Peptic Ulcer Disease

Anderson, M: *Helicobacter pylori* infection: When and in whom is treatment important? Postgrad Med 96:40, 1994.
Beam, E: *Helicobacter pylori* and peptic ulcer disease: Understanding this latest pathogen. Clinician Reviews 5:51, 1995.
Cerda, JJ, et al: A revolution in peptic ulcer disease. Patient Care 28:19, 1994.
Clearfield, H: *Helicobacter pylori:* Aggressor or innocent bystander? Med Clin North Am 75:815, 1991.
Fennerty, MB, and Higbee, M: Drug therapy of gastrointestinal disease. In Bressler, R, and Katz, M (eds): Geriatric Pharmacology. McGraw-Hill, New York, 1993.
Fitzgerald, M: Diagnosis and treatment of *Helicobacter pylori* infection in peptic ulcer disease. Journal of the American Academy of Nurse Practitioners 7:233, 1995.
Hunt, RH: Helicobacter pylori: From theory to practice. Proceeding of a symposium. Am J Med (5A) (suppl), 1996.
Raskin, JB, et al: Miscoprostol dosage in the prevention of nonsteroidal anti-inflammatory drug induced gastric and duodenal ulcers: A comparison of three regimens. Ann Intern Med 123:344, 1995.

Gastric Cancer

Abrams, W, Beers, MH, and Berkow, R: The Merck Manuel of Geriatrics, ed. 2. Merck Research Laboratories, Whitehouse Station, NJ, 1995.
Brady, M, and Cella, D: Helping patients live with their cancer. Patient Care 29:41, 1995.
Eckhardt, VF, et al: Clinical and morphological characteristics of early gastric cancer. Gastroenterology 98:708, 1990.
Foltz, A: Nutritional factors in the prevention of gastrointestinal cancer. Semin Oncol Nurs, 1988.
Goodwin, C: Commentary: Gastric cancer and *Helicobacter pylori:* The whispering killer? Lancet 342:507, 1993.
Normura A, et al: *Helicobacter pylori* infection and gastric carcinoma among Japanese Americans in Hawaii. N Engl J Med 325:1132, 1991.

CHAPTER **11**

REPRODUCTIVE

DISORDERS

Changes in the female reproductive system occur well before the life stage of older adulthood, considering that the average age of menopause is 51 years. However, a plethora of choices are now available to women in this age group for prevention and management of postmenopausal problems such as atrophic vaginitis, incontinence, osteoporosis, hyperlipidemia, and cardiac problems. The gerontological nurse practitioner (GNP) or health-care provider will likely encounter a variety of physical findings during assessment of the older female patient, based on these emerging choices. A comprehensive medication history is very important, to identify medications or dietary supplements that affect the reproductive system, including hormone replacement therapy and vaginal applications. Equally important is a thorough history, including family history of breast or reproductive organ cancer in a first-degree family member, or in the patient herself. The patient should be questioned about any prior breast surgery, including surgery for breast augmentation or reduction. Annual mammograms and gynecologic examination with Pap smear (unless the patient has had a total hysterectomy, including removal of the cervical cuff) should be included in the assessment process. Does the patient do breast self-examination on a regular basis? Has she ever discovered a lump or had a biopsy or ultrasound? The patient should also be questioned about breast pain, nipple discharge, rash, trauma, or swelling.

289

Normal aging changes in the female breast include the atrophy of glandular breast tissue and replacement with connective tissue. There may be a decrease in breast size or breasts may become pendulous and flabby owing to loss of elasticity. Areolar nipple ducts may be palpable, feeling stringy and firm. Nipple retraction may result from breast atrophy; however, the possibility of malignant changes causing nipple retraction must be ruled out. The inframammary ridge assumes more prominence. Axillary hair decreases.

Physical examination of the female breasts includes inspection for symmetry, lumps, dimpling, or nipple retraction. Optimally, the patient should be sitting, with her hands placed on her hips, raising them over her head during the inspection. Patients with large, pendulous breasts should lean forward, so the examiner can observe for attachment to chest wall or retraction; a bimanual hand technique can be used to examine their breasts at this time also. While the patient's arms are at her sides, the examiner palpates the axillary area for lymphadenopathy, probing deeply while manipulating the patient's arm for maximal access. The patient is then positioned supine with a small towel or pillow under the side to be examined and the corresponding arm placed over the head. Using the finger pads, the examiner palpates in one of three patterns:

Concentrically from the nipple to the periphery, including the breast tail.
Extending out from the nipple in a pattern similar to spokes on a wheel.
In a linear pattern from top to bottom, starting medially and moving more laterally with each line.

Breast self-examination technique may be taught at this time also.

Age-related changes in the male breast include gynecomastia in some patients. Examination of the male breast and axillary areas follows the same sequence as for the female breast but in an abbreviated format, because less breast tissue exists.

Assessment of the reproductive system of older men and women includes a sexual history. Sexual preference, patterns of sexual expression, current or desired activity, protective practices to avoid transmission of sexually transmitted diseases including human immunodeficiency virus (HIV), and problems with expression of sexuality should be explored. Review of the medication regimen for potential effects on libido and impotence is important.

If the patient is in a community living situation, are opportunities provided for privacy and intimacy? If medications or medical problems interfere with sexual expression, what interventions are possible? Age-related changes in the reproductive system of both sexes do not interfere with libido and sexual satisfaction, although physiologic response time is slower and more prolonged and orgasmic response is more generalized.

Assessment of the genitoreproductive system of the older female patient includes historical elements such as menarche, obstetrical history, menopause, history of sexually transmitted diseases (STDs) including herpes or condyloma, surgeries, or malignancies. Medication history and sexual history were discussed previously. The patient should be questioned about urinary symptoms and about any vulvovaginal itching, discharge, or bleeding.

Normal aging changes in the female genitoreproductive system include atrophic changes in most structures. Pubic hair becomes gray and sparse, and the labia flatten. Vaginal epithelium is thinner, drier, and itchy, with less rugae; decreased secretions and alkalinity predispose patients to painful intercourse, friability, and vaginitis. The vagina becomes shorter, narrower, and less elastic; tissue is pale pink and shiny. Sexual abstinence or infrequent intercourse intensifies atrophic changes. Undergarments often irritate sensitive external structures. The uterus shrinks, and ovaries, which atrophy, are not palpable. The pelvic floor muscles, sacral ligaments, and other supporting structures relax, frequently leading to organ (bladder, rectum, uterus) prolapse.

Examination of the female genitoreproductive system is the same in older patients as in younger patients. With an older patient, before positioning her in the lithotomy position with stirrups, external inspection may be performed by having the patient flex one knee and abduct it. Patients with arthritis may be helped by taking pain medication before the examination. Equipment should be assembled and ready, to limit time spent in the stirrups. Lubrication of the speculum with water before insertion is important for comfort. The choice of speculum is an individual one; the Pederson speculum, with narrow blades, is frequently chosen for virginal or postmenopausal women with a narrow introitus. Examination may reveal relaxation of internal organs, including a cystocele or rectocele. The cervix, which appears pale and shiny, may be flush with the vaginal mucosa or may protrude into the vagina with uterine prolapse. On bimanual examination, the ovaries should not be palpable and the uterus is small and firm.

Patients who have had a hysterectomy with removal of the cervix should undergo routine gynecologic care, with a sample taken from the vagina and vaginal pool for analysis.

The genitourinary and reproductive systems of the older male patient undergo more gradual changes than those of the older female patient. Pubic hair turns gray and becomes sparse. Penile size decreases slightly. Scrotal contents hang lower; the testes decrease in size and firmness, and less sperm are produced owing to the increase in connective tissue in the tubules. Testosterone production declines slowly, resulting in slower arousal and more prolonged erection prior to ejaculation. Ejaculation is less intense, and shorter, with less seminal fluid and rapid detumescence. Prostatic tissue enlargement is common, frequently resulting in nocturia, urinary hesitancy, decreased urine flow, retention (sometimes with overflow incontinence), and less forceful ejaculation.

When taking the history related to the genitourinary and reproductive systems of the older male patient, ask about difficulty urinating, hesitancy, decreased force of stream, frequency with decreased amount, dribbling, or nocturia. If nocturia is present, establish its onset and frequency, and explore possible contributing factors other than prostatic enlargement. These include diuretics, caffeine or alcohol ingestion, increased fluid consumption in the evening, habit, or mild heart failure or dependent edema. Other pertinent questions concern urinary symptoms such as frequency, urgency, dysuria, hematuria, or documented urinary tract infection.

Examination of the reproductive system of the older male patient is essentially the same as for a younger male patient. The normal changes of aging have been described earlier. Examination of the prostate is conducted with the rectal examination, which begins with inspection and palpation of the genitalia for lesions, proceeding to palpation of the inguinal canal for hernia and then to palpation of the inguinofemoral areas for lymphadenopathy. For examination of the prostate through the rectum, the patient is placed in the left lateral decubitus position, or standing and leaning forward over the examination table with toes pointed inward, for easier access to the anorectal area. The examiner uses a well-lubricated, gloved finger, advanced above the anal canal, to palpate the anterior wall of the rectum for the prostate gland. The gland is normally heart-shaped with a central groove that can be felt. The normal surface is smooth, elastic, and nontender on palpation. Absence of the central groove in a smooth gland or protrusion of the gland more than 1 cm into the rectum is typical of benign prostatic hypertrophy. A hard, irregular nodule may indicate carcinoma. Either finding requires further workup.

Atrophic Vaginitis

Atrophic vaginitis, also called adhesive vaginitis, is a noninfectious postmenopausal process in which the female genital tissue thins and becomes fragile.

Etiology: Many years of estrogen deprivation lead to atrophy of the vaginal and vulvar epithelium. Atrophic vaginitis, a common disorder in postmenopausal women, can be surgically induced, created by the natural aging process, or brought on through primary ovarian failure.

Occurrence: This disorder will affect all women, to some degree, unless estrogen replacement therapy (ERT) is provided.

Age: Atrophic vagnitis is predominantly a problem of the postmenopausal woman. The average age of natural menopause in the United States is 52.5 years.

Ethnicity: Not significant.

Gender: Occurs in women only.

Contributing Factors: Estrogen-deficient states accompanying metabolic disorders and changes of normal aging create the risk of atrophic vaginitis. In addition, changes in vaginal epithelium and pH caused by estrogen deficiency provide an environment in which pathogenic bacteria and fungi can flourish. Drugs may also alter vaginal secretions and clinical findings. For example, estrogen therapy alters the maturation index, and digoxin has estrogen-like properties.

Another drug, tamoxifen (Nolvadex) can produce menopause-type symptoms but can also act on genital tissue as a weak estrogen agonist. Finally, drugs used to treat endometriosis or uterine bleeding can produce a reversible pseudo-menopause.

Signs and Symptoms: Atrophic vaginitis is characterized by itching, discomfort, burning, dyspareunia, and, at times, a thin blood-tinged vaginal discharge or bleeding after intercourse as the epithelium thins. Vaginal dryness as vaginal secretions decrease can be another bothersome symptom. Complaints of urinary frequency, urgency, and stress incontinence are not uncommon. Upon physical examination, signs include pale, dry, nonrugated vaginal walls with patches of erythema and/or petechiae. A watery white vaginal discharge without foul odor may be found. Estrogen deficiency can lead to loss of uterine support and subsequent uterine descensus (Fig. 11–1).

Diagnostic Tests:

- If urinary symptoms are present, a urinalysis should be done to rule out urinary tract infection (UTI).
- Examination of the vagina and the vulva, as well as collection of specimens for potassium hydroxide and saline vaginal wet prep studies, is done to rule out other causes of vaginitis.
- Findings of increased white blood cells (WBCs) and decreased Lactobacillus suggest atrophic vaginitis.
- A diagnostic smear of the vaginal wall maturation index has been used but is not universally recommended.
- Serum study of follicle-stimulating hormone (FSH) level can confirm menopause if FSH is elevated; the estradiol level would reflect decreased circulating estrogens.

Differential Diagnosis: Malignancy, vulvar dystrophies, UTI and other infections with organisms such as *Candida albicans*, bacterial vaginosis, trichomoniasis, gonorrhea, and chlamydia mimic atrophic vaginitis.

Treatment: Short intermittent courses of hormone replacement therapy (HRT) are usually adequate. This treatment regimen includes estrogen cream (Premarin cream) or estradiol (Estrace cream) 1/2 (2 g) to 1 (4 g) applicator every night for 1–2 weeks, followed by every-other-night application for 1–2 weeks, then gradually tapering frequency of administration and dosage, until finally discontinuing the treatment. This regimen can then be repeated as needed. Continuous HRT may be initiated with Premarin 0.625 mg PO daily or Estrace 1 mg PO daily, or Estraderm patch 0.05 mg changed twice weekly. If the uterus is not removed and HRT continues for more than 2 months, the addition of cyclical progesterone should be considered, in the form of Provera 2.5 mg PO daily or Provera 10 mg for 10 days of each month. Contraindications to continuous HRT include a history of breast or uterine cancer of estrogen-positive tumor receptors. Nonpharmaceutical measures, which may or may not

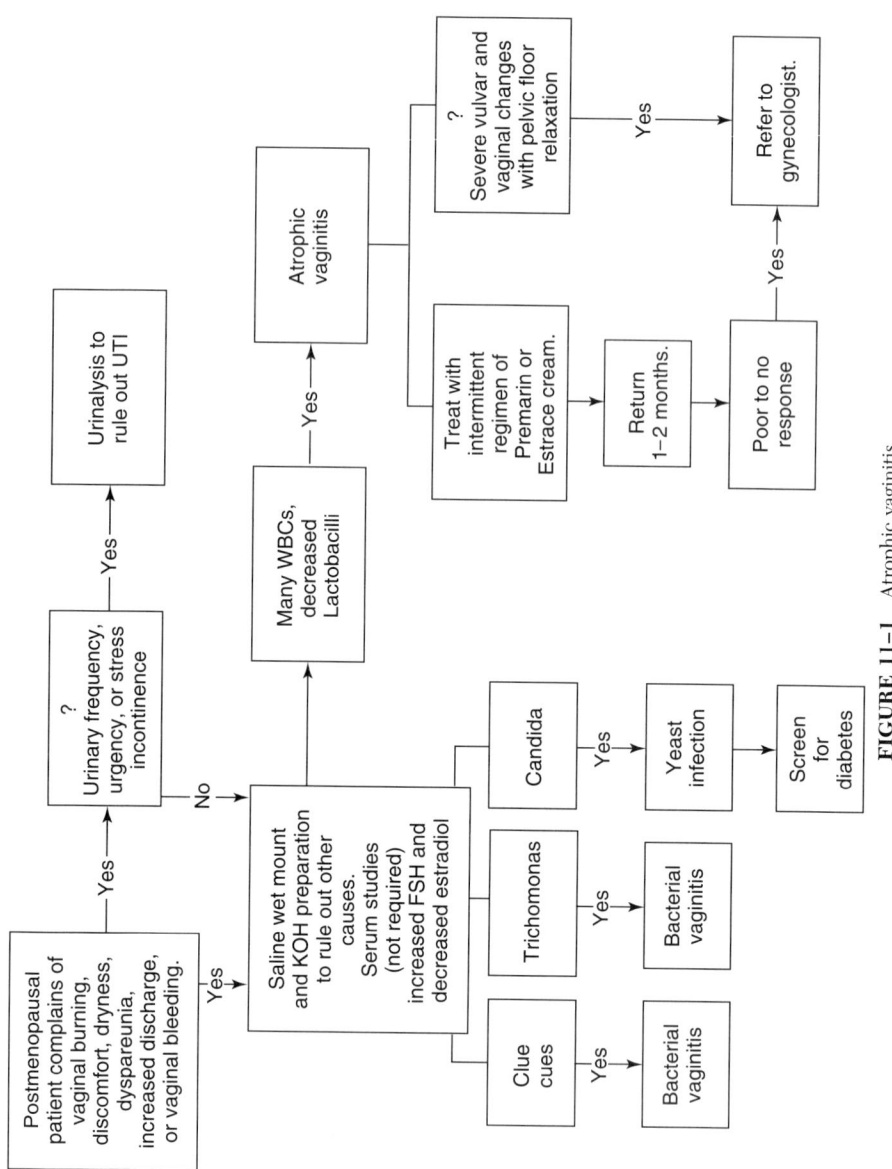

FIGURE 11–1 Atrophic vaginitis.

be helpful, include taking Sitz baths, wearing cotton underwear, and applying yogurt douches.

Follow-up: Expected response is quick, with resolution of symptoms within 30–60 days. If this does not occur, the patient should be reevaluated and reexamined for other causes of symptoms. Because topical estrogen cream is absorbed and can cause systemic effects, patients should have a follow-up visit 1–2 months after beginning oral or vaginal drug therapy. Patients treated with continuous HRT need regular return visits every 3–6 months to check side effects, blood pressure (BP), and response to therapy. Annual visits are necessary for complete history and physical examination.

Sequelae: With changes in the vaginal pH of postmenopausal women (pH greater than 5.0), and this loss of normal acidity, bacterial species grow in the vagina that are not commonly found there. Infections can become frequent and chronic.

Prevention/Prophylaxis: Recognition of early signs and symptoms of atrophic vaginitis can lead to the individual's seeking treatment to prevent atrophy, dryness, infections, urinary and urethral problems, and sexual dysfunction. Intermittent use of topical vaginal estrogen can prevent recurrence of atrophic vaginitis, provide adequate levels of hormone, and give soothing relief.

Referral: Refer to a gynecologist patients who do not respond to ERT. Those who present with severe estrogen depletion evidenced by marked perineal and vaginal changes, along with pelvic floor relaxation, need gynecologic referral before initiating topical treatment.

Education: Use water-soluble lubricants for patients with atrophic vaginitis. Counsel the patient regarding benefits of regular sexual activity. Identify each age-related difficulty associated with intravaginal application of creams. Address these needs with sensitivity.

Benign Prostatic Hypertrophy

Benign prostatic hypertrophy (BPH) is the benign growth of the prostate that may lead to obstruction of the bladder outlet.

Etiology: The causes of BPH are unknown. One hypothesis relates BPH to changes in androgen hormones, whereas another alludes to a second growth phase for prostatic tissue. BPH originates in the transitional and periurethral zones.

Occurrence: BPH occurs universally in older men; genetics is thought to play a part in those who develop it at a younger age.

Age: BPH is seen in 50% of men over age 50, and in 80% of men over age 70.

Ethnicity: Not significant.

Gender: BPH occurs in men only.

Contributing Factors: Risk factors include male gender, age over 40 years, and intact testes.

Signs and Symptoms: Symptoms are frequently categorized as irritative or obstructive. Irritative symptoms arise from involuntary bladder muscle contractions possibly involving hypersensitivity of the bladder wall. The patient may report frequency, urgency, burning or pain on urination, nocturia, or incontinence. Typical obstructive symtoms include straining to urinate, hesitancy, weak or intermittent stream, dribbling, or a sensation of incomplete emptying. These symptoms are related to direct pressure from impingement of prostatic tissue on the urethra or to contraction of muscle fibers in the prostate gland, capsule, and bladder neck from α-adrenergic tone.

The American Urologic Association (AUA) has developed a self-administered symptom questionnaire that addresses the occurrence over the past month of the symptoms mentioned here. This questionnaire, contained in the Agency for Health Care Policy and Research (AHCPR) guidelines, is helpful in quantifying symptoms, although not specific for BPH.

Upon physical examination, the prostate may be enlarged or normal-sized. It should feel smooth, with a rubbery consistency. Nodularity or extreme hardness raise suspicions of malignancy. Prostate size does not correlate with degree of obstruction or severity of symptoms. The suggested rationale for this is that rectal examination is limited to palpation of the peripheral zone of the prostate and does not reach the periurethral zone where symptoms originate. In cases of advanced obstruction, the bladder may be palpated upon examination. Focal neurologic examination assessing the sacral nerve roots is also helpful.

Diagnostic Tests: Urinalysis is recommended to rule out infection (pyuria or bacteriuria) or malignancy (suggested by hematuria). If the urinalysis is positive for bacteria, culture and sensitivity testing is indicated. Urea nitrogen and creatinine are elevated when renal insufficiency or obstructive uropathy is present. Prostate-specific antigen (PSA) testing may be done but is not required. Because the PSA may be elevated in BPH, prostatitis, acute urinary retention, or prostatic infarction, as well as in prostatic cancer, this test is of questionable value in diagnosing BPH. Finasteride will elevate the PSA.

Specialized tests such as intravenous pyelogram (IVP), uroflowmetry, postvoid residual measurement, pressure-flow studies, transrectal ultrasound, and cystourethroscopy are not routinely indicated. In specific instances, they may be performed as a guide to therapy choices or to rule out other conditions.

Differential Diagnosis: Differential diagnosis includes prostate cancer (may coexist with BPH), urethral stricture, neurogenic bladder, medication-induced BPH, prostatitis, detrusor muscle failure, and bladder neck contracture.

Treatment: For patients with minimal symptoms, a program of watchful waiting, with instruction to avoid medications known to worsen symptoms, is prescribed. Medication groups to be avoided include decongestants and other sympathomimetics and anticholinergics such as antipsychotics, tricyclic antidepressants, antispasmodics, and antihistamines.

For mild to moderate symptoms, α-1-adrenergic blockers relax smooth muscle of the bladder neck and prostate. Terazosin (Hytrin), beginning with 1 mg PO hs and increasing as needed up to 10 mg PO hs, is the most frequently prescribed agent. Other agents include prazosin (Minipress) and doxazosin (Cardura). Hypotension, the primary side effect, is minimized by taking the medication at bedtime. Recently, a new medication in this class, tamsulosin HCl (Flomax), has been introduced specifically for BPH treatment; dosage is 0.4 mg or 0.8 mg PO daily.

Another medication frequently used is finasteride (Proscar), a 5-α reductase inhibitor that blocks the conversion of testosterone to dihydrotestosterone, the major intraprostatic androgen in men. Dosage is 5 mg PO daily. Side effects include decreased libido, ejaculatory dysfunction, and impotence. Proscar and an alpha-blocker are sometimes used concurrently.

For severe BPH, surgical treatment may be the primary option. In the past few years, many treatments have proliferated in this category. Transurethral resection of the prostate (TURP) has been the standard for years. Other treatments include open prostatectomy for glands of more than 40 g, transurethral incision of the prostate (TUIP) for gland enlargement of less than 10 g, transurethral needle-aspiration albation of prostate (TUNA), transurethral electrovaporization of the prostate (TVAP), transurethral (TULIP) or visual (VLAP) laser-assisted prostatectomy, insertion of a urethral stent, and transurethral microwave therapy (TUMT).

Follow-up: Scheduling of follow-up depends on the course of treatment. Advise watchful waiting, and evaluate with the AUA symptoms index every 6–12 months. Patients receiving drug therapy should be evaluated for symptoms and side effects every 6 months. Annual digital rectal examination for prostate cancer, and usually PSA testing and urinalysis, is indicated.

Sequelae: Complications of BPH include urinary retention requiring catheterization, renal insufficiency, urinary tract infections, bladder stones, gross hematuria, prostatitis, treatment complications and side effects, and possibily treatment-induced impotence.

Prevention/Prophylaxis: No preventive measures are known; BPH occurs with aging.

Referral: Patients may be referred to a urologist if comorbid conditions exist, if the surgical option is feasible or desirable, for initial evaluation for drug therapy, and to rule out acute prostatitis of prostate cancer. Consider collaborative management for drug therapy.

Education: Educate patient about the condition and its treatment options and their side effects. Instruct patient to avoid spicy foods and any drugs that can increase retention or cause symptoms to flare up, including caffeine, alcohol, sedatives, over-the-counter (OTC) sleeping pills, and OTC cold and allergy remedies. Instruct patient to report hematuria, UTI symptoms, or increased retention.

Breast Cancer

Breast cancer is a malignant neoplasm of the breast.

Etiology: Breast cancer is caused by mutations in critical genes. Approximately 80% of breast cancers are ductal adenocarcinomas.

Occurrence. Breast cancer accounts for 25%–35% of malignancies diagnosed in the United States. It is the third most common cancer. American women have a one-in-nine lifetime risk of developing the disease, the highest breast cancer rate in the world. Approximately 27% of 100,000 individuals diagnosed with breast cancer die from the disease.

Age: The incidence of breast cancer increases dramatically with age. At age 25, 5 in 100,000 women develop breast cancer; at age 50 the incidence increases to 150 in 100,000 and at age 75 to 200 in 100,000.

Ethnicity: White women have a 12.86% lifetime risk of developing breast cancer; black women have an 8.8% risk. Black women tend to have a much lower five-year survival rate (64%) than do white women (81%) who are diagnosed with breast cancer. Only Asian-American women develop breast cancer at statistically lower rates than other American ethnic groups.

Gender: Breast cancer occurs predominantly in women; less than 1% of new cases occur in men.

Contributing Factors: A history of multiple family members, from the same side of the family, with breast or ovarian cancer increases the risk of developing breast cancer, especially for women under age 40. Any primary relative with a history of the disease may be considered a risk factor. The physiologic changes of aging contribute to the development of the disease.

Hormonal factors associated with the development of breast cancer include early menarche, menopause beginning later than 55 years old, child-bearing delayed until after age 30, and nulliparous status. The effect of hormone replacement therapy (HRT) on the development of the disease remains controversial with several studies showing a small but statistically significant increase in breast cancer among women receiving HRT. High dietary fat intake and alcohol consumption are associated with the development of breast cancer. Radiation exposure has been strongly associated with its development. Half of all women diagnosed with breast cancer have no identifiable risk factors.

Signs and Symptoms: The chief symptom is the finding of a breast mass or lump. Up to 80% of these are discovered by the individuals themselves. Symptoms of new breast asymmetry, protrusion, dimpling of the skin, nipple inversion, or a scaly rash around the nipple should be further evaluated. Nipple discharge and breast pain are less common symptoms of malignant disease. Cervical axillary adenopathy can occur.

Physical examination of the breast involves visualization and palpation of the neck, breasts, and axillary regions. When masses are identified, note the location, consistency, regular or irregular boarders, size, and whether the mass is fixed or movable. Skin and nipple changes in the breast are important to note. Compare one breast to the other.

Diagnostic Tests: In addition to eliciting signs and symptoms, focus the medical history on the age of the individual, family health history, reproductive and menstrual history, prior breast biopsies, dietary intake of fats, alcohol consumption, and previous exposure to radiation.

Mammogram and biopsy are indicated for all new or suspicious masses. Biospy may be excisional, incisional, or by fine needle aspiration to allow for histologic evaluation and the estrogen-progesterone receptor (ER/PR) status of the mass. Chest x-ray examination, bone scan, and occasionally liver scan may be indicated. Breast cancer is staged, according to tumor type, node involvement, and metastasis (TNM), using the results of these tests (Fig. 11–2). Obtain blood for complete blood count (CBC), liver function tests, and calcium and phosphorus levels. Tumor markers, CEA and CA 15-3, are found in blood tests that may be used to evaluate the response of the tumor treatment.

Differential Diagnosis: Fibrocystic disease, intraductal papilloma, benign fibroadenoma, calcified fibroadenoma, lymphadenitis, mastitis, posttraumatic fat necrosis, and superficial thrombophlebitis can mimic breast cancer.

Treatment: Surgical intervention may vary from a simple lumpectomy to a mastectomy with an axillary node dissection. Radiation therapy often follows surgery. Hormonal therapy is effective in estrogen receptor–positive tumors, which are more common in older women and have a much better prognosis. Chemotherapy, including high-dose chemotherapy with augologous bone marrow transplant, is used in younger patients with high-risk disease.

Follow-up: During the first year following diagnosis, see the patient with breast cancer every three months for a focused history and physical examination. Perform a complete history and physical examination, chest x-ray examination, mammogram, and CBC, and determine serum levels of calcium, alkaline phosphatase, and lactate dehydrogenase (LDH) at 12 months. Some experts recommended that these be done every 6 months during the first year. Repeat bone and liver scans yearly when indicated. Follow-up is recommended every 6 months during years 2 through 5, including the same yearly tests as listed previously. Yearly routine examinations should suffice thereafter.

Sequelae: Recurrence of disease is the main sequela of breast cancer. Metastasis to lymph nodes, lungs, liver, bones, pleura, adrenals, brain, and less commonly to the ovaries, endometrium, or colon, may occur. Psychological and emotional

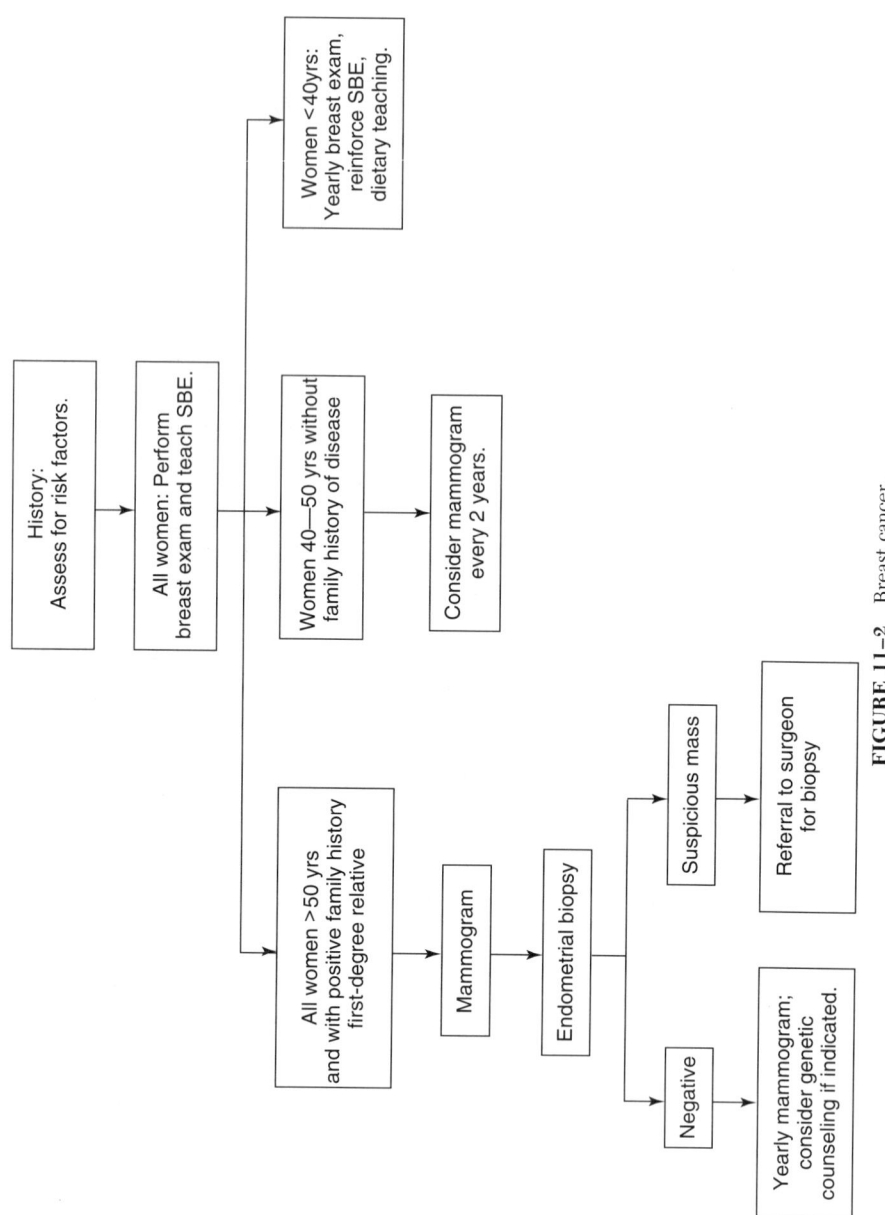

FIGURE 11–2   Breast cancer.

problems may develop related to diagnosis, disfiguring surgery, or reconstructive surgery. Lymphadema may occur in the upper extremity on the operative side. Skin complications related to radiation therapy may be present. Hypercalcemia and bone pain may occur in metastatic disease.

Prevention/Prophylaxis: Encourage all women to perform a breast self-examination (BSE) monthly and have a breast examination by a health-care provider annually. Annual mammograms are recommended for all women over age 50. Many experts recommended annual mammograms for women over age 40, but this is controversial. Prophylactic mastectomy may be advised for women with a strong family history of the disease.

Referral: Refer patients to a surgeon, oncologist, radiologist, genetic counselor, and support group, as appropriate.

Education: Teach BSE to all adult female patients and reinforce the technique at annual examinations. Teach women to perform BSE at the same time each month. BSE "hang tags" are available from the American Cancer Society; patients can leave these in the shower as a reminder to perform BSE. Teach about decreasing dietary fat intake, and explain the risks of excessive alcohol intake.

Drug-Induced Impotence

Impotence, in the strictest sense of the word, is the consistent inability to achieve and maintain erection sufficient for sexual intercourse; it is also referred to as erectile dysfunction. In a broader sense, impotence encompasses problems with arousal, libido, orgasm, sensation, and relationships. Drug-induced impotence refers to that which is caused by a drug or drugs.

Etiology: Drug-induced impotence may be caused by a number of medications and/or medication interactions (see Contributing Factors section).

Occurrence: An estimated 10–15 million American men experience the problem of impotence on a chronic basis.

Age: Incidence rises with age. Approximately 5% of men have a problem with impotence at age 40. At age 65, 15%–25% experience impotence. Because the condition is frequently underreported, the actual percentage is probably higher. In one source, which broke down the percentage by cause, drug-induced impotence was listed as causing 4% of erectile failure among older men.

Ethnicity: Not significant.

Gender: Drug-induced impotence affects only men.

Contributing Factors: The following may contribute to drug-induced impotence:

Stress.

Alcohol use.

Tobacco use.

Recreational drug use.

Certain categories of prescribed medications such as anticholinergics, antiandrogens, antidepressants (including some of the newer serotonin-stimulating reuptake inhibitors [SSRIs]), antipsychotics, central-acting depressants (sedatives/hypnotics, tranquilizers, opiates).

Stimulants such as amphetamines.

Chemotherapeutic agents.

Antihypertensives.

Various processes are involved including effect on libido, neurochemical mediation, and drug side effects.

Signs and Symptoms: There may be no reported symptoms unless the provider includes a sexual history, is aware of the potential for impotence when prescribing certain medications, and asks about baseline sexual activity at that time, then periodically reassesses this during follow-up visits. The patient should be asked about sexual interest, sexual ability, and sexual activity. Also, if a provider detects noncompliance to a prescribed medication regimen in an otherwise cooperative patient, inquire whether impotence occurs when the medication is taken. Drug-induced impotence, which has an acute onset, can be associated with starting a new medication.

Medication history including over-the-counter (OTC) remedies, alcohol use, tobacco use, and use of recreational drugs is also important. The CAGE test for alcoholism, a screening questionnaire for depression, or other psychological screens as needed may be included as part of the history. A history of surgical procedures, especially of those involving the prostate, bladder, or colorectal area, and including the lymphatic channels, may reveal potential sources of impotence.

Physical examination is performed to rule out other causes of impotence; the cause may be multifactorial, especially in the older patient. Evaluate the patient's overall appearance and mobility, and then assess the vital signs, specifically checking for orthostatic hypotension. Palpation of the thyroid may reveal a goiter. Gynecomastia may be related to certain drugs such as cimetidine. Abdominal or femoral bruits may highlight an abdominal aortic aneurysm or vascular obstruction at the bifurcation of the abdominal aorta.

Diminished peripheral pulses suggest a circulatory problem. Lack of sensation or inability to discriminate between sharp and dull may indicate peripheral neuropathy, especially if the history is positive for diabetes. Abnormal reflexes point to a neurologic problem. Decreased mobility may indicate a neurologic or musculoskeletal problem contributing to impotence. Examination of the genital area may reveal testicular atrophy or penile plaques, as seen in those with Peyronie's disease, or an enlarged prostate. Assess for the bulbocavernosus reflex; absense of this reflex indicates penile neuropathy.

Diagnostic Tests: Diagnostic testing is not indicated specifically for drug-induced impotence, but it is performed to eliminate other possible causes of impotence especially vascular and neurologic causes, which are the most common. Testing, specific to the etiology suspected, may include a fasting glucose tolerance test, chemistry panel with blood urea nitrogen (BUN) and creatinine, thyroid-stimulating hormone (TSH) test, lipid panel, complete blood count (CBC), urinalysis, or testing for specific hormonal markers.

Differential Diagnosis: Differential diagnosis includes vascular, endocrine, neurologic, neurovascular, substance abuse, end-organ disease, psychogenic, or social causes. As stated previously, impotence in elderly persons is frequently multifactorial.

Treatment: Whenever possible, eliminate the medication or substitute another medication from available drugs that do not cause impotence. If this is not possible, or if the patient continues to experience the problem after these changes have been made, consider other treatment measures. Counsel the patient regarding alcohol, recreational drug, and tobacco use.

Other treatment measures include Kegel exercises to improve circulation; testosterone replacement therapy by intramuscular injection or transdermal patch, for testosterone deficiency; reconstructive surgery for patients with Peyronie's disease, in whom penile scar tissue interferes with erection; a support sleeve that fits over the penis; and a hand-powered vacuum pump. Medication therapy for impotence has included papaverine and trazodone, neither of which were proven efficacious by research. More recent developments include Caverject, with the active agent alprostadil (PGE_1 synthetic hormone), injected into the corpus cavernosum of the penis before intercourse. This drug relaxes smooth muscle tissue to improve blood flow to the penis. It cannot be used if a vascular problem exists, or if scarring or priapism (abnormally prolonged erection) results. Caverject is also available in a vehicle called the medicated urethral system for erection (MUSE), which uses a tiny plunger instead of a needle to deliver the drug via the penile tip. Hypotension and syncope have occurred when it was used in patients receiving antihypertensive therapy. There are local side effects and precautions for use in pregnancy. Female partners may experience vaginal itching or burning.

Sildenafil citrate (Viagra) is a new selective inhibitor of cyclic guanosine monophosphate (cGMP)–specific phosphodiesterase type 5. During sexual stimulation, nitric acid is released into the corpus cavernosum, resulting in increased cGMP levels, which prevents smooth muscle relaxation and increases blood flow to the penis. Viagra enhances this effect by inhibiting an enzyme that degrades cGMP in the corpus cavernosum. The starting dose for older patients is 25 mg PO 1 hr before sexual activity, up to once daily. It is contraindicated with nitrates; cytochrome influences include increased plasma levels with inhibitors of CYP3A4 or CYP2D9 and decreased plasma levels with inducers of CYP3A4. Side effects include headache, flushing urinary tract infection (UTI), abnormal vision (blue-green, blurring, photosensitivity), nasal congestion, diarrhea, dizziness, and rash. It was effective in clinical trials for drug-induced impotence in patients taking antidepressants/antipsychotics and antihypertensives/diuretics. Agents similar to Viagra are being developed.

This monograph is not intended to be a comprehensive drug reference source; the individual provider must be familiar with all aspects of a drug before prescribing it.

Irreversible penile implants are also used in the treatment of impotence. Because they require invasive implantation, advise the patient to consider all aspects of the procedure before instituting treatment.

Follow-up: Individualize treatment by cause and treatment. Periodic reassessment of treatment for recurrence of the problems is helpful. For medication treatment, monitor for side effects and response.

Sequelae: Disruption of sexual function may result in depression or relationship problems. Complications may arise from treatment.

Prevention/Prophylaxis: Whenever possible, avoid prescribing medications with a high risk for causing impotence, and include a sexual history in routine history and physical examination whenever prescribing a new medication with impotence as a potential side effect.

Referral: Refer patients to a urologist to evaluate for other causes or multifactoral causes of impotence. Refer to a support group those patients experiencing the problem. Refer for psychological services when indicated.

Education: Teach the patient about medication side effects. Have the patient report sexual dysfunction. Educate the patient about normal age-related changes in sexual functioning and how to adapt.

Endometrial Cancer

Endometrial cancer is an abnormal proliferation and neoplastic transformation of endometrial tissues.

Etiology: Endometrial cancer is caused by excessive endogenous or unopposed exogenous estrogenic stimulation of uterine tissues. Ninety percent of endometrial cancers are epithelial tumors affecting the uterine lining.

Occurrence: This is the most common gynecologic cancer, affecting 34,000–36,000 women in the United States, causing 4000–5000 deaths annually.

Age: Less than 5% of endometrial cancers are diagnosed before age 40. The average age of onset is in the sixth and seventh decades of life.

Ethnicity: White women have a higher relative risk than nonwhite women of developing endometrial carcinoma.

Gender: Only women are affected.

Contributing Factors: Obesity, nulliparity, early menarche, long periods of amenorrhea, and late menopause are associated with development of this disease. There is a strong association between the use of unopposed estrogen replacement therapy (ERT) and development of endometrial cancer. Rare familial cancer syndromes and estrogen-secreting tumors are related to development of this type of cancer. A few studies have implied an association between tamoxifen and endometrial cancer, but this is still being researched.

Signs and Symptoms: Abnormal vaginal bleeding is the most common presenting complaint. Often asymptomatic, endometrial cancer is frequently discovered during a routine gynecologic examination (Fig. 11–3).

Diagnostic Tests: Bimanual pelvic examinations may reveal suspicious masses. Endometrial biopsy or biopsy of tissue obtained by dilatation and curettage of the uterus is the definitive diagnostic test. Transvaginal or pelvic ultrasound, computed tomography (CT) scan, or magnetic resonance imaging (MRI) can be useful but are rarely definitive. Complete blood count (CBC), routine chemistries, thyroid-stimulating hormone (TSH) testing, and chest x-ray examinations are recommended. To rule out other causes of abnormal bleeding, patients should be tested for pregnancy (when indicated), for prothrombin time, and for bleeding time. Obtain Pap smear and cultures for sexually transmitted diseases (STDs). Less than 50%, and by some estimates only 10%, of endometrial cancers are discovered by a Pap smear. Serum for the tumor marker CA-125 may help to monitor the response to therapy in metastatic disease.

Differential Diagnosis: Leiomyoma; endometrial polyps; cancer of the cervix, vagina, vulva, or ovary; thyroid disease; bleeding disorders; hepatic or renal failure; genital tract injury; foreign body; and sexually transmitted diseases may mimick endometrial cancer.

Treatment: Surgical resection and operative staging occasionally accompanied by preoperative radiation therapy (usually intracavity) or postoperative radiation. Adjuvant therapy may be hormonal or chemotherapy. Endometrial carcinoma has an excellent prognosis, with nearly 90% of women disease free at 5 years after diagnosis.

Follow-Up: During the first year, see the patient every 3 months for a focused history and physical examination, which should include the pelvic, rectal, and abdominal areas; the breasts; and the lower extremities. Pap smear should be performed and stool tested for guaiac at the same intervals. These visits can stretch out to every 4 months the second year and every 6 months the third year. Yearly examinations may follow therafter. Perform serum testing for CA-125 as indicated.

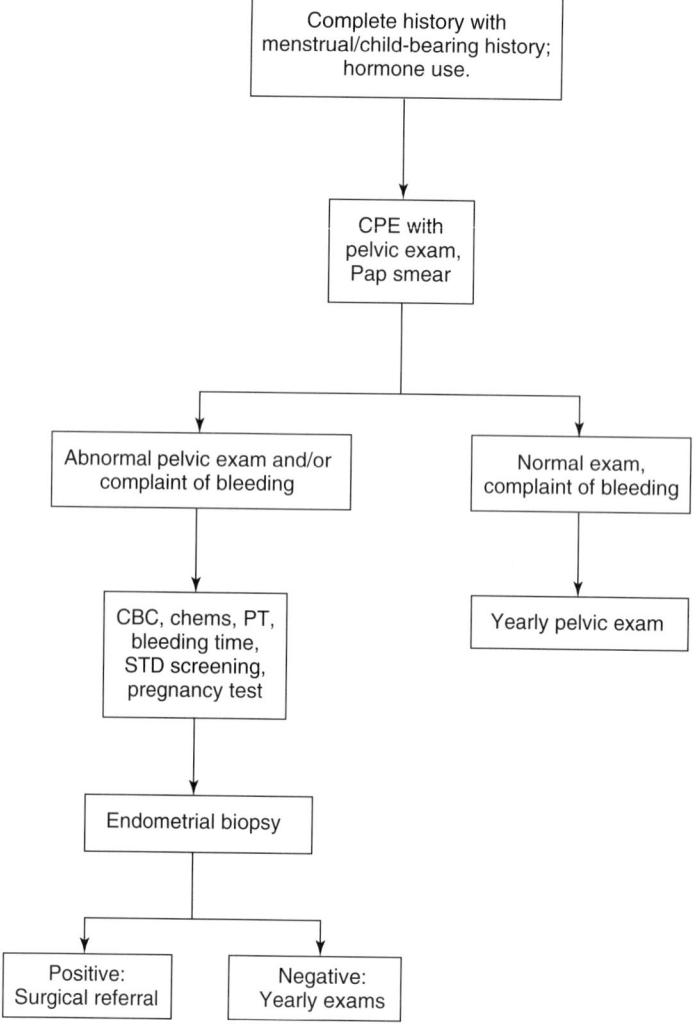

FIGURE 11–3   Endometrial cancer.

Sequelae: Because after surgery the patient will no longer be able to bear children, some patients require emotional support. Rare complications of surgery may include urinary incontinence and sexual dysfunction.

Prevention/Prophylaxis: Encourage obese patients to lose weight. Avoid the use of unopposed estrogen therapy in individuals with an intact uterus.

Referral: Refer patients to a surgeon, oncologist, and cancer support groups. Inform patient and family about hospice resources in the area.

Education: Recommend that older women discuss the need for periodic pelvic examinations. These may be individualized, depending on comorbidities and risk factors. Teach about the connection between high-fat diets and cancer.

Prostate Cancer

Prostate cancer is a malignant neoplasm of the prostate. Ninety-five percent of prostate cancers are adenocarcinoma occurring in the peripheral areas of the prostate.

Etiology: Genetic and environmental factors are believed to influence the development of prostate cancer. Although testosterone is a tumor promoter, its role in the development of prostate cancer is poorly understood.

Occurrence: Carcinoma of the prostate is the most frequently diagnosed cancer in the United States, and it accounts for 13% of all cancer deaths. In men age 55 and older, this cancer is the second leading cause of cancer deaths. In 1995, there were 244,000 new cases of prostate cancer and 40,000 deaths attributable to it. Because of aging of the American population, it is estimated that the incidence of prostate cancer will double by the year 2000. Asymptomatic, previously undiagnosed prostate cancer is seen during autopsy in approximately 30% of American men.

Ethnicity: In the United States, black men have a 30% higher incidence of prostate cancer than white men. Prostate cancer tends to be more advanced and poorly differentiated at the time of diagnosis in black and Hispanic men than in their white counterparts.

Gender: Prostate cancer occurs only in men.

Age: The mean age at diagnosis is age 71; 83% of cases are found in men over age 64.

Contributing Factors: Increasing age contributes to the development of carcinoma of the prostate. A family history of the disease increases the risk for prostate cancer twofold to threefold. Some studies have found a higher incidence of the disease among men who have had vasectomies. Diets high in animal fats, sun exposure, and a history of agricultural work are also associated with the development of prostate cancer.

Signs and Symptoms: Prostate cancer is often asymptomatic in early stages. Nonspecific complaints that may suggest prostate cancer include dysuria, difficulty voiding, urinary frequency, urinary obstruction, back or hip pain, hematuria, hematospermia, and impotence. Occasionally deep vein thrombosis, pulmonary embolus, lower extremity lymphadema, or spinal cord compression may be due to advanced metastatic prostate cancer (Fig. 11–4).

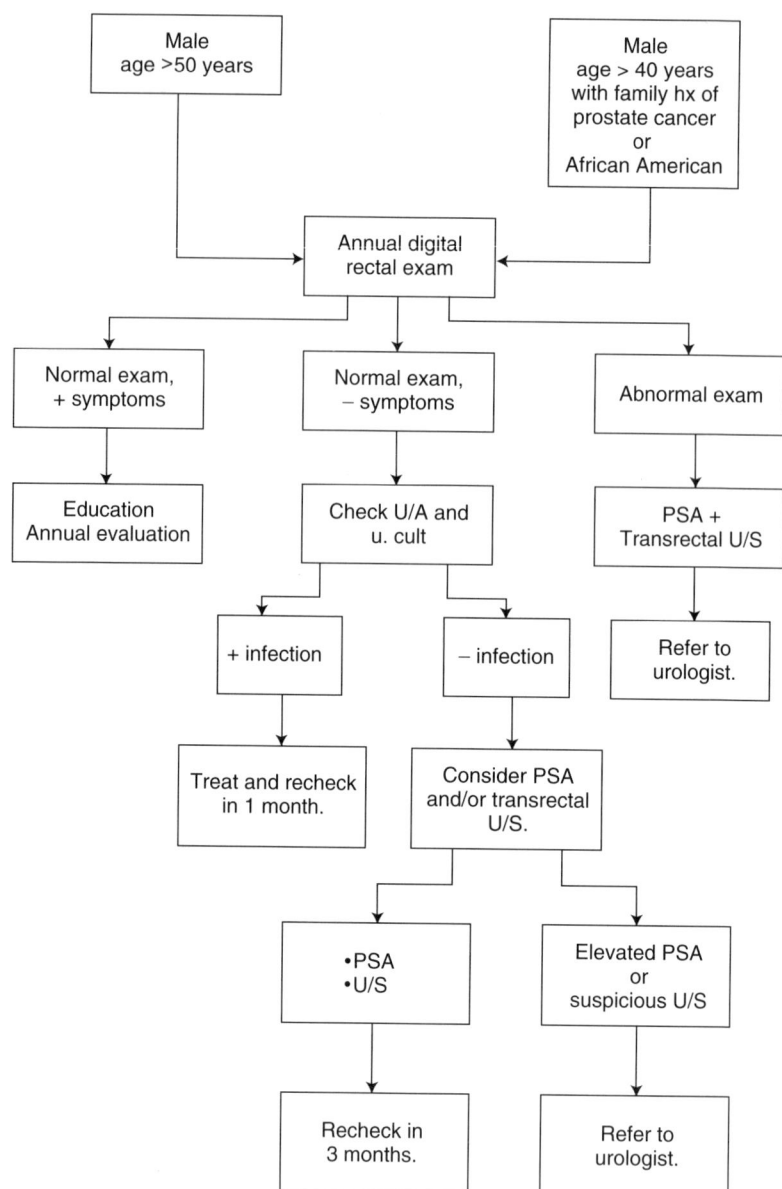

FIGURE 11–4 Prostate cancer.

Diagnostic Procedures

- Digital rectal examination (DRE) allows for palpation of the prostate; cancerous tumors are often felt as hard, irregular nodules.
- Transrectal ultrasound of the prostate is recommended in individuals with a suspicious DRE.
- The use of prostate-specific antigen (PSA) has increased the detection of prostate cancer; this test is neither sensitive nor specific, however, and has a 30% false-negative rare.
- Generally PSA screening should be confirmed to individuals at increased risk for the disease or a suspicious DRE.
- Fine needle aspiration or core needle biopsy of the prostate, usually during ultrasound, enables the collection of cells or tissue for histologic examination and a definitive diagnosis of prostate cancer.

Differential Diagnosis: Differential diagnosis includes benign prostatic hyperplasia, prostatitis, prostatic information, and urethral obstruction.

Treatment: Surgery, radical prostatectomy with or without a pelvic lymphadenectomy, is usually the treatment of choice for prostate cancer confirmed by the histologic examination of a biopsy specimen. Radiation treatment may be used as a primary or adjuvant treatment. Cryotherapy under ultrasound is performed in older patients at 150 centers in the United States. Hormonal therapy and chemotherapies may be used to treat metastatic disease. With well-differentiated, low-grade tumors, watchful waiting may be the treatment of choice in men who have a life expectancy of less than 10 years.

Follow-up: Serial PSA testing, at 3 weeks, 6 weeks, and every 4 months during the first year, every 6 months in years two through five, and yearly thereafter, is recommended following surgical resection or radiation treatment. At the same intervals patients should be evaluated for recurrent or new symptoms and for any complications of treatment, including a focused physical examination.

Sequelae: Complications of treatment may include impotence, incontinence, and radiation cystitis. Metastasis by direct extension may cause obstruction or damage to the seminal vesicles, rectum, bladder, and bowel. Lymphatic metastasis may result in lymphadema and thrombosis. Vascular metastasis to the bones of the axial skeleton is the most common metastasis, but the lungs, colon, or bladder may also become involved.

Prevention/Prophylaxis: Screening should focus on high-risk groups, including black men and all men age 40 and older with a family history of prostate cancer. Other men over age 50 should be screened annually. Screening for prostate cancer includes a symptom review and DRE yearly. Because the role of annual PSA testing for screening purposes is controversial, the test may not be reimbursed by a patient's medical insurance. There are currently no definitive recommendations for PSA testing in screening. Men should avoid the use of androgen supplements.

Referral: Refer patients to a urologist, oncologist, and radiologist.

Education: Review risk factors with patients and encourage yearly screening. Teach dietary guidelines covering the increased risk for cancer associated with a high-fat diet.

Prostatitis

Prostatitis, the inflammation or infection of the prostate gland, may occur in four common forms: acute bacterial, chronic bacterial, nonbacterial, and prostatodynia.

Etiology: The most common causes of acute bacterial and chronic bacterial prostatitis are gram-negative organisms such as *Escherichia coli, Klebsiella pneumoniae, Proteus mirabilis, Enterococcus faecalis,* or *Staphylococcus aureus. Chlamydia trachomatis* and *Ureaplasma* have been linked to the development of nonbacterial prostatitis. A small percentage of men are infected with two or more pathogens at one time.

Occurrence: It is estimated that 25%–50% of all men are diagnosed with prostatitis at least once in their lifetime.

Age: Prostatitis is common in sexually active men; chronic prostatitis is more common in men over age 50.

Ethnicity: Not significant.

Gender: Prostatitis occurs only in men.

Contributing Factors: Patients with a history of urinary tract infections (UTIs) are at risk for developing prostatitis. Other factors that have also been linked to the development of prostatitis include noncircumcision, anal intercourse, urologic procedures, chronic bladder catheterization, and sexually transmitted diseases (STDs). Patients with neuromuscular dysfunction that includes ejaculatory dysfunction, abnormalities of urinary flow (especially a pulsating flow), and urinary hesitancy are also at risk for developing prostatitis.

Signs and Symptoms: In older men, frequency, dribbling, hesitancy, and urgency may be the presenting symptoms, although dysuria can also occur. Question patients about the quality of their urinary flow; a pulsating flow is common in patients with prostatodynia. Inquire if the patient has had penile discharge, painful ejaculations, or hematuria. Irritative voiding is common in chronic prostatitis. It is important to discern if the patient has a history of UTIs; in patients with nonbacterial prostatitis and prostatodynia, a history of UTIs is rare. In acute prostatitis, fever and severe pain may also occur. Patients may complain of myalgia or arthralgia, especially in the lower back, perineum, groin, scrotum, or suprapubic area. Physical examination of patients presenting with symptoms of prostatitis may reveal suprapubic tenderness. Percuss the bladder to note if there is distension. A digital examination should be avoided in men presenting with acute symptoms, to minimize pain for the patient. In examination for chronic prostatitis, the prostate may feel tender or boggy.

Diagnostic Tests: A complete blood count (CBC) with differential may show leukocytosis in acute bacterial prostatitis. Urinalysis may show pyuria, hematuria, and bacteriuria in acute prostatitis and is generally negative in chronic bacterial prostatitis, nonbacterial prostatitis, and prostatodynia. Urine culture should show positive for pathogens in acute prostatitis. Fractional urine examination or prostatic localization studies should be ordered to determine if the patient has chronic prostatitis. Expressed prostatic secretions are also examined for presence of white blood cells (WBCs), oval fat bodies, and reduced lecithin granules. In chronic prostatitis, the number of leukocytes is increased (greater than 10 per high-power field). The bacterial counts need to be at least 10 times higher in the prostatic secretions and the postmassage urine specimens than in the urethral and bladder specimens collected, to make the diagnosis of chronic prostatitis. In nonbacterial prostatitis, the number of leukocytes is increased but the cultures are negative. No abnormal laboratory findings are evident in prostatodynia.

Differential Diagnosis: As part of the clinical workup for prostatitis, consider the following conditions in the differential diagnosis: urethral or bladder infection, interstitial cystitis, diverticulitis, pylenophritis, prostatic abscess, benign prostatic hypertrophy, urethral stricture, neurogenic bladder, and bladder or prostatic carcinoma.

Treatment: Patients presenting with high fever, leukocytosis, or delirium should be hospitalized for hydration and empiric broad-spectrum intravenous (IV) antibiotics; amnoglycosides should be used with caution in the older adult. Once the patient is stabilized, oral antibiotic therapy should be continued. Patients not requiring hospitalization for acute prostatitis should be given trimethoprim/sulfamethoxazole 160 mg/800 mg q 12 hr for 30 days, ciprofloxin HCl 250–500 mg q 12 hr, or norfloxacin 400 mg q 12 hr for least 3 weeks (adjust dosage for creatinine clearance and renal function). Patients can also be instructed to use Sitz baths two to three times a day as needed. Evaluate the need for stool softeners and analgesics. If there is no relief of symptoms within 48 hr, refer patient to a urologist for further evaluation. Treat patients with chronic prostatitis with trimethoprim/sulfamethoxazole, ciprofloxin HCl, or norfloxacin for 1–3 months (again adjusting the dosage as needed for renal function). Those with nonbacterial prostatitis can be given tetracycline 250–500 mg or doxycycline hyclate 100–200 mg in divided doses for 2 weeks. Patients with prostatodynia should be referred to a urologist.

Follow-up: For patients with acute prostatitis, a repeat culture and prostate examination are recommended after completion of the antibiotic regimen. Patients with chronic prostatitis who have a relapse should continue receiving prolonged therapy. Consider suppression therapy of low-dose antibiotics if the infection is not eradicated and repeating the prostatic localization cultures in 6 months to 1 year.

Sequelae: Unresolved acute prostatitis can lead to bacteremia or pyelonephritis. Patients with chronic infection may develop small prostatic stones.

Referral: Refer patients who also have symptoms of benign prostatic hypertrophy or an intractable infection to a urologist. Patients with suspected prostatodynia should always be referred to a urologist.

Education: Inform patients of the importance of increasing fluid intake during symptomatic periods. Emphasize the need to complete the antibiotic regimen to eradicate the organism. Symptomatic patients should avoid bladder irritants such as alcohol and caffeine. The use of certain medications such as anticholinergics should be also restricted while the patient is symptomatic. Patients should be advised that prostatitis can recur and to report symptoms when detected.

BIBLIOGRAPHY

Assessment

Abrams, WB, Beers, MH, and Berkow, R: The Merck Manual of Geriatrics, ed 2. Merck Research Laboratories, Whitehouse Station, NJ, 1995.

Bates, B, Bickley, LS, and Hoekelman, RA: A Guide to Physical Examination and History Taking, ed 6. JB Lippincott, Philadelphia, 1995.

Ebersole, P, and Hess, P: Toward Healthy Aging, ed 4. CV Mosby, St Louis, 1994.

Eliopoulos, C: Health Assessment of the Older Adult, ed 2. Addison-Wesley Nursing, Redwood City, CA, 1990.

Jarvis, CA: Physical Examination and Health Assessment, ed 2. WB Saunders, Philadelphia, 1996.

Mezey, MD, Rauckhorst, LH, and Stakes, SA: Health Assessment of the Older Individual, ed 2. Springer, New York, 1993.

Atrophic Vaginitis

Abrams, W, Beers, MH, and Berkow, R: The Merck Manual of Geriatrics, ed 2. Merck Research Laboratories, Whitehouse Station, NJ, 1995.

Ahronheim, JC: Handbook of Prescribing Medications for Geriatric Patients, ed 1. Little, Brown, Boston, 1992.

Berkow, R, and Fletcher, A (eds): The Merck Manual of Diagnosis and Therapy, ed 16. Merck Research Laboratories, Rahway, NJ, 1992.

Brocklehurst, JC, Tallis, RC, and Fillit, HM (eds): Textbook of Geriatric Medicine and Gerontology, ed 4. Churchill Livingstone, Edinburgh, 1992.

Cassel, CK, Risenberg, DE, Sorensen, LB, and Walsh, JR (eds): Geriatric Medicine, ed 2. Springer-Verlag, New York, 1990.

Dambro, MR, and Griffith, JA (eds): Griffith's 5 Minute Clinical Consult. Williams & Wilkins, Baltimore, 1996.

DeGowin, RL: DeGowin and DeGowin's Diagnostic Examination, ed 6. McGraw-Hill, New York, 1994.

Hazzard, W, et al (eds): Principles of Geriatric Medicine and Gerontology, ed 3. McGraw-Hill, New York, 1994.

Hofland, S, and Powers, J: Sexual dysfunction in the menopausal woman: Hormonal causes and management issues. Geriatr Nurs 17:4, 1996.

Scott, JR, Disaia, PJ, Hammond, CB, and Spellacy, WN (eds): Danforth's Obstetrics and Gynecology, ed 7. JB Lippincott, Philadelphia, 1994.

Uphold, CR, and Graham, MV: Clinical Guidelines in Adult Health. Barmarrae, Gainesville, FL, 1993.

Benign Prostatic Hypertrophy

Dambro, MR: Griffith's 5 Minute Clinical Consult. Williams & Wilkins, Baltimore, 1997.
Hall, NK: Benign prostatic hyperplasia. In Rakel, RE: Saunders Manual of Medical Practice. WB Saunders, Philadelphia, 1996.
Presti, JC, Stoller, ML, and Carroll, PR: Urology. In Tierney, LM, McPhee, SJ, and Papadakis, MA (eds): Current Medical Diagnosis and Treatment, ed 36. Appleton & Lange, Norwalk, CT, 1997.
US Department of Health and Human Services, Public Health Service, Agency for Health Care Policy and Research: Clinical Practice Guideline Number 8, February 1994. Benign Prostatic Hyperplasia: Diagnosis and Treatment. AHCPR Publication No 94-0583, Rockville, MD, 1994.

Breast Cancer

Barron, RH, and Borgen, PI: Genetic susceptibility for breast cancer: Testing and primary prevention options. Oncol Nurs Forum 24:461, 1997.
Clinical guidelines: Adult cancer detection screening by physical examination. Nurse Pract 21:85, 1996.
Fischer, DS: Follow Up of Cancer: A Handbook for Physicians. Lippincott-Raven, Philadelphia, 1996.
Forbes, JF: The incidence of breast cancer: The global burden, public health concerns. Semin Oncol 24(Suppl 1):20, 1997.
Harris, J, Morrow, M, and Norton, L: Malignant tumors of the breast. In DeVita, VT, Hellman, S, and Rosenberg, SA (eds): Cancer Principles of Practice and Oncology. Vol. 2. Lippincott-Raven, Philadelphia, 1997.
Haskell, CM, and Casciato, DA: Breast cancer. In Casciato, DA, and Lowitz, BB (eds): Manual of Clinical Oncology, ed 3. Little, Brown, Boston, 1995.
Henderson, IC: Breast cancer. In Isselbacher, KJ, et al (eds): Harrison's Principles of Internal Medicine, ed 13. McGraw-Hill, New York, 1994.
Jennings, K: Getting black women to screen for cancer: Incorporating health beliefs into practice. JAANP 8:53, 1996.
Townsend, CM: Treatment of breast cancer. Clinical Symposia 49:3, 1997.
Van Dijck, JA, Broeders, JM, and Verbeek AL: Mammographic screening in older women. Is it worthwhile? Drugs Aging 10:69, 1997.

Drug-Induced Impotence

Black, JM, and Matassarin-Jacobs, E: Luckmann and Sorensen's Medical-Surgical Nursing, ed 4. WB Saunders, Philadelphia, 1993.
Darrow, MD: Impotence. In Rakel, RE: Saunders Manual of Medical Practice. WB Saunders, Philadelphia, 1996.
Douglas, V: Sexuality and aging. Focus on Geriatric Care and Rehabilitation, 4(7):1–8, 1991.
Gerchufsky, M: Impotence: The problem men don't talk about. ADVANCE for Nurse Practitioners 3(3):13–16, 1995.
Godschalk, MF, and Mulligan, M: Sexual dysfunction. In Yoshikawa, TT, Cobbs, EL, and Brummel-Smith, K: Practical Ambulatory Geriatrics, ed 2. CV Mosby, St Louis, 1998.
Lerner, SE, Melman A, and Christ, GJ: A review of erectile dysfunction: New insights and more questions. J Urol 149:1246–1255, 1993.
National Institutes of Health: Impotence. NIH Consensus Statement 10(4):1–33, 1992.
Wilson, B: The effect of drugs on male sexual function and fertility. Nurse Practitioner 16(9):12–22, 1991.

Endometrial Cancer

Apgar, BS: Dysmenorrhea and dysfunctional uterine bleeding. Primary Care: Clinics in Office Practice 24:161, 1997.

Burke, TW, Eifel, PJ, and Muggia, FM: Cancer of the uterine body. In DeVita, VT, Hellman, S, Rosenberg, SA (eds): Cancer Principles of Practice and Oncology. Vol 1. Lippincott-Raven, Philadelphia, 1997.

Creasman, MT: Endometrial cancer: Incidence, prognostic factors, diagnosis, and treatment. Semin Oncol 24(Suppl 1):00, 1997.

Farias-Eisner, RP, Walker, DL, and Berek, JS: Gynecological cancers. In Casciato, DA, and Lowitz, BB (eds): Manual of Clinical Oncology, ed 3. Little, Brown, Boston, 1995.

Fischer, DS: Follow-up of Cancer: A Handbook for Physicians. Lippincott-Raven, Philadelphia, 1996.

Gorroll, AH, May, LA, and Mulley, AG: Primary Care Medicine: Office Evaluation of the Adult Patient, ed 3. JB Lippincott, Philadelphia, 1995.

Melnikow, J: Cancer prevention and screening in women. Primary Care: Clinics in Office Practice 24:15, 1997.

Plaxe, SC. Impact of ethnicity on the incidence of high-risk endometrical cancer. Gynecologic Oncology 65:8, 1997.

Prostate Cancer

Bauer, JJ, and Mcleod, DG: Prostate cancer: Diagnosis, treatment, and experience at one tertiary-care military medical center, 1989 and 1994. Military Medicine 161:646, 1996.

Clinical guidelines: Adult cancer detection screening by physical examination. Nurse Practitioner 21:85, 1996.

Collins, M: Increasing prostate cancer awareness in African American men. Oncol Nurs Forum 24:91, 1997.

Fischer, DS: Follow-up of Cancer: A Handbook for Physicians. Lippincott-Raven, Philadelphia, 1996.

Garnick, MB: Prostate cancer: Emerging concepts. Ann Intern Med 125:118, 1996.

Oesterling, J, Fuks, Z, Lee, CT, and Scher, HI: Prostate cancer. In DeVita, VT, Hellman, S, Rosenberg, SA (eds): Cancer Principles of Practice and Oncology. Vol 1. Lippincott-Raven, Philadelphia, 1997.

Sagalowsky, AI, and Wilson, JD: Hyperplasia of the prostate. In Isselbacher, KJ, et al (eds): Harrison's Principles of Internal Medicine, ed 13. McGraw-Hill, New York, 1994.

Sandock, DS, and Resnick, MI: Diseases and imaging of the prostate. In Resnick, MI, and Older, RA (eds): Diagnosis of Genitourinary Disease, ed 2. Thieme, New York, 1997.

Small, EJ: Prostate cancer: Who to screen, and what the results mean. Geriatrics 48:28, 1993.

Zimmerman, SM: Factors influencing Hispanic participation in prostate cancer screening. Oncol Nurs Forum 24:499, 1997.

Prostatitis

Abrams, AB, Beers, MH, and Berkow, R (eds): The Merck Manual of Geriatrics, ed 2. Merck Research Laboratories, Whitehouse Station, NJ, 1995.

Criste, G, Gray, D, and Gallo B: Prostatis: A review of diagnosis and management. Nurse Pract 19(7):32–38, 1994.

Donovan, DA, and Nicholas, PK: Prostatitis: Diagnosis and treatment in primary care. Nurse Pract 22(4):144–156, 1997.

Griffith, HW, and Dambo, MR: The Five Minute Clinical Consultant. Lea & Febiger, Philadelphia, 1994.

Moul, JW: Sorting out the different causes. Post Grad Med 94:191, 1993.

CHAPTER **12**

MUSCULOSKELETAL

DISORDERS

To make an accurate assessment of the musculoskeletal system in the older adult, the nurse practitioner needs to be familiar with changes in the musculoskeletal system caused by aging. For example, aging often brings about a decrease in height, resulting from a decrease in the length of the trunk with respect to the length of the extremities. An older person may tilt the head backward to compensate for the bend in the thoracic spine, producing the typical posture of those in this age group. Because of the loss of subcutaneous fat caused by aging, bony prominences became more noticeable. Some absolute loss of muscle mass occurs, with some muscles diminishing and others atrophying. Without continued use, muscles stiffen and range of motion becomes impaired as an older person ages.

Often when an older person experiences a limitation in functional ability resulting from pain, weakness, or physical impairment, he or she seeks medical attention. To obtain an accurate history of musculoskeletal problems, question the patient about any pain, swelling, stiffness, change in temperature perception (hot or cold), limitation of movement, weakness, body deformity, or paralysis. When a patient complains of one or more of the symptoms, however, the condition may actually be a neurological or systemic disorder. Determine the sequence of events that triggered the onset of each symptom and inquire about precipitating factors. Other symptoms the patient may describe, such as constitutional symptoms of fever or malaise, may be clustered to form a differential diagnosis.

When a patient complains of pain or stiffness with movement, the history of the complaint should be discerned. Has the patient experienced any severe trauma in the past that may be now manifesting itself as an articular degeneration? Because patients who have had a structural deformity or amputation typically place excessive strain on the joints for years, as older individuals they may now experience degeneration of the bone and surrounding musculature. An overextension or a recent increase in activity may lead to muscle soreness, followed by disuse, atrophy, and chronic pain. (adhesive capsulitis). Knowing the history of the presenting symptom may help you distinguish between a local inflammation and a systemic problem. Questioning the patient about the time of day the symptoms of pain and stiffness occur can be helpful too. Rheumatic disease is associated with pain upon waking, whereas osteoarthritic pain and stiffness worsen as the day progresses.

Patients with musculoskeletal problems often complain of weakness and paralysis. Determine whether the disability is local or generalized, constant or intermittent. Local weakness or paralysis may be due to disuse because of pain, trauma, or a neurological problem. Generalized weakness may indicate a systemic disorder. Patients with an underlying thyroid disorder may have constant weakness, whereas those with rheumatoid arthritis may experience weakness intermittently. Muscular weakness should always be differentiated from fatigue.

Generally, proximal weakness results from a myopathy, distal weakness from a neuropathy. The patient should be asked about his or her ability to carry out certain activities of daily living. Does the patient have difficulty combing the hair? Can he or she lift objects? Does the patient have any trouble standing up after sitting in a chair? Patients with a proximal weakness of the upper extremities may have difficulty grooming the hair or lifting objects. Those with a proximal weakness of a lower extremity may have trouble crossing the legs at the knees or walking. If a patient reports difficulty fastening buttons or turning doorknobs, a neuropathy involving the upper extremity is likely.

Another common complaint in patients with a musculoskeletal disorder is deformity. In obtaining the history from a patient with a deformity, the examiner needs to know how long the patient has noticed the deformity. Did it occur suddenly? Was it the result of trauma? Has there been any change in the deformity since its onset?

The overall physical examination of the musculoskeletal disorder begins with observing the patient's gait. Any gait abnormalities or problems in maintaining balance should be noted. The patient's ability to sit in and rise from a chair should be observed. Examine the patient while the patient is standing erect, to note any changes in the spinal curvature. In older adults, kyphosis of the thoracic spine is accentuated. While looking at the older person from the side, the examiner may note that the spine appears to form the number 3. If the curve appears more to be a sharp angle, this is called a gibbus. A gibbus resulting from a vertebral fracture may be the first evidence of osteoporosis.

Patients presenting with a functional limitation should be asked to demonstrate active range of motion (ROM). Active ROM should be performed smoothly and effortlessly. Remember that joint movements include flexion, extension, abduction, adduction, and external rotation. If the patient has limited active ROM, passive ROM should be performed. If the passive range exceeds the active range, the limitation is due to a muscle weakness. Patients may resist passive ROM because of fear, a neurological disorder, or a joint abnormality.

When examining the patient's joints, the joints should be inspected in a relaxed position, and then in flexion and in extension. Abnormalities of the position or carrying angle, joint deformity, erythema, swellings, nodularity, and muscle changes should be assessed. In an older patient with muscle changes, the limb or portion of the body will appear thinner, which indicates atrophy. To determine whether bone structure changes have occurred, appearance and symmetry should be observed. Enlargement, excessive curvature, and irregularity may indicate sequelae of childhood rickets, osteoporotic fractures, Paget's disease, osteoarthritis, or bone tumors. Crepitation or a crackling noise may be heard when the joints are put through ROM. Crepitation is produced by the rubbing together of bone or irregular cartilage surfaces.

A patient presenting with a musculoskeletal deformity may experience one or more of the following: erythema, nodularity, and swelling. Inquire about the duration of any swelling, presence of pain, limitation of movement, evidence of erythema, and locking or buckling of the joint. Erythema is usually associated with active inflammation and accompanied by swelling. An example of joint nodularity is the nodules found in the interphalangeal joints in patients with rheumatoid arthritis and osteoarthritis:

- Heberden's nodes: nodules of the distal interphalangeal joints.
- Bouchard's nodes: nodules of the proximal joints.
- Rheumatoid nodule: often a firm nodule on the dorsum of the wrist.
- Haygarth's nodes: spindle-shaped enlargements of the middle interphalangeal joints that occur in rheumatoid arthritis.

Any joint deformity should be palpated to determine whether it fluctuates because of fluid or is firm because of a thickening or enlargement. If there is fluid, the cause may be recent trauma, inflammation, or joint infection. An articular enlargement of rheumatoid arthritis is usually soft, whereas a joint deformity found in osteoarthritis is usually firm. If the joint swelling persists for more than 3 days, this may indicate an arthritic condition.

Also examine the bursal areas around the joints, palpating for swelling, tenderness, ganglions, and nodularity. A ganglion is usually a soft cystlike swelling, often found near joints. Swelling of the bursae is usually tender upon palpation. All masses should be measured across their greatest diameter.

For the patient complaining of muscle weakness, inspect for evidence of muscle atrophy and palpate the muscles during contraction and rest. Any fluttering of the muscles should be noted. To determine if a patient is having true muscle weakness, the patient should perform against the examiner's resistance. One side should be compared with the other and a numerical value for tested muscle strength recorded. Flexor and extensor muscles should be tested for strength.

Fractures

Fractures or breakage of bone or cartilage are a common cause of disability in older adults. A compound fracture or open fracture occurs when fragments of the bone pierce the skin or mucosa; an impacted fracture occurs when bone fragment is forced into another bone. In older adults, common sites for fractures include:

- Proximal humerus.
- Distal radius.
- Pelvic ramus.
- Proximal femur.
- Proximal tibia.
- Thoracic and lumbar vertebral bodies.

Etiology: Most fractures can be traced to an injury. Vertebral fractures may result from an activity such as lifting or bending that puts great stress on the spine. A relationship exists between the severity of bone mineral loss and the chance of sustaining a fall. In a pathological fracture caused by multiple myeloma, bone marrow is replaced by malignant plasma cells and bone is destroyed.

Occurrence: Estimates show 30% of people age 65 and over fall each year; of that group, 5% of the falls result in fractures. Specifically, 1 million fractures in the United States have been associated with a diagnosis of osteoporosis.

Age: Women over age 50 have a 15% chance of suffering a hip fracture; by age 90, one out of three women and one out of six men suffer a hip fracture.

Ethnicity: White and Asian-American women have a higher prevalence of fractures than African-American women because of the risk of osteoporosis in these two groups.

Gender: The prevalence for fracture is higher in women because of the higher incidence of osteoporosis in women.

Contributing Factors: Factors that can contribute to the incidence of fractures in older adults include

- Advanced age.
- Female gender.
- Osteoporosis.
- Family history of osteoporosis.
- Osteopenia.
- Confusion.

- Parkinson's disease.
- Prolonged bed rest.
- Motor vehicle trauma.
- Cerebrovascular accident (CVA).
- Urinary retention.
- Peripheral neuropathy.
- Peripheral edema.
- Bone metastases.

Additional factors that are all known contributors to falls in older adults include environmental hazards, reduced visual acuity, change in depth perception, vestibular dysfunction, postural hypotension, and certain medications that include alcohol.

Signs and Symptoms: Patients present with a history of recent injury to the affected area. For vertebral compression fractures, however, trauma may not be necessary for the insult to occur. Generally, for any type of fracture, an older adult may report pain, pressure, spasms, and swelling in the injured area. A patient with a femoral neck fracture may report groin pain. Physical examination reveals soft tissue swelling, ecchymosis, local tenderness and pain with any motion. In a hip fracture, the affected leg appears shorter than the other leg and externally rotated (Fig. 12–1).

Diagnostic Tests: Radiographs of the affected area are standard procedure in diagnosing a fracture. A complete blood count (CBC) is necessary to determine if there has been internal blood loss when there has been major trauma. Erythrocyte sedimentation rate is assessed to rule out an infectious or neoplastic process.

Differential Diagnosis: When radiographs diagnose a fracture, the clinician needs to determine if the cause of the fracture is an infectious or a neoplastic process. Vertebral fractures involving the thoracic spine are thought to be a result of osteoporosis, whereas lumbar fractures have been related to infectious processes such as osteomyelitis or neoplastic disease such as multiple myeloma.

Treatment: For the pain related to the fracture, analgesics and non-steroid anti-inflammatory drugs (NSAIDs), if not prohibited, are helpful. Depending on the site of the fracture, casting, elastic wrapping, splints, immobilization, traction, or surgical intervention may be used. The most common surgical intervention for a fractured hip is open reduction internal rotation (ORIF), especially for fractures of the intertrochanteric or subtrochanteric region.

Follow-up: The long-term management of a patient with a fracture depends not only on the location of the fracture, but also on the etiology of the fracture, whether osteoporosis, an infectious process, or neoplasia. Patients may have return appointments with an orthopedist, physical therapy, or both. Patients should be questioned about any muscle weakness or paresthesia following the incident. The function of the affected area should be evaluated. Determine what impact the injury had on the patient's instrumental activities of daily living (IADLs) and activities of daily living (ADLs).

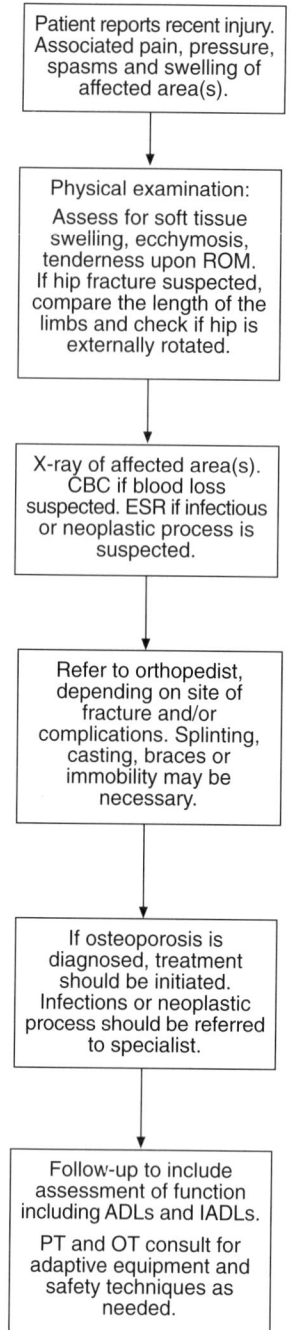

FIGURE 12-1 Fractures.

Sequelae: The complications resulting from a fracture depend on a number of factors such as comorbidities, health status of the patient prior to the injury, and the location of the fracture. Patients are susceptible to hypovolemic shock, infection, incontinence, decubiti, subdural hematoma, dehydration, electrolyte imbalance, hypothermia, and phlebitis after sustaining the injury and throughout the recovery period. For hip fractures, approximately 10%–17% of patients will be readmitted to the hospital during the first 6 months. There is also a high mortality rate associated with hip fractures. Loss of physical and social function may also follow an injury.

Prevention/Prophylaxis: Related to osteoporosis, estrogen replacement therapy reduces the incidence of hip fractures as much as 50%–75%. Exercise programs, and cataract surgery in patients whose vision is impaired, reduce the number of fractures. The modification of the patient's environment to remove hazards such as throw rugs and small pieces of furniture, improvements in lighting, and installation of grab bars, raised toilet seats, and ramps helps prevent injuries.

Referral: Depending on the radiographic findings and location of the fracture, patients may need to be referred immediately to orthopedist. A physical therapy consultation is often necessary to teach patients exercises to improve or maintain function. The patient should be referred to an occupational therapist for recommendations for the need for adaptive equipment such as grabbers, reachers, and elevated toilet seats when the patient has suffered loss of function.

Education: Following an injury, older adults are often hesitant or afraid to repeat the activity that led to the incident. Patients with osteoporosis need to be instructed on safe practices for lifting, bending, and reaching for objects. If the injury occurred after a fall, assessment of the home environment and consideration of adaptive equipment are suggested.

Gout

Gout, an inflammatory disease associated with malfunctioning metabolism of purine, leading to overproduction or underexcretion of uric acid, results in deposits of sodium urate crystals in the joints, periarticular tissues, subcutaneous tissues, and kidneys. Primary gout is the clinical disease caused by hyperuricemia; secondary gout usually occurs as a result of extended use of agents that decrease uric acid excretion.

Etiology: Clinically, hyperuricemia is defined when the serum urate level is greater than 7 mg/dL. With levels above 10 mg/dL, the chance of an acute attack of gout is greater than 90%. In 70%–95% of patients with diagnosed gout, underexcretion of urate rather than a metabolic overproduction causes elevation of the plasma urate level.

Occurrence: For every 100,000 people in the United States, 100 cases of gout occur.

Age: Primary gout usually begins in the fourth to sixth decade, whereas a new presentation of gout in the elderly occurs in the sixth to seventh decade.

Ethnicity: Not significant.

Gender: Primary gout is 20 times more prevalent in men than in women; however, among the elderly population, gout occurs predominantly in women.

Contributing Factors: Factors associated with primary gout in men include positive family history, obesity, trauma, hyperlipidemia, alcohol consumption, fasting, binge-eating, analgesic nephropathy, nephrolithiasis, and polycystic kidney disease. In women or men over age 60, with a first-time presentation of gout, a relationship between long-term use of thiazide diuretics, salicylate use, hypertension, and renal insufficiency is observed. Patients taking nicotinic acid, cyclosporine, and ethambutol are also at risk for gout. Acute gout attacks have also been linked to stressors such as surgery or illness. Certain malignancies such as hemolytic anemia, lymphoreticular cancers, and leukemias can lead to secondary gout because of the accelerated turnover of cells that occurs with these conditions, leading to increased purine biosynthesis. Lead intoxication and consumption of illegal or "moonshine" whiskey has been found to be a contributor to saturnine gout.

Signs and Symptoms: Review the patient's history for evidence of excessive alcohol consumption, dietary habits, medical diagnosis of gout, family history of gout, exposure to lead, consumption of illicit whiskey, trauma, and all medication use. The following questions are helpful to ask the patient, to understand the presentation of symptoms:

- Did the pain occur suddenly or become noticeable gradually?
- Has the pain ever occurred before?
- If so, how long did it last and was the swelling in the same joint(s)?

In middle-aged men, the classic presentation of an acute gout attack is a hot, swollen metatarsophalangeal (MTP) joint of the great toe. Usually, in the first presentation of gout in middle-aged men, joint involvement is monarticular. In elderly women, joint involvement with gout is usually polyarticular. The proximal interphalangeal (PIP) joints and the distal interphalangeal joints should be examined and the instep, heel, ankle, knee, wrist, and olecranon bursa palpated for signs of swelling and tenderness. Tophi, subcutaneous deposits of sodium urate, are common in chronic gout. Examine the helix of the ear, olecranon bursa, prepatellar bursa, Achilles tendon, over the Heberden's nodes, and finger pads for signs of tophi. Fever may be present. Refer to Fig. 12–2.

Diagnostic Tests: Evidence of monosodium urate crystals in joint aspirates is the "gold standard" in diagnosing gout and rules out sepsis in the joint(s). A 24-hr urine test for uric acid is ordered to differentiate between an overproducer or underexcretor of uric acid. If the 24-hr urinary uric acid level is greater than

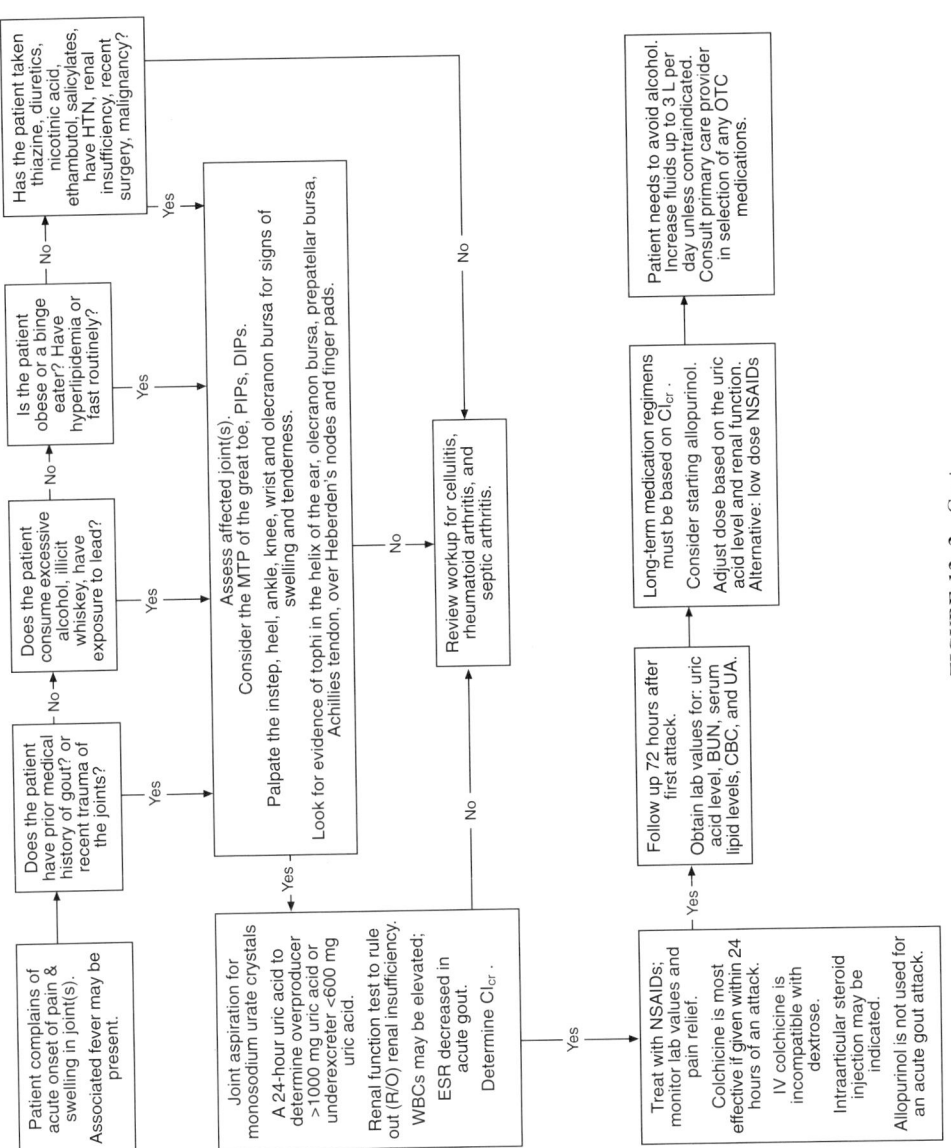

FIGURE 12–2 Gout.

1000 mg, the patient is overproducing uric acid. If the urinary uric acid level is less than 600 mg in 24 hr, the patient is underexcreting. Underexcretion can be seen in patients taking diuretics and salicylates. Serum uric acid levels are often normal in patients with acute gout. A renal function test should be ordered in older adults because renal insufficiency is a complication of gout. Initial radiographic changes will show soft tissue swelling; later, as the disease progresses, oval punched-out erosions will be evident. The white blood cell (WBC) count may be elevated during an acute attack; the sedimentation rate may also be increased.

Differential Diagnosis: Often pseudogout, traumatic joint injury, septic arthritis, cellulitis, or hemarthros can mimic the presentation of acute gout. Rheumatoid arthritis is often mistaken for chronic gout when subcutaneous tophi are present.

Treatment: Management of the older adult with gout requires careful monitoring. Elderly persons are susceptible to renal insufficiency, may have other concomitant diseases, and experience hypersensitivity to some of the medications used to treat younger patients with gout. NSAIDs are the drugs of choice for older adults with gout. Indomethacin is effective in the treatment of acute gout; the usual dose is 25–50 mg PO bid to tid until the symptoms cease, which should be in about 3 days. Other NSAIDs such as naproxen, ibuprofen, fenoprofen, and sulindac can be tried. As with any NSAID, renal function must be monitored. NSAIDs can endanger existing renal function, especially when the Cl_{cr} is less than or equal to 30 mL/min. Colchicine can be given for acute gout attacks either intravenously (IV) or orally. It is most effective if given within 24 hr of an attack. IV dosage is 1 to 2 mg in 10–20 mL of normal saline IV, followed by 1 mg once or twice more at 4-hr intervals. **Note:** Colchicine is incompatible with dextrose because precipitation will occur. The oral colchicine dose is 0.5 mg every 2 hr until relief is felt; gastrointestinal (GI) toxicity commonly precedes a therapeutic response. Because oral colchicine is associated with more side effects than IV colchicine is, it should not be administered to patients with impaired renal or hepatic function or GI disease or to postoperative patients because of the potential for vomiting. Patients for whom both colchicine and NSAIDs are contraindicated may be given intra-auricular steroid injections. Allopurinol and uricosuric drugs should not be prescribed for an acute gout attack.

Follow-up: Patients experiencing a first acute attack of gout should be followed up 72 hr after initiating treatment to determine effectiveness and presence of any side effects. Patients who have more than three attacks of gout in a year are considered to have chronic disease. Before initiating a long-term medication regimen, uric acid level, blood urea nitrogen (BUN), and serum lipid levels, CBC, and urinalysis should be ordered.

Patients with chronic gout may require a uric acid–lowering agent such as allopurinol. The starting dose for allopurinol is 100 mg/day, to be increased until the desired uric acid level is achieved (less than 6.5 mg/dL). The dose may need to be increased gradually to 600 mg/day for severe gout and adjusted based on renal function. A dose of 200 mg/dL is probably the maximum dose that should be prescribed if the Cl_{cr} is 50–60 mL/min. The usefulness of probenecid in the older adult is limited because it is only effective when the Cl_{cr} is less than 50 mL/min. Alternative treatment for chronic gout includes indomethacin 25 mg bid or another low-dose NSAID, reducing the dose in patients with documented hepatic or renal disease.

Sequelae: Older adults who have preexisting hypertension or primary renal disease or who use NSAIDs and diuretics are at risk for developing renal insufficiency, urate nephropathy, and acute hyperuricemia nephropathy. Uric acid nephrolithiasis is also a complication of gout. Untreated chronic gout may lead to multilobular, tender subcutaneous tophaceous gout, which can be deforming and impair ADLs.

Prevention/Prophylaxis: Thiazide diuretics and salicylates should be avoided in patients with gout.

Referral: Patients may need a referral to a rheumatologist if they require intraarticular injections of steroids or joint aspiration, have complications from treatment, or have unusual presentation of the disease.

Education: Patients need to be informed that during an acute attack they should rest the affected area and limit weight bearing if the first MTP joint is involved. Intake of fluids to up to 3 L/day is recommended unless contraindicated. The use of alcohol should be discouraged. Patients should consult their primary care provider regarding selection of any over-the-counter medications.

Osteoarthritis

Osteoarthritis (OA), still also referred to as degenerative joint disease, is a degenerative disease of the joint cartilage. It is the leading cause of disability in older adults in the United States. OA most commonly affects the distal and proximal interphalangeal joints of the hand, the hips, the knees, and the cervical and lumbar spine.

Etiology: The etiology of OA is unknown; however, it is known that OA is not age-dependent. Conditions that change joint mechanics, such as untreated hip dislocation, may predispose an individual to osteoarthritis.

Occurrence: Approximately 60 million people in the United States are afflicted with OA.

Age: OA is very common in older adults. An estimated 33%–90% of the population over age 65 are thought to have OA.

Ethnicity: OA of the knee is more common in African-American women than in white women. Also, the prevalence of OA in male and female Alaskan natives is considerably lower than in white Americans.

Gender: In adults age 55 and older, women are affected more often than men.

Contributing Factors: Increasing age, obesity, and previous joint injury, occupation, hobby, or prolonged sport activity involving the weight-bearing joints contribute to the development of OA. Other factors include calcium pyrophosphate or uric acid crystal deposits in the joints, Wilson's disease, acromegaly, hyperparathyroidism, and diabetes mellitus.

Signs and Symptoms: Complaints of morning stiffness, lasting less than 30 minutes or stiffness that improves with activity, as well as accompanying muscle spasms, may indicate OA. Persistent pain and limitation of motion in the affected joint may also be reported. Bouchard's nodes (nontender nodules of the PIP joints), Heberden's nodes (nontender nodules of the distal interphalangeal [DIP] joints of the hands and/or feet), or both, may be found. In women, inflammatory OA often occurs in the PIPs and DIPs, manifesting red, tender joints. MTP joints may also be involved.

Upon examination, patients with OA of the hip and knee may present with an antalgic gait. Crepitus of the affected joint is common. Internal and external hip rotation may be reduced. Some patients may complain of knee-locking and unsteadiness.

Patients with OA of the cervical spine often complain of paresthesias and numbness in the arms, waking them from their sleep; this sensation generally improves when the limb is shaken. Examination of the cervical spine may show some restricted joint movement and muscle tenderness.

When OA affects the lumbosacral spine, patients may report pain across the lower back with radiation to the buttocks and posterior thigh; if nerve root compression has occurred, patients may complain of pain in the lower leg. Refer to Fig. 12–3.

Diagnostic Tests: In determining the presence of systemic inflammation, results of erythrocyte sedimentation rate (ESR), C-reactive protein, and blood counts are usually normal in a person with OA. Routine radiographs confirm the diagnosis of OA; joint space narrowing, proliferative spurs, subchondral cysts, and subchondral bony sclerosis may be noted. Patients with spinal OA may require computerized tomography (CT) or magnetic resonance imaging (MRI) to rule out other spinal disorders and to determine if there is nerve entrapment.

Differential Diagnosis: When the spine is involved, osteoporosis, metastatic disease, and multiple myeloma need to be ruled out.

Treatment: In patients with no evidence of inflammation, acetaminophen is the medication of choice in doses of 2.6–4 g/day. Nonpharmacological therapies such as walking can also be beneficial. For patients not getting relief from

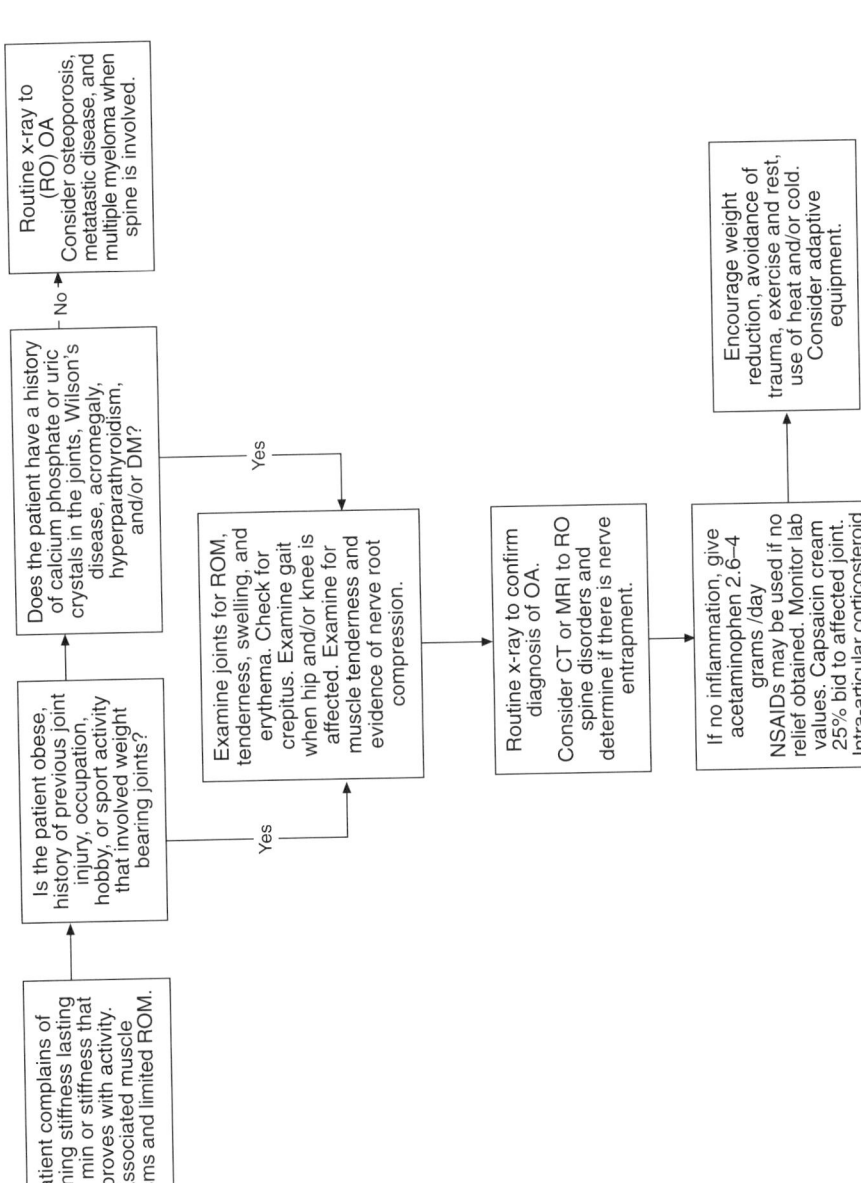

FIGURE 12–3 Osteoarthritis (OA).

acetaminophen and exercise, other NSAIDs can be tried. Selection of an NSAID should be based on dosing frequency, toxicity potential, and cost to the patient. Older adults should be started on a low dose of an NSAID, increasing the dose gradually. Capsaicin cream 25%, applied twice daily to the affected joint(s), has also been shown to reduce pain. When only one or a few joints are inflamed, intra-articular corticosteroid injections may be beneficial; however, use of such injections should be limited to only a couple of times each year. Patients with severe pain and restricted mobility may benefit from surgical intervention or reconstructive joint surgery.

Follow-up: Patients should be reevaluated in about 2–3 weeks initially, to determine the effectiveness of the treatment. At this time, the patient should be weighed if obesity is a contributing factor; diet and exercise should be reviewed. The patient should be asked about benefits received from heat, cold, massage, and so forth. Response to pharmacological measures can be reevaluated in patients who have been prescribed NSAIDs. A CBC and creatinine clearance and liver function tests should be ordered at this time, and then every 3 months. Question the patient about any new onset of dyspepsia, abdominal pain, and/or bleeding.

Sequelae: Because OA is a slowly progressive disease, joint deformity and functional disability may occur in individuals who have difficulty responding to the therapeutic regimen.

Prevention/Prophylaxis: Weight reduction and avoidance of joint trauma may prevent further joint deformity in persons with OA.

Referral: Patients may need a referral to a rheumatologist if they have complications from treatment or an unusual presentation of the disease. Patients with involved joint deformities should be referred to an orthopedic surgeon for possible joint replacement.

Education: Patients should be given a treatment plan that includes information about the importance of exercise, scheduled rest periods, weight reduction, the safe use of heat, cold, and medication to control or alleviate pain. Information should be provided about acquiring necessary adaptive equipment such as walkers, canes, elevated toilet seats, and any orthotics needed. Patients may require instruction on how to use these devices safely.

Osteoporosis

Osteoporosis is a systemic skeletal disease resulting in a reduction in bone mass and microarchitectural deterioration of bone tissue, which increases susceptibility to fractures. Fractures are common in the vertebrae, the proximal femur, and the distal forearm.

Etiology: Osteoporosis results from an imbalance between bone resorption and bone formation, causing a reduction in bone tissue. Two types of primary osteoporosis are type I, which occurs mainly in postmenopausal women and is characterized by increased in bone resorption, reduced production of parathyroid hormone, and a decreased activation of vitamin D; and type II, or senile osteoporosis, which develops in persons age 70 and older. In type I osteoporosis, trabecular bone loss is accelerated. Women who have estrogen deficiency due to early natural or surgical menopause are at risk for developing this type of osteoporosis. In type II osteoporosis, trabecular and cortical bone loss occurs. Type I and type II osteoporosis may overlap. Secondary osteoporosis may result from hormone excess, malignancy, genetic disorders, chronic disease, and certain medications.

Occurrence: More than 25 million Americans have osteoporosis, 80% of whom are women.

Age: Type I osteoporosis is found in persons age 55–75; type II, in those age 70–85.

Ethnicity: The risk for osteoporosis is twice as great in white women than in African-American women. Asian-American women are also at a high risk. About 15% of Mexican-American women have osteoporosis. White men are also at greater risk for developing osteoporosis than African-American men.

Gender: The ratio of women to men for developing type I osteoporosis is 6 : 1; the ratio decreases to 2 : 1 for type II osteoporosis.

Contributing Factors: A number of risk factors predispose individuals to osteoporosis including female gender, white or Asian race, small body structure, light hair and complexion, and family history of the disease. A history of tobacco abuse and excessive alcohol and caffeine intake increase the risk of developing osteoporosis. A diet that limits calcium and vitamin D but contains large quantities of protein and phosphorus may also put patients at greater risk. Patients taking certain medications such as corticosteroids, thyroid hormones, anticonvulsants (e.g., phenytoin), anticoagulants, lithium, certain chemotherapeutic agents, aluminum antacids, and tetracyclines are at increased risk. Individuals diagnosed with hyperthyroidism, type I diabetes mellitus, rheumatoid arthritis, chronic renal failure, liver disease, epilepsy, alcholism, malabsorption states, anorexia nervosa, and those having menopause before age 40 without hormonal replacement, hyperparathyroidism, and those who are immobile, are also susceptible to osteoporosis. A history of fracture or of a tendency to fall puts the person at risk for sustaining an osteoporotic fracture.

Signs and Symptoms: People with osteoporosis may be asymptomatic. Patients need to be questioned about all of the risk factors for osteoporosis. Inquire about family history of fractures and get a thorough menstrual history in women; questions about libido and potency in men are important. The person's height should be measured at initial visit and yearly. The mouth should be examined to assess dentition and any evidence of oral bone loss, and the thyroid gland should be palpated. The spine should be examined in detail, including configuration. Any tenderness to palpation over the spinous processes, evidence of swelling, tenderness, and ecchymosis present at the sight of the injury should be noted. ROM should be determined, noting limitations or painful movement. An abdominal examination will reveal whether the abdomen is protuberant from spinal changes; the distance between the rib cage and the anterior iliac crest should be recorded. Physical examination may reveal loss of height with associated kyphosis of the spine. The most common site for vertebral fractures in patients with osteoporosis is the lower thoracic (T12) or upper lumbar (L1) region. Gait should be assessed objectively and the patient's body mechanics observed at this time.

Diagnostic Tests: Baseline laboratory studies should include CBC, thyroid-stimulating hormone (TSH) level, urinalysis for markers of bone loss, and blood chemistries, including calcium, phosphorus, creatinine, and electrolyte levels. Other laboratory tests may be ordered, based on the patient's history and physical examination. Bone mass measurements accurately reflect fracture risk for patients with osteoporosis; however, widespread screening for osteoporosis in asymptomatic women is not yet recommended. Bone densitometry is also indicated in special cases to monitor the treatment program for osteoporosis. Dual-energy x-ray absortiometry (DEXA) is the most effective means of bone densitometry. If the bone density is greater than or equal to 2.5 standard deviations (SDs) below the young adult mean at the same site in a person of the same sex, osteoporosis is said to be technically present.

Differential Diagnosis: In establishing a diagnosis of osteoporosis, secondary causes of the disease must be ruled out. Other diseases associated with low bone mass include multiple myeloma, hyperparathyroidism, osteomalacia, hyperthyroidism, and Cushing's syndrome. Multiple myeloma may be detected by using urinalysis or serum protein electrophoresis, and hyperparathyroidism by measuring serum calcium and parathyroid hormone levels. Osteomalacia can be implicated with an elevated alkaline phosphatase level. Hyperthyroidism can be determined by testing a serum TSH level, and Cushing's syndrome through a 24-hour urine-free cortisol test.

Treatment: The management of osteoporosis is comprehensive. Patients should be educated on the importance of preventing injury and altering changeable risk factors. Dietary adjustments should include supplementation with 1500 mg of elemental calcium for patients not receiving hormone replacement therapy or 1000 mg of calcium for those who are receiving this treatment, unless the patient has hypercalciuria. Calcium carbonate is 40% elemental calcium by weight but may cause constipation; calcium citrate, which is 22% elemental calcium by weight, is better absorbed and has fewer GI side effects. Recommend elimination of tobacco, excessive alcohol and caffeine, and a reduction in the amount of high-phosphorus foods. Patients should engage in regular weight-bearing exercises. Measures to enhance safety in the home and surrounding environment should be emphasized. Options for pharmacological measures to treat osteoporosis in postmenopausal women include estrogen replacement therapy (ESR), vitamin D, biophosphonates, calcitonin, and fluoride. Treatment plans must be individualized. Unless contraindicated, conjugated equine estrogen or its equivalent 625 μg daily or cycled, or transdermal estrogen by patch 0.05–0.1 μg daily or cycled. A woman with an intact uterus may be given medroxyprogesterone 2.5–10 mg the last 10–13 days of estrogen dosing each month or daily. An intake of 250–400 units/day of vitamin D in the form of a multivitamin or fortified dairy products is recommended. Salmon calcitonin is available as an injection or a nasal spray for patients who cannot tolerate estrogen, with the dosage being 50 IU three times weekly to 100 IU daily subcutaneously (SC) or intramuscularly (IM). The dosage for the nasal spray is one puff daily (0.09 mL, 200 IU), in alternating nostrils. Another option for the postmenopausal woman is alendronate 10 mg once daily in the morning swallowed whole with 8 oz of plain water; the patient must remain fully upright for 30 minutes and when at least that amount of time has elapsed, consume the first meal of the day. Alendronate is not recommended for patients with creatinine clearance greater than 35 mL/min.

Follow-up: For persons at risk for osteoporosis, monitor the patient's height, exercise patterns, habits, and diet; review the safety measures for the home and proper body mechanics; and evaluate the need for adaptive equipment. Repeat bone densitometry may be indicated. For patients receiving pharmacological therapy, review the medication regimen, assess for side effects, and repeat laboratory tests as indicated. The patient should also be assessed for fractures and for the need for analgesics.

Sequelae: Osteoporosis-related fractures are major complications of the disease. Of the 250,000 people who sustain a hip fracture yearly, 12%–20% will die within the first year after the injury and more than half of the patients will require long-term care. Because patients often have a fear of falling and injury, a loss of social and physical function may occur.

Prevention/Prophylaxis: As part of the routine examination, patients should be screened to determine their level of risk for the development of osteoporosis. Dietary history, exercise patterns, and habits should be reviewed with patients. A measurement of height should be recorded at least yearly for all adults. The benefits of changing lifestyle patterns should be emphasized to patients even in advanced age. For patients with identifiable risk factors for osteoporosis, bone mass measurement should be considered. Dual-photon and dual-energy x-ray absorptiometry and quantitative CT scans can determine whether a patient has lost enough bone mass to be at risk for fracture.

Referral: Women who will be beginning hormone replacement therapy may be referred to a gynecologist. For patients who have sustained a fracture, depending on its location, an immediate referral to an orthopedist is recommended. Patients may require referral for physical therapy to be evaluated for weight-bearing exercises and for demonstration of safe transferring, lifting, and bending. Patients with functional limitations need instruction on the use of adaptive equipment (e.g., walkers, reacher-grabbers).

Education: Patients can contact the National Osteoporosis Foundation at 2100 M Street, N.W., Suite 602, Washington, DC 20037 (202-223-2226), for educational materials. Patients should also be given information about local support groups for persons with osteoporosis, senior exercise classes, and dietary counseling.

Polymyalgia Rheumatica

Polymyalgia rheumatica (PMR) is a clinical syndrome characterized by fatigue, pain, and stiffness primarily in the neck, shoulders, hips, and pelvic girdle, occurring primarily in older adults. An elevated Westergren ESR is essential in the diagnosis of PMR.

Etiology: The etiology of PMR is unknown. A relationship between the presence of the HLA-DR4 haplotype and presentation of PMR has been suggested.

Occurrence: PMR affects 1 in 1000 persons age 50 and older in the United States.

Age: This disease occurs predominantly in adults over age 50. For older adults over age 80, PMR and temporal arteritis (TA) occur 10 times more frequently than in adults under age 60.

Ethnicity: PMR is six times more common in whites than in African-Americans. A genetic factor, the HLA-DR4 haplotype, is found in persons with PMR.

Gender: PMR occurs twice as often in women as in men.

Contributing Factors: Advanced age and a possible genetic disposition are thought to contribute to the development of PMR.

Signs and Symptoms: Patients often complain of fatigue and generalized malaise. Fever is common; patients may report night sweating. Additionally, patients usually have bilateral, proximal aching and stiffness in the neck, shoulders, upper arms, hips, thighs, and lower back. Stiffness occurs in the morning and may last longer than 30 minutes. Anorexia, weight loss, apathy, fear, and depression are also constitutional symptoms of PMR. Musculoskeletal pain and related symptoms have lasted about a month. Muscle weakness usually is not elicited upon physical examination. Tenderness may be elicited upon palpation to the muscle groups mentioned earlier. Check for signs of carpal tunnel syndrome, such as paresthesia of the thumb and index and middle fingers. Patients may complain of numbness and tingling in the fingers and a decreased ability to grasp small objects. Diagnostic studies may reveal anemia, and checking for signs of pallor is important. Because TA is associated with PMR, the work-up should also include questions to evaluate for TA, such as complaints of occipital or temporal headaches, transient visual disturbances, jaw or ear pain, sore throat, hoarseness, and cough. Assess for tender temporal arteries and visual acuity. Fundoscopic examination may reveal retinal hemorrhages, "cotton wool" patches, and edema of the optic disk. Refer to Fig. 12–4.

Diagnostic Tests

- The laboratory hallmark for PMR is an elevated Westergren ESR. Findings of greater than 50 mm/hr are common and readings may exeed 100 mm/hr.
- A CBC with indices may show a normocytic normochromic anemia in half of the patients with PMR.
- Other immunologic studies, such as those for RA factor and antinuclear antibodies (ANA), often show elevated levels in older adults; thus, these studies would be of little benefit when establishing a differential diagnosis.

Differential Diagnosis: PMR can be differentiated from rheumatoid arthritis by the absence of synovitis in PMR. It is distinguished from polymyositis by the finding of normal muscle enzymes and muscle biopsy. Other diseases to consider in the differential diagnosis are fibromyalgia, hypothyroidism, OA, and depression. Older patients with carcinomatosis can present with symptoms that mimic PMR.

Treatment: If the patient presents with signs and symptoms only of PMR, the treatment is to start low-dose prednisone (5–15 mg/day). Symptoms should begin to resolve after 24 hr, and the ESR rate should normalize in 7–10 days. The prednisone is tapered off slowly, continuing over months, once the symptoms have resolved and the ESR rate is within normal limits. NSAIDs such as ibuprofen may be used instead of the steroids once the patient is stable. Patients presenting with visual disturbances or other symptoms of TA need a higher dose of oral corticosteroids; prednisone 40–60 mg/day is the suggested starting dose, again with a gradual tapering depending on symptoms and laboratory values. Treatment may last from 6 months to a year.

Follow-up: For patients with polymyalgia rheumatica, the ESR is monitored until it falls and previously reported symptoms resolve. Patients also presenting with TA need to be monitored in the same way, with repeated eye examinations as warranted. Because patients with TA are at risk for developing aortic aneurysm, follow-up abdominal examination for aortic aneurysm is needed.

Sequelae: The diagnosis of PMR is confirmed when a response to the corticosteroid is noted. Usually the patient begins to exhibit a reduction in symptoms within 24 hr after starting treatment. Patients should be alerted to the signs of TA. Patients with untreated TA are at risk for blindness. Patients should be informed they must complete all of the prescribed medication to avoid a relapse.

Prevention/Prophylaxis: No preventive measures exist for PMR, but, because the disease can recur, patients should be advised to contact their health-care providers when any of the prevailing signs and symptoms reappear.

Referral: For patients with signs of visual disturbance, fundoscopic changes, or both, referral to an ophthalmologist is warranted if the patient can be evaluated

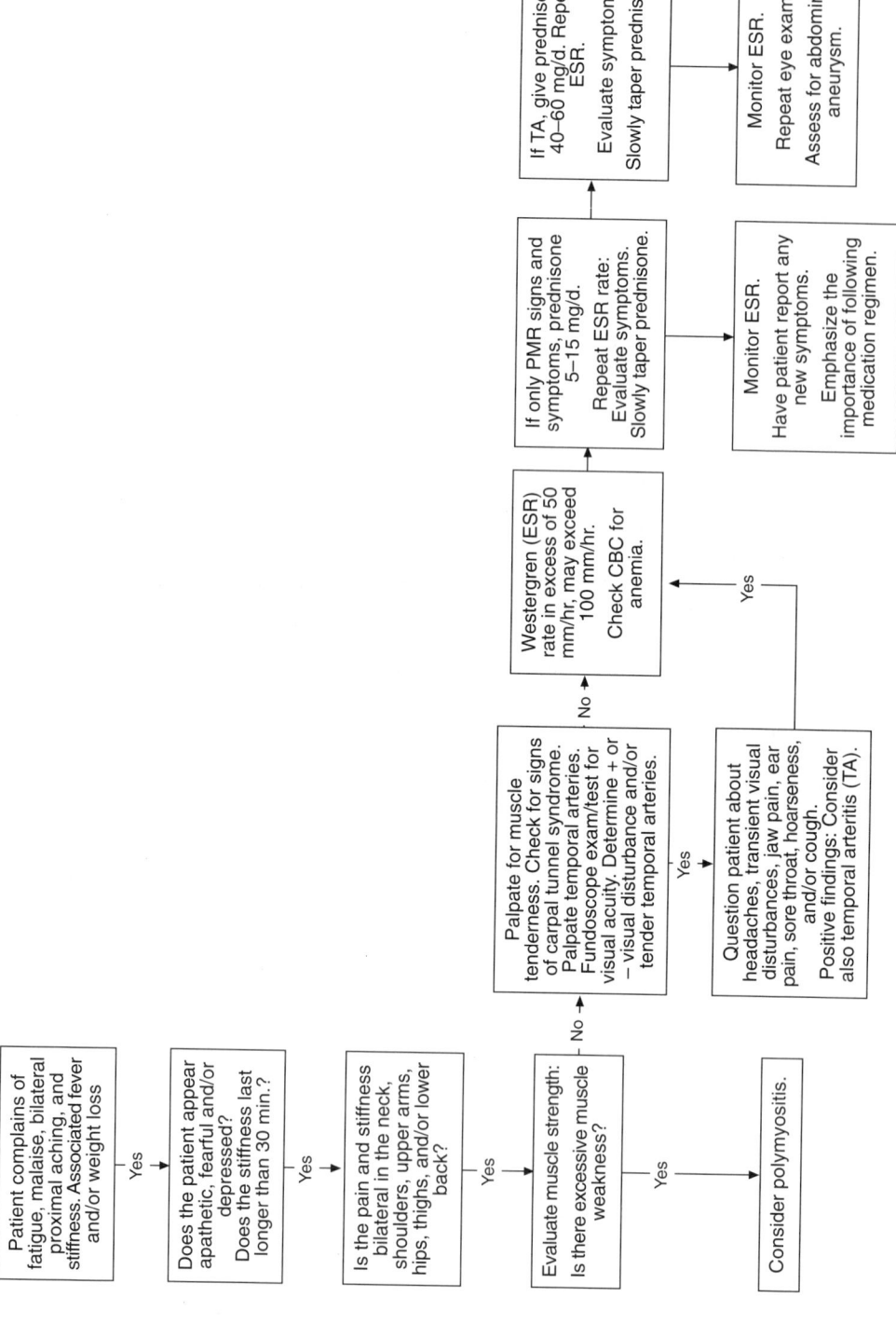

FIGURE 12-4 Polymyalgia rheumatica (PMR).

immediately. If not, these patients should be referred to an emergency room for immediate evaluation. Consultation with a rheumatologist is beneficial for persons who have TA or who do not respond to treatment for PMR.

Education: Patients should be taught the precautions needed when steroids are being taken. They should be instructed to include an adequate amount of calcium in their diets. Patients who do not have TA should be alerted to potential symptoms such as visual disturbance, headache, temporal tenderness, and jaw pain.

Rheumatoid Arthritis

Rheumatoid arthritis (RA) is a chronic systemic inflammatory process evidenced by symmetrical polyarthritis. Patients generally experience episodes of remission and acute exacerbations of the disease. Extraarticular presentations of RA can include vasculitis, rheumatoid nodules, scleritis, pericarditis, neuropathy, interstitial fibrosis, Sjögren's syndrome, and Felty's syndrome.

Etiology: The cause for RA remains unknown. Susceptibility to the disease is genetic; a relationship between presence of class II human leukocyte antigen (HLA) and RA has been identified.

Occurrence: Rheumatoid arthritis occurs in 0.3%–1.5% of the population in the United States.

Age: The usual age of onset is 20–60 years, and initial presentation of the disease peaks between ages 35 and 45. Elderly-onset RA (EORA) begins after age 60.

Ethnicity: RA in Native Americans have a prevalence of 3.5%–5.3%. A familial tendency also exists.

Gender: RA affects women two to three times more frequently than it affects men.

Contributing Factors: Factors associated with the development of RA include family history of RA, female gender, Native American ethnic background, and presence of the HLA haplotype.

Signs and Symptoms: The clinical presentation for patients with longstanding RA before age 60 reflects the duration of the individual's disease and concomitant conditions. For patients with EORA, the initial presentation may be a gradual onset of morning stiffness, swelling, and pain in multiple joints. In others, the first attack may be more acute. In older adults constitutional symptoms with RA may include low-grade fever, anorexia, weight loss, malaise, and depression. In EORA, larger joints such as the shoulders are often involved more frequently than in patients with earlier-onset RA, in whom smaller joints are usually affected. Joint deformities prevalent in patients with a history of RA include

Hyperflexion of the PIP joints and flexion of the DIP joints (known as a swan-neck deformity).

Flexion of the PIP joints and extension of the DIP joints (known as a bouton-
nière deformity).
Ulnar deviation of the MCP joint.
Knee and ankle effusions.

The MCP, wrist, PIP, MTP, shoulder, ankle, and elbow joints should be examined for ROM, tenderness, erythema, warmth, and swelling. The skin should
be checked for subcutaneous nodules, which are generally less than 1–3 cm in
diameter and feel firm and fixed upon palpation; these are often found proximal
to the elbow. Systemic evaluation also includes an eye examination to check
for keratoconjunctivitis, scleritis, and corneal ulcers. The lungs are evaluated
to determine if pleuritis or pneumonitis is present. Pericarditis, a possible
manifestation of RA, warrants a cardiac examination. The clinician should also
examine the patient for evidence of nerve entrapment and sensory neuropathy.
All patients should be questioned about the impact of RA on their lifestyle and
current ability to carry out ADLs. Refer to Fig. 12–5.

Diagnostic Tests: A CBC may reveal a normochromic, normocytic anemia, mild
leukocytosis, and thrombocytosis. The ESR is elevated in RA. Rheumatoid
factor is positive in about 50% of all cases, although an elevated rheumatoid
titer can also be present in healthy persons of advanced age. If the synovial
fluids are examined in an acute inflammatory stage of RA, a high concentration
of white blood cells is found. Radiographic examination in patients with EORA
may first indicate only soft tissue swelling, but eventually symmetrical joint
space narrowing, subluxations, and erosions will become evident.

Differential Diagnosis: In individuals over age 60, conditions that can mimic
RA include erosive OA, PMR, polyarticular gout, pseudogout, chronic infection,
and occult malignancy. Other conditions to consider include Sjögren's syndrome,
systemic lupus erythematosus or drug-induced lupus, scleroderma, and polymyositis.

Treatment: For patients who have been treated for years for RA, modifications
in the drug regimen may be necessary to protect against renal toxicity, NSAID-
induced gastritis, and central nervous system (CNS) toxicity. The three classes of
drugs used to treat RA are the NSAIDs, corticosteroids, and disease-modifying
antirheumatic drugs (DMARDs). When using NSAIDs to treat older adults
with RA, the NSAID selection should be based on the medications' half-lives,
giving favor to those with short half-lives, using the lowest effective dose. Low-
dose oral corticosteroids may provide relief, starting with doses of less than 10
mg and then tapering off to determine the lowest effective dose. The DMARDs
used for treating RA include injectable gold salts, oral gold, hydroxychloroquine,
sulfasalazine, and D-penicillamine. Consultation with a rheumatologist is recommended for the proper management of RA.

Follow-up: Routine evaluations for patients with RA should include the patient's
response to the pharmacological and nonpharmacological therapy. Medications

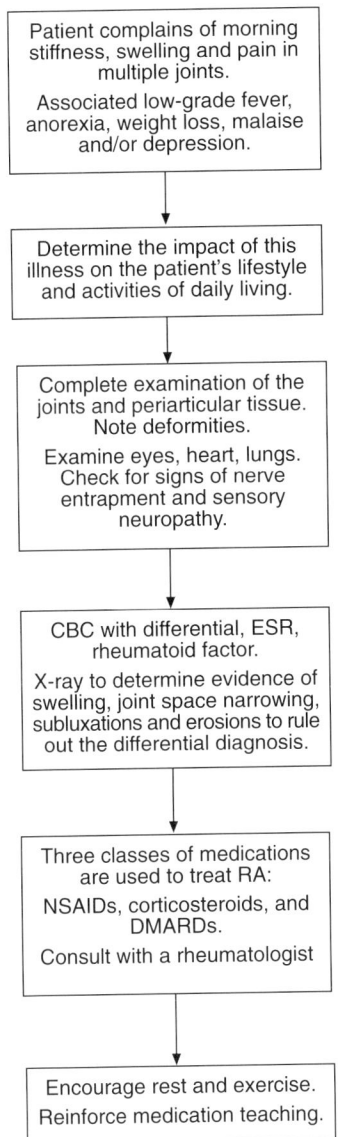

Patient complains of morning
stiffness, swelling and pain in
multiple joints.

Associated low-grade fever,
anorexia, weight loss, malaise
and/or depression.

↓

Determine the impact of this
illness on the patient's lifestyle
and activities of daily living.

↓

Complete examination of the
joints and periarticular tissue.
Note deformities.

Examine eyes, heart, lungs.
Check for signs of nerve
entrapment and sensory
neuropathy.

↓

CBC with differential, ESR,
rheumatoid factor.

X-ray to determine evidence of
swelling, joint space narrowing,
subluxations and erosions to rule
out the differential diagnosis.

↓

Three classes of medications
are used to treat RA:

NSAIDs, corticosteroids, and
DMARDs.

Consult with a rheumatologist

↓

Encourage rest and exercise.
Reinforce medication teaching.

FIGURE 12–5 Rheumatoid arthritis (RA).

should be adjusted if the patient does not obtain symptomatic relief from the current therapy. Progression of the articular and extra-articular disease should be monitored through physical examination. Any change in the patient's ability to carry out ADLs, as well as his or her psychosocial status, should be evaluated at each visit.

Sequelae: Older adults who have had RA for years eventually experience more severe disease with increased joint deformities. Comorbidities such as septic arthritis, Sjögren's syndrome, Felty's syndrome, and pericarditis may exist in patients with a history of RA. Patients with EORA may tend to have a milder course of the disease, with periods of remission; however, patients experiencing a more rapid decline have also been reported. Complications from the medication regimen need to be considered.

Prevention/Prophylaxis: Although RA cannot be prevented, a program of gentle ROM exercises can help maintain function and muscle strength.

Referral: Patients experiencing a period of prolonged inflammation despite therapy or one of the comorbidities mentioned earlier should be referred to a rheumatologist. Patients can also benefit from referral to a physical therapist and an occupational therapist, to assist them in their exercise programs, splinting needs, and adaptive equipment requirements, all aimed at maintaining function and independence for as long as possible.

Education: Patients should be taught the importance of incorporating periods of rest and exercise into their daily lives. Medication education is important in RA because of the potential for side effects associated with a complicated drug regimen. Because there is no cure for RA, patients must be skeptical about "antidotes" promised for RA and check with their health-care providers if they have any concerns about treatments. Patients can contact the Arthritis Foundation (800-282-7800) for information; a booklet, "Overcoming Rheumatoid Arthritis," is available.

BIBLIOGRAPHY

General

Abrams, W, Beers, MH, and Berkow, R: The Merck Manual of Geriatrics, ed 2. Merck Research Laboratories, Whitehouse Station, NJ, 1995.
Affable, RA, and Ettinger, WH: Musculoskeletal disease in the aged: Diagnosis and management. Drug Therapy 3:49, 1993.
Berg, D: Handbook of Primary Care Medicine. JB Lippincott, Philadelphia, 1993.
DeGowin, RL: DeGowin & DeGowin's Bedside Diagnostic Examination, ed. 5. McGraw-Hill, New York, 1987.
McConnell, E, and Linton, AD (eds): Gerontological Nursing Concepts and Practice, ed 2. WB Saunders, Philadelphia, 1996.
Pincus, T: A pragmatic approach to cost-effective use of laboratory tests and imaging procedures in patients with musculoskeletal symptoms. Prim Care 20:795, 1993.

Assessment

DeGowin, R: DeGowin and DeGowin's Bedside Diagnostic Examination. McGraw-Hill, New York, 1987.
Lueckennotte, A: Pocket Guide to Gerontological Assessment, ed 2. Mosby, St. Louis, 1994.
Matteson, MA: Age-related changes in the musculoskeletal system. In Matteson, MA, Mezey, M, Rauckhorst, LH, and Stokes, SA: Health Assessment of the Older Individual. ed 2. Springer Publishing Co, New York, 1993.

Wilms, JL, Schneiderman, HS, and Algranti, PS: Physical Diagnosis: Evaluation of Diagnosis and Function. Williams & Wilkins, Baltimore, 1994.

Fractures

Birge, S: Osteoporosis and hip fracture. Clinics in Ger Med 9:69, 1993.
Birge, S, Morrow-Howell, N, and Proctor, EK: Hip fracture. Clinics in Ger Med 10:589, 1994.
Onieal, M-E: The adult knee. Advance for Nur Pract 3:13, 1995.
Pellino,TA: How to manage hip fracture. AJN 94:46, 1994.
Perry, CR: Intracapsular fracture of the proximal femur. Clinics in Ger Med 10:647, 1994.

Gout

Agarwal, AK: Gout and pseudogout. Prim Care 20:839, 1993.
Cohen, PR, Schmidt, WA, and Rapini, RA: Chronic tophaceous gout with severely deforming arthritis: A case report with emphasis on histopathologic considerations.
Collo, MB, Johnson, JL, Finch, WR, and Felicetta, JV: Evaluating arthritic complaints. Nurse Pract 16:9, 1991.
Giansiracusa, DF: Crystal-induced rheumatic disorders. In Noble, J (ed): Textbook of Primary Care Medicine. CV Mosby, St. Louis, 1996.

Osteoarthritis

Blechman, WJ, Roth, SH, and Wilske, K: Osteoarthritis: Are you up to date? Patient Care 26:99, 1992.
Collo, MB, Johnson, JL, Finch, WR, and Felicetta, JV: Evaluating arthritic complaints. Nurse Pract 16:9, 1991.
de Bock, GH, van Marwijk, HWJ, Kaptein, AA, and Mulder, JD: Osteoarthritis pain assessment in family practice. Arthritis Care and Research 7:40, 1994.
Hamerman, D: Aging and osteoarthritis: Basic mechanisms. J Am Geriatr Soc 41:760, 1993.
Jacobson, EW: Osteoarthritis. In Noble, J (ed): Textbook of Primary Care Medicine. CV Mosby, St. Louis, 1996.
Nesher, G, and Moore, MD: Clinical presentation and treatment of arthritis in the aged. Clin Geriatr Med 10:659, 1994.
Peyron, JG, and Altam, RD: The epidemiology of osteoarthritis. In Moskowitz RW, Howell, DS, Goldberg, VM, and Mankin, HJ (eds): Osteoarthritis: Diagnosis and Medical/Surgical Management, ed 2. WB Saunders, Philadelphia, 1992.
Reinhard, JD, and Calkins, E: Geriatric issues in the diagnosis and management of patients with rheumatic disorders. Primary Care 20:911, 1993.
Scott, DL: Guidelines for the diagnosis, investigation and management of osteoarthritis of the hip and knee. J R Coll Physicians Lond 27:391, 1993.
Swedberg, JA: Osteoarthritis. Am Fam Physician 45:557, 1992.

Osteoporosis

Birge, S: Osteoporosis and hip fracture. Clin Geriatr Med 9:69, 1993.
Brager, R: Alendronate treatment for osteoporosis. Advance for Nurse Practitioners 5:28, 1997.
Gamble, CL: Osteoporosis: Drug and nondrug therapies for the patient at risk. Geriatrics 50:39, 1995.
Kessenich, CR: Update on pharmacologic therapies for osteoporosis. Nurse Prac 21:19, 1996.
Lonergan, ET, and Harris, ST: Osteoporosis. In Lonergan, ET (ed): Geriatrics, ed 1. Appleton & Lange, Stamford, CT, 1996.
Nordin, BEC, Need, AG, Horowitz, M, and Morris, H: Treatment of osteoporosis in the elderly. Clin Geriatr Med 10:625, 1994.

Polymyalgia Rheumatica

Carpenter, DR, and Hudacek, S: Polymyalgia rheumatica: A comprehensive review of this debilitating disease. Nurse Pract 19:51, 1994.

Collo, MB, Johnson, JL, Finch, WR, and Felicetta, JV: Evaluating arthritic complaints. Nurse Pract 16:9, 1991.

Evans, JM, O'Fallon, WM, and Hunder, GG: Increased incidence of aortic aneurysm and dissection in giant cell (temporal) arteritis. Ann Intern Med 122:502, 1995.

Goroll, AH: Approach to the patient with polymyalgia rheumatica or temporal arteritis. In Goroll, AH, May, LA, and Mulley, AG (eds): Primary Care Medicine: Office Evaluation of the Adult Patient, ed 3. JB Lippincott, Philadelphia, 1995.

Nesher, G, and Moore,TL: Clinical presentation and treatment of arthritis in the aged. Clin Geriatr Med 10:659, 1994.

Pincus, T: A pragmatic approach to cost-effective use of laboratory tests and imaging procedures in patients with musculoskeletal symptoms. Prim Care 20:795, 1993.

Reinhard, JD, and Calkins, E: Geriatric issues in the diagnosis and management of patients with rheumatic disorders. Prim Care 20:911, 1993.

Rheumatoid Arthritis

Collo, MB, Johnson, JL, Finch, WR, and Felicetta, JV: Evaluating arthritis complaints. Nurse Pract 16:9, 1991.

Nesher, G, and Moore, TL: Clinical presentation and treatment of arthritis in the aged. Clin Geriatr Med 10:659, 1994.

Pagano, MP: Rheumatoid arthritis: An update. Clin Rev 6:65, 1996.

Stevens, MB: Rheumatoid arthritis. In Stobo, JD, et al (eds): The Principles and Practice of Medicine, ed 23, Appleton & Lange, Stamford, CT, 1996.

CHAPTER **13**

CENTRAL AND

PERIPHERAL NERVOUS

SYSTEM DISORDERS

The neurologic assessment of the older adult begins with assessment of mental status. The interview should begin with an assessment of level of consciousness, speech pattern, mood and affect, concentration ability, short-term memory, and orientation. This information can usually be obtained during the course of a standard interview. If any questions regarding mental status arise, family members may be asked for additional information to investigate the patient's cognitive abilities further.

The focused interview for a neurologic complaint should include asking about the following signs and symptoms:

- Loss of consciousness or presyncope (full description of any episodes and their precipitating factors).
- Episodes of seizures, weakness or paralysis, tremors, involuntary movements, pain, numbness, parasthesias, gait problems, or restlessness of the legs.
- All medications, diet, and sleep patterns.

After the interview, the examiner may perform a focused neurologic examination, beginning with an examination of cranial nerve (CN) function.

Cranial Nerve Function

CN I (Olfactory)   Make sure to test one nostril at a time using familiar scents. This sense may be lessened or absent because of nasal disease, head trauma, smoking, use of cocaine, or normal aging. It may also be congenitally absent.

CN II (Optic)   Funduscopic examination will reveal disc or small vessel abnormalities. Assess pupillary reactions to light and visual fields.

CN III, IV, and VI (Oculomotor, Trochlear, and Abducens)   These nerves may be examined together by testing extraocular movements and convergence. Inspect for ptosis.

CN V (Trigeminal)   The motor function of this nerve can be assessed by palpating the temporal and masseter muscles. If the patient has no teeth, this test may be difficult to interpret. The sensory function of this nerve should be tested with sharp and dull stimuli in all three branches: ophthalmic, maxillary, and mandibular. If any abnormalities are noted, light touch and temperature sensation should also be assessed. The corneal reflex should be assessed using a wisp of cotton. Patients who wear contact lenses may have diminished corneal reflexes.

CN VII (Facial)   Observe the patient's face at rest and continue to observe throughout the examination for any asymmetry. Motor function may be tested by asking the patient to smile, frown, raise both eyebrows, close eyes tightly and resist the examiner's attempts to open them, and puffing out both cheeks. A peripheral injury to this nerve, such as Bell's palsy, may affect both the upper and the lower face, whereas a central lesion mainly affects the lower face.

CN VIII (Acoustic)   Assess auditory acuity using the whisper test. If hearing loss is present, test for lateralization using Weber's test and for air versus bone conduction using Rinne's test.

CN IX and X (Glossopharyngeal and Vagus)   Observe the quality of the patient's voice. Hoarseness may indicate vocal cord paralysis; a nasal quality may indicate paralysis of the palate. Difficulty in swallowing could indicate palatal or pharyngeal weakness. Inspect movement of the palate and pharynx when the patient swallows. With a bilateral lesion of the nerve, the palate will fail to rise. With unilateral lesion, one side of the palate will fail to rise and will be pulled, along with the uvula, to the normal side. Test the gag reflex by stimulating the back of the throat on each side.

CN XI (Spinal Accessory)   Observe for atrophy or fasciculations in the trapezius muscles. Test motor strength bilaterally with a shoulder shrug.

CN XII (Hypoglossal)   Inspect for fasciculations of the tongue at rest. Look for asymmetry of movement, atrophy, or deviation from midline. Atrophy or fasciculations suggest peripheral lesions. With unilateral lesions, the protruded tongue will deviate toward the affected side.

Motor Function

Assessment of motor function should focus on inspection of body position and involuntary movements (tremors, tics, or fasciculations). Note that the incidence of benign essential tremor increases with aging.

Inspect the patient's muscle bulk, comparing sizes and contours of muscles. Pay particular attention to the hands, shoulders, and thighs. Atrophy of the hand muscles may occur with normal aging. Muscular atrophy may also result from diseases of the peripheral nervous system, motor neuron disease, rheumatoid arthritis, muscle disuse, and malnutrition.

Motor assessment also includes inspection of muscle tone, best assessed by the patient's resistance to passive stretch. Inspect tone in all extremities during flexion and extension. Increased tone that is worst at extremes of the range is known as spasticity; resistance that persists throughout and in both directions is known as lead-pipe rigidity. Decreased resistance suggests peripheral nervous system disease, cerebellar disease, or the acute stage of spinal cord injury.

Assess muscle strength against resistance in all major muscle groups and grade on a scale from 0–5, with 5 being active movement against full resistance. Test the biceps and triceps; grip strength; finger abductions; opposition of the thumb; trunk strength; flexion, extension, abduction, and adduction at the hip; flexion and extension at the knee; and dorsiflexion and plantarflexion of the foot during passive range-of-motion exercises. If you note weakness, assess strength against gravity alone or with gravity eliminated. Many clinicians make further distinctions by using + or − signs toward the stronger end of the scale.

Test coordination using rapid alternating movements of the hands, fingers, and feet and point-to-point movements. Gait function should be tested; assess tandem gait, walking on toes and heels, hopping in place, and shallow kneebends on each side. Romberg's test is to evaluate position sense and is performed with the patient's feet together and eyes closed for 20–30 sec without support. Normally, only minimal swaying should occur. This test may be combined with the pronator drift test, in which the patient stands with eyes closed and both arms straight forward, palms up. Normally, this position may be held for 20–30 sec. After instructing the patient to maintain this position, tap the patient's arms briskly downward. The arms should return smoothly to the horizontal position; a downward drift indicates muscle weakness.

Allow extra time for the elderly patient to perform gait and coordination maneuvers.

Sensory Function

Assessment of sensory function helps to establish a lesion of the sensory cortex, the level of a spinal cord lesion or the location of a peripheral lesion. Sensory function is tested using pain and temperature (spinothalamic tract), position and vibration (posterior column), and touch (posterior horn). When you locate an area of hypersensitivity or sensory loss, map out its boundaries in detail. Unilateral sensory loss suggests a lesion in the spinal cord or higher pathways; a symmetric sensory loss suggests a neuropathy such as that experienced by persons with diabetes. Touch and vibratory sensations may diminish as a result of normal aging.

Discriminative sensations test the ability of the sensory cortex to analyze and interpret stimuli. These techniques include stereognosis, number identification, two-point discrimination, point localization, and extinction.

Reflexes

During assessment of the reflexes, the patient should be relaxed, with limbs positioned symmetrically. Palpate the tendon to locate position, and make sure the tendon is slightly stretched. Strike the tendon briskly, and note the speed, force, and amplitude of response. Grade on a scale from 0–4+, with the normal response at 2+. The older adult may have diminished or absent reflexes, usually affecting lower extremities before upper extremities.

If the response is asymmetric, check the force and location of the strike. If the response is symmetrically diminished, the examiner may use reinforcement, in which isometric contraction of other muscles may increase reflex activity. Ask the patient to clench the teeth when testing upper extremities, and to lock hands together and pull hands against each other when testing lower extremities.

Assess all reflexes: biceps (C5, C6); triceps (C6, C7); brachioradialis (C5, C6); patellar (L2, L3, L4); and ankle (S1). Assess the abdominal reflex by stroking each side of the abdomen both above (T8, T9, T10) and below (T10, T11, T12) the umbilicus. Evaluate the plantar response by stimulating the lateral aspect of the sole of the foot from the heel to the ball of the foot, curving medially across the ball. Look for flexion of the toes as a normal response. If dorsiflexion of the big toe and fanning of the other toes is noted, this constitutes a positive Babinski response, indicating a central nervous system (CNS) lesion. This response may also be noted in certain unconscious states (e.g., drug or alcohol intoxication, postictal state).

Make sure to document completely all findings of the neurologic examination, especially if additional diagnostic testing is indicated.

Alzheimer's Disease

Alzheimer's disease, a progressive neurodegenerative disease of the brain, ultimately results in significant dementia and dependence. The most common type of dementia, Alzheimer's disease is defined by diminished cognitive function accompanied by affective and behavioral disturbances, manifested by memory loss, and an inability to calculate and determine visuospatial orientation. Alzheimer's disease is one of the leading contributing causes of death and premature institutionalization among older adults.

Etiology: The etiology of Alzheimer's disease is unknown, and disease progression varies. Alzheimer's disease is characterized by the presence of neurofibrillary tangles and neuritic plaques. The process of the neuron destruction is unknown. The degeneration of the neurons is believed to occur first in the hippocampus, spreading from there to other parts of the brain.

Occurrence: An estimated 10% of individuals age 65 and over are afflicted with Alzheimer's disease, increasing to 47% for those over age 85.

Age: The prevalence of Alzheimer's disease increases with age. Onset can occur as early as the fourth decade.

Ethnicity: Not significant.

Gender: Alzheimer's disease is twice as common in women as in men.

Contributing Factors: Family history of a first-degree relative with Alzheimer's disease, genetic predisposition, and Down syndrome have been shown to increase the risk of developing Alzheimer's disease. The presence of apolipoprotein E-e4, infrequent use of nonsteroidal anti-inflammatory drugs (NSAIDs), little or no use of postmenopausal estrogen replacement, deficiency of antioxidant nutrients, history of head injury with loss of consciousness, and family history of Down syndrome may also increase the risk.

Signs and Symptoms: Patients and/or family members report difficulty with errors of judgment and subtle memory loss. The ability to comprehend, assimilate, and interpret new information is impaired, and attention to usual social amenities is decreased. Ask the patient and family if there has been a change in performance, difficulty with language, difficulty with orientation to time or place, or any personality or mood changes, including depression. Determine whether these occurrences have been gradual or sudden.

Review all medications with the patient and family. A nutritional history is also important to determine presence of nutritional deficiencies and malnutrition.

Administer the Mini Mental Status Examination (MMSE) or other objective test of cognition to obtain baseline information. Also determine the patient's baseline functional status. The Functional Activities Questionnaire (FAQ) can be used to evaluate the patient's performance of 10 complex activities. The Hachinski Ischemic Score can be used to differentiate between multi-infarct dementia and Alzheimer's disease. A score of 7 or higher on the scale suggests multi-infarct dementia; below 7 indicates Alzheimer's disease. In addition, stages of functional decline of patients with Alzheimer's disease can be determined by using the Functional Assessment Scale (FAST), which divides Alzheimer's disease into 16 stages.

Direct the physical examination toward looking for primary causes of dementia and determining if any coexisting conditions may be contributing to the patient's decline in mental or functional status. In the absence of concomitant disease processes, findings on the overall physical examination are usually normal. Pay particular attention to the vascular and neurologic parts of the examination. In general, the cranial nerves, sensation, and motor function are intact. Special neurologic examination techniques may elicit primitive reflexes such as the palmar grasp reflex; the glabellar reflex, in which a patient with dementia continues to blink after the examiner has stopped tapping on the patient's forehead, and the plantar reflex. Patient's with Alzheimer's disease can lose the sense of taste and smell, so these senses should be evaluated. In the early stages of Alzheimer's disease, the patient may have difficulty initiating ambulation. There may be some muscle rigidity as a result of increased muscle tone.

Diagnostic Tests: Patients who present with changes in cognitive status should have the following diagnostic tests:

Complete blood count (CBC) to determine if infection or anemia is present.

Vitamin B_{12} and folate level measurement, depending on the CBC results.

Creatinine, blood urea nitrogen (BUN), and urinalysis, to determine if any kidney impairment is contributing to the dementia.

Thyroid-stimulating hormone (TSH) level, to consider hypothyroidism.

Serologic tests for syphilis.

Human immunodeficiency virus-1 (HIV-1) titer to diagnosis AIDS dementia complex.

Serum electrolytes and fasting glucose, to determine electrolyte imbalance.

Screening for heavy metals, such as lead.

Electrocardiogram (ECG) and chest x-ray examination, if indicated by the patient's history.

Computed tomography (CT) or magnetic resonance imaging (MRI) to determine if brain tumor, stroke, or normal pressure hydrocephalus is present.

Electroencephalography to determine if the patient has Creutzfeldt-Jakob disease.

Lumbar puncture for analysis of cerebrospinal fluid if neurosyphilis or neoplastic meningitis is suspected.

Differential Diagnosis: A number of different dementia syndromes must be considered in the differential diagnosis, including multi-infarct dementia; dementia associated with Parkinson's disease; Pick's disease; progressive supranuclear palsy; metabolic, endocrine, and nutritional dementia; dementia associated with long-term alcoholism; early-stage depression; Creutzfeldt-Jakob disease; cerebral tumors; subdural hematoma; head injuries; encephalitis; syphilis; and AIDS. Toxic disorders to consider include heavy metal exposure, pollutants, drugs, alcohol, and carbon monoxide.

Treatment: Treatment of Alzheimer's disease consists of first optimizing the patient's environment by maintaining safety and consistency, fostering or preserving independence with activities of daily living (ADLs), and minimizing restraint for behaviors that do not represent a danger to the patient or others. Any behavioral change requires medical evaluation to address the intervening illness.

Pharmacologic treatment for patients with Alzheimer's disease is not curative. The benefit of patients with Alzheimer's disease taking vitamin E 800 units a day is supported by some. The cholinesterase inhibitor donepezil HCl has been shown to delay cognitive decline. Initial starting dose is 5 mg daily before bedtime. Patients can be reevaluated 4–6 weeks after initial dose to determine efficacy, presence of side effects, and whether an increase to 10 mg a day is warranted.

Follow-up: Patients should be seen every 3–6 months from the time of diagnosis of Alzheimer's disease, depending partly on the patient's physical, mental, and emotional status. At follow-up appointments, the patient's competence to drive (if applicable) and to manage household responsibilities and finances should be assessed. Periodic reevaluation of mental status, ADLs, and instrumental activities of daily living (IADLs) is recommended. An annual decrease of four points in the MMSE is expected in a person with Alzheimer's disease. Determine whether the patient is having any episodes of aggression, sleep disturbances, wandering, communication difficulties, depression, or failure to recognize familiar surroundings or family members.

At each follow-up visit, review the patient's diet, monitor the patient for weight loss, and obtain a history of change in continence of bowel and bladder. A rectal examination is performed to determine the competency of the internal and external sphincters and to test for occult blood. All concurrent medical illnesses should be managed to avoid further compromising the patient's cognitive function. Dehydration, infection, anemia, and respiratory, cardiovascular, and endocrine disorders should be treated to maintain the patient's quality of life. Determine the current ability of family members to provide care for the person with Alzheimer's disease if he or she is residing at home. Family members should be informed of the prognosis of the disease.

Sequelae: Survival for persons with Alzheimer's disease has been estimated to be 2–20 years from time of diagnosis. The numerous complications that can arise in the patient with Alzheimer's disease have been categorized as behavioral, psychiatric, and metabolic. Patients can exhibit behavioral and psychiatric changes throughout the course of the disease. Depression and anxiety may develop early in the disease. Hostility, wandering, and agitation may occur at a later stage. The sudden onset of a behavioral and/or psychiatric change may indicate an underlying infection or metabolic disturbance. Some patients experience evening confusion or "sundowning." Ambulatory patients with Alzheimer's disease are at risk for sustaining injuries such as falls, burns, or accidental poisoning. In the final stages of Alzheimer's disease, patients are unable to communicate verbally or ambulate. Bowel and bladder incontinence occurs, and patients may be unable to swallow and eat. These individuals are at risk for malnutrition, aspiration pneumonia, and decubitus ulcers. Death occurs usually from an unresolved infection.

Prevention/Prophylaxis: No primary prevention measures are known for Alzheimer's disease; prevention measures for those who already have Alzheimer's disease include providing a safe environment with consistent structure and routine.

Referral: After reversible causes of dementia have been excluded, patients with abnormal mental status examination findings but without functional changes or the reverse should have further neuropsychologic testing. Patients who are not responding to medications, who are experiencing symptoms of paranoia or psychosis, who have complex comorbidity, and who suffer severe impairment may also be referred for specialist management. The National Alzheimer's Association's toll-free telephone number is 1-800-272-3900. Families can ask for information about programs closest to their area; every state has at least one local chapter. The national office is located at 919 North Michigan Avenue, Chicago, IL 60611. A nationwide directory assistance service also helps older adults and families locate resources; the toll-free number is 800-677-1116.

Education: In the early stages of Alzheimer's disease, the patient and the family need to be provided with information on how to create a safe, nonthreatening environment for the victim. Reminder aids and reinforcing cues such as large signs and calendars can help patients maintain orientation.

When Alzheimer's disease is diagnosed early, patients and family members have time to plan household responsibility management, retirement from the work force, and resolution of transportation issues. As the disease progresses, the family should consider acquiring special identification cards and bracelet for the patient, especially if wandering has become problematic. For additional information, encourage the family to contact The Alzheimer's Disease Education and Referral Center, P.O. Box 8250, Silver Spring, MD 20907; the telephone number is 301-495-3311.

Brain Tumor

A brain tumor is a malignant or benign neoplasm of the brain or its supportive structures, which may arise from glial cells, blood vessels, connective tissue, meninges, pituitary, or pineal glands. The most common primary brain tumor in adults is glial neoplasm, which arises from the astrocytes. Other types of primary brain tumors include oligodendroglioma, arising from the oligodendrocytes; central nervous system (CNS) lymphoma, from lymphocytes; meningioma, from the meninges; ganglioma, from the neurons; and ependymoma from the ependyma.

Etiology: Brain tumor etiology remains largely unknown. Hereditary syndromes do exist.

Occurrence: Since 1984, there has been a 50% increase in the incidence of primary brain tumors. Approximately 17,900 new cases were diagnosed in 1996, accounting for 1% of the cancers in the United States. Brain tumors occur most commonly in children under age 15 and in adults in the fifth and sixth decades of life. Gliomas account for 65% of the brain tumors seen in adults; pituitary adenoma, acoustic neuroma, and menigiomas also occur in adults but almost never in children. The incidence of CNS lymphoma among adults is increasing.

Ethnicity: Not significant.

Gender: Brain tumors occur equally among males and females.

Contributing Factors: No association between environmental factors and primary tumors of the brain, except that of vinylchloride exposure and gliomas, has been proven. Some association does exist between Epstein-Barr virus (EBV) and CNS lymphoma. Prior radiation and chemotherapy are also associated with brain tumors.

Signs and Symptoms: Constant or paroxysmal headaches may be due to tumor infiltration of nervous tissue, displacement of brain structures by tumor mass, or increased intercranial pressure (ICP). These headaches tend to be more severe in the morning, when upright, and with position changes. They may be relieved by analgesics and rarely interfere with sleep. Headaches related to brain tumors may be accompanied by vomiting, which often occurs without nausea. Brain tumor should be part of the differential diagnosis for any headaches of recent onset, differing from the patient's usual pattern of headaches, or accompanied by a migraine-like aura that persists after the pain is gone. Nausea, appetite changes, and hiccups occur less frequently.

Partial motor, sensory, or grand mal seizures occur in 20%–30% of patients with brain tumors. New-onset focal seizures in people over age 40 are suspicious for brain tumor until proven otherwise. Psychomotor function may slow down in patients with primary brain tumors. Personality changes may be marked or subtle, including changes in mood, concentration, and intellectual functions.

Focal neurologic changes are related to the area of the brain invaded by tumor. Frontal and parietal lobe tumors may cause changes in memory, behavior, and cognitive function. Memory, hearing, vision, and emotions are most often affected by temporal lobe tumors. Symptoms of temporal lobe tumors may mimic those of affective or psychotic thought disorders. Visual changes can occur with occipital lobe tumors, in addition to speech, motor, and sensory changes for left-sided occipital masses and an inability to grasp abstract concepts for right-sided occipital masses. Lesions in the cerebellum affect balance and coordination. Pituitary tumors may present with the symptoms of hypothyroidism, hypocortisolism, diabetes insipidus, or visual changes (Fig. 13–1).

Diagnostic Tests: A careful history of symptoms is invaluable. Complete physical examination should include:

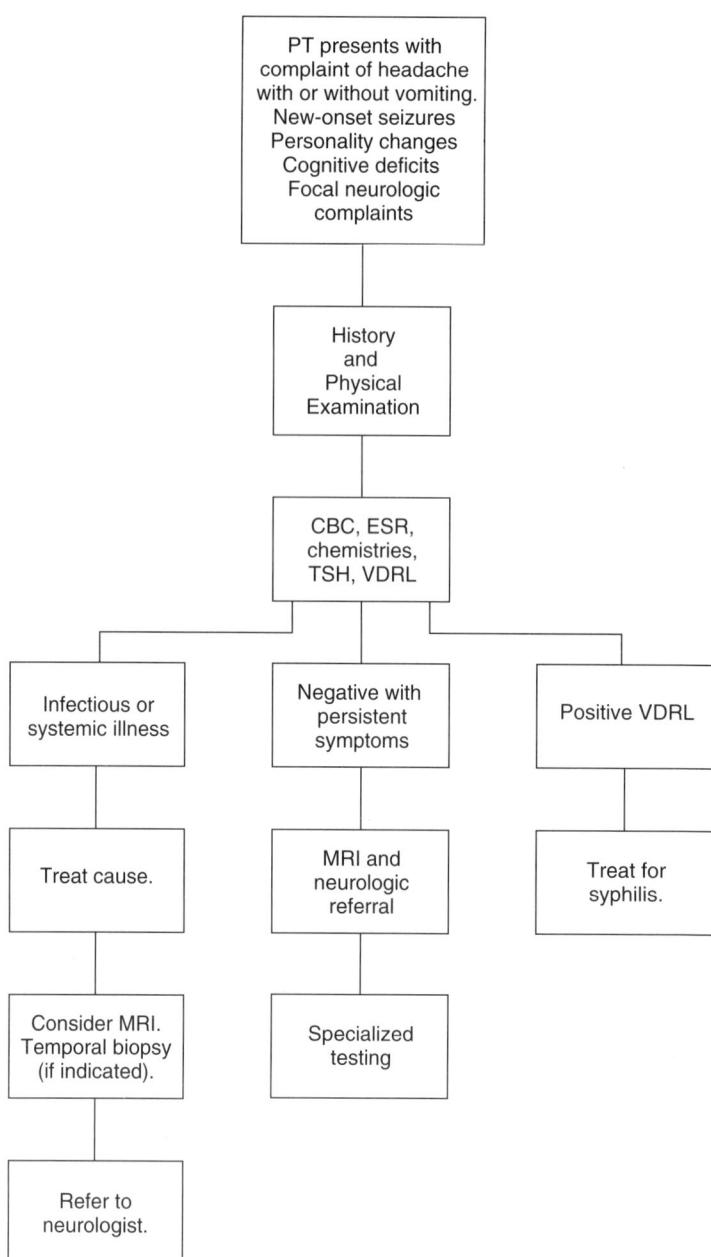

FIGURE 13–1 Brain tumor.

- Skin survey for stigmata of neurocutaneous syndromes or melanoma.
- Lymph node examination.
- Abdominal examination for hepatomegaly or splenomegaly.
- Rectal examination with guaiac stool testing.
- Breast and pelvic examination in women.
- Cardiopulmonary examination.

The neurologic evaluation should include a mental status evaluation, testing for cognitive deficits or memory loss, and assessment for personality changes. Family members may be able to provide clues about subtle personality changes. Ophthalmic examination is essential to assess for papilledema. Test also for asymmetry of strength, sensation, visual fields, reflex activity, cranial nerve function, and radicular signs.

Laboratory studies should include complete blood count (CBC), erythrocyte sedimentation rate (ESR), blood chemistry analyses, thyroid-stimulating hormone (TSH) levels, and venereal (VDRL) to rule out infectious, inflammatory, or systemic illnesses. Magnetic resonance imaging (MRI) of the brain, with or without contrast, is the recommended diagnostic examination for suspected brain tumor. Computed tomography (CT) scan with contrast is acceptable in special circumstances, such as when a patient is uncooperative or MRI is unavailable. Lumbar puncture (LP) should not be performed before MRI or CT scan because of the potential for fatal brain herniation to result. LP can yield pressure readings and fluid for cytology, protein, glucose, and tumor markers. Testing blood for tumor markers, α-fetoprotein, or beta human chorionic gonadotrophic hormone (HCG) is useful for the diagnosis of some brain tumors. Histologic examination of brain tissue through a biopsy may be required.

Differential Diagnosis: Cerebral vascular accident (CVA), aneurysm, arteriovenous malformation, meningitis, abscess, syphilis, human immunodeficiency virus (HIV), subdural hematoma, postconcussion syndrome, trauma, temporal arteritis, normal pressure hydrocephalus, multi-infarct dementia, Alzheimer's disease, chemical poisoning, and migraine or other headache syndromes can mimic brain tumor.

Treatment: Treatment of brain tumor includes surgery, radiation, and chemotherapy.

Follow-up: Prognosis depends on the tumor type. During the first year after treatment, the patient should have a focused history and physical examination, including a neurologic and fundoscopic examination every 3 months. MRI of the head is recommended at the same intervals during the first year. The patient should be seen every 6 months during years two through five, with a yearly MRI. Patients receiving palliative care should be seen as necessary for pain and symptom control; hospice care is recommended for these individuals.

Sequelae: Various neurologic deficits, personality changes, seizure disorders, and chronic head pain can result from brain tumor. Paraplegia, hemiplegia, and quadraplegia are also consequences of brain tumor. Bradycardia, hypertension, and respiratory arrest can occur with increased ICP. Brain herniation is a life-threatening emergent complication.

Prevention/Prophylaxis: Instruct patients to avoid radiation exposure.

Referral: Refer patients to a neurosurgeon, oncologist, radiation oncologist, and hospice, as appropriate.

Education: Genetic counseling is warranted in hereditary syndromes of brain tumor.

Cerebrovascular Accident (Stroke)

A cerebrovascular accident (CVA), or stroke, occurs when a disruption in blood flow to the brain leads to brain tissue ischemia and infarction. The consequent impairment depends on the location and extent of the infarction.

Etiology: The two major types of strokes are *ischemic,* which can result from a thrombus or embolus, small vessel disease, or a hypotensive episode; and *hemorrhagic.* Ischemic events account for approximately 80% of all strokes. In an ischemic stroke, an atherosclerotic plaque breaks off from a vessel wall, usually the carotid, and occludes a cerebral artery or one of its branches. Cardiac arrhythmias and dysfunctional cardiac valves are also a frequent source of emboli. Hemorrhagic strokes result from trauma or a hypertensive episode when a weak area of an intracranial vessel ruptures.

Occurrence: CVA, or stroke, the leading neurologic cause of death and disability in the United States, affecting an estimated 500,000 people each year.

Age: Stroke occurs mostly in persons over age 65; the incidence increases exponentially with advancing age.

Ethnicity: A higher incidence of stroke has been noted in the American black population, but this may be due to the concurrent higher incidence of hypertension and other cardiovascular diseases found in this group.

Gender: CVA occurs equally in men and women.

Contributing Factors: Risk factors for stroke include: hypertension, hypercholesterolemia, diabetes, family history of stroke, smoking, alcohol abuse, and obesity.

Signs and Symptoms: History may indicate a prior transient ischemic attack (TIA). Patients may report any of the following symptoms, usually with a sudden onset: weakness, numbness, or paralysis in the face, arm, or leg (usually unilateral); difficulty speaking or understanding verbal communication; blurred or decreased monocular or binocular vision; loss of balance or coordination, and severe headache. Physical signs may include one or more of the following:
Decreased visual acuity or field cut.
Diplopia.

Slurred speech.

Hemiparesis or sensory changes of the face, arm, or leg.

A decrease in coordination or balance.

Acute confusional state.

Elevated blood pressure.

Physical examination should include repeated measures of vital signs and examination of the head and neck for signs of trauma and infection, checks of the peripheral and carotid pulses, auscultation of the neck for bruits, and a complete neurologic examination for focal abnormalities (Fig. 13–2).

Diagnostic Tests: A cranial computed tomography (CCT) scan or magnetic resonance imagery (MRI) will reveal a hemorrhagic stroke immediately. Ischemic events may not be visible on scan for 24–48 hours and may be noted anywhere in the cerebral cortex, cerebellum, or brainstem.

- Laboratory tests should include an electrocardiogram (ECG), chest x-ray examination, complete blood count (CBC), platelet count, prothrombin time (PT), partial thromboplastin time (PTT), serum electrolytes, and blood glucose level.
- If a hemorrhagic stroke is confirmed, immediately refer the patient for angiography to identify the bleeding source.

Differential Diagnosis: Temporal arteritis, vertebral disk disease, migraine, head trauma, brain tumor, and a CNS or meningeal infection may cause symptoms that mimic those of a CVA. Distinctions may usually be found in the history of onset of symptoms and physical examination.

Treatment: Hypertension associated with stroke usually resolves spontaneously over the first 24 hours; aggressive use of antihypertensives may further reduce cerebral perfusion. Elevated blood pressure in the presence of ischemic stroke should be reduced if:

- Systolic blood pressure (SBP) is greater than 220 mmHg or diastolic blood pressure (DBP) is greater than 115 mmHg.
- Cardiac ischemia or failure is noted.
- Thrombolytic therapy is used.

Initiate anticoagulant therapy if the workup reveals a risk of recurrent embolization. If the patient presents within 3 hours of the onset of symptoms and a hemorrhagic event is ruled out, tissue plasminogen activator (tPA), a thrombolytic agent, may minimize the size of the infarct. Experimental trials with several other neuroprotective agents are currently ongoing. Hemorrhagic events are treated surgically. Control of any other comorbid disease is also indicated.

Follow-up: Indications for follow-up depend on the type and extent of the infarct. Referral to inpatient rehabilitation is usually indicated for individualized therapy: physical, occupational, speech, or cognitive retraining with the focus on restoring optimal levels of function. After a stroke, patients should be followed regularly

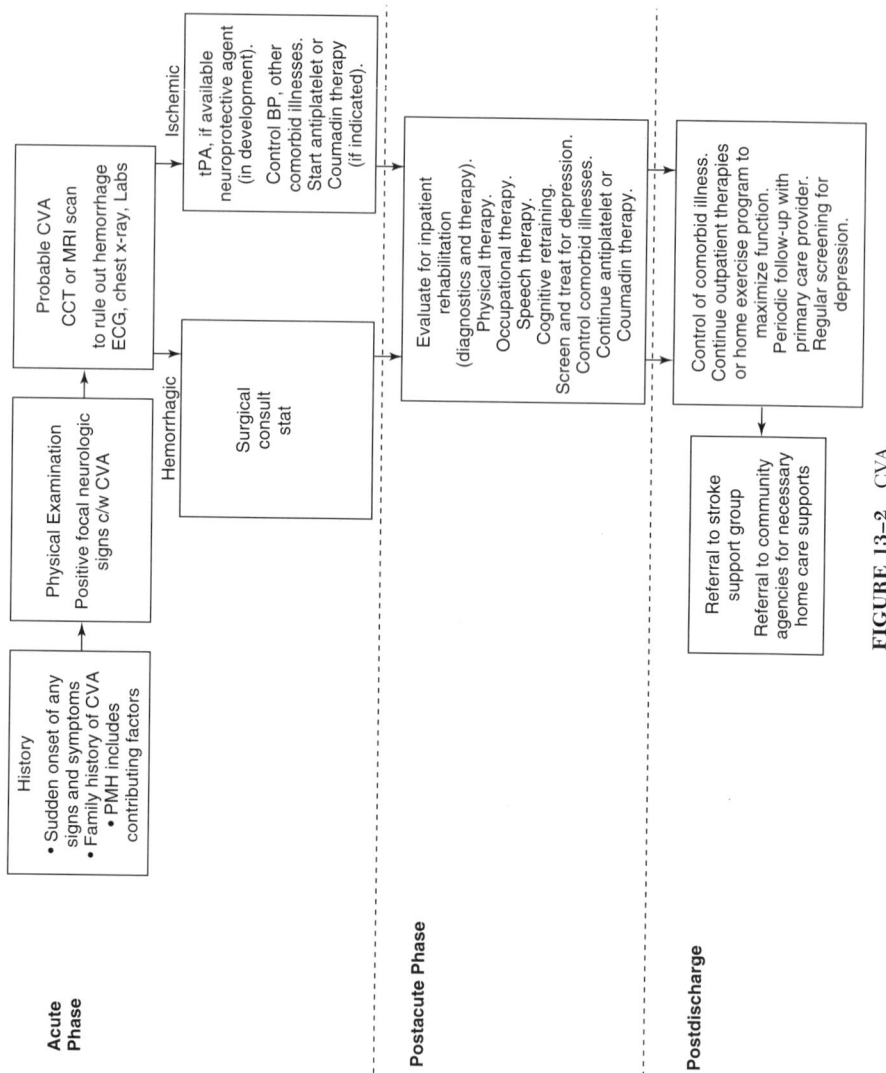

Acute Phase

History
• Sudden onset of any signs and symptoms
• Family history of CVA
• PMH includes contributing factors

Physical Examination
Positive focal neurologic signs c/w CVA

Probable CVA
CCT or MRI scan
to rule out hemorrhage
ECG, chest x-ray, Labs

Hemorrhagic
Surgical consult stat

Ischemic
tPA, if available
neuroprotective agent (in development).
Control BP, other comorbid illnesses.
Start antiplatelet or Coumadin therapy (if indicated).

Postacute Phase

Evaluate for inpatient rehabilitation (diagnostics and therapy).
Physical therapy.
Occupational therapy.
Speech therapy.
Cognitive retraining.
Screen and treat for depression.
Control comorbid illnesses.
Continue antiplatelet or Coumadin therapy.

Control of comorbid illness.
Continue outpatient therapies or home exercise program to maximize function.
Periodic follow-up with primary care provider.
Regular screening for depression.

Postdischarge

Referral to stroke support group
Referral to community agencies for necessary home care supports

FIGURE 13-2 CVA.

by a primary care provider to periodically assess changes in level of function and to control comorbid illnesses.

Sequelae: Stroke survivors are most commonly at high risk for complications related to immobility such as skin breakdown, loss of muscle strength and pulmonary compromise. Speech and swallowing difficulties may also persist after a stroke. Depression is also a common consequence of stroke. Patients are at highest risk for depression during the first 2 years after stroke; however, because it may occur at any time, screen patients for depression regularly and treat as indicated.

Prevention/Prophylaxis: Strategies to prevent stroke are similar to those used to prevent other cardiovascular diseases. Control hypertension, diabetes, hypercholesterolemia and cardiac disease, if present. Encourage patients to lose weight and stop smoking. Prophylactic treatment with antiplatelet agents such as aspirin or ticlopidine (Ticlid) is recommended, unless contraindicated. Prophylactic warfarin (Coumadin) therapy is recommended in patients with known arrhythmias, but the international normalized ratio (INR) must be monitored regularly and kept within the range of 2.0–3.0.

Referral: Referrals depend on the type and severity of impairment from the stroke and the influence of any comorbid illnesses. Referrals to physiatry (rehabilitation medicine), neurology, and cardiology for consultation are common.

Education: Education for patients after a stroke should emphasize:

- Cause of the stroke.
- Limitation of risk factors to prevent future events.
- Introduction of a home exercise program or other therapies to maintain or improve functional levels.
- Access to support groups for patients and caregivers.
- The importance of periodic follow-up with the primary care provider.

Parkinson's Disease

Parkinson's disease, a gradually degenerative condition, results in a loss of melanin-containing dopaminergic nerve cells in the substantia nigra and a progressive loss of the inhibitory neurotransmitter dopamine. The imbalance between dopamine and acetylcholine is primarily responsible for an overall worsening of symptoms leading to immobility and debilitation. The cardinal features of Parkinson's disease include resting tremor, rigidity, bradykinesia, and gait disturbances. Between 60% and 80% of the substantia nigra neurons and striatal dopamine must be lost before clinical features become evident. Subtle motor impairment may precede by many years the development of overt clinical signs and symptoms.

Etiology: The cause of idiopathic primary Parkinson's disease is unknown. Secondary Parkinson's disease (Parkinson's syndrome) may be caused by toxins, drug-induced and other conditions (e.g., those that follow head trauma or encephalitis), Shy-Drager syndrome, progressive supranuclear palsy, hypoparathyroidism, and Wilson's disease.

Occurrence: Approximately 1% of the population, or 100–150 cases in 100,000 individuals, are diagnosed with Parkinson's disease.

Age: Parkinson's disease is found predominantly in older adults; however, 15% of newly diagnosed cases occur before age 49.

Ethnicity: Parkinson's disease can be found in all cultures; however, it is less prevalent in blacks in the United States and in the Japanese than in the general population.

Gender: The ratio of Parkinson's disease in men and women is 1.4 : 1, indicating an almost-equal prevalence in gender.

Contributing Factors: Some evidence exists linking environmental toxins, viral infections, and a possible genetic tendency to the development of Parkinson's disease.

Signs and Symptoms: An initial clinical symptom of Parkinson's disease is a resting tremor, often initially unilateral, that disappears with movement. Tremor is also noted in the lips, chin, and tongue. Patients may also make a motion of the thumb and forefinger known as "pill rolling." Although common, tremor is not present in every patient with Parkinson's disease. Rigidity, as demonstrated by increased resistance to passive range of motion, is a classic sign. Cogwheel rigidity can be noted in the wrists and elbows. Patients experience a slowing of movements known as bradykinesia. Patients also report having difficulty initiating movement. Autonomic movements, such as the normal pattern of arm swinging during ambulation, are decreased.

Other associated manifestations include masked facial expression, decreased blinking, and delayed ability to demonstrate facial expressions. Patients also experience an associated softening of the voice, hypophonia, and drooling. The size of the patient's handwriting changes (micrographia). Flexed posture is common, with a bowed head, kyphotic back, and a trunk that leans forward. The gait may become faster, with the body propelled forward (festination). Ask the patient about associated presentations such as constipation, seborrhea, myalgia, impotence, and urinary incontinence. Depression and dementia are also very common in patients with Parkinson's disease. Patients and family members may report mood swings, hallucinations, and insomnia.

Clinical examination should begin with observation of the patient's stature to note any kyphosis and bending of the head forward. Have the patient ambulate and observe the gait, including arm swing. Test the patient for postural instability while standing, by gently pushing the patient forward and then backward and noting whether the postural reflexes are absent. Check the patient's ocular movements; impairment of upward or downward gaze is common in progressive supranuclear palsy and not in Parkinson's disease. Examine the patient's upper and lower extremities. Test for range of motion and strength, noting any cogwheel rigidity. Strength generally does not deteriorate despite the rigidity. Tendon reflexes are almost always normal. To test for tremor, have the patient rest the arms on the legs while seated. Note the frequency and amplitude of the tremor. The patient's blood pressure should be checked on every visit since hypotension is common in patients with Parkinson's disease.

Diagnostic Tests: No histologic markers can establish the diagnosis of Parkinson's disease. Magnetic resonance imagery (MRI) may be ordered by a neurologist to rule out suspected brain lesions or abnormalities such as normal-pressure hydrocephalus.

Differential Diagnosis: Several clinical syndromes can mimic the presentation of Parkinson's disease, including essential (benign familial) tremor, Huntington's disease, Shy-Drager syndrome, progressive supranuclear palsy, Creutzfeldt-Jakob disease, and normal-pressure hydrocephalus. In the early stages of the disease, depression may resemble Parkinson's disease.

Treatment: Drug therapy (Table 13–1; Fig. 13–3) focuses on correcting the imbalance of dopamine and acetylcholine. Patients with mild disease with no interference with activities of daily living (ADLs) may not require treatment. When tremors and rigidity cause impairment of the patient's ability to perform ADLs, and disability level is mild to moderate, treatment may include amantidine which is thought to augment dopamine release from presynaptic nerve terminals or to inhibit dopamine reuptake. Initial dose is usually 100 mg with breakfast. In 5–7 days, add amantadine 100 mg with lunch, and then increase daily dose to 300 mg. Additionally, anticholinergics are used to block acetylcholine. Procyclidine 10–25 mg/day or trihexyphenidyl 10–25 mg/day may be started in small doses and increased in small incremental dosages every 3–5 days.

Patients with severe disability may require carbidopa and levodopa therapy alone to replenish the depleted dopamine in the brain by increasing the dopamine precursor, levodopa, or (in combination with a dopamine agonist such as bromocriptine or pergolide) to stimulate dopamine receptors. Carbidopa and levodopa can be started using Sinemet 25–100 (carbidopa 25 mg, levodopa 100 mg) 2 tablets once a day. Dosage can be increased by 2 tablets every 3–5 days until the total daily dose is 3 doses of 2 tablets of Sinemet 25–100.

Daily therapy with bromocriptine 1.25 mg or pergolide 0.125 mg can be started, increasing dose every 5 days, to a total daily dose of 30 mg of bromocriptine or 3 mg of pergolide.

Selegiline, a monoamine oxidase-B inhibitor, inhibits the enzyme responsible for inactivating dopamine. Adding selegiline 5 mg/day (increasing to 10 mg/day within 1 week) can improve the "wearing-off" effect of levodopa.

Follow-up: Ask the patient if any medications seem to be "wearing off."

TABLE 13–1 COMMONLY USED MEDICATIONS FOR PATIENTS WITH PARKINSON'S DISEASE

Medication/generic	Medication/brand	Class of medication	Use/target symptoms	Clinically effective dosage commonly prescribed
Amantadine HCl	Symmetrel	Glutamate antagonist?	All PD symptomatology	100 mg bid–tid
Apomorphine (1)	Brittaject	Dopamine agonist (D1, D2)	Wearing off	1–5 mg SQ q 3–4 hr
Benztropine	Cogentin	Anticholinergic	All PD symptomatology	0.5–1 mg qid/tid
Bromocriptine mesytate	Parlodel	Agonist (D2); antagonist/agonist (D1)	All PD symptomatology	2.5–10 mg tid/qid
Carbidopa (2)	Lodosyn	Amino acid decarboxylase inhibitor	Antiemetic	25 mg tid/qid
Carbidopa/levodopa	Sinemet	Dopamine agonist	All PD symptomatology	See notes (3)
Clonazepam	Klonopin	Benzodiazepine	Anxiety	0.25–0.50 mg qid/bid
Clozapine	Clozaril	Antipsychotic	Psychosis, anxiety, insomnia	6.25–75 mg/d
Domperidone (1)	Motilium	D2 receptor antagonist (peripheral)	Antiemetic, GI hypomotility	10 mg tid
Donepezil	Aricept	Acetyl cholinesterase inhibitor	Cognitive impairment, ? abulia	5–10 mg qid
Entacapone (1)	Comtan	COMT inhibitor	Wearing off	100–200 mg with levodopa dose
Fludrocortisone acetate	Florinef	Adrenocortical steroid	Orthostatic hypotension	0.1–0.6 mg/d
Fluoxetuen HCl	Prozac	SSRI	Depression	10–20 mg qid
Lorazepam	Ativan	Benzodiazepine	Anxiety	0.5 mg bid/tid
Midodrine	Pro Amatine	Alpha-1 adrenergic agonist (peripheral)	Orthostatic hypotension	2.5–10 mg q 4 hr
Mirtazapine	Remeron	5HT, H1 and alpha-2 antagonist	Depression	7.5–15 mg qhs
Olanzapine	Zyprexa	Antipsychotic	Psychosis	2.5–5 mg qhs
Paroxetine	Paxil	SSRI	Depression, anxiety	10–20 mg qid
Pergolide	Permax	Dopamine agonist (D1, D2, D3)	All PD symptomatology	0.25 mg–1 mg tid/qid
Pramipexole	Mirapex	Dopamine agonist (D2, D3)	All PD symptomatology	0.5 mg–1.5 mg tid/qid
Procyclidine HCl	Kemadrin	Anticholinergic	All PD symptomatology	2.5–5 mg qid/tid
Ropinirole	Requip	Dopamine agonist (D2, D3)	All PD symptomatology	1–5 mg tid/qid
Selegiline HCl	Eldepryl, Deprenyl	MAO-B inhibitor	All PD symptomatology	5–10 mg/d
Sertraline	Zoloft	SSRI	Depression, anxiety	25–50 mg qid
Tolcapone	Tasmar	COMT inhibitor	Wearing off	200 mg tid
Trihexyphenidyl	Artane	Anticholinergic	All PD symptomatology	1–5 mg qid/tid

GI = gastrointestinal

PD = Parkinson's disease

SSRI = selective serotonin reuptake inhibitor

COMT = catechol-O-methyl transferase

1. Not currently available in United States.

2. Available directly from DuPont Pharma.

3. Varying proportions of levodopa and carbidopa: levodopa dose 100–1000 mg/d; carbidopa 25–250 mg/d.

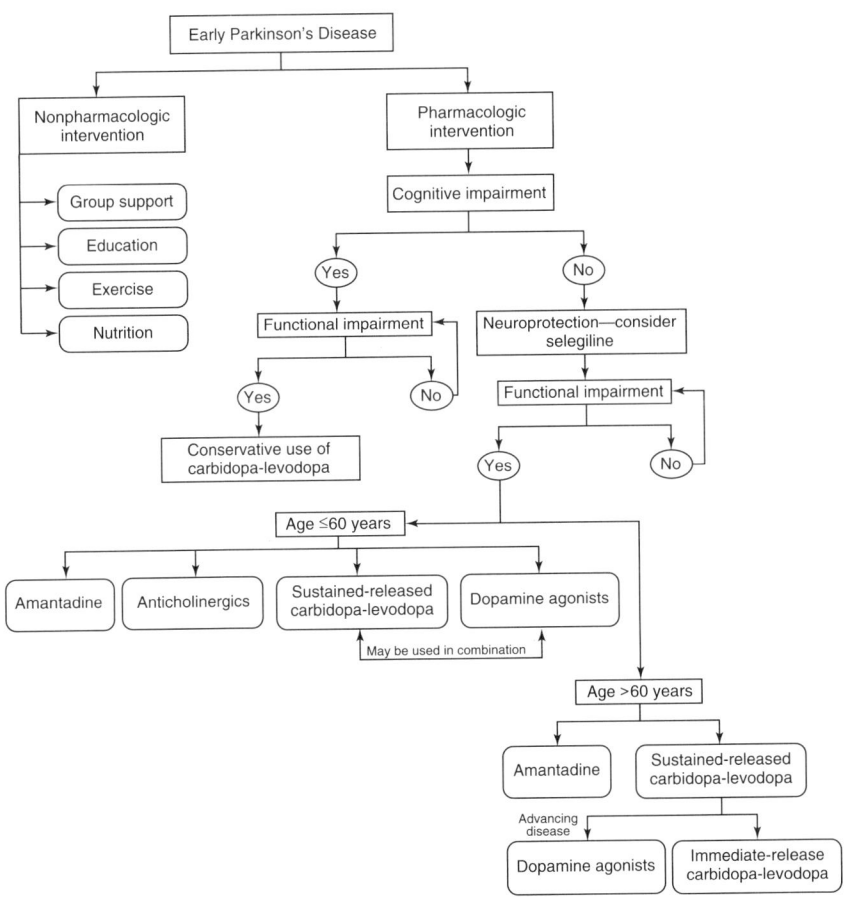

FIGURE 13–3   Parkinson's disease.

Sequelae: As Parkinson's disease is chronic and progressive, the patient with advanced illness is susceptible to developing injury resulting from falls, infection, inanition related to problems with gastric motility, and respiratory complications such as pulmonary embolism. With the advancement of medical therapeutics, the life expectancy of a patient with Parkinson's disease is about 15 years after diagnosis.

Prevention/Prophylaxis: No preventive measures exist for idiopathic Parkinson's disease.

Referral: Refer to a neurologist any patients with unusual presentation or sustained complications of the illness and those who do not respond to the initial medication regimen. Patients may also benefit from physical and occupational therapy to assist with adaptive equipment and techniques to enhance independence while maintaining a safe environment. Refer patients with voice changes or difficulty swallowing to a speech therapist. Those receiving levodopa therapy may benefit from a dietary consultation.

Education: Provide patients and family members with written information about Parkinson's disease, including information about local support groups. The following list of national organizations can be contacted for educational resources:

American Parkinson's Disease Association
Staten Island, New York
800-223-2732

National Parkinson's Foundation
Miami, Florida
800-327-4545

Parkinson's Disease Foundation
New York, New York
800-457-6676

United Parkinson Foundation
Chicago, Illinois
312-733-1893

Transient Ischemic Attack

A transient ischemic attack (TIA) is a neurologic impairment of presumed ischemic origin, lasting less than 24 hours. Attacks usually last less than 10 minutes.

Etiology: TIAs result from the temporary occlusion of an artery in the brain, caused by a thrombus or an embolus. The majority are due to emboli of platelets and fibrin breaking off a vessel wall, usually the carotid artery, or originating from a cardiac lesion. Transient hypotension, in conjunction with significant carotid stenosis, may also cause a TIA.

Occurrence: In the United States the incidence of TIA is estimated at 160 in 100,000. Because most TIAs are diagnosed by history only, and many more go unreported, the actual incidence is probably considerably higher.

Age: TIAs can occur at any age but are most prevalent in the elderly population.

Ethnicity: The incidence is almost equal among all ethnic groups in the United States, with a slight increase in blacks, which may be because concurrent hypertension and other cardiovascular disorders are more common in blacks.

Gender: Sources are divided on the incidence of TIA among men and women. Because many episodes go unreported, the incidence is probably equal between the sexes.

Contributing Factors: Risk factors for TIAs include advanced age, hypertension, hypercholesterolemia, diabetes, family history of stroke, smoking, alcohol abuse, antiphospholipid antibodies, and obesity.

Signs and Symptoms: TIAs are often diagnosed on the basis of history alone because symptoms usually resolve before a patient can seek health care. Patients report a sudden onset of symptoms that can last up to 24 hours but usually less than 10 minutes. TIAs can be divided into those that indicate disease in the carotid circulation and those indicating disease in the vertebrobasilar area. Clues to carotid disease include monocular blindness, weakness or numbness of the hand or leg, and disturbed speech. Vertebrobasilar disease is suggested by binocular visual disturbance, vertigo, paresthesia, ataxia, diplopia, dysarthria, lightheadedness, generalized weakness, or loss of consciousness. Cardiac physical examination may reveal a carotid bruit, cardiac arrhythmia, or heart murmur during auscultation. Blood pressure may be elevated (Fig. 13–4).

Diagnostic Tests:

- Arteriography is the "gold standard" to evaluate the condition of cerebral arteries.
- Carotid and transcranial Doppler studies are most helpful in cases of very high grade stenosis. Studies indicate that for mild to moderate carotid stenosis Doppler results may be misleading.
- A computed tomography (CT) or magnetic resonance imagery (MRI) scan of the brain should be performed to detect silent or prior infarction, unsuspected hemorrhage, or tumor.
- Echocardiography and Holter monitoring may be useful in detecting cardiac problems. An electroencephalogram (EEG) is helpful if a seizure is suspected.

Differential Diagnosis: Focal seizures, migraine, cervical disk osteophyte, hyperventilation, and carpal tunnel syndrome may produce symptoms that mimic those of TIA.

Treatment: Treatment for TIA focuses on prevention of stroke. Carotid endarterectomy is recommended for patients with high-grade stenosis. Antiplatelet agents (aspirin, ticlopidine) are given alternatively to patients with mild to moderate stenosis or to those who are not suitable candidates for surgery. If cardiac evaluation reveals a possible source of emboli, warfarin (Coumadin) therapy should be instituted, and INR monitored closely and maintained within a range of 2.0–3.0.

Follow-up: Monitor patients periodically for continuation of symptoms and for control of any comorbid illnesses.

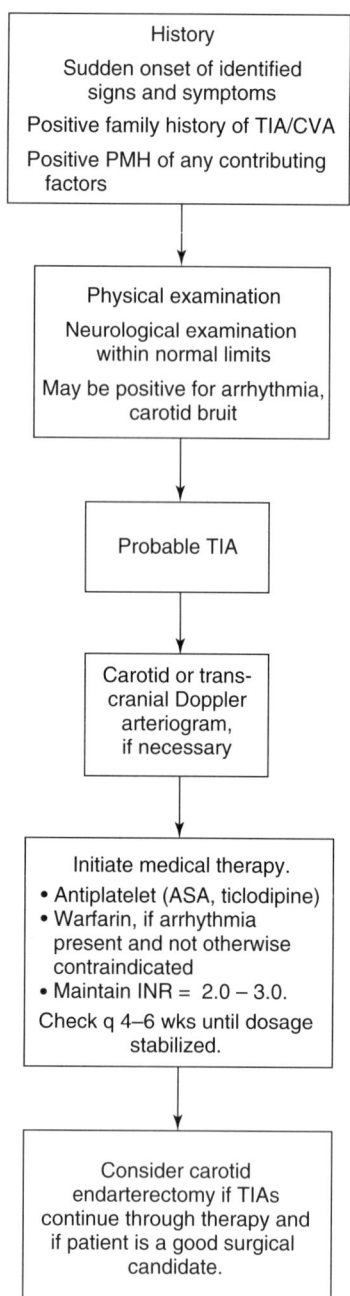

FIGURE 13–4 TIA.

Sequelae: In addition to being at risk for another TIA, all patients are at risk for stroke. Of those who go on to suffer a stroke, 50% do so within 1 year after the TIA, while 20% occur within one month. A higher risk of myocardial infarction is also noted in this population.

Prevention/Prophylaxis: See Treatment above.

Referral: Patients who suffer drop attacks or vertigo or who have a focal neurologic finding are referred to neurology for further work up. An ophthalmologist may be consulted for patients whose complaints include transient monocular blindness. Patients with any gross cardiac abnormalities should be referred to a cardiologist.

Education: Focus patient education on the cause of the TIA, and explain the increased risk of stroke, appropriate prevention modalities, and modification of risk factors.

BIBLIOGRAPHY

Assessment

Bates, B, Bickley, LS, and Hoekelman, RA: A Guide to Physical Examination and History Taking, ed 6. JB Lippincott, Philadelphia, 1995.
Willms, JL, Schneiderman, H, and Algranati, PS: Physical Diagnosis: Bedside Evaluation of Diagnosis and Function. Williams & Wilkins, Baltimore, 1994.

Alzheimer's Disease

Abraham, IL, et al: Multidisciplinary assessment of patients with Alzheimer's disease. Nurs Clin North Am 29(1):113–127, 1994.
Abrams, W, et al: The Merck Manual of Geriatrics, ed 2. Merck Research Laboratories, Whitehouse Station, NJ, 1995.
Bennett, DA, and Knopman, DS: Alzheimer's disease: A comprehensive approach to patient management. Geriatrics 49(8):20–26, 1994.
Costa PT Jr, et al: Early Identification of Alzheimer's Disease and Related Dementias. Clinical Practice Guideline, Quick Reference Guide for Clinicians, No. 19. US Department of Health and Human Services, Agency for Health Care Policy and Research. AHCPR Publications No. 97-0703. Rockville, Md, 1996.
Filley, CM: Alzheimer's disease: It's irreversible but not untreatable. Geriatrics 50(7):18–23, 1995.
Hachinski, VC, et al: Cerebral blood flow in dementia. Arch Neurol 32:632–637, 1975.
Hendrie, HC: Epidemiology of Alzheimer's disease. Geriatrics 52:4–8, 1997.
Morris, JC: Alzheimer's disease: A review of clinical assessment and management issues. Geriatrics 52:22–25, 1997.
Pfeffer, RI, et al: Measurement of functional activities of older adults in the community. J Gerontol 37:323–329, 1982.
Sano, M, et al: A standardized technique for establishing onset and duration of symptoms of Alzheimer's disease. Arch Neurol 52:961, 1995.
Small, GW, et al: Diagnosis and treatment of Alzheimer's disease and related disorders. JAMA 278:1363–1371, 1997.
Stephenson, J: More evidence links NSAIDs, estrogen with reduced Alzheimer's risk. JAMA 275:1389, 1996.
Thal, LJ: Potential prevention strategies for Alzheimer's disease. Alzheimer's Disease and Associated Disorders 10(Suppl 1):6–8, 1996.

Brain Tumor

Armstrong, TS, and Gilbert, MR: Glial neoplasms: Classification, treatment, and pathways for the future. Oncol Nurs Forum 23:615, 1996.

Berger, MS, et al: Primary central nervous system tumors of the supratentorial compartment. In Levin, VA: Cancer in the Nervous System. Churchill Livingstone, New York, 1996.

Bullock, BL, and Rosendahl, PP: Pathophysiology: Adaptations and Alterations in Function. Scott, Foresman, Glenview, Ill, 1988.

DeGowin, RL: DeGowin and DeGowin's Diagnostic Examination. McGraw-Hill, New York, 1994.

Hochberg, F, and Pruitt, A: Neoplastic diseases of the central nervous system. In Isselbacher, KJ, et al (eds): Harrison's Principles of Internal Medicine, ed 13. McGraw-Hill, New York, 1994.

Levin, VA, Leibel, SA, and Gutin, PH: Neoplasms of the central nervous system. In DeVita, VT, Hellman, S, Rosenberg, SA (eds): Cancer Principles of Practice and Oncology. Vol. 2. Lippincott-Raven, Philadelphia, 1997.

Newton, C, and Matoe, MA: Uncertainty: Strategies for patients with brain tumors and their families. Cancer Nurs 17(2):137–140, 1994.

Posner, JB: Central nervous system cancer. In Fischer, DS: Follow-up of Cancer: A Handbook for Physicians. Lippincott-Raven, Philadelphia, 1996.

Pruitt, AA: Evaluation of dementia. In Goroll, AH, May, LA, and Mulley, AG: Primary Care Medicine. JB Lippincott, Philadelphia, 1995.

Pruitt, AA: Approach to the patient with headache. In Goroll, AH, May, LA, and Mulley, AG: Primary Care Medicine. JB Lippincott, Philadelphia, 1995.

CVA

Agency for Health Care Policy and Research: Carotid Endarterectomy, Number 5, DHHS Publication #(PHS)91-3472. Government Printing Office, Washington, DC, 1990.

Gorelick, PB: Cerebrovascular disease: Pathophysiology and diagnosis. Nurs Clin North Am 21(2):275–288, 1986.

Goroll, AH, May, LA, and Mulley, AG: Primary Care Medicine, ed 3. JB Lippincott, Philadelphia, 1995.

Hazzard, WR, et al: Principles of Geriatric Medicine and Gerontology. McGraw-Hill, New York, 1994.

McCabe, ML: Cerebrovascular disease. In Taylor, RB (ed): Family Medicine Principles and Practice, ed 4. Springer-Verlag, New York, 1992.

National Stroke Association: Stroke: The First Hours—Emergency Evaluation and Treatment—Consensus Statement. National Stroke Association, Englewood, Colo, 1997.

Oertel, LB: International normalized ratio (INR): An improved way to monitor anticoagulant therapy. Nurse Pract 20(9):15–22, 1995.

Rosenbaum, D: Early treatment of ischemic stroke with a calcium channel agonist. Stroke 22(4):437–441, 1991.

Parkinson's Disease

Abrams, W, Beers, MH, and Berkow, R: The Merck Manual of Geriatrics, ed 2. Merck Research Laboratories, Whitehouse Station, NJ, 1995.

Aminoff, MJ: Parkinsonism. In Tiery, LM, McPhee, SJ, Papadakis, MA (eds): Current Medical Diagnosis and Treatment 1997. Appleton & Lange, Stamford, Conn, 1996, pp. 919–921.

Imke, S: Parkinson's disease: A medical management update. Adv Nurse Pract 6(1):24–28, 1998.

Tapper, VJ: Pathophysiology, assessment, and treatment of Parkinson's disease. Nurse Pract 22(7):76–95, 1997.

Unger, J: Diagnosis and management of Parkinson's disease. The Clinical Advisor 1:26, 1998.

Transient Ischemic Attack

Agency for Health Care Policy and Research: Carotid Endarterectomy. Number 5, DHHS Publication #(PHS)91-3472. Government Printing Office, Washington, DC, 1990.

Gorelick, PB: Cerebrovascular disease: Pathophysiology and diagnosis. Nurs Clin North Am 21(2):275–288, 1986.

Goroll, AH, May, LA, and Mulley, AG: Primary Care Medicine, ed 3. JB Lippincott, Philadelphia, 1995.

Hazzard, WR, et al: Principles of Geriatric Medicine and Gerontology. McGraw-Hill, New York, 1994.

National Stroke Association: Stroke: The First Hours—Emergency Evaluation and Treatment—Consensus Statement. National Stroke Association, Englewood, Colo, 1997.

Oertel, LB: International normalized ratio (INR): An improved way to monitor anticoagulant therapy. Nurse Pract 20(9):15–22, 1995.

CHAPTER **14**

ENDOCRINE,

METABOLIC,

AND NUTRITIONAL

DISORDERS

Accurate history taking of complaints associated with endocrine disease is essential in completing the examination of the older adult. Because changes in the endocrine system may appear subtle to the older person, it may be difficult to pinpoint the onset of the presentation. Reevaluate the patient's family history for endocrine disease. Explore with the patient any difficulty with decreased heat or increased cold intolerance and any changes in the texture or distribution of body hair or in skin temperature or texture. Review with the patient any episodes of unexplained weight loss or gain, fatigue, weakness, palpitations, or shortness of breath. Ask the patient or significant other(s) if there has been any acute memory impairment.

Does the patient offer any complaints of paresthesia or carpal tunnel syndrome symptoms?

Has the patient noticed excessive thirst, appetite, or urination?

Has the patient experienced repeated yeast infections?

Has the patient had a skin ulcer that has failed to heal?

Has the patient noticed a new onset of constipation?

Have there been any changes in the patient's tone of voice?

Has the patient experienced vertigo or gait disturbances?

Are there any other symptoms that could be clustered to form a differential diagnosis?

It is important to determine from the patient what therapeutic measures have been initiated or prescribed in the past to alleviate any of these symptoms.

The physical examination should focus on the presentation of signs of common diseases of older adults (i.e., diabetes mellitus, hypothyroidism, hyperthyroidism). Examine the skin for changes in texture, temperature, evidence of infection, or open wounds. Inspect the hair distribution and note any dryness, coarseness, or brittleness of the hair. Has the hair distribution of the eyebrows changed? Eye examination includes ruling out cataracts and/or diabetic retinopathy or exophthalmia. Any reported changes in hearing or tinnitus warrant an ear examination. During the examination of the mouth, look for changes in the oral mucosal membrane and note if any tremor of the tongue is present. In the older adult the thyroid gland can be found in a lower position relative to the clavicles because of age-related changes in height and in the neck. The thyroid gland is more flexible and thyroid nodules are more common in an older person. Goiters are frequently found in older patients with thyroid disease. Focus the cardiac examination on determining the presence of arrhythmias and abnormal heart sounds. An S_3 is often found in older adults with congestive heart failure. Examine the extremities for evidence of weakness, tremor, and peripheral neuropathies. A diminished patellar and Achilles tendon reflex may accompany diabetes mellitus in an older adult. Evaluate the patient's gait for disturbances.

Chronic Pancreatitis

Chronic pancreatitis is chronic inflammation of the pancreas associated with fibrotic changes and calcification, leading to functional and structural damage of the organ.

Etiology: Pancreatic insufficiency resulting from a long history of alcohol abuse, vascular disease, pancreatic carcinoma, and abdominal radiation therapy can result in chronic pancreatitis.

Occurrence: About 15 of 100,000 persons will develop chronic pancreatitis.

Age: The prevalence of chronic pancreatitis is low in older adults because people with alcoholism usually do not live into old age. The peak age of occurrence of this disease is age 35–45.

Ethnicity: Countries known to have high rates of alcoholism such as the United States, Australia, and South Africa have higher rates of chronic pancreatitis than those that do not.

Gender: Chronic pancreatitis occurs equally in men and women.

Contributing Factor: The most significant factor contributing to the development of chronic pancreatitis is alcoholism. Patients who are addicted to narcotics are also susceptible to developing chronic pancreatitis. Elderly women with a history of cholelithiasis are at risk for recurring pancreatitis. Other diseases that may contribute to chronic pancreatitis are hyperparathyroidism; hyperlipidemia; peptic ulcer disease; obstruction of the main pancreatic duct because of carcinoma, stone, or stenosis; biliary tract disease; and systemic lupus erythematosus. Severe malnutrition is another cause of chronic pancreatitis.

Signs and Symptoms: Older patients with chronic pancreatitis may or may not experience pain. Severe epigastric pain may occur in the upper abdominal area, radiating to the back; the origin of the pain may be difficult to discern. Weight loss occurs because of either anorexia or malabsorption. Physical examination may reveal mild fever, hypotension, tachycardia, and tachypnea. Auscultation of the lungs may indicate basilar atelectasis; the clinician should have the patient cough deeply and reassess to determine if the atelectasis is still present. Jaundice may be present. Bowel sounds may be diminished or absent. Epigastric tenderness may be elicited and the abdomen may be rigid. The gallbladder is not usually palpable. If there is a bluish discoloration around the umbilicus (Cullen's sign) and at the flank (Turner's sign), hemorrhagic necrotizing pancreatitis should be suspected.

Diagnostic Tests: The serum amylase level is usually elevated in the early stage of an attack; however, in subsequent episodes of pancreatitis, the serum amylase level decreases. Levels of serum lipase, alkaline phosphatase, and bilirubin may also be elevated with common bile duct compression. Glycosuria may be present. Abdominal films may show pancreatic calcification. Abdominal computed tomography (CT) may reveal dilated ducts, presence of pseudocyst, and an enlarged pancreas. To further evaluate pancreatic duct function, endoscopic retrograde cholangiopancreatography (ERCP) may be ordered by a specialist. Patients experiencing steatorrhea should have fecal fat content analyzed.

Differential Diagnosis: In diagnosing chronic pancreatitis, the following diagnoses may mimic a similar presentation: choledocholithiasis, pancreatitis, duodenal neoplasms, choledochal cyst, pancreatic pseudocyst, and biliary tract stricture.

Treatment: Patients with chronic pancreatitis must avoid all alcoholic products. Pain control should be managed without the use of narcotics; nonnarcotic analgesics can be tried unless contraindicated. Tricyclic antidepressants are also useful in controlling this type of pain. A low-fat diet should be prescribed. Refer patients with steatorrhea to a gastroenterologist for consideration of pancreatic supplements. Diabetes mellitus will need to be managed. Refer to a specialist patients who may benefit from surgical intervention to alleviate pain. When chronic pancreatitis can be attributed to cholelithiasis, hyperparathyroidism, peptic ulcer disease, or hyperlipidemia, these conditions should be treated, after which the symptoms from the pancreatic attacks should lessen or cease.

Follow-up: On return visits, ask patients about their diet, pain control, and compliance with abstaining from alcohol. Patients who have developed diabetes mellitus, hyperlipidemia, hyperparathyroidism, or peptic ulcer disease need continued evaluation.

Sequelae: Diabetes mellitus, pancreatic pseudocyst or abscess, peptic ulcer disease, and bile duct stricture may be complications of recurring pancreatitis.

Prevention/Prophylaxis: Cessation of alcohol consumption is critical to the prognosis of chronic pancreatitis.

Referral: Refer patients with complicated chronic pancreatitis to a gastroenterologist. Surgical intervention may also be recommended. Refer anyone presenting with a severe pancreatic attack (i.e., those who are dehydrated or febrile, have tachycardia, or have elevated amylase greater than 1000 mg/dL) to a gastroenterologist for possible hospital admission.

Education: Instruct patients to eliminate all alcohol consumption. Recommend an alcohol treatment program and provide the telephone number for the nearest chapter of Alcoholics Anonymous. Additional organizations that may be beneficial to the patient with alcoholism include Secular Organization for Sobriety (301-821-8430) and Rational Recovery Systems (916-621-4374).

Diabetes Mellitus

The diagnosis of diabetes mellitus in elderly persons involves a constellation of signs and symptoms. The disease has several forms, however, the focus of this chapter is insulin-dependent diabetes mellitus (IDDM, or type 1) and non–insulin-dependent diabetes mellitus (NIDDM, or type 2), which are most specific to the elderly patient. IDDM occurs when more than 90% of the islet beta cells have been destroyed. The cause of NIDDM, which may indeed be linked to various etiologies, is being investigated. Both forms, especially when uncontrolled, have a negative impact on the anatomy; drain the patient financially, psychologically, and socially; and impair function, lifestyle, and longevity. Consequences of uncontrolled diabetes in adults include blindness, end-stage renal disease, and atraumatic amputations. The estimated cost of diabetes and its related problems (amputations, lost time from work, blindness) in the United States exceeds $92 billion per year, in direct and indirect costs.

A separate diagnostic category, impaired glucose tolerance (IGT) is diagnosed when glucose challenge testing reveals glucose levels that are outside the normal distribution but do not reach the threshold for the diagnosis of diabetes (i.e., 140 mg/dL or higher but no more than 200 mg/dL). Diagnosing IGT and following individuals with this condition is important because they are at greater risk than the general population for developing macrovascular disease (whereas diabetics have microvascular disease) and have a one-in-three chance of developing NIDDM within 10 years of the diagnosis. A new diagnostic category was introduced by the American Diabetic Association in 1997; impaired fasting glucose (IFG). IFG is diagnosed when fasting blood sugar is greater than 110 mg/dL but no more than 126 mg/dL. Diabetes mellitus primarily characterized by abnormal glucose metabolism, is also associated with abnormal regulation of lipid and protein metabolism and with the development of vascular and nervous system disease. Each clinical form of diabetes has a distinct etiology, clinical presentation, and course.

Etiology: Patients with type 1 diabetes, which is associated with reduced pancreatic islet beta cell mass and absolute insulinopenia, are prone to ketosis and need exogenous insulin for immediate survival. In contrast, type 2 diabetes is often associated with significant insulin secretion, but with cellular receptor site or post–cellular receptor site resistance. Persons with type 2 diabetes are not typically prone to ketosis and are not insulin dependent. Both types of diabetes may have genetic, environmental, viral, and immunologic causes. Research continues to discover the exact relationship between each of these factors and onset of the disease.

Occurrence: Type 1 diabetes occurs in 1 in 250 individuals in the United States; 3% of persons with type 1 diabetes are over age 65. Type 2 diabetes is a much more common disease; prevalence studies estimate that NIDDM occurs in 18% of persons over age 65. An estimated 10% of the US population will have NIDDM by age 60. Diabetes is present in 40% of the population over age 80. In elderly individuals, diabetes may be present for up to 7 years before it is diagnosed.

Age: The onset of type 1 diabetes is usually in youth (birth to early 20s). The onset of type 2 diabetes is typically after age 40. However, both types of diabetes can occur at any point in life.

Ethnicity: IDDM is more common in whites than in African-Americans. The prevalence of NIDDM, however, is higher among African-Americans and Hispanics than among whites.

Gender: IDDM occurs equally in men and women, but NIDDM is more common in women.

Contributing Factors: Obesity (occurring in 80% of all NIDDM patients), sedentary lifestyle, family history, stressful occurrences, and pharmaceuticals are all contributors. Drugs that promote insulin resistance and hyperglycemia include diuretics, glucocorticoids, estrogens, nicotinic acid, phenothiazines, phenytoins, sympathomimetic agents, lithium, and sugar-containing medications. Medications that can potentiate hypoglycemia include alcohol, dicumarol, beta-blockers, monoamine oxidase (MAO) inhibitors, phenylbutazone, salicylates (large doses), sulfonamides, sulfonylureas, cimetidine, anabolic steroids, and insulin.

Signs and Symptoms: Elderly individuals with IDDM typically present with relatively acute glycosuria, weight loss, and anorexia for 2 months or less. They are typically thin, with symptoms of ketoacidosis. NIDDM has a more insidious presentation among elderly persons. Recurrent infections, unexplained weight loss, fatigue, and cataracts are often the presenting signs. Degenerative changes in blood vessels and nerves leading to atherosclerotic complications and neuropathy, renal failure, and retinopathy can be found on physical examination.

The classic symptoms of polydipsia, polyuria, and slow wound healing may be attributed to normal aging and therefore may be neglected in the history. Anorexia, cognitive dysfunction, depression, altered sensorium, decreased pain, poor dentition, alterations in gastrointestinal function, microaneurysms, detached retinas, recurrent bacterial or fungal infections, cardiovascular changes (silent ischemia, postural hypotension, stroke, peripheral vascular disease, gangrene), small vessel disease affecting the eyes (hemorrhages, exudates), or kidneys (microalbuminuria, uremia, glomeruloneuropathy), impotency, and bladder atony (overflow incontinence) are also presenting factors. Hyperlipidemia, osteoporosis, history of gestational diabetes, delivery of large babies, past glucose intolerance, and family history are significant findings.

Diagnostic Tests: Note: The classic markers of diabetes may be masked or absent in elderly persons. The criteria for the diagnosis of diabetes mellitus are the same in elderly patients as in younger patients. Fasting plasma glucose (FPG) levels are relatively unaltered by age and are easy to monitor; fasting is defined as no caloric intake for 8 hr. If the FPG is greater than 126 mg/dL, or a random plasma glucose level is 200 mg/dL (11.1 mmol/pL) or greater with signs or symptoms of diabetes (polydipsia, polyuria, polyphagia, or weight loss), the diagnosis for diabetes is firm. Rarely does an individual have a FPG level greater than 126 mg/dL at one testing and then a normal FPG at another time. If there is any reason to doubt the initial results, repeat the FPG test. An oral glucose tolerance test normally is not necessary. When an FPG level is below 126 mg/dL (7.0 mmol/dL) but diabetes is still suspected, two or more sustained elevated FPG levels discovered during at least two glucose tolerance tests confirm the diagnosis. This approach, however, is rarely necessary to establish the diagnosis in older patients. Another consideration for management of questionable readings is to diagnose patient's condition as impaired glucose tolerance and follow the patient's blood glucose levels during maintenance visits.

Differential Diagnosis: Endocrinologic disorders, such as Cushing's disease, pheochromocytoma, acromegaly, pharmacotherapeutic interventions and exogenous insulinopenia may mimic diabetes mellitus.

Treatment: First, consider secondary causes such as certain drugs that promote cellular insulin resistance or potentiate hyperglycemia; these drugs should be avoided. A diet and exercise program modified to meet the patient's lifestyle and ability is preferred prior to treatment with oral agents. A weight loss program should consider the issues of dentition, salivation, altered taste, and cost. Weight loss should be no greater than ½–1 lb/week. The diet should be rich in complex carbohdyrates and fiber. Weight reduction and its maintenance should be considered the cornerstone of NIDDM management in elderly patients. A minimum of two diet instruction sessions, or referral to a registered dietitian, is usually necessary. Exercise is customized according to the individual's current physical capabilities. The purpose of exercise is to increase circulation to make muscles use circulating glucose more effectively.

When diet and exercise fail (determined by a continued FPG level greater than 126 mg/dL), an oral agent should be introduced. Only about half of elderly persons with diabetes require insulin or oral sulfonylureas. The first-generation oral sulfonylureas are highly protein bound for transport; their effectiveness is reduced in hypoalbuminemic states or when other drugs are taken that compete for binding (e.g., dicumarol, or silicylates). Declining renal function or hepatic dysfunction delays sulfonylureas and insulin clearance and potentiates hypoglycemia.

Several sulfonylurea drugs and doses are available. In older adults, short-acting second-generation sulfonylureas (glyburides) appear to have less hypoglycemic effects because they are less likely to be displaced from their protein transport and are therefore more stable. Furthermore, glyburide has benefits over glipizide in that glyburide has dual clearance by the liver and kidneys, which may further reduce the risk for hypoglycemia. Dosing tpically starts at 5 mg taken each morning 30–45 minutes before a meal, increasing to 5 mg twice daily, and then to a maximum of 20 mg daily if FPG levels remain elevated.

The addition of a metformin-type (antiglucose) drug should be done very judiciously with elderly patients. Given the severity of hypoglycemia and the mortality associated with this condition in older adults, such rapid reductions may not be desirable. In addition, individuals with impaired renal function should not use metformin because of fatal and near-fatal metabolic acidosis reported with treatment by agents in this drug family. Chlorpropamide should not be used in elderly patients because it can cause the syndrome of inappropriate antidiuretic hormone secretion (SIADH), hyponatremia, and a deterioration in mental status.

The four basic reasons why oral sulfonylureas fail are:

1. Progression of disease, requiring more than the maximum dose of oral sulfonylureas.
2. Temporary and/or reversible deterioration of glycemic control (i.e., infection, surgery, or other stressor). Insulin is usually required during these periods, but the patient can resume oral therapy after the acute episode.
3. Dietary noncompliance, the most common reason among older persons.
4. In cases of "glucose toxicity," initial therapy may require insulin. Intensive dietary consulting is the only option before turning to insulin for diabetic control.

Newer classes of antidiabetic medications are rapidly becoming available. Briefly, these drugs include acarbose, glimepiride, and troglitazone. Acarbose, which inhibits carbohydrate absorption in the intestine, is associated with gastrointestinal side effects secondary to the increased sugar content of the stool. Use of acarbose is contraindicated in patients with renal dysfunction, inflammatory bowel disease, and ulcerative colitis. Glimepiride, which is used for monotherapy or in combination with insulin, stimulates insulin release from beta cells, increases insulin sensitivity in peripheral tissues, and reduces hepatic glucose production. Hypoglycemia has been noted in patients receiving combination therapy and in those with hepatic or renal impairment. Trogliatzone is indicated for persons with diabetes whose condition cannot be controlled with insulin therapy. Its use enhances the effects of circulating insulin, reduces triglycerides, and lowers blood pressure. Other reported benefits include decreases in hemoglobin, hematocrit, and white blood cells and resumption of ovulation in premenopausal anovulatory patients. Because these promising newer classes of medications have not been tested extensively in elderly patients, their use depends on judicious, individualized decisions, along with close monitoring of blood glucose levels and renal and hepatic tolerances.

Regimens for insulin in older adults are similar to those in the younger population. For elderly persons, however, the attempt to "normalize" should be interpreted differently. There are multiple preparations (porcine, bovine, human) and classifications (short, intermediate, long-acting, and mixed). The goal with an older patient is to introduce insulin to the point at which the patient is asymptomatic of the diabetes (no polyuria, stable weight, no fatigue or polyphagia).

An individual can be inadvertently prescribed insulin injections while still having beta cell function. This may occur for a variety of reasons, including a stressful hospitalization that caused a hyperglycemic state, removal of a pharmaceutical agent, multiple health-care providers, or as part of overall polypharmacy. Therefore, elderly individuals designated as having IDDM may indeed have NIDDM.

Persons currently taking insulin may be carefully weaned on a trial basis. To determine if the capacity to produce insulin exists, blood should be drawn for a C-peptide level. Insulin secretion rates can be estimated from baseline plasma C-peptide levels. Consider referring the patient to an endocrinologist for the initial determination of insulin-producing capacity and recommended wean. The wean from insulin should be strictly monitored. Reducing insulin administration while managing diet and activity, plus the introduction of an oral agent, can precipitate hypoglycemia, the most serious complication of managing diabetes in elderly persons (Fig. 14–1).

Follow-up: Monitoring patients with diabetes involves assessment of diet, activity, medication compliance, and blood glucose level, as well as any financial concerns attributable to diet and medication. The HgA$_{1C}$ is now considered standard follow-up for long-term compliance in most diabetic populations; however, the HgA$_{1C}$ has not been consistently reliable within the elderly population, and the literature findings are inconsistent. The patient may be better managed by obtaining venous samples and listening to the current complaint. The practitioner and the patient should reach a "comfort zone" wherein both determine that the management is effective. Tighter control may be desirable if surgery is planned. Typically, the goal range is between 90–100 mg/dL and 160–170 mg/dL. Visits should be weekly for three visits, then once every 2 weeks twice,

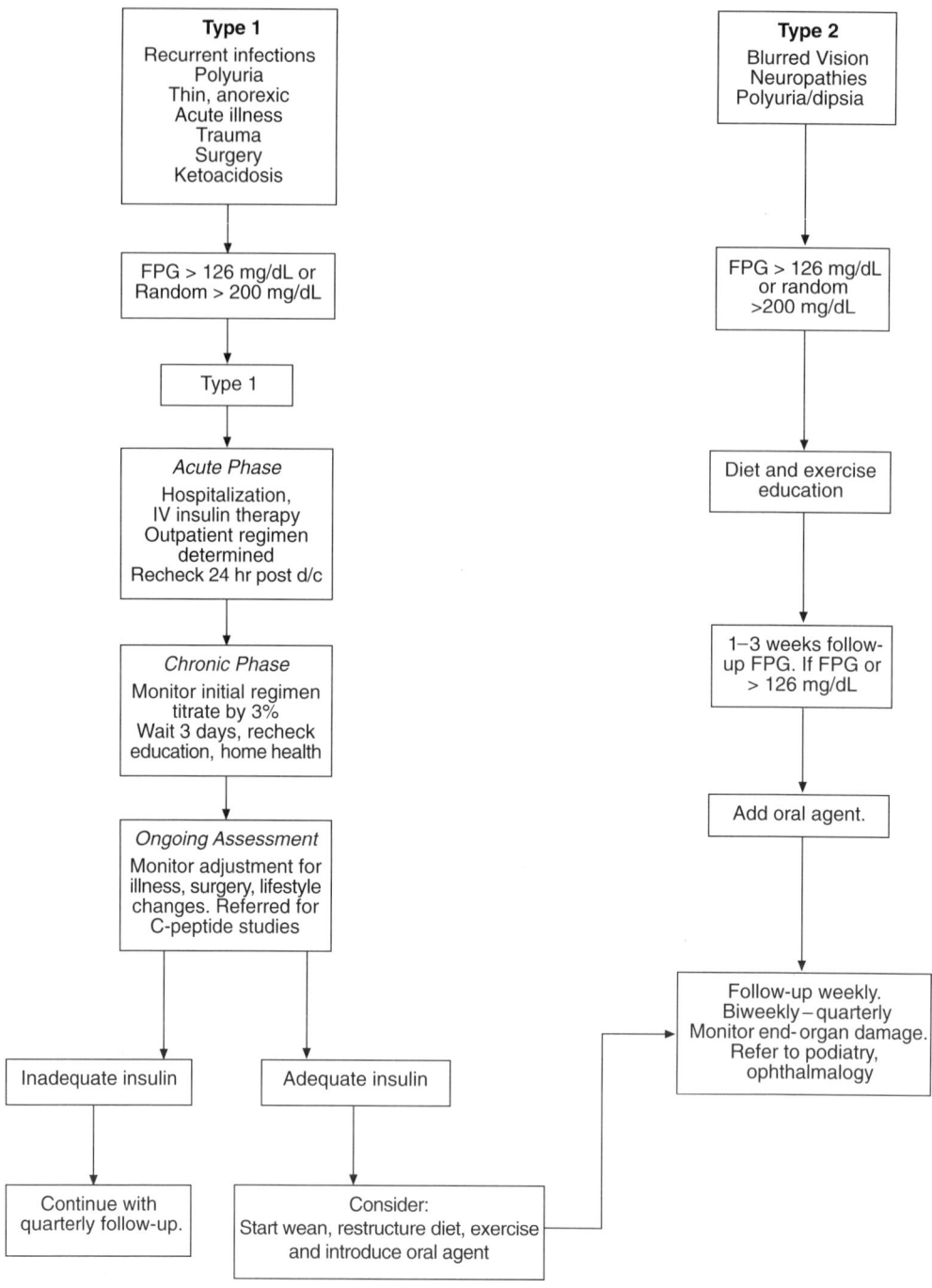

FIGURE 14–1   Diabetes mellitus.

then once every 3 months. Proper eye and foot care is essential, as is constant assessment for related sequelae. Treatment of likely comorbidities like hypertension, hyperlipidemia, and smoking should be concurrent.

Sequelae: Diabetes, by definition, implies both abnormal glucose intolerance levels and long-term vascular complications. Hypertension, hyperlipidemia, neuropathies, and visual changes should be closely monitored. Untreated diabetes progresses to deterioration of the cardiovascular and neurovascular systems, resulting in stroke, myocardial infarction, peripheral vascular disease, gastrointestinal difficulties, blindness, neuropathies, and loss of limb and function.

Prevention/Prophylaxis: The diagnosis of diabetes in elderly persons brings with it the assumption of end-organ damage or at least organ stress. The goal is to halt the rate of damage by controlling blood glucose levels, maintaining proper diet and exercise regimens, increasing circulation, providing education, and by rapidly attending to early signs of organ deterioration (specifically, failing vision and renal function, increased vascular deterioration, and neuropathy).

Referral: Patients with issues such as ophthalmologic and special podiatric concerns (i.e., fitting of shoes or complex foot care) should be referred. Acute life-threatening issues such as ketoacidosis, hypoglycemia, and renal failure are emergent in nature and require the cooperation of a multidisciplinary team. Consult with a geriatrician or endocrinologist when weaning individuals from insulin to oral agents. Consider referring the patient to a registered dietitian or registered nurse who is a Certified Diabetic Educator (CDE) if you are not well versed in the ADA recommendations. The CDE is also a resource for the holistic management of diabetes.

Education: Individuals with diabetes who manage their disease correctly are in turn very knowledgeable about the overall cycle of cause and effect in diabetes. Knowledge of the effect of food intake is essential to the survival of any person diagnosed with diabetes. Monitoring blood glucose, by home health nurses or by the individual with a home glucose monitor, is especially important when medication is initiated or adjusted. Materials for the monitors can be costly; daily monitoring is not necessary with type 2 diabetes once glucose levels have stabilized. Testing urine for ketones is important for patients with type 1 diabetes, especially when they first develop symptoms of a cold, flu, nausea, vomiting, abdominal pain, or polyuria, or if a high plasma glucose level is found through glucose monitoring. Medication and its timing must become second nature. Knowledge of the signs and symptoms of hypoglycemia and hyperglycemia is critical. Any changes in vision, integument, or sensation, or an intuitive clue that "something is not right" should be brought to the attention of the practitioner. In essence, any biologic or social system that is not functioning at an optimal level must be considered to be affected by diabetes and may benefit from intervention. Families of individuals with diabetes should be made aware that diabetes has a hereditary factor (patient permitting), so that health care can be managed accordingly.

Hyperlipidemia

Elevated levels of circulating lipoproteins, or hyperlipidemia, can result from an increase in their synthesis owing to a diet high in saturated fats or from a genetically determined reduction in the amount removed from the circulation. This causes an increase in the concentration of cholesterol and/or triglycerides in the plasma.

> The definition of hyperlipoproteinemia (HLP) is levels of plasma, cholesterol, and triglycerides exceeding the 95th percentile for adjusted age and gender. According to the National Cholesterol Education Program (NCEP), a cholesterol level less than 200 mg/dL is desirable.
> Triglycerides should be 40–150 mg/100 mL.

Occurrence: More than 120 million people in the United States have a total cholesterol level of 200 mg/dL or more, with 60 million people having a level greater than 240 mg/dL.

Age: Most common onset for hyperlipidemia is in the sixth decade.

Ethnicity: Hyperlipidemia is more common in whites than in African-Americans.

Gender: This condition is more prevalent in men than in women.

Contributing Factors: Factors contributing to development of hyperlipidemia are coronary heart disease, a high-fat diet, nephrotic syndrome, hypothyroidism, severe obesity (greater than 50 lb over ideal body weight [IBW]), pancreatitis, hypertension, family history of coronary heart disease, obstructive liver disease, excessive alcohol intake, renal failure, smoking, certain diuretics, anabolic steroids, sedentary lifestyle, and diabetes. Caffeine intake may increase cholesterol levels.

Signs and Symptoms: Most patients do not present with physical complaints. Routine physical examination, however, may reveal xanthomata, xanthelasma, arterial bruits, and evidence of claudication. Corneal arcus found in patients under age 50 often indicates hyperlipidemia.

Diagnostic Tests: After the patient has been fasting for a minimum of 12 hours, the following tests should be done:

Serum cholesterol.
Low-density lipoprotein (LDL) cholesterol.
Very low density lipoprotein (VLDL) cholesterol.
High-density lipoprotein (HDL) cholesterol.
Triglycerides (TG).

Significant findings include:

Total cholesterol greater than 200 mg/dL.
LDL cholesterol greater than 130 mg/dL.
TG greater than 250 mg/dL.

LDL can be determined using the following calculation when the triglyceride level is less than 400 mg/dL.

LDL cholesterol = Total cholesterol − (HDL cholesterol + TG/5).

Thyroid-stimulating hormone (TSH) level should be measured if hyperthyroidism is a suspected contributor to the hyperlipidemia.

Differential Diagnosis: Diagnosis of hyperlipidemia is determined by elevated serum cholesterol levels of greater than 200 mg/dL and/or triglycerides of greater than 150 mg/100 mL.

Treatment: Changing dietary habits is essential to lowering cholesterol level. Dietary restrictions of cholesterol (300 mg), along with a restriction of foods with saturated fats to less than 10% of total calories daily is recommended to reduce LDL cholesterol. For the frail older adult, secondary measures such as smoking cessation and control of hypertension may be more advantageous because malnutrition may occur inadvertently if certain foods are restricted, which is often a problem in older adults wih limited resources. Weight loss, aerobic exercise, and stress reduction may also be recommended for the stable, ambulatory older adult. Diet therapy with exercise and stress reduction should be initiated first for a 6-month trial period before initiating medications. If a patient's LDL is greater than 160 and additional risk factors exist or the LDL is greater than 190 with or without additional risk factors, then medication can be initiated. Lovastatin is recommended for use in older adults because of its low side effects. The initial dose is 20 mg with the evening meal, as tolerated. The dose may be increased, depending on the results of the follow-up cholesterol level, but should not exceed 80 mg/day. Liver function tests should be performed prior to the initial dose and then every 4–6 weeks during the first 12–15 months of treatment. Other HMG CoA Reductase agents include pravastatin (starting dose 10 mg) and simvastatin (starting dose 5 mg). Other cholesterol-lowering agents such as bile acid sequestrants and nicotinic acid, which are costly, have been found to interact with many common medications and require multiple doses throughout the day, are not recommended as first-line drug therapy in the older adult. Drug therapy is contraindicated in very advanced age and in patients in a debilitated state.

Follow-up: Inform patients and family members that medication therapy, laboratory testing, and lifestyle changes will become a way of life after the diagnosis of hyperlipidemia. Dietary changes should be monitored with repeat blood work first in 4–6 weeks and then at 3 months. If no improvement is found, drug therapy should be added. Monitoring laboratory studies should be done at 3-month intervals for the first year of therapy and every 6 months thereafter.

Sequelae: If dietary and lifestyle changes are made and adhered to, prognosis is good for reduction of serum cholesterol. If drug therapy is used, results are just as promising.

Prevention/Prophylaxis: Having lifelong dietary habits including less than 20 g of fat per day and following a moderate exercise regimen are the best prevention. The need for monitoring of total cholesterol levels throughout the patient's lifespan is emphasized.

Referral: Patients may benefit from a self-help group for dietary guidance such as Weight Watchers or TOPS.

Education: Patient and family require dietary instruction, exercise parameters, and stress reduction information.

Hyperthyroidism

Hyperthyroidism is an excessive amount of thyroid hormone in the body tissue.

Etiology: The most common cause of a new onset of hyperthyroidism in older adults is a toxic nodular goiter followed by Graves' disease and toxic adenoma. The multiple nodules of a toxic multinodular goiter are thought to produce thyroid hormone without TSH, resulting in thyrotoxicosis. Graves' disease, an autoimmune disease of unknown origin, is familial.

Occurrence: Less than 5% of people in the United States have hyperthyroidism.

Age: Of all cases of hyperthyroidism, 15%–25% occur in people 65 and older; People over age 60 compose about 10%–15% of individuals with hyperthyroidism.

Ethnicity: No significant evidence of ethnic prevalence exists.

Gender: Hyperthyroidism is more prevalent in women than in men. Although it has been shown that by age 70, the prevalence of the disease among men and women is almost equal.

Contributing Factors: Patients with other autoimmune problems are at risk for developing hyperthyroidism. A familial tendency for developing hyperthyroidism exists. Patients taking amiodarone or radiographic contrast media can develop iodine-induced hyperthyroidism.

Signs and Symptoms: Older patients may report weight loss, apathy, heat intolerance, weakness, insomnia, palpitations, nervousness, and anxiety. When questioned about their bowel habits, patients may report that they are no longer constipated. A reduction or increase in appetite may be revealed. Photophobia and blurred and/or double vision may be noted. Upon physical examination, ophthalmologic changes in the elderly such as exophthalmos are not as common. Lid lag is a more common finding. An enlarged thyroid occurs only in 20%–40% of patients age 70 and older. The examiner needs to remember that the thyroid is found lower in the neck and substernal in older adults than in a younger person. Because cardiac findings are very prevalent in older adults with hyperthyroidism, a thorough examination is essential. Tachycardia, atrial fibrillation, and congestive heart failure are common manifestations of untreated hyperthyroidism. A reduction in muscle mass may be detected, so muscle strength should be tested. Ask patients to demonstrate their ability to stand up from a seated position. A coarse tremor may be evident. Assess for signs of anemia such as pallor (Fig. 14–2).

Diagnostic Tests: In patients with hyperthyroidism, the TSH will be lower. The sensitive third-generation assay is a valuable screening test. If the test result for TSH is decreased, then a free T_4 test can be ordered; in hyperthyroidism, an elevation can be expected. If the T_4 test result is normal following a decreased TSH, then a serum T_3 test should be ordered. This value is sometimes increased, indicating T_3 toxicosis. If the T_3 result is also normal, then the patient is said to have subclinical disease. Radioactive iodine uptake (RAIU) is ordered to differentiate the cause of the thyrotoxicosis; this test result is usually elevated in the presence of hyperthyroidism. Other initial tests to consider include an electrolyte panel, blood urea nitrogen (BUN), and fasting glucose to look for electrolyte disturbances and a complete blood count (CBC) to determine the presence of anemia. Patients presenting with cardiac changes need an electrocardiogram (ECG).

Differential Diagnosis: Anxiety, diabetes mellitus, certain endocrine malignancies, and adrenal insufficiency are all probable candidates for the differential diagnosis of hyperthyroidism. Patients presenting with atrial fibrillation should be evaluated for thyroid disease.

Treatment: Hyperthyroidism needs immediate attention in older adults because it is usually associated with involvement of other organ systems, especially cardiac. Radioisotope therapy is the treatment of choice for toxic thyroid nodules and Graves' disease; however, patients should be in a euthyroid state before receiving radioactive iodine treatment. Patients may be treated with antithyroid agents initially. Beta-blockers are indicated in the early treatment of hyperthyroidism to control the cardiac symptoms of palpitations and tachycardia. Beta-blockers are not recommended for patients with bronchospasm, congestive heart failure, or insulin-dependent diabetics. Patients should be referred to an endocrinologist for treatment of hyperthyroidism.

Follow-up: Patients with hyperthyroidism require monitoring during the course of treatment to include thyroid studies, cardiac status, and changes in mental status. The patient must be aware of changes to note impending hypothyroidism once treatment has been initiated. Diagnostic studies, usually ordered by the patient's endocrinologist, include free T_4 and serum T_3 monitored every 6–8 weeks until a euthyroid state is achieved, and then TSH levels every 3 months for the first year, and twice yearly thereafter until the patient's condition is stable and he or she is asymptomatic for thyroid disease. Underlying anemia present when the patient was hyperthyroid needs reevaluation.

Sequelae: Complications that can develop in patients with hyperthyroidism include underlying ischemic heart disease, angina, cardiac arrhythmia, myocardial

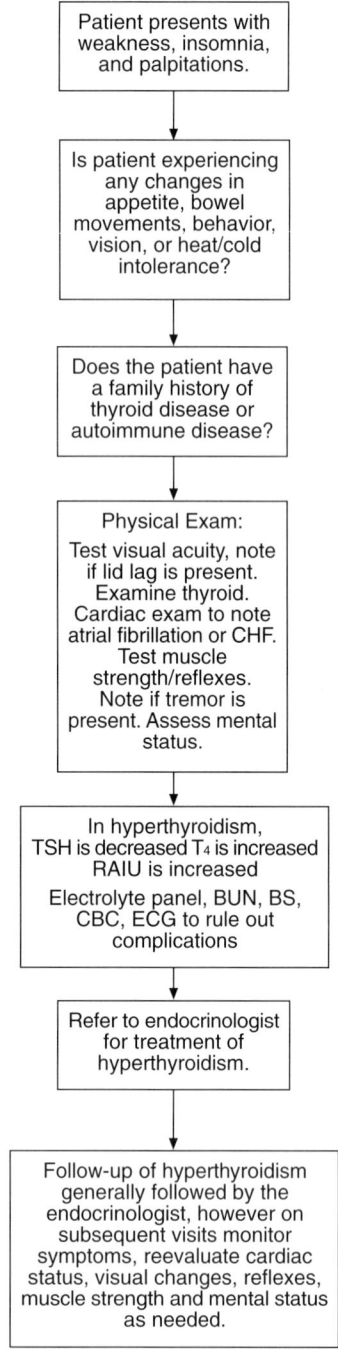

Patient presents with weakness, insomnia, and palpitations.

Is patient experiencing any changes in appetite, bowel movements, behavior, vision, or heat/cold intolerance?

Does the patient have a family history of thyroid disease or autoimmune disease?

Physical Exam:

Test visual acuity, note if lid lag is present. Examine thyroid. Cardiac exam to note atrial fibrillation or CHF. Test muscle strength/reflexes. Note if tremor is present. Assess mental status.

In hyperthyroidism, TSH is decreased T_4 is increased RAIU is increased

Electrolyte panel, BUN, BS, CBC, ECG to rule out complications

Refer to endocrinologist for treatment of hyperthyroidism.

Follow-up of hyperthyroidism generally followed by the endocrinologist, however on subsequent visits monitor symptoms, reevaluate cardiac status, visual changes, reflexes, muscle strength and mental status as needed.

FIGURE 14–2 Hyperthyroidism.

infarction, and congestive heart failure. Bone density may decrease also, rendering the patient susceptible to the development of osteoporosis.

Prevention/Prophylaxis: Hyperthyroidism is not known to be preventable. However, as thyroid disease is prevalent in the elderly, regular screening for signs and symptoms of hyperthyroidism is essential for older adults, especially those with a history of rheumatoid arthritis and other collagen diseases and diabetes mellitus.

Referral: Patients need to be referred to a radiotherapist for calculation of the dose of I_{131}. Patients with complicated hyperthyroidism should be treated by an endocrinologist, especially in the presence of atrial fibrillation and thyroid storm; these patients usually require hospitalization.

Education: Patients should note a change in their overall behavior following the initial treatment. Thus, patients must realize that they will need to take the prescribed medication daily and to continue with the radioactive iodine treatment. After patients have achieved the euthyroid state and received the radioactive iodine treatment, have them report to their health-care provider if they experience signs and symptoms of hypothyroidism or hyperthyroidism.

Hypothyroidism

Hypothyroidism occurs when the body tissues are subjected to subnormal amounts of thyroid hormone.

Etiology: Autoimmune thyroiditis is the most common cause of hypothyroidism in older adults. Persons who have had prior thyroid surgery or ablation of the thyroid are also susceptible to hypothyroidism.

Occurrence: Six percent of adults age 65 and over have hypothyroidism; however, up to 20% have subclinical hypothyroidism.

Age: Hypothyroidism predominantly begins at age 40, although the age of onset can continue through old age.

Ethnicity: No significant evidence of ethnic prevalence exists.

Gender: Hypothyroidism is more prevalent in women than in men.

Contributing Factors: Patients who have had extensive neck surgery or radiation or prior thyroid surgery without proper follow-up often develop hypothyroidism. Hypothyroidism can also result from pituitary disease and certain infiltrative diseases such as sarcoidosis and scleroderma. A relationship exists between contact with some environmental pollutants (e.g., fire retardation materials), fungicides, and coal conversion products and the development of hypothyroidism. Long-term lithium use can also be a contributor to the disease. Patients with first-degree relatives with thyroid disease are also at risk. Patients with insulin-dependent diabetes, rheumatoid arthritis, or Addison's disease should be routinely screened for thyroid disease.

Signs and Symptoms: Patients often present with weakness, myalgias, arthralgias, fatigue, cold intolerance, constipation, hair loss, leg cramps, hoarseness, tinnitus, paresthesia, reported weight changes, and depression. Patients or family members may report impaired memory or the inability to concentrate. If the disease has progressed untreated, patients appear apathetic and debilitated, with possible psychosis.

On physical examination, the overall appearance of the patient may reveal brittle nails, puffiness of the face and eyelids, thinning of the outer halves of the eyebrows, and dry skin. During the thyroid examination, the examiner should first observe the thyroid while the patient swallows and then proceed to the hands-on examination. If the thyroid gland is very tender to touch, the patient may have thyroiditis. A goiter may be present that feels rubbery, is not tender, and is possibly nodular. Thyroid nodules, which are very common in older adults, are benign if they feel smooth and easy to manipulate, whereas malignant nodules are hard, irregular, fixed, and tender on palpation. Bradycardia and cardiac enlargement may be detected during the cardiac examination; the diastolic blood pressure may be elevated. Bowel sounds may be diminished. A change in reflexes may be present, notably normal upstroke with a delay in the relaxation phase. Nonpitting edema may be found in the lower extremities. Patients should be examined for signs of carpal tunnel disease and cerebellar dysfunction to check for ataxia. Patients with secondary hypothyroidism may have diminished body hair and postural hypotension. A screening mental status examination should be performed. Note: Patients may be asymptomatic, with hypothyroidism discovered only during diagnostic testing (Fig. 14–3).

Diagnostic Tests: In patients with hypothyroidism, the TSH level is elevated. The sensitive third-generation assay is a valuable screening test. If the test result indicates increased TSH, then a free T_4 test can be ordered; in hypothyroidism, a decrease can be expected. If the T_4 result is normal following an increased TSH, then a serum T_3 test should be ordered. This result is sometimes decreased. If the T_3 result is also normal, then the patient is said to have subclinical disease. An RAIU test is not necessary in the workup for hypothyroidism. The presence of thyroid antibodies are useful in the diagnoses of subclinical hypothyroidism or goiter and Hashimoto's thyroiditis. An ECG typically shows sinus bradycardia, prolonged QT intervals, and possibly atrioventricular block and conduction disturbances.

Differential Diagnosis: In determining whether or not a patient has hypothyroidism, the first thing to consider is whether the disease is primary or secondary hypothyroidism. Hashimoto's thyroiditis, postirradiation disease, subacute thyroiditis, iodide deficiency, and subtotal thyroidectomy can cause primary hypothyroidism. People who have pituitary hyposecretion, pituitary tumors, and

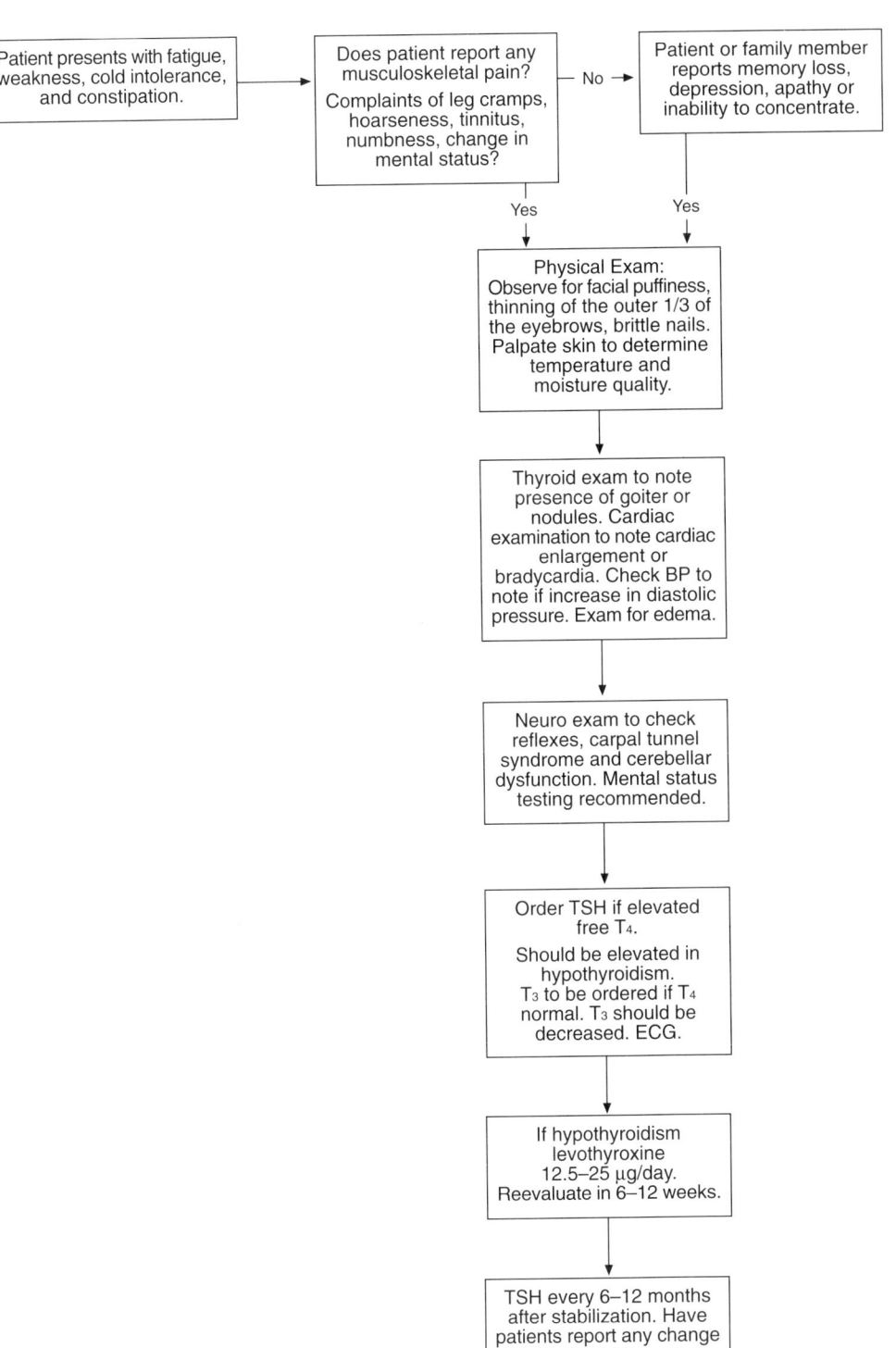

FIGURE 14–3 Hypothyroidism.

some infiltrative diseases (e.g., sarcoidosis) are susceptible to secondary hypothyroidism. In the older adult, when there are numerous signs and symptoms of hypothyroidism, an increased number of these clinical findings point to thyroid disease. However, consider dementia, anemia, and depression, among other conditions, when making the diagnosis.

Treatment: Older adults with an underactive thyroid are prescribed levothyroxine for lifelong treatment. The starting dose in older adults is 12.5–25 μg/day. Patients should then be reevaluated in 8–12 weeks for assessment of clinical presentation and TSH level. Patients may continue to have increased TSH levels, yet show signs of clinical improvement. Excessive doses of levothyroxine induce osteoporosis. Older adults with cardiac disease should receive no more than 25 μg/day. A thorough medication history is necessary when prescribing levothyroxine; cholestyramine, ferrous sulfate, sucralfate, and antacids, containing aluminum hydroxide can reduce the effectiveness of this medication. Phenytoin, carbamazepine, rifampin, and anticoagulants may increase the drug metabolism. Patients taking any of these medications with levothyroxine should allow a 4- to 6-hr interval between the medications. Dietary fiber can also interfere with absorption so suggest taking the levothyroxine on an empty stomach in the morning.

Follow-up: Patients should have a routine TSH evaluation every 6–12 months after stabilization. Patients with secondary hypothyroidism need a free T_4 test. Monitor clinical signs in all patients.

Sequelae: Patients with untreated hypothyroidism may develop coronary artery disease because of the increase in low-density lipoprotein and triglyceride levels associated with this disorder. Megacolon may occur in patients with a long history of untreated hypothyroidism. Myxedema coma with hypothermia and hypotension is a complication of severe untreated hypothyroidism.

Prevention/Prophylaxis: Regular screening for thyroid disease is advocated for people age 60 and older, especially those with insulin-dependent diabetes, rheumatoid arthritis and other collagen-related disorders, and with a family history of thyroid disease.

Referral: If the patient has numerous complications or is not responding to treatment despite compliance, refer him or her to an endocrinologist.

Education: Because patients should note an improvement in their overall behavior following the initial treatment, they should realize that they need to take the prescribed medication daily. Tell patients not to increase their dosage even if they are experiencing symptoms of hypothyroidism; rather they should contact their health-care provider. Any unexplained weight gain of 5 lb or more should be reported. Encourage patients to increase their activity level. Alert patients to contact their health-care provider if they experience signs and symptoms of hypothyroidism or hyperthyroidism.

Malnutrition

Protein-calorie malnutrition is diagnosed when a patient's serum albumin level is less than 3.5 g/dL.

Etiology: Although a number of factors can lead to malnutrition in older adults, certain age-associated factors are precursors to malnutrition in persons 85 and over, including reduced food and micronutrient intake, decreased absorption of ingested food, and the increased bodily demands for protein, calories, or micronutrients because of physiologic stressors. Decreases in metabolic rate, physical activity, and sensory input can also contribute to malnutrition.

Occurrence: More than 6 million older adults are at high risk for malnutrition.

Age: Malnutrition can occur at any age. Frail older adults and people over age 80 are at the highest risk for malnutrition.

Ethnicity: Because the reasons for malnutrition vary, no specific ethnic prevalence is known.

Gender: Malnutrition in people age 85 and over is more prevalent in women because of the higher number of women than men in this age bracket.

Contributing Factors: Any of several factors may contribute to malnutrition in older adults: poverty, decreased olfactory sensitivity, loss of taste buds, being edentulous, certain chronic diseases such as intestinal ischemia, hyperthyroidism, depression, chronic obstructive pulmonary disease, alcoholism, chronic impaction, malabsorption syndromes, dementia, obesity, and cholelithiasis. Hospitalization with a restricted diet, drug-nutrient interactions related to polypharmacy, and social isolation also may contribute to malnutrition.

Signs and Symptoms: Assessment of malnutrition is complex because it involves investigation of physiologic, psychological, pathologic, functional, and financial parameters to determine the possible causes of the malnutrition. In patients with suspected malnutrition, all risk factors for poor nutritional status should be assessed using objective measures as indicated (i.e., depression scales, mental status scales, functional status tests). It is important to determine a patient's educational level and financial situation. Review medications to determine if the patient is taking any substance that can cause anorexia such as digoxin, quinidine, or hydralazine. During the physical examination, discern if the malnutrition is related to cardiac, respiratory, intestinal, endocrine, hepatic, neurological, or renal impairment. Look for specific signs of nutritional deficiencies such as nail abnormalities, brittle hair, bruises, skin color (jaundice, pallor), cheilosis, glossitis, loss of subcutaneous body fat, muscle wasting, and edema. Explore any unexplained weight loss to rule out treatable causes of malnutrition. If a patient is found to be 15% or more below body weight or had a recent loss of 10% under baseline weight, consider protein-calorie malnutrition. Body mass index (weight in kg/height in m^2) should range from 24–27 kg/m^2 in healthy older adults; below 20 kg/m² indicates a serious caloric deficit. In older adults, mid-arm circumference (MAC) and triceps skinfold (TSF) measurement is not an accurate means for testing for malnutrition; however, as an estimate, a MAC or TSF measurement below the 10th percentile indicates poor nutritional status.

Diagnostic Tests: If a specific nutritional deficiency is suspected, direct measurement of the serum vitamin or mineral (e.g., serum folate, iron) can be ordered. In screening for malnutrition, laboratory values should be considered only as an indirect measurement. A complete blood count should be ordered to determine any protein, iron, folate, and/or vitamin B_{12} deficiencies. Total lymphocyte counts less than 1500 cells/mm³ are found in mild to moderate malnutrition; a total of less than 1000 cells/mm³ is associated with immune paralysis. Serum albumin levels less than 3.5 mg/dL indicate protein depletion. Serum albumin levels can be skewed in patients experiencing urinary loss from the nephrotic syndrome or in those receiving intravenous fluids. Because the half-life of albumin is 18 days, serum albumin levels rise slowly following nutritional supplementation. A decrease in the serum transferrin levels also points to malnutrition. In patients with coexisting iron-deficiency anemia, however, the results will be misleading (normal to elevated serum transferrin). Total cholesterol levels below 160 mg/dL are also considered a marker for malnutrition.

Differential Diagnosis: When determining if a person is suffering from malnutrition, discern if any of the following conditions coexist: dental problems, dementia, depression, chronic infection, neoplasia, or failure to thrive.

Treatment: Identifying the contributing factors to malnutrition in each individual patient is essential to treating this condition. When possible, a diet history should be obtained to determine the severity of the nutritional deprivation. All medications that can cause drug-induced malnutrition should be discontinued or reconsidered or an alternative should be used. Any fecal impaction should be removed. Because not all factors, such as alterations in sensory input, can be treated, dietary consultation should be ordered to assist in the diagnosis of malnutrition and planning of diet supplementation. Any older person experiencing a physiologic stressor such as surgery, infection, or trauma usually requires an increase in protein, calories, and micronutrients. If the patient has been diagnosed with protein-energy undernutrition (PEU), nutritional support will depend on the patient's medical condition and the degree of the PEU.

Follow-up: Patients who are hospitalized for malnutrition or who develop malnutrition secondary to an acute-care hospitalization should be monitored daily for response to the nutritional supplementation. The patient's weight should be monitored closely until the malnutrition has been corrected. If a psychosocial factor contributed to the malnutrition, periodic review of the patient's improvement is warranted. Community-dwelling older adults may benefit from a nurse case manager to follow their progress in the home.

Sequelae: An older person's initial reaction to prescribed nutrient supplements may result in electrolyte abnormalities, hyperglycemia, hypotension, and aspiration pneumonia. Long-term malnutrition increases the risk of morbidity and mortality. Careful assessment is necessary to determine if a patient is suffering from failure to thrive.

Prevention/Prophylaxis: Given the number of older adults who are at risk for malnutrition, the health-care provider must periodically screen patients for nutritional deficits. In 1991 the Nutritional Initiative Program developed a patient self-assessment checklist. The nine-item DETERMINE Your Nutritional Health Checklist can be completed by coherent older adults. The letters in DETERMINE stand for:

Disease.
Eating poorly.
Tooth loss and mouth pain.
Economic hardship.
Reduced social contact.
Multiple medicines.
Involuntary weight loss or gain.
Needs assistance in self-care.
Elder years greater than age 80.

There are 21 total points on the checklist. A score of 3–5 indicates a moderate nutritional risk; a score of 6 or more places the patient at high nutritional risk. If the score on the DETERMINE checklist indicates a need for further assessment, or if the patient is unable to complete the DETERMINE checklist, then the level I and level II screening tests may be used.

Referral: Referring patients who are malnourished to a specialist depends on the identifiable cause of the nutrition depletion. A dietitian should be consulted for a nutritional support evaluation. Refer patients who need long-term enteral support to a gastroenterologist for consideration of a percutaneous endoscopic gastrostomy or, in some cases, a feeding jejunostomy. Arrangements can be made for the community-dwelling older adult to receive Meals on Wheels. Provide information on the location of centers for congregate meals sites. For the patient diagnosed with a terminal illness, discuss the patient's and family's decision on nutritional support before beginning any intervention. If social isolation, low income, and/or functional status contributed to the development of malnutrition, the patient should be referred for social services and/or discharge planning.

Education: For the alert ambulatory older adult, review the Dietary Guidelines for Americans and the Food Pyramid (see Fig. 2–1). Teach family members caring for cognitively impaired or physically disabled older adults about dietary requirements and nutritional supplementation.

Obesity

Obesity is most often defined as being 20% above IBW; severe or morbid obesity, as 40% above IBW.

Etiology: The etiology of obesity is unknown. Obesity is highly familial and hereditary, involving constitutional and psychological factors.

Occurrence: Obesity is the most common nutritional disorder in the United States. In the United States 34 million people are obese and 13 million morbidly obese.

Age: Obesity rarely begins in the older adult; it is usually a lifelong process.

Ethnicity: African-American women have more of a tendency to be obese than do white women.

Gender: Obesity is more prevalent in women than in men.

Contributing Factors: Familial tendency, sedentary lifestyle, lack of dietary instruction, social impetus to eat, mood and hormone fluctuation, environmental stressors, metabolism, endocrine disorders, boredom, medications, and preexisting diseases may contribute to the development of obesity.

Signs and Symptoms: Obesity is recognized when a patient's weight is 20% above IBW. A thorough nutritional assessment is warranted. Symptoms resulting from obesity include arthralgia, lethargy, headaches, and alopecia. As part of the physical examination, determine the degree and distribution of the patient's body fat. Look for secondary causes of obesity, such as hypothyroidism or Cushing's syndrome.

Diagnostic Tests: Lipid profile and fasting glucose levels should be obtained for all obese patients. If an endocrine disorder is suspected:

TSH levels should be ordered to rule out hypothyroidism.

Dexamethasone suppression testing is suggested to determine presence of Cushing's syndrome.

Differential Diagnosis: Determine the IBW for height: Patients 20% above IBW are considered obese; those 40% above IBW are morbidly obese.

Treatment: Weight loss, with reductions of salt, fat, and carbohydrates in the diet is recommended. Patients should increase their activity level and participate in group therapy or self-help groups (i.e., Weight Watchers, TOPS, Diet Center). Diet suppressants are not recommended for older adults.

Follow-up: Return visits should occur as often as needed to monitor weight reduction and achieve the goal set for the patient.

Sequelae: Coronary artery disease, diabetes, and hypertension are all much more prevalent in obese individuals.

Prevention/Prophylaxis: A low-fat nutritionally adequate diet and regular exercise help prevent and/or treat obesity.

Referral: Morbidly obese patients may require surgical intervention, but most obese persons can be treated by primary care practitioners. Patients may be referred to the local Weight Watchers or TOPS organization.

Education: Teach patients and significant others meal preparation, calorie counts, and fat gram calculation. Elimination of alcohol and fatty foods is essential. Encourage patients to begin a safe exercise regimen.

Pancreatic Cancer

Pancreatic cancer, found primarily in older adults, is one of the leading causes of death in this population. Eighty percent of exocrine neoplasms of the pancreas occur in the head of the pancreas, with the remaining 20% occurring in the body and tail. The types of pancreatic cancer are as follows:

- Ductal cell adenocarcinoma, accounting for more than 75% of all types of pancreatic cancers.
- Giant cell carcinoma, which is highly malignant.
- Adenosquamous carcinoma, common in patients with a history of radiation treatment.
- Cystadenocarcinoma.

Etiology: Although the etiology of pancreatic cancer is unknown, a number of predisposing factors such as cigarette smoking, carcinogens in the environment (e.g., coal tar derivatives), diabetes mellitus, and heredity may be precursors to pancreatic cancer.

Occurrence: Pancreatic cancer is the fourth most common cause of death from cancer, accounting for 13% of gastrointestinal malignancies. The incidence of pancreatic cancer appears to be highest in people from urban areas and in the lower socioeconomic classes.

Age: Pancreatic cancer usually appears in persons age 60–80, with the peak time of onset in the ninth decade.

Ethnicity: Exocrine pancreatic cancer is higher in African-Americans and in people of Hawaiian descent than in whites.

Gender: Pancreatic cancer is more prevalent in men than in women.

Contributing Factors: Pancreatic cancer is more common in heavy cigarette smokers than in nonsmokers. Persons with a history of familial colorectal cancer, polyposis syndrome, and diabetes mellitus are susceptible to pancreatic cancer.

Signs and Symptoms: Older adults with pancreatic cancer often present with anorexia, weight loss, anxiety, diarrhea, and depression and may report that these symptoms have existed for the past 3–6 months. Complaints of epigastric pain radiating to the back, unexplained weight loss, and in some cases steatorrhea are common. Jaundice appears with progression of the disease, and patients may complain of itching. Symptoms of diabetes may appear or worsen. During the abdominal examination, you may find a palpable gallbladder (Courvoisier's sign), hepatomegaly, overall abdominal tenderness, and possibly evidence of ascites. Thrombophlebitis occurs in a small percentage of patients (Fig. 14–4).

Diagnostic Tests: Laboratory findings for pancreatic cancer may include a mild anemia, and, in 10%–20% of cases, signs of diabetes mellitus such as glycosuria and hyperglycemia. Liver function test results may be abnormal, suggesting obstructive jaundice. The serum amylase level may be elevated. CT of the abdomen is recommended as the first imaging test to diagnose pancreatic cancer. CT or magnetic resonance imaging (MRI) can detect a mass in about 80% of cases. The mass is then confirmed using a CT-guided needle aspiration biopsy of the pancreas. If the mass is located at the pancreaticobiliary junction, an endoscopic retrograde cholangiopancreatography (ERCP) may verify a biliary or ampullary tumor.

Differential Diagnosis: The following conditions may mimic the presentation of pancreatic cancer: choledocholithiasis, pancreatitis, duodenal neoplasms, choledochal cyst, pancreatic pseudocyst, and biliary tract stricture.

Treatment: Given the poor prognosis of pancreatic cancer combined with the advanced age of the patient, treatment is usually limited to palliative measures. For patients with nonmetastatic lesions located in the head of the pancreas, pancreatoduodenectomy (Whipple's procedure) may be recommended. In some cases, a specialist may recommend use of a biliary stent to reduce the jaundice and itching. Control of pain is essential; analgesics and oral narcotics should be ordered. An antihistamine can be prescribed to control the pruritus.

Follow-up: Emotional support and pain control are critical for patients with pancreatic cancer. Because the progression of the disease can be quite rapid, patients and their families may need assistance in preparing for end-of-life decisions.

Sequelae: The prognosis of pancreatic cancer in older adults is very grim. The mortality rate for adenocarcinoma of the pancreas is very high shortly after diagnosis.

Prevention/Prophylaxis: Cessation of alcohol consumption and cigarette smoking is recommended.

Referral: Refer to an oncologist when the diagnosis of pancreatic cancer is suspected. Contact local hospice care services for the patient and family.

Education: For their nutritional needs, advise patients to consume six small meals a day instead of the usual three. Patients may prefer nutritional supplements

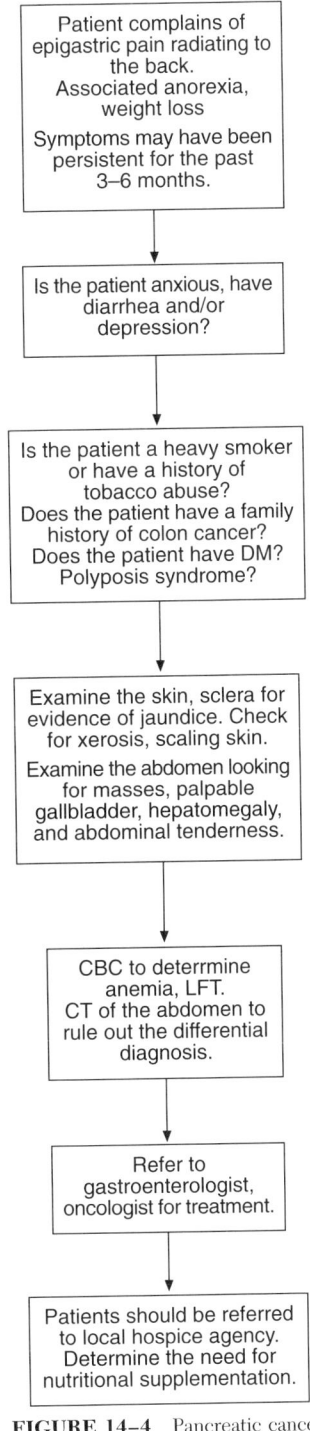

FIGURE 14–4 Pancreatic cancer.

in place of one or more of these meals each day. When the disease has reached the terminal stage, assure the patient that you will collaborate with the hospice agency to provide for the patient's comfort throughout the disease process.

BIBLIOGRAPHY

General

Abrams, W, Beers, MH, and Berkow, R: The Merck Manual of Geriatrics, ed 2. Merck Research Laboratories, Whitehouse Station, NJ, 1995.

Bullock, BL, and Rosendal, PP: Pathophysiology: Adaptations and Alterations in Function, ed 3. JB Lippincott, Philadelphia, 1992.

DeGowin, R: DeGowin and DeGowin's Bedside Diagnostic Examination. McGraw-Hill, New York, 1987.

Duespoke, TA: Nursing Diagnosis Manual for the Well and Ill Client. WB Saunders, Philadelphia, 1989.

Kane, R, et al: Essentials of Clinical Geriatrics, ed 2. McGraw-Hill, Philadelphia, 1989.

Lueckennotte, A: Pocket Guide to Gerontological Assessment, ed 2. CV Mosby, St Louis, 1994.

Schroeder, S, et al: Current Medical Diagnosis and Treatment. Appleton and Lange, Stamford, CT, 1991.

Semla, TP, Beizer, JL, and Higbee, MD: Geriatric Dosage Handbook: 1995–1996, ed 2. Lexi-Comp Inc, Hudson, OH, 1995.

Staab, AS, and Lyles, MF: Manual of Geriatric Nursing. Scott, Foresman/Little Brown Higher Education, 1993.

Wilson, JD, Martin, JB, Fauci, A, and Kasper, D (eds): Harrison's Principles of Internal Medicine, ed 13. McGraw-Hill, New York, 1994.

Assessment

Linton, AD, Lee, P, and Matteson, MA: Age-related changes in the endocrine system. In Matteson, MA, McConnell, ES, and Linton, AD (eds): Gerontological Nursing Concepts and Practice, ed 2. WB Saunders, Philadelphia, 1996.

Chronic Pancreatitis

Richter, JR: Management of pancreatitis. In Goroll, AH, May, LA, and Mulley, AG (eds): Primary Care Medicine: Office Evaluation of the Adult Patient, ed 3. JB Lippincott, Philadelphia, 1995.

Diabetes

American Diabetes Association Publications, July 1997.

Goldberg, AP, Andres, R, and Bierman, EL: Diabetes Mellitus in the Elderly. In Hazzard, WR, Andres R, Bierman, EL, and Blass, JP (eds): Principle of Geriatric Medicine and Geronotology, ed 2. McGraw-Hill, New York, 1990.

Reed, RL, and Mooradian, AD: Treatment of diabetes in the elderly. Am Fam Physician 44:3, 1991.

Palmer, CF: Special Issues in the Management of the Elderly Patient with Diabetes, Mt Sinai J Of Scientific American, Inc. Diabetes Mellitus, chap IV, 1993.

Hyperlipidemia

Ball, M, and Mann, J: Lipids and Heart Disease: A Guide for the Primary Care Team, ed 2. Oxford University Press, 1994.

Braunwald, E: Heart Disease: A Textbook of Cardiovascular Medicine. WB Saunders, Philadephia, 1988.

Glueck, C, et al: Using two-drug therapy safely for refractory mixed hyperlipidemia. Cardiology Board Review 10:6, 1993.

Kreisberg, RA: Low high density lipoprotein cholesterol: What does it mean, what can we do about it, and what should we do about it? Am J Med 94:1, 1993.
Manninen, V, et al: Identifying high-risk hyperlipidemia likely to respond to drug treatment. Cardiology Board Review 9:12, 1992.
Robinson, JG, and Hunninghake, DB: Practical management for hyperlipidemia. Contemporary Internal Medicine 7:15, 1995.
Stein, Y: The hyperlipidemic subject with multiple risk factors: A comprehensive approach. Am J Med 96:6A, 1994.
Wilson, JD, Martin, JB, Fauci, A, and Kasper, D (eds): Harrison's Principles of Internal Medicine, ed 13. McGraw-Hill, New York, 1994.

Hyperthyroidism

Aronow, WS: The heart and thyroid disease. Clin Geriatr Med 11:219, 1995.
Begancy, T: Thyroid disease: When to screen, when to treat. Patient Care 18, 1997.
Clutter, WE: Endocrine diseases. In Carey, CF, Lee, HH, and Woeltje, KT (eds): The Washington Manual of Therapeutics, ed 29. Lippincott-Raven, Philadelphia, 1998.
Gambert, S: Hyperthyroidism in the elderly. Clin Geriatr Med 11:181, 1995.
Garcia, M, et al: AACE clinical practice guidelines for the evaluation and treatment of hyperthyroidism and hypothyroidism. Endocr Pract 1:56, 1995.
Singer, PA, et al: Treatment guidelines for patients with hyperthyroidism and hypothyroidism. JAMA 273:802, 1995.
Wheeler, SF: Thyroid disease. In Mengel, MB, and Schwiebert, LP (eds): Ambulatory Medicine: The Primary Care of Families, ed 2. Appleton and Lange, Stamford, CT, 1996.

Hypothyroidism

Aronow, WS: The heart and thyroid disease. Clin Geriatr Med 11:219, 1995.
Barzel, US: Hypothyroidism: Diagnosis and management. Clin Geriatr Med 11:239, 1995.
Begancy, T: Thyroid disease: When to screen, when to treat. Patient Care 18, 1997.
Garcia, M, et al: AACE clinical practice guidelines for the evaluation and treatment of hyperthyroidism and hypothyroidism. Endocr Pract 1:56, 1995.
Goroll, AH: Approach to the patient with hypothyroidism. In Goroll, AH, May, LA, and Mulley, AG (eds): Primary Care Medicine: Office Evaluation of the Adult Patient, ed 3. JB Lippincott, Philadelphia, 1995.
Sawain, CT: Subclinical hypothyroidism in older persons. Clin Geriatr Med 11:239, 1995.
Singer, PA, et al: Treatment guidelines for patients with hyperthyroidism and hypothyroidism. JAMA 273:802, 1995.
Wheeler, SF: Thyroid disease. In Mengel, MB, and Schwiebert, LP (eds): Ambulatory Medicine: The Primary Care of Families, ed 2. Appleton and Lange, Stamford, Conn, 1996.

Malnutrition

Barrocas, A, Belcher, D, Champagne, C, and Jastram, C: Nutritional assessment practical approaches. Clin Geriatr Med 11:675, 1995.
Ham, RJ: The signs and symptoms of poor nutritional status. Prim Care 21:33, 1994.
Lipschitz, DA: Approaches to the nutritional support of the older patient. Clin Geriatr Med 11:715, 1995.
Longergan, ET, and Sweeny-Soiffer, MS: Nutrition. In Lonergan, ET (ed): Geriatrics, ed 1. Appleton and Lange. Stamford, Conn, 1996.
Roubenoff, R, and Roubenoff, R: Nutritional issues in acute illness. In Stobo, JD, et al (eds): The principles and practice of medicine, ed 23. Appleton and Lange, Stamford, Conn, 1996.
The Nutrition Screening Initiative: Incorporating nutrition screening and interventions into medical practice: A monograph for physicians. The Nutrition Screening Initiative, Washington, DC, 1994.

Obesity

Baron, RS: Nutrition. In Tierney, LM, McPhee, SJ, and Papadakis, MA (eds): Current Medical Diagnosis and Treatment, ed 36. Appleton and Lange, Stamford, CT, 1997.

Bodenheimer, T, et al: Helping your patients control their weight. Intern Med 15:6, 1994.

Pancreatic Cancer

Bresalier, RS, and Duh, Q-Y: Gastrointestinal neoplasms. In Lonergan, ET (ed): Geriatrics, ed 1. Appleton and Lange, Stamford, CT, 1996.

Everhart, J, and Wright, D: Diabetes mellitus as a risk factor for pancreatic cancer: A meta-analysis. JAMA 273:1605, 1995.

Hammel, P, et al: Preoperative cyst fluid analysis is useful for the differential diagnosis of cystic lesions of the pancreas. Gastroenterology 108:1230, 1995.

Mercer, L, and Saltzstein, EC: Pancreatic cancer: Exocrine. In Griffith, HW, and Dambro, MR (eds): The 5 Minute Clinical Consultant, ed 2. Lea & Febiger, Philadelphia, 1994.

CHAPTER 15

HEMATOLOGIC AND

IMMUNE SYSTEM

DISORDERS

Many factors affect patients' hemolytic and immune status. The assessment process includes a detailed history, physical examination, and diagnostic testing. The presenting symptom of hemolytic deficiency can include excessive bruising, petechiae, unexplained bleeding (epistaxis), or inflamed lymph nodes. Elderly patients with severe anemia may complain of fatigue, dizziness, heart palpitation, headache, shortness of breath with exertion, exercise intolerance, confusion (alteration in mental status), depression, and cold intolerance.

The medical history obtained from the patient should include past history of anemia, hemoglobin abnormalities (thalassemia), vitamin C or K deficiency, recent surgery or blood transfusion, and clotting disorders. Also inquire about any occupational or other known exposure to toxic agents or radiation, family history of anemia, current medications, and any other chronic disease.

Some of the most common causes of hemolytic disease in the elderly include iron-deficiency anemia, anemia of chronic disease, and pernicious anemia (vitamin B_{12} deficiency, which has an increased incidence in patients over age 60). Systemic disease and severe clotting disorders need to be included in the differential diagnosis.

The physical examination should be complete and thorough. Assess the eyes for pale conjunctivae and icteric sclera, which occur with pernicious anemia. Inspect the color of the skin, noting any ashen or yellow changes. Check for petechiae, bruising, and pale mucous membranes. Assess the nails for the presence of concave "spoon" nails, seen with iron deficiency. A red, painful, beefy tongue

395

can be present with pernicious anemia. Palpate the abdomen for any splenomegaly or tenderness. Tachypnea and tachycardia can be seen with severe anemia. Auscultate the heart for any systolic murmurs. If blood loss is suspected and the history warrants, a rectal examination to assess for guaiac-positive stools is performed. Finally, determine whether any mental status changes have occurred; do a complete neurologic examination, checking cranial nerve function and deep tendon reflexes. The absence or presence of physical findings on examination helps to narrow the clinical diagnosis.

Diagnostic tests done to complete the hemolytic assessment include the following:

- Complete blood count (CBC) with differential; check red blood cells (RBCs), hemoglobin (Hgb), hematocrit (Hct), mean corpuscular volume (MCV), mean corpuscular hemoglobin concentration (MCHC).
- Iron, total iron-binding capacity (TIBC), ferritin if iron-deficiency or microcytic anemia is considered.
- Reticulocyte count to assess for the blood loss or blood cell destruction.
- Hbg electrophoresis to assess for hemoglobin abnormalities or thalassemia.
- Vitamin B_{12} and folate levels to rule out pernicious anemia.

The presentation or complaints of immunologic disease may be vague and nonspecific. Elderly patients may present with chronic fatigue, frequent or recurrent illness, weight loss, lymphadenopathy, depression, or recurrent infections. As stated earlier, a complete medical history should be obtained. Inquire about past history of any sexually transmitted diseases (STDs) such as syphilis, recent travel, tick bite, risk factors for human immunodeficiency virus (HIV), recent immunization or surgery, and medication use. The general physical examination should note any weight loss or wasting, skin changes, or lymphadenopathy. The history and physical examination provides the baseline for the plan of care and necessary diagnostic testing. The general laboratory tests ordered should include a CBC with differential (platelet count), urinalysis, electrolyte panel (random or fasting glucose levels to assess for diabetes), erythrocyte sedimentation rate (ESR), and rapid plasma reagin (RPR). Tests to rule out more specific disease include titers for HIV, Lyme disease, Epstein-Barr virus (EBV), toxoplasmosis, and cytomegalovirus (CMV). Clinical consultation with a physician or experienced nurse practitioner may be necessary to work up the elderly patient with suspected immunologic suppression or disease.

This assessment can be complex requiring a thorough examination and diagnostic testing. Consultation and referral may be needed to ensure that the appropriate diagnosis is made.

Human Immunodeficiency Virus

Human immunodeficiency virus (HIV), a human retrovirus, is the infectious agent that causes acquired immune deficiency syndrome (AIDS). Two types of HIV have been identified: HIV-1 and HIV-2. Even though the viruses share similar epidemiologic traits, they are serologically and geographically distinct. HIV-1, the more pathogenic of the two, is found worldwide, with infection being most prevalent in the sub-Saharan regions of Africa, the Americas, Western Europe, and South and Southeast Asia. The HIV-2 virus resides primarily in West Africa; cases in other areas have been epidemiologically linked to West Africa.

Etiology: HIV, the etiologic agent for AIDS, is spread by contact with parenteral and body fluids. The three known modes of transmission are:

Contact with blood and blood products: needle sharing, transfusions.
Sexual transmission: anal, oral, or vaginal intercourse.
Perinatal transmission: in utero, during delivery, through breast-feeding.

Occurrence: HIV occurs worldwide; the World Health Organization (WHO) estimates that more than 10 million people have HIV. The United States has reported the largest number of cases, with approximately 500,000 full-blown AIDS cases by 1995. An estimated 1.5 million people with HIV in the United States are asymptomatic.

Age: HIV occurs in all age groups; 11% of all AIDS cases reported to the Centers for Disease Control (CDC) have involved patients over age 50, with 3% being over age 60. Older patients with AIDS are likely to die sooner from the disease; in a recent study, 37% of patients over age 80 died within a month after diagnosis.

Ethnicity: Not significant.

Gender: More men than women have HIV; however, the largest rate of increase in reported AIDS cases is currently in women.

Contributing Factors: High-risk behaviors such as engaging in unprotected heterosexual or homosexual sex can lead to HIV infection. The older patient is much less likely to use a condom because there is no fear of pregnancy. The frequency of sexual contact and number of sexual partners also affect an individual's risk for getting HIV. Postmenopausal women are more likely to have lesions of vaginal mucous membranes, owing to atrophic changes. Intravenous (IV) drug use is a risk factor, particularly with shared needles. Blood transfusion with contaminated blood is another contributing factor. Possibly, the immune system changes that occur with aging may render older patients more susceptible to contracting the virus once they have encountered it.

Signs and Symptoms: In the initial asymptomatic phase of HIV infection, the patient does not have any symptoms. In the older patient, the first sign may be confusion or AIDS-related dementia. Vague signs and symptoms such as weight loss, dehydration, ataxic gait, fatigue, or withdrawal may go unnoticed or be attributed to other illnesses. Because the index of suspicion is generally low in the older patient, the diagnosis may never be made. A sexual history is critical in exposing risk factors. Once the possibility has been established, permission for diagnostic testing should be obtained. The presence of disseminated herpes zoster, vaginal or oral candidiasis, or tuberculosis should raise the index of suspicion for HIV.

Diagnostic Tests: HIV diagnosis requires a positive enzyme-linked immunosorbent assay (ELISA) test result, followed by a confirmatory positive Western blot test result. Once the diagnosis has been confirmed, a pretreatment plasma HIV RNA level and a CD4+ T-cell count should be obtained (see Treatment; Table 15–1).

Differential Diagnosis: Differential diagnosis in the older patient with HIV includes Alzheimer's dementia, influenza, depression, malabsorption, malnutrition, occult malignancy, tuberculosis, and pneumonia.

Treatment: Although every attempt has been made to offer accurate and complete information, because of the rapidly changing nature of HIV treatment practitioners should seek out the latest guidelines before starting therapy. No specific

TABLE 15–1   INDICATIONS FOR PLASMA HIV RNA TESTING*

Clinical Indication	Information	Use
Syndrome consistent with acute HIV infection	Establishes diagnosis when HIV antibody test result is negative or indeterminate	Diagnosis†
Initial evaluation of newly diagnosed HIV infection	Baseline viral load "set-point"	Decision to start or defer therapy
Every 3–4 months in patients not receiving therapy	Changes in viral load	Decision to start therapy
4–8 weeks after initiation of antiretroviral therapy	Initial assessment of drug efficacy	Decision to continue or change therapy
3–4 months after start of therapy	Maximal effect of therapy	Decision to continue or change therapy
Every 3–4 months in patients receiving therapy	Durability of antiretroviral effect	Decision to continue or change therapy
Clinical event or significant decline in CD4+ T cells	Association with changing or stable viral load	Decision to continue, initiate, or change therapy

° Acute illness (e.g., bacterial pneumonia, tuberculosis, herpes simplex virus (HSV), *Pneumonia carinii* pneumonia [PCP], and so on) and immunizations can cause increases in plasma HIV RNA for 2–4 weeks; viral load testing should not be performed during this time. Plasma HIV RNA results should usually be verified with a repeat determination before starting or making changes in therapy. HIV RNA determinations should always be measured using the same laboratoy and the same assay.

† Diagnosis of HIV infection made by HIV RNA testing should be confirmed by standard methods such as Western blot serology performed 2–4 months after the initial indeterminate or negative test result.

Source: Centers for Disease Control and Prevention: Report of the NIH Panel to Define Principles of Therapy of HIV Infection and Guidelines for the Use of Antiretroviral Agents in HIV-infected Adults and Adolescents. MMWR 47 (No. RR-5): 75. US Government Printing Office, Washington, DC, 1998.

guidelines exist at present for treatment specific to the older adult with HIV. Adult and adolescent guidelines are used.

Before treatment, obtain a HIV RNA level (baseline viral load set-point) and a CD4+ T-cell count, preferably on two different occasions, using the same laboratory both times, to ensure accuracy and consistency. Patients presenting with advanced disease should be treated after the initial measurement. If the patient is not treated, HIV RNA levels should continue to be measured every 3–4 months; CD4+ T cells should be measured every 3–6 months.

Patients are divided into two categories for discussion: asymptomatic infection or symptomatic disease including AIDS. All patients with symptomatic disease should be offered antiretroviral therapy. Treatment of asymptomatic patients presents a complex situation. Studies have shown that antiretroviral therapy is clinically beneficial to HIV-infected patients with advanced disease and immunosuppression. However, the treatment options available that offer the maximum benefit are medically complex, with a high incidence of side effects and interactions. The challenge, then, is achieving patient compliance. The HIV specialist and the patient must consider many factors before deciding on treatment during this asymptomatic stage. (Complete guidelines for further information in this area can be found on the CDC website.)

Once a decision has been made to initiate therapy in either category, the following studies should be performed:

Complete history and physical examination.
CBC, chemistry profile.
CD4+ T lymphocyte count.
Plasma HIV RNA measurement.

Routine studies pertinent to prevention of opportunistic infections include:

Venereal disease research laboratory (VDRL) test, purified protein derivative (PPD), and toxoplasma IgG.
Possible chest x-ray examination.
Hepatitis C serology.
Cytomegalovirus (CMV) serology.
Hepatitis B serology.

For older patients, perform liver function and creatinine clearance studies. The two approaches for asymptomatic patients are:

Aggressive
Give early treatment, based on awareness of HIV's progressive nature.

- Begin treatment before development of significant immunosuppression and treat to achieve undetectable viremia.
- Treat all patients with fewer than 500 CD4+ T cells/mm^3.
- Treat all patients with higher CD4+ T cell levels whose plasma viral load is greater than 10,000 (bDNA) or 20,000 (RT-PCR).

Conservative

Delay therapy because risk of clinically significant progression and other factors weigh in favor of observation and delay.

- Patients with fewer than 500 CD4+ T cells/mm^3 and low levels of viremia.
- Patients with CD4+ T-cell counts greater than 500/mm^3.
- Exceptions include those with a high viral load, regardless of CD4+ T-cell count, who have a high probability of developing an AIDS-defining complication of HIV within 3 years.

Therapy is begun with a regimen that reduces viral replication to undetectable levels. This is accomplished by using two nucleoside analogues (NRTIs) and one powerful protease inhibitor (PI) (see drug information in Tables 15–2 and 15–3). These tables are provided as informational guides and are not intended as comprehensive guidelines for treatment.

Starting Therapy in Patients with Advanced HIV

Advanced HIV is any condition that meets the 1993 CDC definition of AIDS. These patients require treatment with antiretroviral agents, despite plasma viral levels, as do patients who have symptomatic HIV without AIDS, defined by presence of thrush or unexplained fever. Even though many of these patients have opportunistic infections, malignancy, wasting, or dementia when initially diagnosed, drug therapy is still needed as outlined (Tables 15–4 through 15–7). The provider must consider the whole picture, including drug toxicity, treatment compliance, drug interactions, and laboratory findings, before beginning treatment with a powerful and efficacious regimen such as two NRTIs and a PI. Strict criteria for discontinuation of therapy should be adhered to, despite acute situations; problems with drug toxicity, intolerance, or interactions are valid considerations. The complexity of the drug treatment regimen and the potential for drug interactions and toxicities are impressive. Additionally, the PIs and NNRTIs involve the cytochrome P450 enzymatic pathway. Interactive communication about drug treatment and avoidance of over-the-counter (OTC) and other drugs without first consulting the HIV professional are essential. If interruption of antiretroviral drug therapy is necessary, all agents should be discontinued simultaneously to minimize the development of resistant strains.

You must distinguish between drug failure and drug toxicity causing a need to change therapy. A multiplicity of factors must be considered before making a change, including plasma HIV RNA levels measured on two different occasions, CD4+ T lymphocyte count, treatment options, compliance and complexity of regimen, mental health issues, pharmacokinetics, patient education, and toxicity (Table 15–8). Three groups of patients should be considered for treatment change:

- Patients receiving incompletely suppressive antiretroviral therapy.
- Patients receiving powerful combination therapy, including a PI, with initially suppressed but now detectable viremia.

TABLE 15–2   CHARACTERISTICS OF NRTIs

Generic Name Trade Name	Zidovudine (AZT, ZDV) Retrovir	Didanosine (ddI) Videx	Zalcitabine (ddC) HIVID	Stavudine (d4T) Zerit	Lamivudine (3TC) Epivir
Dosing recommendations	200 mg tid or 300 mg bid or with 3TC as Combivir, 1 bid	Tablets >60 kg: 200 mg bid <60 kg: 125 mg bid	0.75 mg tid	>60 kg: 40 mg bid <60 kg: 30 mg bid	150 mg bid <50 kg: 2 mg/kg bid or with ZDV as Combivir, 1 bid
Oral bioavailability	60%	Tablet: 40% Powder: 30%	85%	86%	86%
Serum half-life Intracellular half-life	1.1 hr 3 hr	1.6 hr 25–40 hr	1.2 hr 3 hr	1.0 hr 3.5 hr	3–6 hr 12 hr
Elimination	Metabolized to AZT glucuronide (GAZT); renal excretion of GAZT	Renal excretion 50%	Renal excretion 70%	Renal excretion 50%	Renal excretion unchanged
Adverse events	Bone marrow suppression: Anemia and/or neutropenia Subjective complaints: GI intolerance, headache, insomnia, asthenia	Pancreatitis, peripheral neuropathy, nausea, diarrhea	Peripheral neuropathy, stomatitis	Peripheral neuropathy	Minimal toxicity

Source: Guidelines for the Use of Antiretroviral Agents in HIV Infected Adults and Adolescents, developed for Department of Health and Human Services and the Henry J. Kaiser Family Foundation by the Panel on Clinical Practices for Treatment of HIV Infection.

TABLE 15–3   NNRTIs

Generic Name *Trade Name*	Nevirapine *Viramune*	Delavirdine *Rescriptor*
Form	200 mg tabs	100 mg tabs
Dosing recommenda-tions	200 mg PO qid × 14 days, then 200 mg PO bid	400 mg PO tid (Four 100 mg tabs in ≥3 oz water to produce slurry)
Oral bioavailability	>90%	85%
Serum half-life	25–30 hr	5.8 hr
Elimination	Metabolized by cytochrome P450; 80% excreted in urine (glu-curonidated metabolites, <5% unchanged), 10% in feces	Metabolized by cytochrome P450; 51% excreted in urine (<5% unchanged), 44% in feces
Drug interactions	Induces cytochrome P450 enzymes (The following drugs have suspected interactions that require careful monitoring if co-administered with nevirapine: rifampin, rifabutin, oral contraceptives, protease inhibitors, triazolam and midazolam.)	Inhibits cytochrome P450 enzymes • Not recommended for concurrent use with terfenadine, astemizole, alprazolam, midazolam, cisapride, rifabutin, rifampin, triazolam, ergot drivatives, amphetamines, nifedipine, anticonvulsants (phenytoin, carbamazepine, phenobarbitol) • Delaviridine increases levels of clarithromycin, dapsone, quinidine, warfarin, indinavir, saquinavir • Antacids and didanosine: separate administration by ≥1 hr
Adverse events	Rash, increased transaminase levels, hepatitis	Rash, headaches

Source: Guidelines for the Use of Antiretroviral Agents in HIV Infected Adults and Adolescents, developed for Department of Health and Human Services and the Henry J. Kaiser Family Foundation by the Panel on Clinical Practices for Treatment of HIV Infection.

• Patients receiving powerful combination therapy, including a PI, who never had viremic suppression to below detectable limits.

Goal of antiretroviral therapy is improvement of length and quality of life by maximal suppression of viral replication to undetectable levels (fewer than 500 copies/mL) early enough to preserve immune function. If this is not accomplished with one regimen, then a change is indicated. Plasma HIV RNA level is the key parameter indicating response to therapy. (Refer to reference list for more in-depth information in this area).

Follow-up: Planned follow-up by HIV specialist includes plasma HIV RNA and CD4+ T cell counts as specified earlier, self-monitoring, and development of good self-care habits. If a patient's sexual contact is the source of the infection, encourage that person to undergo testing. Report disease to proper public health authority; reporting of HIV is mandatory. Close monitoring of the patient for medication side effects and toxicity is especially needed with older patients.

Sequelae: HIV has many possible complications, including opportunistic infections.

Prevention/Prophylaxis: Patients can prevent HIV infection through avoidance of unprotected sex and IV drug use, and by considering autologous blood transfusion for any planned surgery. Immunization of HIV-positive individuals with pneumococcal and influenza vaccines is indicated, unless the patient is allergic to these vaccines. Health-care personnel should use universal precautions and proper handling and disposal of contaminated needles and blood collection equipment.

Referral: Upon diagnosis refer patients to an HIV specialty nurse practitioner (NP) or other health-care specialist in HIV; whenever possible, management should be done by someone who specializes in this area. Collaborative management is indicated during stable periods. Refer patients to a nutritionist for dietary guidance for weight loss or wasting. Refer community-dwelling older adults to home health services when appropriate. Refer to support group if patient desires.

Education: Teach patient and family or caregivers about disease transmission, precautions, treatment options, self-care measures, and "safe sex" to prevent transmission to others. Teach patient not to take any other medications or OTC preparations without first clearing it with the health-care provider because of the potential for interactions with cytochrome P450 drugs.

Iron-Deficiency Anemia

Iron-deficiency anemia is a microcytic anemia caused by reduced iron stores. The onset may be acute, reflecting rapid blood loss, or chronic with slow blood loss and poor nutrition. Many authorities recommend 12 g/dL as the lower-normal hemoglobin value for older adults of both sexes.

Etiology: Potential causes of iron-deficiency anemia include inadequate ingestion and increased requirements, decreased absorption or utilization, or blood loss. The etiology may be multifactorial.

Occurrence: Iron-deficiency anemia is the most common type of anemia in the United States, affecting 10%–30% of the adult population.

Age: Iron-deficiency anemia affects all ages. It accounts for 60% of anemia in people over age 65.

Ethnicity: Not significant.

TABLE 15–4 CHARACTERISTICS OF PROTEASE INHIBITORS (PIs)

Generic Name / Trade Name	Indinavir / Crixivan	Ritonavir / Norvir	Saquinavir / Invirase	Fortovase	Nelfinavi / Viracept
Form	200, 400 mg caps	100 mg caps; 600 mg/7.5 ml PO solution	200 mg caps	200 mg caps	250 mg tablets; 50 mg/g of powder
Dosing recommendations	800 mg q8h; Take 1 hr before or 2 hr after meals; may take with skim milk or low-fat meal	600 mg q12 hr°; Take with food	600 mg tid; Take with high-fat meal	1200 mg tid; Take with large meal	750 mg tid; Take with food (meal, light snack)
Oral bioavailability	30%	Not determined	Hard gel capsule: 4%, erratic	Soft-gel capsule (not determined)	20–80%
Serum half-life	1.5–2 hr	3–5 hr	1–2 hr	1–2 hr	3.5–5 hr
Route of metabolism	P450 cytochrome 3A4	P450 cytochrome 3A4 > 2D6	P450 cytochrome 3A4	P450 cytochrome 3A4	P450 cytochrome 3A4
Storage	Room temperature	Refrigerate capsules; refrigeration for oral solution is preferred but not required if used within 30 days	Room temperature	Refrigerate or store at room temperature (up to 3 mo)	Room temperature
Adverse effects	• Nephrolithiasis • GI intolerance • Lab: increased indirect bilirubinemia (inconsequential) • Misc: headache, asthenia, blurred vision, dizziness, rash, metallic taste, thrombocytopenia Hyperglycemia§	• GI intolerance, nausea, vomiting, diarrhea • Paresthesias-circumoral and extremities • Hepatitis • Asthenia • Taste perversion • Lab: Triglycerides increase >200%, transaminase elevation, elevated creatine phosphatase (CPK) and uric acid Hyperglycemia§	• GI intolerance, nausea, diarrhea • Headache • Elevated transaminase enzymes Hyperglycemia§	• GI intolerance, nausea, diarrhea, abdominal pain and dyspepsia • Headache • Elevated transaminase enzymes Hyperglycemia§	• Diarrhea Hyperglycemia§

Drug interactions				
• Inhibits cytochrome P450 (less than ritonavir) • Not recommended for concurrent use: rifampin, terfenadine, astemizole, cisapride, trazolam, midazolam, ergot alkaloids • Indinavir levels increased by ketoconazole,‡ delavirdine • Indinavir levels reduced by rifampin, rifabutin, grapefruit juice, nevirapine • Didanosine reduces indinavir absorption unless taken >2 hr apart	• Inhibits cytochrome P450 (potent inhibitor) • Ritonavir increases levels of multiple drugs that are not recommended for concurrent use† • Didanosine: may cause reduced absorption of both drugs; should be taken >2 hr apart • Ritonavir decreases levels of ethinyl estradiol, theophylline, sulfamethoxazole, and zidovudine • Ritonavir increases levels of clarithromycin and desipramine	• Inhibits cytochrome P450 • Saquinavir levels increased by: ritonavir, ketoconazole, grapefruit juice, nelfinavir, delavirdine • Saquinavir levels reduced by: rifampin, rifabutin and possibly the following; phenobarbital, phenytoin, dexamethasone, carbamezepine, and nevirapine • Not recommended for concurrent use: terfenadine, astemizole, cisapride, ergot alkaloids	• Inhibits cytochrome P450 • Saquinavir levels increased by: ritonavir, ketoconazole, grapefruit juice, nelfinavir, delavirdine • Saquinavir levels reduced by: rifampin, rifabutin and possibly the following: phenobarbital, phenytoin, dexamethasone, carbamezepine, and nevirapine • Not recommended for concurrent use: terfenadine, astemizole, cisapride, ergot alkaloids	• Inhibits cytochrome P450 (less than ritonavir) • Nelfinavir levels reduced by rifampin, rifabutin • Not recommended for concurrent use: rifampin, triazolam, midazolam, ergot alkaloid, terfenadine, astemizole, cisapride • Nelfinavir decreases astemizole, cisapride levels of ethinyl estradiol and norethindrone • Nelfinavir increases levels of rifabutin, saquinavir, and indinavir

°Dose escalation for ritonavir: Day 1–2: 300 mg bid; day 3–5: 400 mg bid; day 6–13: 500 mg bid; day 14: 600 mg bid. Combination treatment regimen with saquinavir (400–600 mg PO bid) plus ritonavir (400–600 mg PO bid).

†Drugs contraindicated for concurrent use with ritonavir: amiodarone (Cordarone), astemizole (Hismanal), bepridil (Vascar), bupropion (Wellbutin), cisapride (Propulsid), clorazepate (Tranxene), clozapine (Clozaril), diazepam (Valium), encainide (Enkaid), estazolam (ProSom), flecainide (Tambocor), flurazepam (Dalmane), meperidine (Demerol), midazolam (Versed), piroxicam (Feldene), propoxyphene (Darvon), propafenone (Rythmol), quinidine, rifabutin, terfenadine (Seldane), triazolam (Halcion), zolpidem (Ambien), ergot alkaloids.

‡Decrease indinavir to 600 mg q8h.

§Cases of new-onset hyperglycemia have been reported in association with the use of all PIs.

TABLE 15–5 DRUGS THAT SHOULD NOT BE USED WITH PIs

Drug Category	Indinavir	Ritonavir*	Saquinavir (given as Invirase or Fortovase)	Nelfinavir	Alternatives
Analgesics	None	Meperidine, piroxicam, propoxyphene	None	None	Aspirin, oxycodon, acetaminophen
Cardiac	None	Amioderone Encainide Flecainide Propafenone Quinidine	None	None	Limited experience
Antimycobacterial	Rifampin	Rifabutin†	Rifampin Rifabutin	Rifampin	For rifabutin (as alternative for MAI treatment): clarithromycin, ethambutol (treatment, not prophylaxis), or azithromycin

Ca++ channel blocker	None	Bepridil	None	None	Limited experience
Antihistimine	Astemizole, terfenadine	Astemizole, terfenadine	Astemizole, terfen-adine	Astemizole, terfenadine	Loratadine
GI	Cisapride	Cisapride	Cisapride	Cisapride	Limited experience
Antidepressant	None	Bupropion	None	None	Fluoxetine, desipramine
Neuroleptic	None	Clozapine, pimozide	None	None	Limited experience
Psychotropic	Midazolam, triazolam	Clorazepate, Diazepam, Estazolam, Flurazepam, Midazolam, Triazolam, Zolpidem	None	Midazolam (Versed), triazolam (Halcion)	Temazepam, lorazepam
Ergot alkaloid (Vasoconstrictor)		Dihydroergotamine (DHE 45), ergotamine‡ (various forms)		Dihydroergotamine (DHE 45), ergotamine‡ (various forms)	

*Reduce rifabutin dose to one quarter of the standard dose.

†The contraindicated drugs listed are based on theoretical considerations. Thus, drugs with low therapeutic indices yet with suspected major metabolic contribution from cytochrome P450 3A, CYP2D6, or unknown pathways are included in this table. Actual interactions may or may not occur in patients.

‡This is likely a class effect.

TABLE 15–6 DRUG INTERACTIONS REQUIRING DOSE MODIFICATIONS

	Indinavir	Ritonavir	Saquinavir	Nelfinavir
Fluconazole	No dose change	No dose change	No data	No change
Ketoconazole	Decrease dose to 600 mg q8h	Increases ketoconazole more than threefold; dose adjustment required	Increases saquinavir levels threefold; no dose change	No change
Rifabutin	Reduce rifabutin to half dose: 150 mg qd	Consider alternative drug	Not recommended with either Invirase or Fortovase	Reduce rifabutin to half dose: 150 mg qd
Rifampin	Contraindicated	Unknown	Not recommended with either Invirase or Fortovase°	Not recommended
Oral contraceptives	Modest increase Ortho-Novum levels; no dose change	Ethinyl estradiol levels decreased; use alternative or additional contraceptive method	No data	Ethinyl estradiol and norethindrone levels decreased; use alternative or additional contraceptive method
Miscellaneous	Grapefruit juice reduces indinavir levels by 26%	• Desipramine increased 145%: reduce dose • Theophylline levels decreased: increase dose	Grapefruit juice increases saquinavir levels†	

°Several drug interaction studies have been completed with saquinavir given as Invirase or Fortovase. Results from studies conducted with Invirase may not be applicable to Fortovase

†Conducted with Fortovase. Rifampin reduces ritonavir 35%. Increased ritonavir dose or use of ritonavir in combination therapy is strongly recommended. The effect of ritonavir on rifampin is unknown. Used concurrently, liver toxicity may increase. Therefore, patients taking ritonavir and rifampin should be monitored closely.

TABLE 15–7 DRUG INTERACTIONS: EFFECT OF PIs AND NNRTIs ON LEVELS AND DOSE

Drug Affected	Indinavir	Ritonavir	Saquinavir*	Nelfinavir	Nevirapine	Delavirdine
Indinavir (IDV)	°	No data	Levels: IDV no effect; SQV ↑ 4–7×‡ Dose: No data	Levels: IDV ↑ 50% NFV: ↑ 80% Dose: No data	Levels: IDV ↓ 28% Dose: standard	Levels: IDV ↑ 40% Dose: IDV 600 mg q8h
Ritonavir (RTV)	No data	°	Levels: RTV no effect; SQV ↑ 20×†‡ Dose: Invirase or Fortovase 400 mg bid† RTV: 400 mg bid	Levels: RTV no effect; NFV ↑ 1.5× Dose: No data	Levels RTV ↓ 11% Dose: standard	Levels: RTV 70% Dose: No data
Saquinavir (SQV)	Levels: SQV ↑ 4–7×; IDV no effect‡ Dose: no data	Levels: SQV ↑ 20×,†‡; RTV no effect Dose: Invirase or Fortovase 400 mg bid† RTV 400 mg bid	°	Levels: SQV ↑ 3–5×; NFV ↑ 20%‡ Dose: standard NFV Fortovase 800 mg tid	Levels: SQV ↓ 25%† Dose: no data	Levels: SQV ↑ 5× Dose: standard for Invirase Monitor transaminase levels
Nelfinavir (NFV)	Levels: NFV ↑ 80% IDV ↑ 50% Dose: no data	Levels: NFV ↑ 1.5× RTV no effect Dose: no data	Levels: NFV ↑ 20%; SQV ↑ 3–5×‡ Dose: standard (no dose adjustments needed with hard gel formulation)	°	Levels: NFV 10% Dose: standard	Levels: NFV ↑ 2× DLV ↓ 50% Dose: standard (monitor for neutropenic complications)
Nevirapine (NVP)	Levels: IDV ↓ 28% Dose: standard	Levels: RTV ↓ 11% Dose: standard	Levels: SQV ↓ 25%, Dose: No data	Levels: NFV 10% Dose: standard	°	Do not use together.
Delavirdine (DLV)	Levels: IDV ↑ 40% Dose: IDV 600 q8h	Levels: RTV ↑ 70% Dose: no data	Levels: SQV ↑ 5×† Dose: standard for Invirase (monitor transaminase levels)	Levels: NFV ↑ 2× DLV ↓ 50% Dose: standard (monitor for neutropenic complications)	Do not use together.	°

° Several drug interaction studies have been completed with saquinavir given as Invirase or Fortovase. Results from studies conducted with Invirase may not be applicable to Fortovase.

† Conducted with Invirase.

‡ Conducted with Fortovase.

TABLE 15–8   ACUTE RETROVIRAL SYNDROME:
ASSOCIATED SIGNS AND SYMPTOMS

Fever (96%), lymphadenopathy (74%), phar-
  yngitis (70%), rash (70%)
  Erythematous maculopapular with lesions
    on face and trunk and sometimes extrem-
    ities, including palms and soles
  Mucocutaneous ulceration involving mouth,
    esophagus, or genitals
• Myalgia or arthralgia (54%)
• Diarrhea (32%)
• Headache (32%)
• Nausea and vomiting (27%)

• Hepatosplenomegaly (14%)
• Thrush (12%)
• Weight loss
• Neurologic symptoms (12%)
  Meningoencephalitis or aseptic meningitis
  Peripheral neuropathy or radiculopathy
  Facial palsy
  Guillain-Barré syndrome
  Brachial neuritis
  Cognitive impairment or psychosis

Gender: More women than men are affected.

Contributing Factors: In the older adult patient, decreased oral intake, partial gastrectomy, malabsorption syndromes, low socioeconomic status, medications, combination of medication and alcohol, or chronic blood loss (most frequently from the gastrointestinal [GI] tract), are contributing factors for iron-deficiency anemia. Some GI causes include peptic ulcer disease, gastritis, hiatal hernia with mucosal ulceration, neoplasms, diverticular disease, or bleeding caused by inflammatory bowel disease. In patients with prosthetic heart valves, intravascular hemolysis may lead to iron-deficiency anemia related to increased hemosiderin loss in the urine. Epistaxis, hematuria, uterine bleeding, or bleeding diathesis are other possible contributing factors.

Signs and Symptoms: The presentation of iron-deficiency anemia is vague, frequently going unnoticed in older patients. It may be an incidental blood study finding, prompting further investigation. Fatigue, weakness, lethargy, tachycardia, palpitations, dyspnea on exertion, headache, irritability, inability to concentrate, neuralgia, sore tongue, paresthesias, and susceptibility to infection are other possible symptoms. Dizziness, faintness, claudication, exercise intolerance, or angina may also present. In some cases, symptoms may reflect the underlying cause (e.g., stomach discomfort with peptic ulcer disease).

Physical examination may be unremarkable. Pallor, common in patients with significant anemia, is also common with aging, and may be discounted as a normal age-related finding. Conjunctival pallor, bluish discoloration of the sclerae, cheilosis, glossitis, brittle ridged nails, or "spoon" nails (koilonychia) may also be present.

Cardiovascular and respiratory examination may reveal tachycardia, systolic murmur, or signs of congestive heart failure (CHF). In some patients, splenomegaly may be present owing to hemolysis of iron-deficient red blood cells.

Diagnostic Tests: Complete blood count (CBC) done initially will reveal a low hemoglobin, less than 12 g/dL. Peripheral smear will demonstrate microcytosis, poikilocytosis, and hypochromia as iron deficiency progresses (usually at hemoglobin less than 8 g/dL). Documented absence of or decrease in iron stores, necessary to establish diagnosis, is usually accomplished by measuring serum iron, total iron-binding capacity (TIBC), and ferritin. Serum iron is reduced; this also occurs with infection, malignancy, or acute or chronic inflammation. TIBC is increased and serum ferritin is low; transferrin saturation is also low. Bone marrow iron stain is usually unnecessary, unless there are confounding factors. Diagnostic studies related to the possible cause of the iron deficiency must also be undertaken.

Differential Diagnosis: Differential diagnosis includes other causes of hypochromic, microcytic anemia: thallasemia, glucose-6-dehydrogenase (G6PD) deficiency, sideroblastic anemia or secondary sideroblastic anemia related to lead intoxication, or toxic effects of isoniazid and/or pyrazinamide therapy for tuberculosis. Defective iron reutilization such as seen with infection, chronic diseases, cancer, or inflammation is another differential diagnosis. Decreased erythropoetin from renal failure, hypothyroidism, and other hypoproliferative states must also be considered.

Treatment: Besides relieving symptoms, treatment must also treat the underlying disorder whenever possible. Transfusion with packed red blood cells may be necessary initially, if blood loss threatens to damage vital organs. Oral iron supplementation should be instituted with ferrous sulfate 325 mg PO bid or tid for 6 months, on an empty stomach, if tolerated. Ascorbic acid taken with the medication enhances absorption. Medication effect should be demonstrated after 2 weeks of therapy. If follow-up laboratory studies fail to show increases in hematocrit after 6–8 weeks, reevaluate the patient for noncompliance, malabsorption, ongoing bleeding, or missed diagnosis.

Medication therapy may cause significant GI side effects in 20%–25% of patients, including constipation, diarrhea, nausea, or abdominal cramping. Ferrous gluconate or fumarate may be better tolerated; alternatively, consider a reduction in ferrous sulfate dosage to once daily over a 1-year period. In some cases, taking the medication with food may be necessary. Milk, antacids, and tetracycline should not be administered within 2 hours of oral iron therapy. For patients who are unable to take oral iron preparations, parenteral therapy with iron dextran must be considered. This costly alternative, associated with a high incidence of tissue toxicity, requires individualization of dosage. Dietary measures to treat iron deficiency include inclusion of meat, beans, and green, leafy vegetables. An increase in dietary fiber may help to prevent constipation from oral iron therapy. Patients' activity levels should be adjusted as tolerated for safety.

Follow-up: Hemoglobin should be reevaluated for response after 6–8 weeks of therapy. The patient should be seen to reassess symptoms or side effects from the treatment regimen. Emphasize the need to continue treatment. If the patient is stable, reevaluate in 3–6 months.

Sequelae: Possible complications include failure to identify an occult bleeding source, especially a bleeding malignancy.

Prevention/Prophylaxis: Iron-deficiency anemia can be prevented by following good nutrition guidelines, with adequate iron intake and through prompt evaluation of symptoms or any bleeding.

Referral: Refer patients to a specialist in the area where anemia is suspected to originate (e.g., a gastroenterologist for diagnostic studies, a hematologist or oncologist if malignancy is suspected). Collaborative management is appropriate if many confounding factors are present or medication regimen is complex. Refer patients to a nutritionist for evaluation of dietary inadequacies and assistance with meal planning or with congregate or home-delivered meals.

Education: Teach the patient about the mechanism of anemia, its possible causes, and the need for workup. Patients need to continue their medication regimen until discontinued by the health-care provider. Instruction should include dietary sources of iron.

BIBLIOGRAPHY

Assessment

Bates, B: A Guide to Physical Examination and History Taking, ed 5. JB Lippincott, Philadelphia, 1991.
Barker LR, Burton JR, and Zieve PD: Principles of Ambulatory Medicine, ed 3. Williams & Wilkins, Baltimore, 1991.
DeGowin: Bedside Diagnostic Examination, ed 5. Macmillan, New York, 1987.
Jarvis, C: Physical Examination and Health Assessment. WB Saunders, Philadelphia, 1992.
Schwartz, M: Textbook of Physical Diagnosis, ed 2. WB Saunders, Philadelphia, 1994.

Human Immunodeficiency Virus

Bartlett, JA (ed): Care and Management of Patients With HIV Infection. Glaxo Wellcome, Durham, NC, 1997.
Berenson, AS (ed): Control of Communicable Diseases Manual, ed 16. Washington, DC, American Public Health Association, 1995.
Centers for Disease Control and Prevention: Report of the NIH Panel to Define Principles of Therapy of HIV Infection and Guidelines for the Use of Antiretroviral Agents in HIV-infected Adults and Adolescents. MMWR 47 (No. RR-5): 75. US Government Printing Office, Washington, DC, 1998.
Feldman, M, et al: The growing risk of AIDS in older patients. Patient Care. 28(17):61–71, 1994.
Johnson, PC: Late symptomatic HIV infection. In Rakel, RE: Saunders Manual of Medical Practice. WB Saunders, Philadelphia, 1996.
Krishna, L: Early symptomatic HIV infection. In Rakel, RE: Saunders Manual of Medical Practice. WB Saunders, Philadelphia, 1996.
Patterson, J, et al: Basic and clinical considerations of HIV infection in the elderly. Clin Geriatr 3(10):21–34, 1995.
Tatum, NO: Asymptomatic HIV infection. In Rakel, RE: Saunders Manual of Medical Practice. WB Saunders, Philadelphia, 1996.
Whipple, B, and Scura, KW: The overlooked epidemic: HIV in older adults. AJN 96(2):23–29, 1996.

Iron-Deficiency Anemia

Dambro, MR: Griffith's 5 Minute Clinical Consult. Williams & Wilkins, Baltimore, 1997.

Lee, TC: Iron deficiency anemia. In Rakel, RE: Saunders Manual of Medical Practice. WB Saunders, Philadelphia, 1996.

Mansouri, A, and Lipschitz, DA: Anemia in the elderly patient. Med Clin North Am 76(3):619–630, 1992.

Massey, A: Microcytic anemia: Differential diagnosis and management of iron deficiency anemia. Med Clin North Am 76(3):549–565, 1992.

Small, EJ, and Damon, LE: Blood. In Lonergan, ET (ed): Geriatrics. Appleton & Lange, Stamford, Conn, 1996.

Yoshikawa, TT, and Lipschitz, DA: Anemia. In Yoshikawa, TT, Cobbs, EL, and Brummel-Smith, K: Practical Ambulatory Geriatrics, ed 2. CV Mosby, St Louis, 1998.

CHAPTER **16**

PSYCHOSOCIAL

DISORDERS

Psychosocial assessment of the older adult is the systematic review and evaluation of patient, family, and environment.

Rationale

The psychosocial assessment provides the foundation for developing and implementing a comprehensive plan of care and means for evaluating its effectiveness. The practitioner must understand what happens during the aging process because this knowledge allows differentiation between symptoms that are normal and those considered abnormal. For the older adult, physical health, mental health, and environmental and social problems all interact to complicate the life and function of the older patient, caregiver, and family.

The psychosocial assessment of the older adult entails evaluation of the following basic needs:

- Autonomy and independence.
- Dignity, credibility, and respect.
- Identity and individuality.
- Communication.
- Belonging.
- Touch.

An accurate psychosocial assessment is an interactive process between the practitioner and the older adult that creates an awareness of risks, limitations, and functional changes. This enables the older adult to make appropriate lifestyle changes to accommodate these changes and maintain autonomy, independence, and dignity.

The psychosocial assessment should be performed on initial examination and annually thereafter for all older adults. Reassessment is appropriate whenever a patient's health status changes.

Ethnicity

Ethnicity may be defined as affiliation with a group whose members share a common social and cultural heritage that is passed on to successive generations and provides a sense of identity. To provide culturally competent care, the nurse practitioner should perform a cultural assessment within the psychosocial assessment for a multicultural society. Giger and Davidhizar's Transcultural Assessment Model (1991; Fig. 16–1) shows guidelines for an assessment of six cultural phenomena that are evident in all cultural groups:

- Communication.
- Space.
- Social organization.
- Time.
- Environmental control.
- Biologic variations.

Contributing Factors

A positive correlation exists between social supports and the use of health-care services by older adults. Older adults who are alone and lonely, depressed, or having difficulty adapting to change appear in their practitioner's office more frequently than those with adequate support systems. Social networks are an important aspect of a patient's social functions as are work, hobbies, and interests. Older adults may be reluctant to reveal social or emotional concerns and, in some cultures, may feel that it is unacceptable to share personal problems with outsiders. However, they may feel comfortable discussing a physical manifestation, such as pain or sleeplessness, with a health-care provider.

Risk Factors

The older adult population is not a homogeneous group, because of the diversity in health, social and environmental supports, financial security, and cultural and

CULTURALLY UNIQUE INDIVIDUAL
1. Place of birth
2. Cultural definition: What is ...
3. Race: What is ...
4. Length of time in country (if appropriate)

COMMUNICATION
1. Voice quality
   A. Strong, resonant
   B. Soft
   C. Average
   D. Shrill
2. Pronunciation and enunciation
   A. Clear
   B. Slurred
   C. Dialect (geographical)
3. Use of silence
   A. Infrequent
   B. Often
   C. Length
      (1) Brief
      (2) Moderate
      (3) Long
      (4) Not observed
4. Use of nonverbal
   A. Hand movement
   B. Eye movement
   C. Kinesics (gestures, expressions, or stances)
5. Touch
   A. Startles or withdraws when touched
   B. Accepts touch without difficulty
   C. Touches others without difficulty
6. Ask these and similar questions
   A. How do you get your point across to others?
   B. Do you like communicating with family, friends, acquaintances?
   C. When asked a question, do you usually respond (in words or body movement, or both)?
   D. If you have something important to discuss with your family, how would you approach them?

SPACE
1. Degree of comfort
   A. Moves when space invaded
   B. Does not move when space invaded
2. Distance in conversations
   A. 0 to 18 inches
   B. 18 inches to 3 feet
   C. 3 feet or more
3. Definition of space
   A. Describe degree of comfort with closeness when talking with or standing near others
   B. How do objects (e.g., furniture) in the environment affect your sense of space?
4. Ask these and similar questions:
   A. When you talk to family members how close do you stand?
   B. When you communicate with coworkers and other acquaintances, how close do you stand?
   C. If a loved stranger touches you, how do you react or feel?
   D. If a loved one touches you, how do you react or feel?
   E. Are you comfortable with the distance between us now?

FIGURE 16–1 Giger and Davidhizar's Transcultural Assessment Model.

SOCIAL ORGANIZATION
1. Normal state of health
    A. Poor
    B. Fair
    C. Good
    D. Excellent
2. Marital status
3. Number of children
4. Parents living or deceased?
5. Ask these and similar questions:
    A. How do you define social activities?
    B. What are some activities that you enjoy?
    C. What are your hobbies, or what do you do when you have free time?
    D. Do you believe in a Supreme Being?
    E. How do you worship that Supreme Being?
    F. What is your function (what do you do) in your family unit/system?
    G. What is your role in your family unit/system (father, mother, child, advisor)?
    H. When you were a child, what or who influenced you the most?
    I. What is/was your relationship with your siblings and parents?
    J. What does work mean to you?
    K. Describe your past, present, and future jobs.
    L. What are your political views?
    M. How have your political views influenced your attitude toward health and illness?

TIME
1. Orientation to time:
    A. Past-oriented
    B. Present-oriented
    C. Future-oriented
2. View of time
    A. Social time
    B. Clock-oriented
3. Physiochemical reaction to time
    A. Sleeps at least 8 hours a night
    B. Goes to sleep and wakes up on a consistent schedule
    C. Understands the importance of taking medication and other treatments on schedule
4. Ask these and similar questions:
    A. What kind of timepiece do you wear daily?
    B. If you have an appointment at 2 PM, what time is acceptable to arrive?
    C. If a nurse tells you that you will receive a medication in "about a half hour," realistically, how much time will you allow before calling the nurses' station?

ENVIRONMENTAL CONTROL
1. Locus-of-control
    A. Internal locus-of-control (believes that the power to affect change lies within)
    B. External locus-of-control (believes that fate, luck, and chance have a great deal to do with how things turn out)
2. Value orientation
    A. Believes in supernatural forces
    B. Relies on magic, witchcraft, and prayer to affect change
    C. Does not believe in supernatural forces

FIGURE 16–1 Continued

ENVIRONMENTAL CONTROL (continued)
  D. Does not rely on magic, witchcraft, and prayer to affect change.
3. Ask these and similar questions:
  A. How often do you have visitors at your home?
  B. Is it acceptable to you to have visitors drop in unexpectedly?
  C. Name some ways your parents or other persons treated your illnesses when you were a child.
  D. Have you or someone else in your immediate surroundings ever used a home remedy that made you sick?
  E. What home remedies have you used that have worked? Will you use them in the future?
  F. What is your definition of "good health"?
  G. What is your definition of illness or "poor health"?

BIOLOGIC VARIATIONS
1. Conduct a complete physical assessment noting:
  A. Body structure (small, medium, or large frame)
  B. Skin color
  C. Unusual skin discoloration
  D. Hair color and distribution
  E. Other visible physical characteristics (e.g., keloids, chloasma)
  F. Weight
  G. Height
  H. Check lab work for variation in hemoglobin, hematocrit, and sickle phenomena if African-American or Mediterranean
2. Ask these and similar questions:
  A. What diseases or illnesses are common in your family?
  B. Describe your family's typical behavior when a family member is ill.
  C. How do you respond when you are angry?
  D. Who (or what) usually helps you to cope during a difficult time?
  E. What foods do you and your family like to eat?
  F. Have you ever had an unusual cravings for:
    (1) White or red clay dirt?
    (2) Laundry starch?
  G. When you were a child what types of foods did you eat?
  H. What foods are family favorites or are considered traditional?

FIGURE 16–1   Continued

personal philosophies. Some distinctive occurrences in the lives of older adults may include:

• Developmental milestones that have an impact on most older adults (i.e., retirement, loss of a spouse).
• Changes in financial and social resources that allow the older adult to cope effectively with age-related phenomena.

Relocation, financial concerns, and lack of social supports may be the impetus for physical and mental health problems. The most common life events that place the older adult at risk for psychosocial dysfunction include:

NURSING ASSESSMENT
1. Note whether the client has become culturally assimilated or observes own culture?
2. Incorporate data into plan of nursing care:
   A. Encourage the client to discuss cultural differences; people from diverse cultures who hold different world-views can enlighten nurses.
   B. Make efforts to accept and understand methods of communication.
   C. Respect the individual's personal need for space.
   D. Respect the rights of clients to honor and worship the Supreme Being of their choice.
   E. Identify a clerical or spirtual person to contact.
   F. Determine whether spiritual practices have implications for health, life, and well-being (e.g., Jehovah's Witnesses may refuse blood and blood derivatives; an Orthodox Jew may eat only kosher food high in sodium and may not drink milk when meat is served).
   G. Identify hobbies, especially when devising interventions for a short or extended convalescence, or for rehabilitation.
   H. Honor time and value orientations and differences in these areas. Allay anxiety and apprehension if adherence to time is necessary.
   I. Provide privacy according to personal need and health status of client (NOTE: the perception and reaction to pain may be culturally related).
   J. Note cultural health practices:
      (1) Identify and encourage efficacious practices.
      (2) Identify and discourage dysfunctional practices.
      (3) Identify and determine whether neutral practices will have a long-term ill effect.
   K. Note food preferences:
      (1) Make as many adjustments in diet as health status and long-term benefits will allow and that dietary department can provide.
      (2) Note dietary practices that may have serious implications for the client.

Source: From Giger, JN, & Davidhizar, RE. *Transcultural Nursing: Assessment and intervention* (1995, 11–13). St. Louis: Mosby. Reprinted with permission.

Guidelines for Relating to Patients from Different Cultures:
1. Assess personal beliefs of persons from different cultures.
2. Assess communication variables from a cultural perspective.
3. Plan care based on the communicated needs and cultural background.
4. Modify communication approaches to meet cultural needs.
5. Understand that respect for the patient and communicated needs is central to the therapeutic relationship.
6. Communicate in a nonthreatening manner.
7. Use validating techniques in communication.
8. Be considerate of reluctance to talk when the subject involves sexual matters.
9. Adopt special approaches when a patient speaks a different language.
10. Use interpreters to improve communication.

From Giger, JN, & Davidhizar, RE. *Transcultural Nursing: Assessment and Intervention* 34–37, St. Louis, Mosby, 1995.

FIGURE 16–1 Continued

- Retirement/role loss.
- Loss of spouse.
- Deaths of close friends.
- Family problems.
- Relocation.
- Financial problems.

Screening Tools

PSYCHOLOGICAL HEALTH

Because older adult patients may hesitate to discuss social or emotional problems with a health-care provider, physical symptoms may be an expression of underlying psychosocial dysfunction. Therefore, measurement of psychological health adds an important component to the older adult assessment. Psychological health is measured based on the two subdomains of *cognition* (mental status) and *affect* (anxiety and depression). The Folstein Mini Mental State Exam (MMSE) is the most commonly used scale for assessing cognitive function in older adults and can be administered efficiently (Fig. 16–2). Scores lower than 24 out of the possible 30 suggest delirium, dementia, or severe depression. The short-form Yesavage Geriatric Depression Scale (Table 16–1) is an easy-to-use widely accepted screening tool for depression in the older adult. Although helpful, screening tools should not replace the interactive relationship between practitioner and patient.

SOCIOENVIRONMENTAL TOOLS

The heterogeneity of socioenvironmental factors precludes the use of a single tool for evaluating the older adult, however, to evaluate this domain the environmental and safety checklist (Fig. 16–3) may be helpful; it may also be used for patient and family education. The information derived from this evaluation will direct the practitioner in areas of education for the patient and family.

Expected Outcomes

Chronic disease, physical disability, pain and suffering, cognitive impairment, accumulated losses, and social isolation may occur when an individual is least able to cope with change. Therefore, a psychosocial assessment provides a foundation for developing and implementing a comprehensive plan of care. The expected outcome for the older adult is an enhanced quality of life.

Folstein MMSE

1. Orientation

		Score	Total
What is the	day	_____ 1	
	date	_____ 1	
	month	_____ 1	
	year	_____ 1	
	season	_____ 1	_____ 5
What is the	city	_____ 1	
	state	_____ 1	
	county	_____ 1	
	building	_____ 1	
	floor	_____ 1	_____ 5

2. Registration
Name three objects and take 1 second to say each. Then ask the patient
To repeat all 3 objects. (Give 1 point for each correct answer. Repeat
until patient can get all 3 objects.) _____ 3

3. Attention and calculation
Serial 7s: Ask the patient to count backward by 7s from 100.
(Stop after 5 answers. Give 1 point for each correct answer.)
Alternate: Spell *world* backward. (Give 1 point for each correctly placed letter.) _____ 5

4. Recall
After 2 minutes, ask for the 3 objects' names in question 2.
(Give 1 point for each correct answer.) _____ 3

5. Language
Point to a pencil and watch. Ask the patient to name each as you point
to them. (Give 1 point for each correct answer.) _____ 2

Ask the patient to repeat the following phrase: "No *ifs, ands,* or *buts.*"
(Give 1 point for the correct answer.) _____ 1

Ask the patient to perform the following three-stage command:
"Take a paper in your right hand, fold it in half, and lay it on the table."
(Give 1 point for each correct step.) _____ 3

Ask the patient to read and carry out the following command:
CLOSE YOUR EYES (Give 1 point for the correct response.) _____ 1

Ask the patient to write a sentence. It must contain a noun and
a verb and make sense. Ignore spelling errors.
(Give 1 point for the correct answer.) _____ 1

Ask the patient to draw 2 interlocking pentagons. There must be
5 sides to each pentagon and 4 interlocking sides. Example:
(Give 1 point for the correct answer.) _____ 1

Total _____ 30

Source: Adapted with permission from Journal of Psychiatric Research (1975; 12: 196-197), Copyright© 1975, Pergamon Journals, Ltd.

FIGURE 16–2 Folstein Mini Mental State Exam (MMSE).

TABLE 16–1   YESAVAGE GERIATRIC DEPRESSION SCALE, SHORT FORM

1. Are you basically satisfied with your life?	Yes	No
2. Have you dropped many of your activities and interests?	Yes	No
3. Do you feel that your life is empty?	Yes	No
4. Do you often get bored?	Yes	No
5. Are you in good spirits most of the time?	Yes	No
6. Are you afraid that something bad is going to happen to you?	Yes	No
7. Do you feel happy most of the time?	Yes	No
8. Do you often feel helpless?	Yes	No
9. Do you prefer to stay at home rather than go out and do new things?	Yes	No
10. Do you feel you have more problems with memory than most?	Yes	No
11. Do you think it is wonderful to be alive now?	Yes	No
12. Do you feel pretty worthless the way you are now?	Yes	No
13. Do you feel full of energy?	Yes	No
14. Do you feel that your situation is hopeless?	Yes	No
15. Do you think that most people are better off than you are?	Yes	No

Score 1 point for: "No" to questions 1, 5, 7, 11, and "Yes" to other questions.
Score°: _____/15 (°A score of 5 or more may indicate depression.)

From Yesavage, JA, Brink, TL: Development and validation of a geriatric depression screening scale: A preliminary report. *J Psychiatr Res* 17:37–49, 1983.

Alcohol Abuse

Alcohol abuse is a pathologic pattern of alcohol use involving social, occupational, or functional impairment that has persisted for at least 1 month or recurred repeatedly over a long period of time.

Etiology: Four models are viewed as explanations for alcohol abuse. The biogenetic model posits that genetic factors influence the metabolism of alcohol, producing changes in the neurotransmitters and receptors. The sociocultural model suggests that external factors such as poverty, social isolation, loss, and culture predispose an older adult to alcohol abuse. The learning theory or behavioral model supports alcohol abuse as a learned behavior that can be reversed. The psychological-psychodynamic model views alcohol abuse as a manifestation of underlying psychopathology.

Occurrence: About 11% of older adults are heavy alcohol users.

Age: More middle-aged adults are currently at risk for developing alcohol-related problems because alcohol use throughout life has been greater in this cohort than in previous cohorts.

Ethnicity: Not significant.

Gender: Men are four times more likely than women to abuse alcohol.

General Household:

Lighting: □ Adequate □ Too dim □ Too direct, creating glare □ Light switches inaccessible □ Other: _____

Carpets, rugs: □ No problem □ Torn □ Slippery □ Scatter rugs □ Comments: _____

Chairs: □ No problem □ Unstable □ Lack of armrests □ Low-back chairs □ Other: _____

Furniture: □ Obstructs walkway □ Cluttered □ Limits or interferes with egress □ Other: _____

Heating: □ Central heat □ Unable to control □ No central heat: (details) _____

Cooling: □ Central air □ Unable to control □ No central cooling: (details) _____

Kitchen:

Cabinets & shelves: □ No problem □ Too high □ Inaccessible R/T _____

Floor: □ Safe, without scatter rugs □ Slippery □ Linoleum irregular Comments: _____

Stove: □ Accessible □ Dial difficult to reach □ Inaccessible R/T _____

Sink: □ Accessible □ Faucets difficult to reach □ Inaccessible R/T _____

Chair: □ Stable with armrests for support □ Unstable □ Lack of armrests □ Low-back chairs □ Other: _____

Table: □ No problem □ Wobbly, unstable □ Inaccessible Comments: _____

Bathroom:

Bathtub: □ Safe for use (pt. demonstrate entry & exit) □ No grab bar or transfer aid □ Slippery, without skid-resistant strips _____

Toilet: □ Safe for use □ Seat too low □ No transfer aid □ Seat unsafe □ Other: _____

Medicine cabinet: □ Adequate lighting, drugs labeled/dated □ Poor lighting □ Drugs improperly labeled □ Other: _____

Door: □ Can be opened from outside □ Lock opens from inside only □ Doorway too narrow for assistive devices

Stairways:

□ Safe for use with rise ~6 inches, sturdy handrail in place, not too steep, not slippery, not cluttered & lighting adequate

□ Cluttered □ Slippery □ Rise too high □ Handrails missing □ Too steep □ Lighting inadequate □ Other: _____

From Stauffer KL: Comprehensive Evaluation of the Older Adult. Lydia HealthCare Consulting, 1997.

FIGURE 16–3 Environmental and safety checklist.

Contributing Factors: Concerns about alcohol consumption in the older adult are primarily directed toward the physiologic changes that accompany aging and the problems posed by regular alcohol consumption. Chemical breakdown of alcohol does not appear to change with aging; however, the changes associated with aging may increase the concentration of alcohol in the blood. These age-related changes include the following:

- Decreased lean muscle mass.
- Decreased amount of body water.
- Changes in liver function.
- Increased nervous system sensitivity to alcohol.

After drinking 1 ounce of 80-proof alcohol, a 60-year-old would have a 20% higher blood alcohol level than a 20-year-old, and a 90-year old would have a 50% higher blood alcohol level than the 20-year-old. Another major concern associated with alcohol abuse in the older adult is the increased occurrence of drug-alcohol interactions. The decreased metabolism of drugs by the liver in older adults yields significantly higher than normal drug levels, and alcohol increases this effect. Alcohol diminishes the effect of oral hypoglycemics, anticoagulants, and anticonvulsants, and unpredictably strengthens the effects of sedatives.

Signs and Symptoms: Alcohol abuse is often overlooked in older adults because medical problems, psychosocial problems, and medication use may obscure the signs of alcoholism. Patterns of alcohol dependence in older adults have been divided into two categories:

- Early onset, which occurs before age 60.
- Late onset, which occurs after age 60.

In older adults, 50%–75% are early-onset alcohol abusers who have a family history of alcoholism, are less well adjusted, and may have experienced alcohol-related legal problems. It is thought that late-onset alcohol abuse is related to the stresses and losses of aging, and may respond more favorably to treatment.

Complaints that may suggest alcohol abuse include the following:

- Inconsistent mild hypertension.
- Insomnia or anxiety.
- Confusion.
- Falls.
- History of pancreatitis without stones.
- Paranoid ideation.

Diagnostic Tests: Diagnostic assessment depends on a thorough history. The CAGE Questions, the screening test of choice for early detection, should be part of every health history (Fig. 16–4). Another approach that may elicit more accurate alcohol-related information is to ask, "Have you ever had a drinking problem?" and "When was your last drink?" (Standard questions such as "How much do you drink?" and "How often do you drink?" often result in dishonesty.)

Have you ever felt the need to **C**ut down on drinking?
Have you ever felt **A**nnoyed by criticism of drinking?
Have you ever had **G**uilty feelings about drinking?
Have you ever taken a morning **E**ye opener?

SCORE:

➤ Two or more positive answers should raise the suspicion of alcohol abuse.
➤ A positive response to one question should prompt further inquiry.

FIGURE 16–4 CAGE Questionnaire.

A psychosocial assessment that includes a mental status examination and a geriatric depression scale should be performed. Also, consider a cultural assessment, if appropriate. During the physical examination, focus on the following:

- Vital signs.
- The abdomen for hepatosplenomegaly; stool guaiac test for occult blood.
- The skin for jaundice, spider angiomata, and bruises on the extremities.
- A complete neurologic examination that includes cranial nerves, gait, sensory, motor, reflexes, and Romberg's test.
- For men, evaluate for gynecomastia, loss of axillary and pubic hair, and testicular atrophy (Fig. 16–5).

Diagnostic Tests

- Complete blood count (CBC) for chronic blood loss or marrow suppression.
- Liver function tests (LFTs), including lactate dehydrogenase (LDH), aspartate aminotransferase (AST) (serum glutamic-oxaloacetic transaminase [SGOT]), alanine aminotransferase (ALT) (serum glutamic-pyruvic transaminase [SGPT]), and alkaline phosphotase for liver function.
- Blood chemistries, particularly glucose and magnesium.
- Electrocardiogram (ECG), suggesting cardiomyopathy.

Differential Diagnoses: Abuse of other psychoactive substances such as opiates, hypnotics, and sedatives can cause symptoms similar to those of alcohol abuse.

Treatment: The goal of treatment is sobriety or total abstinence from alcohol. Patients with symptoms of alcohol withdrawal should be hospitalized. Uncomplicated alcohol abuse can be treated in the outpatient setting. Alcoholics Anonymous (AA) is the most successful group in encouraging ongoing sobriety; however, the self-sufficient spirit often characteristic of older adults reduces the probability of participation. An AA volunteer of the same gender and of an age comparable to the patient's age is usually available to meet with an individual at the clinic site and can assume the role of the patient's sponsor, reducing fear and providing the support that may encourage group participation. For older adults, people who are important in their lives need to be instructed by counselors in ways to encourage the treatment process and decrease behaviors that enable the older adult to abuse alcohol. After consultation with a physician, disulfuram (Antabuse) may be given to help maintain abstinence in healthy patients. For chronic alcoholism, the diet should be supplemented with multivitamins containing folic acid and thiamine 100 mg/day. Magnesium deficiency requires elemental magnesium 240 mg/day or bid. Ferrous sulfate 325 mg/day may be indicated.

Follow-up: Initially, the older adult should be seen weekly to provide continuity in the practitioner-patient relationship and to monitor treatment effectiveness. Once the patient is participating in the treatment protocol, monthly visits should be adequate to monitor progress.

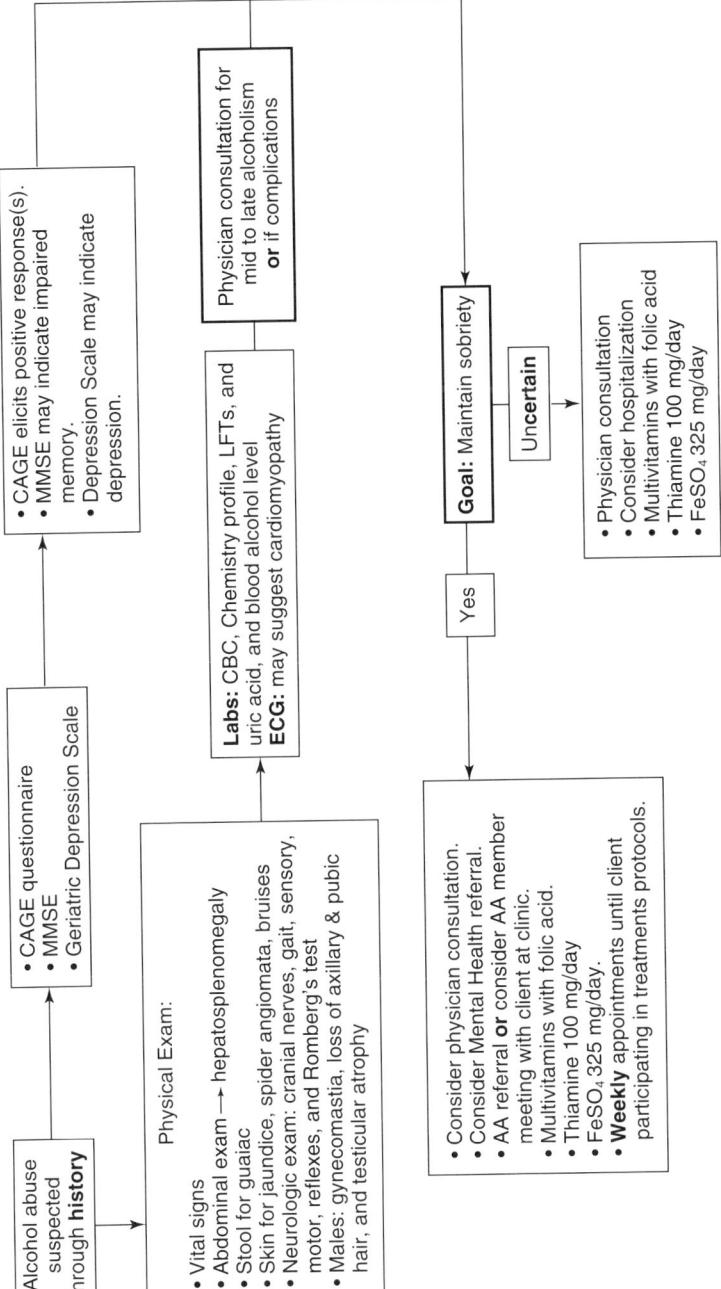

FIGURE 16–5 Alcohol abuse.

Sequelae: Alcohol abuse can lead to gastrointestinal (GI) bleeding, especially if the patient is taking aspirin or arthritis medications. Some other concerns include the following:

- Malnutrition.
- Cirrhosis.
- Decline in cognitive status.
- Addiction and tolerance with concomitant withdrawal symptoms.

The withdrawal symptoms of alcohol include increased anxiety, sleep problems, nausea, and weakness. Without treatment the anxiety and agitation progress to a tremulous state within 1–2 days, followed by increasingly severe symptoms that include hallucinations and withdrawal seizures (delirium tremens).

Prevention/Prophylaxis: Prevention demands more than warning of the dangers of the health hazards of alcohol. Taking a brief drinking history with the yearly evaluation provides the practitioner with an opportunity for patient education.

Referral: Refer for physician consultation patients with mid- to late-stage alcoholism or with suspected complications. Pending physician consultation, consider for inpatient detoxification program. Refer to mental health professional as indicated.

Education: Patients must be encouraged to continue participation in a treatment program, and family members to participate in a support group. Dietary supplements should be taken as ordered.

Anxiety

Anxiety is a subjective state of internal discomfort, dread, and foreboding accompanied by autonomic system arousal.

Etiology: Anxiety tends to occur without conscious stimulus. Many anxiety-producing events occur in the lives of older adults when their mastery and control of changes are diminished. State anxiety, an individual's transitory anxiety response to stressors, appears to increase in later life, whereas trait anxiety, an individual's predisposition to anxiety as a function of a personality disorder, remains relatively constant.

Occurrence: About 10%–15% of older adults seek medical treatment for anxiety.

Age: Anxiety can occur at all ages; however, anxiety states may be more incapacitating to older adults than to persons of other ages.

Ethnicity: Not significant.

Gender: The distribution of anxiety in older adults is slightly higher in women than in men.

Contributing Factors: Prior history of anxiety or related psychosocial problem, physical dependence, lack of control, change in daily routine, environmental change, fear of death, chronic illness, lack of social support, high caffeine intake, use of OTC sympathomimetic drugs; frequently occurs with depression.

Signs and Symptoms: Anxiety is divided into four categories in the *Diagnostic and Statistical Manual of Mental Disorders (DSM-IV)*.

- Motor tension (shakiness, jumpiness, trembling, inability to relax).
- Autonomic hyperactivity (sweating, palpitations, dry mouth, dizziness, hot or cold spells, frequent urination, or diarrhea).
- Apprehensive expectation (worry or anticipation of personal misfortune).
- Vigilance and scanning (distractibility, poor concentration, insomnia, edginess).

The patient must manifest symptoms in at least three of the four categories, and these symptoms should persist for at least 6 months.

Diagnostic Tests: Obtain a complete history, including a careful drug profile that encompasses current and recently discontinued medications, caffeine and alcohol intake, and OTC medications (Fig. 16–6). A psychosocial assessment that includes a mental status examination and a depression scale aids in the evaluation of psychiatric disorders. Assess for medical causes, directing attention toward disorders associated with anxiety. Laboratory tests may include a complete blood count (CBC), chemistry profile, thyroid panel, and an electrocardiogram (ECG).

Differential Diagnoses: The differential diagnosis may include hyperthyroidism, excessive caffeine intake, unstable angina, substance abuse, organic brain syndrome, depression, hypertension, and nutritional insufficiency.

Treatment: After accurately diagnosing generalized anxiety disorder, management requires a strong practitioner-patient relationship, counseling, family support, and appropriate medication. Psychotherapeutic approaches may be useful in alleviating generalized anxiety, especially if it is related to the bereavement process. Behavioral therapy is helpful for specific phobias and panic attacks seen in the older adult. In addition to counseling, the antianxiety drug of choice is buspirone (BuSpar) 5 mg tid, adjusted up to a maximum of 20–30 mg/day. BuSpar is nonaddictive and causes no withdrawal symptoms; however, subjective improvement with this drug takes about 2 weeks of continuous therapy. Another option is a shorter-acting anxiolytic: lorazepam (Ativan) 0.5–1 mg/day at bedtime or oxazepam (Serax) 10 mg at bedtime. It should be understood that the anxiolytics are for short-term (4–6 weeks) or occasional use as needed.

Situations that may contribute to anxiety include:

Postural hypotension from medication: Withdraw drug or reduce dosage.

Major depression: Fluoxetine HCl (Prozac) 10 mg q AM initially, increasing to 20 mg q AM if needed or sertraline HCl (Zoloft) 25 mg q AM initially, increasing weekly to 75–100 mg daily if lower dosage ineffective.

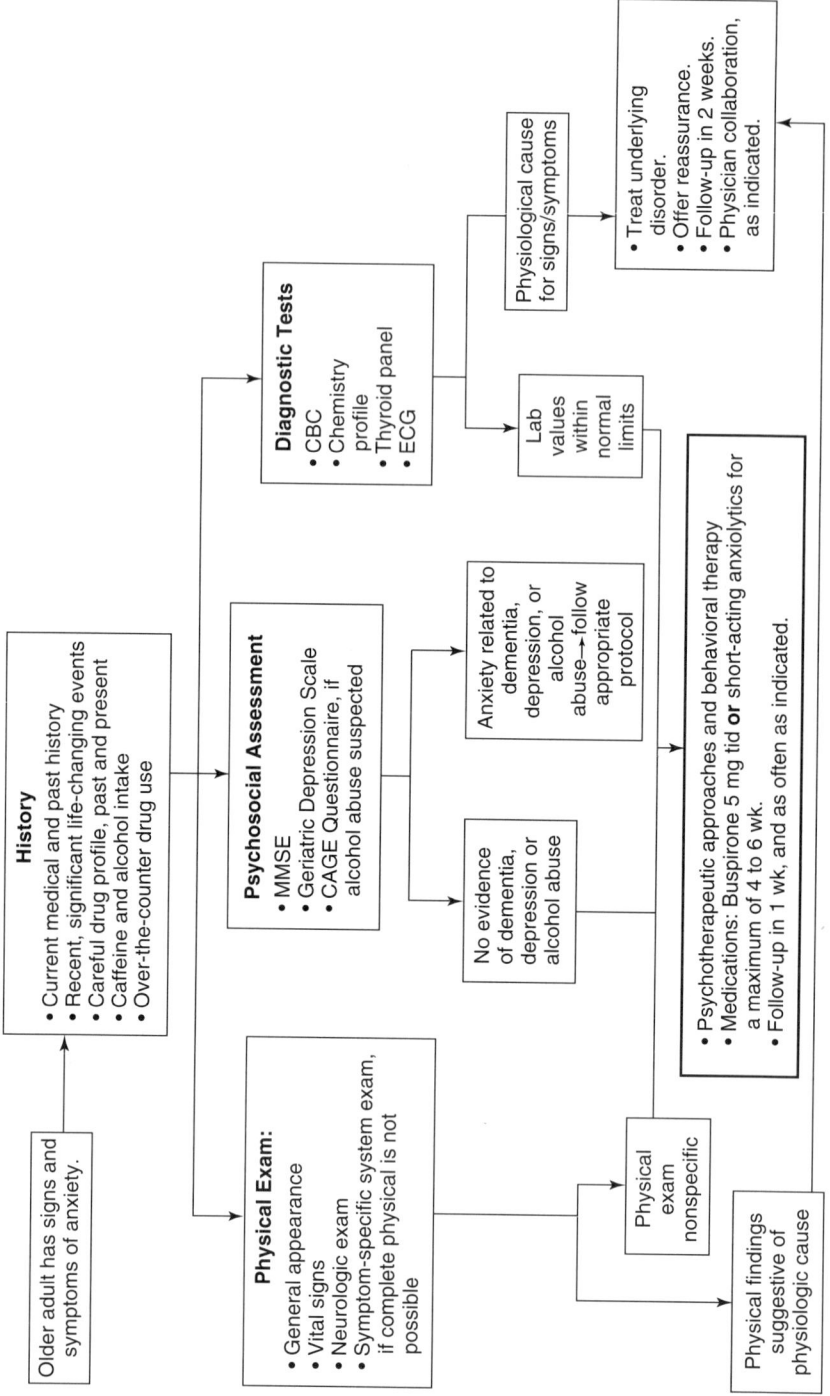

FIGURE 16-6   Anxiety.

Mild to moderate dementia: Emphasize need for more structured environment.

Follow-up: Return visit should be scheduled for 1 week, and as often as necessary to continue supportive therapy.

Sequelae: Reduced quality of life, impaired social interaction patterns.

Prevention: Management of stress, augmentation of social supports, maintenance of daily routines when possible, patient participation in decision affecting cure.

Referral: Patients with evidence of underlying organic or other disease state, including manifestation of a symptom not consistent with generalized anxiety, should be referred to a physician. Mental health referral is indicated if there is evidence of depressant drug abuse, the presenting symptoms are of long standing and not related to a current crisis, and symptoms persist after 2 weeks of treatment.

Education: Most older adults respond best to limited psychotherapy, short-term anxiolytic medication, and interventions that provide greater mastery and control over their physical or environmental stressors.

Depression

Depression is a mood disorder that may be classified as:

1 Major depression.
2 Bipolar disorder.
3 Psychotic depression.
4 Dysthymic disorder.
5 Adjustment disorder with depressed mood.
6 Organic mood disorder or a mood disorder secondary to a medical condition.

Etiology: No single cause of depression has been given. A number of theories exist related to the biologic etiology of depression. Most theories postulate problems with neurotransmitters such as impaired synthesis, lack of neurotransmitter, increased uptake, and increased metabolism or breakdown. Another theory identifies a genetic link for major depression and bipolar disorders. A psychosocial theory of the etiology of depression has also been proposed. The psychoanalytic view of depression is that the individual is mourning symbolic object loss with regard to his or her superego, leading to feelings of worthlessness. According to cognitive theory, depression is a result of habitual reinforcement of negative ideas about oneself, others, and the future. Finally, the environment and social factors contribute to depression when major stressors such as losses occur and social support systems are inadequate.

Occurrence: The prevalence of depression ranges from 8% to 15% of the older adult population; however, the incidence of depression rises to 12% of hospitalized elderly persons and to as high as 30% of older nursing home residents.

Age: Major depression tends to occur more in younger adulthood; the diagnosis of primary depression after age 50 is uncommon. However, the risk for suicide is highest for elderly white men.

Ethnicity: Native Americans have very high rates of depression. Asian Americans have high suicide rates. Elderly white men have the highest suicide rate.

Gender: Depression is more common in women than in men.

Contributing Factors: In older adults, factors that contribute to the development of depression in later life include a change in the environment or admission to a health-care facility; stressful losses, including loss of autonomy, privacy, functional status, a body part, or friend or family member; alcohol or substance abuse; and a history of attempted suicide or psychiatric hospitalizations. A personal or family history of depression also contributes to the onset of depression. Several medical conditions predispose a person to depression: Alzheimer's disease, Parkinson's disease, cerebrovascular accident (CVA), Huntington's disease, progressive supranuclear palsy, heart disease, hypothyroidism, anemia, and neoplasms. Medications associated with a high risk of depression include corticosteroids, antihypertensive agents, cimetidine, nonsteroidal anti-inflammatory drugs (NSAIDs), alcohol, and sedatives.

Signs and Symptoms: Patients who are experiencing depression may be able to tell you if there was a precipitating event before the depression began, as well as what symptoms they have been experiencing.

The DSM-IV criteria for major depression are that five or more of the following symptoms be present during the same 2-week time and must represent a change from the patient's previous level of function (at least one symptom must be either depressed mood or loss of pleasure or interest):

Depressed mood most of the day nearly every day.
Markedly diminished interest or ability to experience pleasure.
Significant weight loss without dieting.
Insomnia or hypersomnia.
Fatigue or loss of energy.
Feeling of worthlessness or excessive guilt.
Difficulty remembering.
Recurrent thoughts of death.

Patients with bipolar disorder experience depression as well as episodes of mania. Adjustment disorder with depressed mood occurs when a maladaptive reaction to an identified stressor has persisted for less than 6 months (acute) or for 6 months or longer (chronic). The onset of the depression must begin within 3 months of the stressor. Psychotic depression includes features of delusions, hallucinations, bizarre behavior, or disorganized thinking patterns.

Dysthmic disorder is chronic, mild depressive disorder with symptoms persisting for less than 2 years. Symptoms are less severe than those of major depression and neurovegetative symptoms.

In addition, older adults may present with a sense of hopelessness, excessive worry, persistent sadness, anxiety, irritability, constipation, and social withdrawal. Clinical examination may reveal a patient with inattention to personal appearance, tearfulness or poor eye contact, and slowed speech and movements. Patients may exhibit hand-wringing and pacing. Patients or family members may report social withdrawal or isolation.

Physical examination to check for any secondary causes of depression is recommended. The neurologic examination should focus on ruling out neurologic causes of depression (e.g., dementia or Parkinson's disease). A standardized depression screening tool such as the Geriatric Depression Rating Scale, can be administered to patients at risk. A score of 11 or more suggests the need for referral for a more detailed evaluation. If the patient seems confused, a mental status examination should be administered.

Differential Diagnosis: Consider the following presentations in the workup of depression in older adults: organic mood disorders secondary to drugs or illness, schizophrenia, grief, substance abuse, hypochondriasis, somatization disorder, sleep disorder, pseudodementia, and dementia. Also, discern if the patient is experiencing melancholic depression or nonmelancholic depression. Symptoms of melancholic depression include marked loss of pleasure, psychomotor retardation, weight loss, and insomnia. Knowing whether the patient is having a psychotic or a nonpsychotic episode will also help determine the treatment plan.

Diagnostic Tests: As depression in older adults can be secondary to physical illness, the following laboratory diagnostic tests are recommended:

Complete blood count (CBC) with differential to rule out anemia or infection.
Urinalysis.
Chest x-ray examination to determine presence of lung carcinoma.
Electrocardiogram (ECG) to establish a baseline before initiation of antidepressant medications.
Blood chemistries.
Thyroid-stimulating hormone (TSH) levels for assessment of thyroid function.
Dexamethasone suppression test: although not diagnostic, may help identify melancholic depression. Postdexamethasone cortisol level of greater than 5 μg/dL) is considered positive.

Treatment: The initial step in treating depression in older adults is to evaluate the present medication regimen and remove and/or change any depressogenic medications. Treat any metabolic or systemic disorder that may have predisposed the patient to depression. Ensure that the patient's nutrition, elimination, sleep, and physical comfort are considered in the treatment plan.

Pharmacotherapy is indicated when the symptoms of depression are moderately severe and/or when patterns of melancholic or endogenous depression are manifested. Antidepressant medications are recommended, considering the patients age and coexisting medical conditions and medications, the drug's side effect profile, and prior response to or failure of a particular drug. Start at a low dosage and monitor response. Agents with little or no anticholinergic effects are recommended. A tricyclic such as nortryptiline 10–25 mg/day at bedtime or desipramine 10–25 mg as the initial dose can be ordered. Selective serotonin reuptake inhibitors (SSRIs) can be prescribed with small initial doses (paroxetine 10–20 mg/day, sertraline 25–50 mg/day, or fluoxetine 10–20 mg/day). Bupropion 50–100 mg/day initially in divided doses, can also be tried.

Psychotherapy, often used in conjunction with pharmacotherapy, tends to be more beneficial to patients with nonmelancholic depression. If the patient is delusional or the condition is rapidly deteriorating, consult a psychiatrist, as electroconvulsive therapy (ECT) may be indicated.

Follow-up: Older adults who present without suicidal ideation should be seen in 2 weeks to evaluate therapeutic response and the possible need to increase medication dosage, then again 6 weeks after the initial trial of medications. If psychotherapy was ordered, then reevaluate in 6–8 weeks to determine if at least partial improvement has occurred and there is symptom relief. By 10–12 weeks a full response to treatment should be expected. If there is no noticeable improvement, a new treatment can be ordered. Then patients should be followed every 4–6 months. Antidepressant medications can be discontinued when no longer needed.

Sequelae: The most critical complication of depression in older adults is suicide. Social isolation, personal neglect, and malnutrition may also occur.

Prevention/Prophylaxis: For primary prevention, select medications that tend not to be depressogenic in older adults, especially for patients with a history of depression. Supporting patients through times of great loss and stressors by providing information about community resources and other educational materials also aids in preventing depression for this vulnerable population. For patients in long-term care facilities, especially for the newly admitted, arrange for participation in group activities such as reminiscence, music, or movement therapy, and if they have a history of having domestic animals, pet therapy if available. For anyone who has sustained a change or loss in physical functioning, arrange for physical or occupational therapy to assist with enhancement of independence as much as possible.

Referral: Refer patients to a specialist if they require acute hospitalization, if they appear actively suicidal, if the presentation is complicated (e.g., patients with severe, recurrent or psychotic depression), if they do not adhere to the prescribed regimen, or if the treatment does not result in a favorable outcome.

Education: Patients need to be informed that the medication will not work right away, and that a change in mood may not occur for some time after initiating therapy. Explain to the patient that understanding the cause of the depression (if known) would be beneficial. Emphasize the need to avoid alcohol as a means of alleviating the depressed mood, and also explain that alcohol is contraindicated when taking antidepressant medications. Provide information about community resources for older adults.

Elder Abuse

Elder mistreatment, defined as the abuse and neglect of older persons, includes physical, psychological and sexual abuse, caregiver and self-neglect, and financial exploitation (Capezuti, Brush, & Lawton, 1997). Physical abuse includes striking, shaking, restraining, or feeding improperly. Psychological abuse inflicts emotional stress or injury through verbal abuse. Sexual abuse is a form of sexual intimacy without consent, or by force, or by threat of force. Financial abuse is the misuse or exploitation of an older adult's possession or financial assets.

Etiology: The major etiologic theories that surface in the literature are: (1) abuser psychopathology, (2) stress, (3) transgenerational violence, and (4) dependency. The theory of abuser psychopathology suggests that the abuser has been hospitalized repeatedly for serious psychiatric disorders and may abuse alcohol and/or drugs. The stress theory posits that the psychological and physical demands placed on the caregiver by a cognitively impaired and/or medically ill elder is expressed through violent acts. Transgenerational violence theory indicates that violence is a learned response to difficult life experiences, and a learned method of expressing anger and frustration. The dependency theory postulates that when older adults are dependent for physical, emotional, and financial support, family members may become resentful and angry, predisposing the elder to abuse and neglect.

Occurrence: Slightly less common than child abuse. Approximately one million older Americans are mistreated annually with an estimated 1 out of 5 cases of elder abuse being reported to the authorities (Brewer, 1989).

Age: Elder abuse is most prevalent in persons over age 75.

Ethnicity: A greater incidence exists among whites.

Contributing Factors: Abuse occurs in all socioeconomic groups; however, it is more likely to occur among the lower class. The typical victim is a white woman over age 75, who lives with a relative and has a physical and/or mental impairment.

Sign and Symptoms: The health-care provider must remain nonjudgmental; however, elder abuse may be suspected when the following indicators are present:
- Pattern of "health-care hopping."
- Series of missed appointments.
- Medication misuse.

- Unexplained injuries such as fractures, welts, bald spots, and bite marks.
- Burns in unusual places.
- Bruises in varying stages of resolution.
- Poor personal hygiene.
- Clothes that are inappropriate for the season (such as a sweater in hot weather).
- Malnutrition and dehydration.
- Sexually transmitted disease and/or unusual genital infections.
- Bruises or bleeding in perineal area.
- Extreme mood changes.
- Depression.
- Fearfulness.
- Sleep disorders.
- Missing prosthetic devices (dentures, hearing aids, eyeglasses).
- Concern with health-care costs (see Fig. 16-7).

Diagnostic Tests: The individual's history and physical examination findings dictate what diagnostic tests to perform.

Differential Diagnosis: Unintended injury and poverty, which may preclude access to food, appropriate shelter, and health care, should be considered in the differential diagnosis.

Treatment: Elder abuse is a multidisciplinary issue that includes health-care providers, social workers, lawyers, law enforcement officers, and psychiatrists. For suspected mistreatment, the health-care professional may enact the following strategy:

1. Report to adult protective services (APS) or other public agency, as mandated by the law. APS must investigate reported elder mistreatment cases by interviewing victims, *despite the victim's wishes,* and others who may be knowledgeable about the case.
2. Determine whether emergency intervention is required. Emergency intervention is mandatory if medical and/or psychiatric care are needed, and if results of mistreatment are life-threatening. A cognitively impaired older adult with malnutrition and dehydration is an example of an appropriate situation for an emergency order of protection and emergency intervention.
3. *If the patient is in immediate danger,* create a safety plan. Options include hospitalization, court protective order, or safe home placement.
4. Perform a full, private, comprehensive assessment. ***Record accurately because this documentation may become part of a court case.*** A psychological history can elicit details about the primary caregiver, the elder-caregiver relationship and supportive relationships, the living situation, and the emotional status of the victim. Give a complete mental status examination to determine if the older adult is a competent consenting victim, a competent nonconsenting victim, or an incompetent victim. Con-

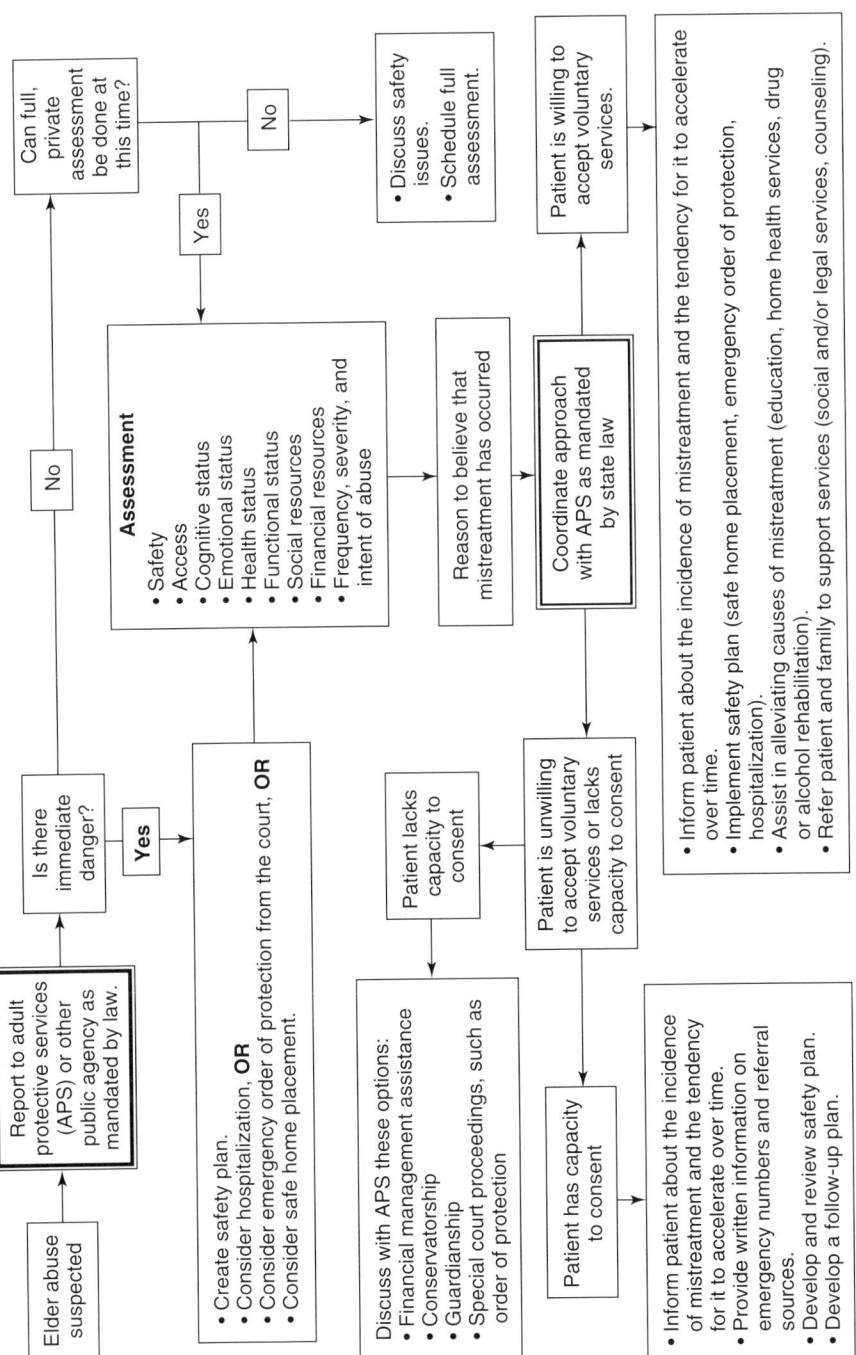

FIGURE 16–7 Elder abuse.

Elder abuse suspected

Report to adult protective services (APS) or other public agency as mandated by law.

Is there immediate danger?

Yes

• Create safety plan.
• Consider hospitalization, **OR**
• Consider emergency order of protection from the court, **OR**
• Consider safe home placement.

No

Can full, private assessment be done at this time?

No

• Discuss safety issues.
• Schedule full assessment.

Yes

Assessment
• Safety
• Access
• Cognitive status
• Emotional status
• Health status
• Functional status
• Social resources
• Financial resources
• Frequency, severity, and intent of abuse

Reason to believe that mistreatment has occurred

Coordinate approach with APS as mandated by state law

Patient is willing to accept voluntary services.

• Inform patient about the incidence of mistreatment and the tendency for it to accelerate over time.
• Implement safety plan (safe home placement, emergency order of protection, hospitalization).
• Assist in alleviating causes of mistreatment (education, home health services, drug or alcohol rehabilitation).
• Refer patient and family to support services (social and/or legal services, counseling).

Patient is unwilling to accept voluntary services or lacks capacity to consent

Patient lacks capacity to consent

Discuss with APS these options:
• Financial management assistance
• Conservatorship
• Guardianship
• Special court proceedings, such as order of protection

Patient has capacity to consent

• Inform patient about the incidence of mistreatment and the tendency for it to accelerate over time.
• Provide written information on emergency numbers and referral sources.
• Develop and review safety plan.
• Develop a follow-up plan.

duct a physical examination that includes functional status. If a physical injury is present, ask detailed questions that describe when and how it happened. An inconsistent or contradictory story should be a "red flag." *Use drawings or photographs, as necessary, to substantiate findings.*
5. Coordinate approach with APS as mandated by state law.

Follow-up: Monitor the outcome of all cases of abuse and neglect that have come to your attention.

Sequelae: The implications for the abused may subsequently result in long-term care placement. For the abuser, the outcome may include legal proceedings (for intentional cases) and immediate relief from the demands of caregiving through assistance from community resources, counseling, and education.

Prevention/Prophylaxis: Prevention of abuse comes from an increased understanding of the complex needs of a dependent older adult, and the support provided for the caregiving family. Prevention interventions may include the following:

- Educate the public about the changes of aging.
- Help families develop and nurture informal support systems.
- Link families with support groups.
- Teach families stress management techniques.
- Ensure that families have the home health support services needed to provide adequate care.
- Encourage the use of respite and adult day care.
- Inform families of community services available for meals and transportation.

Referral: Physician collaboration is necessary, as indicated.

Education: See section on Prevention.

Grief

Grief is a normal emotional response to loss; when the patient is unable to work through it, physical and/or psychological illness may occur.

Etiology: Loss or change perceived as loss.

Occurrence: Approximately 50% of women over age 65 are widows; 13% of men over age 65 are widowers.

Age: Grief may occur at any age.

Ethnicity: Not significant.

Gender: Grief affects more women than men.

Contributing Factors. Varied grief reactions to becoming widowed may be related to the following factors:

- Length of illness.
- Pain of illness.
- Personality deficits before death.
- Quality of the relationship.
- Personality attributes of the survivor.
- Degree of responsibility survivor feels.
- Personal and financial expense of the illness.

Studies have not found a positive correlation between anticipatory grief and adaptation to the loss of a spouse, alerting practitioners to notice varied grief reactions despite the expectancy of death. Widows and widowers with recent disabilities, few friends, and poor relationships with their children were more apt to require counseling.

Signs and Symptoms: Grief is characterized by feelings of depression with associated symptoms of poor appetite and weight loss or compulsive eating and weight gain, sleep disturbance, tearfulness, lack of interest, withdrawal and isolation, emptiness, indecisiveness, and guilt feelings (Fig. 16–8).

Diagnostic Tests: None.

Differential Diagnoses: A major depressive episode may mimic grief.

Treatment: Provide emotional support, allowing the older adult to express feelings. Encourage patients to return to their normal routine as soon as possible, but no more than 2 weeks after the event. Daily physical exercise can help patients cope with the depression that accompanies grief.

Follow-up: Once a month or more often depending on patient needs.

Prevention/Prophylaxis: The goal is to encourage and support the patient in the normal grieving process and prevent dysfunctional grieving. Bereavement groups, activation of social and spiritual support networks, discussion of anticipated loss by participants, and involvement in group activities may be helpful.

Sequelae: In the first 3 months after the death of a spouse for adults over age 65 years, the mortality rate increases 48% in men and 22% in women. Practitioners must be alert to older adults who do not improve in 3 months after the loss. Additionally, a major depressive syndrome that occurs for 2 or more weeks early in the course of bereavement should be taken seriously, and managed accordingly.

Referral: Older adults experiencing abnormal grieving may benefit from a mental health referral. Referral to support groups, such as Widow-to-Widow, may be helpful in the grieving process.

Education: Make patients and their support networks aware of normal grieving stages; alert them to signs of dysfunctional grieving and resources for help.

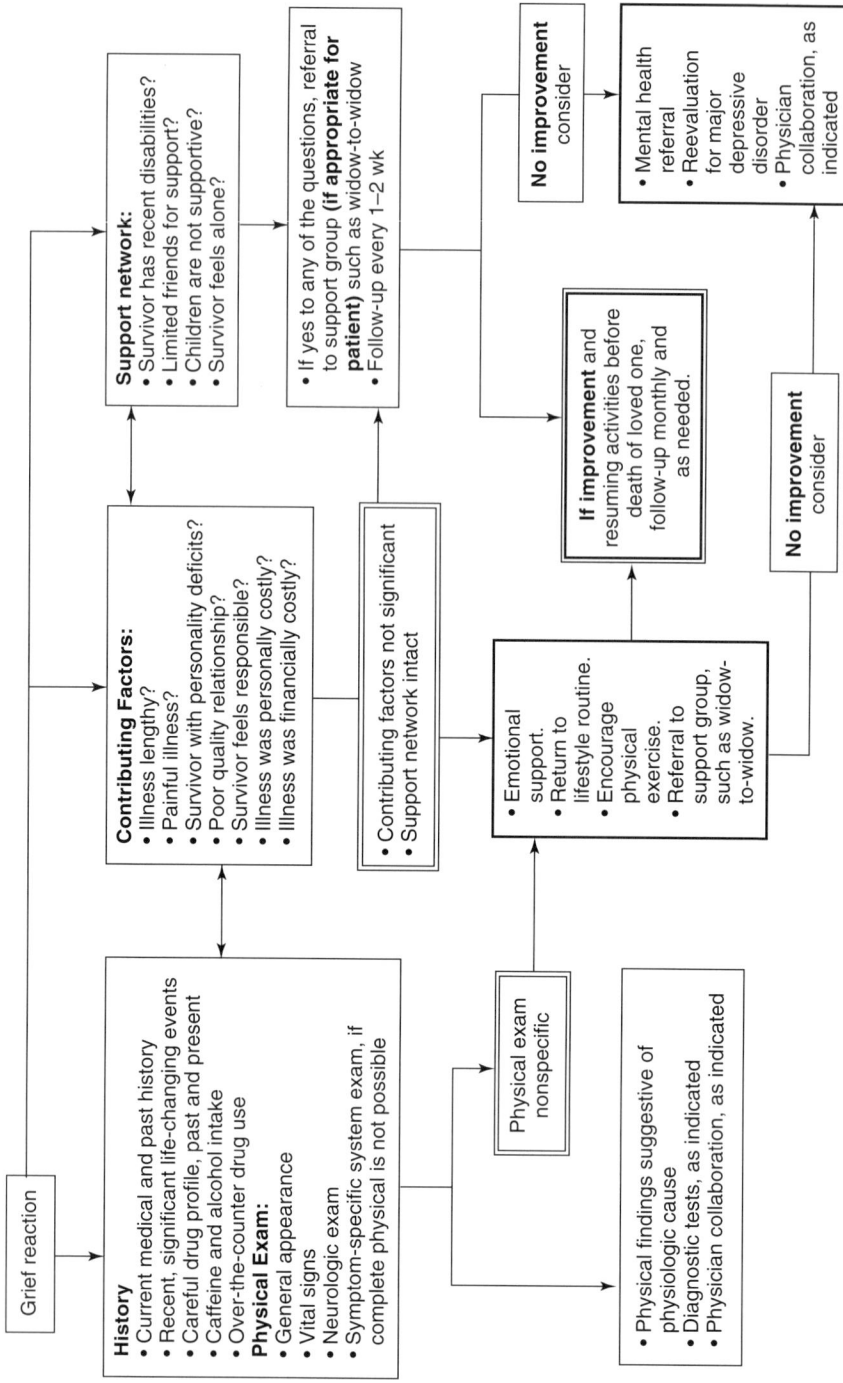

FIGURE 16–8 Grief.

Insomnia

Insomnia is the inability to sleep despite the desire to do so.

Etiology: Sleeping states and sleep schedules change with age, reflecting the aging process and the impact of physical maladies and psychiatric disorders. The most important age-related changes in sleep include:

- Decreased continuity of sleep with an increase in the number of arousals.
- Tendency for the major period of sleep and rapid eye movement (REM) sleep to occur earlier in the night.
- Decrease in the very deepest parts of nonrapid eye movement (NREM) sleep.
- Increased napping during the day.
- Tendency to spend more time in bed.

Transient insomnia, which lasts a few nights, is related to situational stress and usually resolves without medical intervention when the older adult adapts to the change or removes it. *Short-term insomnia,* which is similar to transient insomnia, lasts less than a month and is related to an acute medical or psychological condition or to persistent situational stress. *Chronic insomnia* lasts more than 1 month and results from both age-related changes in sleep and chronic stressors. About one third of patients who suffer from chronic insomnia have psychiatric disorders.

Occurrence: Approximately 35% of people over age 60 suffer from and regularly complain of poor sleep quality.

Age: Insomnia can occur at any age; however, older adults have greater difficulty falling asleep and staying asleep.

Ethnicity: Not significant.

Gender: Older men show poorer sleep maintenance than do older women.

Contributing Factors: Factors that may contribute to insomnia include:

- Restless syndrome.
- Periodic limb movement disorder.
- Sleep apnea.
- Dementia.
- Depression.
- Drugs, including caffeine and alcohol.

Certain medical conditions and drugs used for their treatment may interfere with sleep:

- Musculoskeletal disorders: osteoarthritis, fibromyositis, polymyalgia rheumatica, recent fractures, and flexion contractures.
- Cardiovascular disorders: the drugs for treating hypertension (diuretics, beta-blockers, clonidine, reserpine, and methyldopa), heart failure, and angina.

- Pulmonary disorders: Chronic obstructive pulmonary disease (COPD) and the sympathomimetic bronchodilators used for treating bronchospasm.
- Gastrointestinal (GI) disorders: gastroesophageal reflux disease (GERD) and peptic ulcer disease (PUD).
- Renal disease: renal dialysis, uremia, and prostate enlargement.
- Metabolic disorders: hypothyroidism and hyperthyroidism.
- Neurologic disorders: Parkinson's disease.

Signs and Symptoms: A complete history should reveal a full description of the problems (Fig. 16–9). Patients may complain about difficulty falling asleep and staying asleep, frequent awakenings, early morning awakening and inability to return to sleep, daytime fatigue with unwanted naps, irritability, or difficulty concentrating. Additionally, an older adult may spend 10–12 hours in bed at night trying to sleep. A pertinent physical examination should evaluate the systems associated with any medical conditions listed here. A mental status examination is useful in detecting psychiatric disease.

Diagnostic Tests: None, unless indicated by history and physical examination.

Differential Diagnosis: Anxiety, inadequate sleep hygiene, medical problems, medication-related sleep disorder, depression, alcohol-related sleep disorder, or primary sleep disorder are considerations.

Treatment: Patients should avoid caffeine for up to 12 hours prior to bedtime and discontinue alcohol and unnecessary sleep-interrupting drugs. For transient or short-term insomnia, initiate short-term use of a short-acting sedative-hypnotic such as temazepam (Restoril) 7.5–15 mg 1–2 hr before desired bedtime for no more than 2 to 3 nights. If this is ineffective, reevaluate diagnosis and restructure treatment modalities. For chronic insomnia, the treatment is more complex and includes the following:

- Provide patient education and reassurance, exploring the reasons behind poor sleeping habits and evaluating diet and exercise habits.
- Treat underlying or coexisting disorders.
- Encourage patients to discontinue caffeine and alcohol.
- Initiate short-term use of sedative-hypnotics.
- Treat specific sleep disorder.

Follow-up: Patients should return in 2 weeks. Examine the patient's sleep diary and evaluate the effectiveness of the treatment. If indicated, reevaluate diagnosis and restructure treatment.

Sequelae: Reduced quality of life, increased risk for falls/injury, potential for drug dependence or drug interactions due to use of OTC sleep aids.

Prevention/Prophylaxis: Sleep hygiene suggestions may include the following:

- Establish a regular bedtime and wake-up time.
- Set aside a time each evening for relaxation and thinking.
- Avoid caffeine, alcohol, and nicotine because they all interrupt sleep.
- Minimize awake time in bed, reserving bed for sleep and sexual activity.

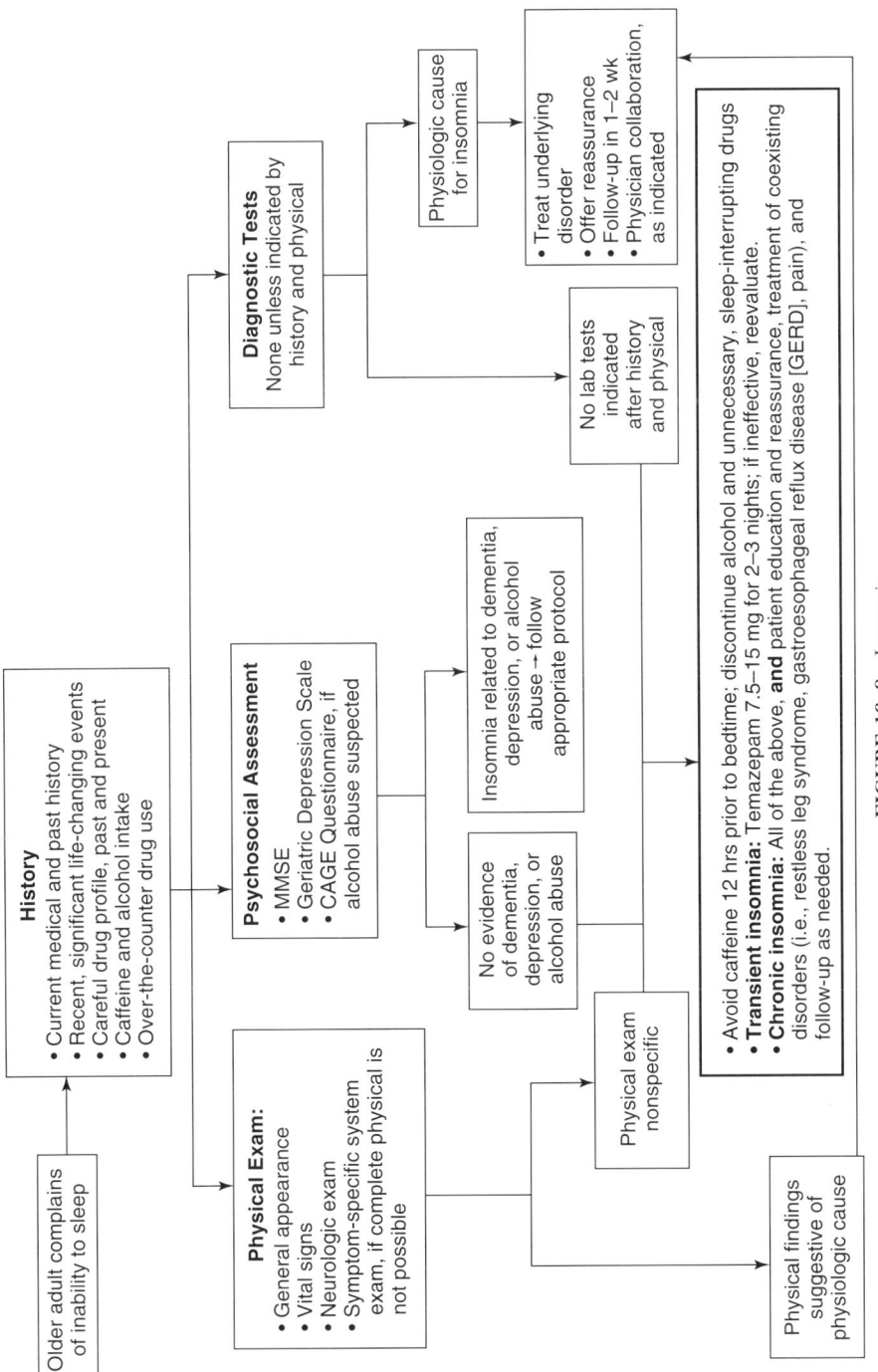

Older adult complains of inability to sleep

History
• Current medical and past history
• Recent, significant life-changing events
• Careful drug profile, past and present
• Caffeine and alcohol intake
• Over-the-counter drug use

Physical Exam:
• General appearance
• Vital signs
• Neurologic exam
• Symptom-specific system exam, if complete physical is not possible

Psychosocial Assessment
• MMSE
• Geriatric Depression Scale
• CAGE Questionnaire, if alcohol abuse suspected

Diagnostic Tests
None unless indicated by history and physical

Physiologic cause for insomnia

• Treat underlying disorder
• Offer reassurance
• Follow-up in 1–2 wk
• Physician collaboration, as indicated

No lab tests indicated after history and physical

Insomnia related to dementia, depression, or alcohol abuse → follow appropriate protocol

No evidence of dementia, depression, or alcohol abuse

Physical exam nonspecific

Physical findings suggestive of physiologic cause

• Avoid caffeine 12 hrs prior to bedtime; discontinue alcohol and unnecessary, sleep-interrupting drugs
• **Transient insomnia:** Temazepam 7.5–15 mg for 2–3 nights; if ineffective, reevaluate.
• **Chronic insomnia:** All of the above, **and** patient education and reassurance, treatment of coexisting disorders (i.e., restless leg syndrome, gastroesophageal reflux disease [GERD], pain), and follow-up as needed.

FIGURE 16–9 Insomnia.

- Create an optimal sleep environment.
- Establish regular eating habits because hunger can interrupt sleep.
- Avoid napping.
- Exercise daily to extent possible, but avoid exercise just prior to bedtime.
- Maximize daytime exposure to bright light.

Referral: If therapy brings no improvement and other underlying causes have been eliminated, refer the patient to a sleep laboratory for evaluation.

Education: Teach the patient to follow the guidelines listed under Prevention.

Wandering

Wandering is "a purposeful behavior that attempts to fulfill a particular need (from the context of the wanderer), is initiated by a cognitively impaired and disoriented individual, and is characterized by excessive ambulation that often leads to safety and/or nuisance-related problems" (Thomas, 1995). Wandering has been viewed as a form of agenda behavior that is directed toward meeting perceived social, emotional, or physical needs. Agenda behavior may be a method for the wanderer to regain feelings of safety and belonging that provided satisfaction in the past.

Etiology: Factors that have been identified with wandering include:

- Cognitive impairment.
- Confusion.
- Darkened or unfamiliar environment.
- Diseases of the central nervous system.
- Stress.
- Tension.
- Anxiety.
- Lack of control.
- Lack of exercise.
- Boredom.
- Cardiac decompensation.

Nocturnal wandering that accompanies "sundowning" appears to be associated with the onset of darkness and related to the individual's loss of spatial relationships in the dark.

Age: Dementia affects 5%–10% of persons over age 65 and approximately 30% of persons over age 85.

Occurrence: The most common type of dementia is Alzheimer's disease, which accounts for 50%–60% of the cases of dementia. Because a positive correlation exists between the frequency of wandering and severity of dementia, the more severe the dementia the greater the probability the person will exhibit wandering behavior. One recent study (Thomas, 1997) found that wanderers were usually diagnosed with Alzheimer's disease, suggesting that the cognitive progression associated with Alzheimer's disease is more likely to produce wandering.

Ethnicity: Not significant.

Gender: Because Alzheimer's disease is twice as common in women as in men (perhaps because women live longer or female gender may be a risk factor), wandering may be more prevalent in women.

Contributing Factors: The cognitive status of wanderers is no worse than that of nonwanderers; however, *wanderers are more likely to have irreversible bases of impairment*. Wandering can be affected by many factors in the person, in the environment, or both. Physiologic factors that may contribute to wandering include:

- Medication interactions and/or use of psychotropic agents.
- Physical discomfort caused by pain, thirst, or hunger.
- Need for toileting.
- Desire to exercise.

Psychological factors suggest wandering may stem from loneliness and separation and may serve to dissipate stress. **Environmental factors** may include an impoverished social climate, restrictive surroundings, an overstimulating climate, or new and unfamiliar situations.

Signs and Symptoms: Wanderers may have greater overall impairment of basic cognitive skills such as memory, orientation, and concentration, as well as impairment of higher-order cognitive skills that include abstract thinking, judgment, language, and spatial skills. Language impairment seems to distinguish the wanderers from the nonwanderers. Behaviors associated with wandering include:

- Pacing.
- Agitation.
- Aggressiveness.
- Incontinence.

Diagnostic Tests: Obtain a complete history (Fig. 16–10), including a careful drug profile that encompasses current and recently discontinued medications, caffeine and alcohol intake, and over-the-counter (OTC) medications. Perform a psychosocial assessment that includes a mental status examination. Assess for medical causes with attention directed toward disorders associated with wandering. Laboratory tests may include complete blood count (CBC), chemistry profile, thyroid panel, and electrocardiogram (ECG).

Differential Diagnosis: Alternative diagnoses may include:

- Medication interactions.
- Inappropriate psychotropic medication use.
- Physical discomfort caused by pain.

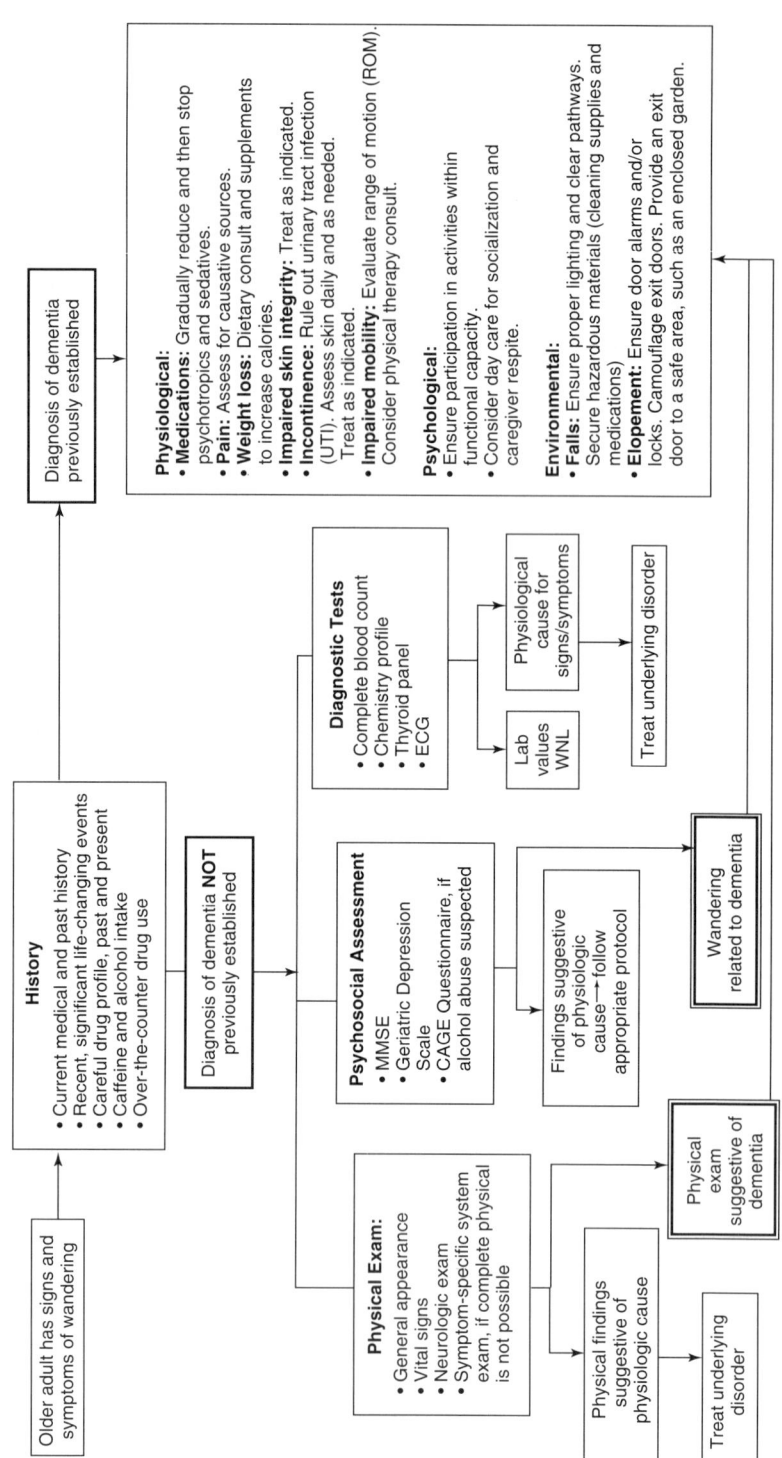

FIGURE 16–10 Wandering.

- Nutritional insufficiency.
- Cardiac decompensation.
- Diseases of the central nervous system (CNS).

Treatment: Many of the management strategies are directed toward caregiver and/or staff education. Some strategies that are directed toward physiologic, psychological, and environmental factors are shown in Table 16–2.

TABLE 16–2 WANDERING MANAGEMENT STRATEGIES

Factor	Etiology	Intervention
Physiologic	Medications	Gradually reduce and then stop psychotropics and sedatives.
		Review medications, including over-the-counter (OTC) products for interactions.
	Pain	Assess for physical sources that may cause pain; treat, initially, with acetaminophen 500 mg qid. Review for effectiveness.
		Assess feet for corns, calluses, and mycotic toenails; treat as indicated. Refer to podiatrist as needed.
		Evaluate footwear for proper fit. Request proper footwear if poor fit.
	Weight loss	Arrange a dietary consult for caloric needs assessment.
		Give supplements to increase calories.
	Impaired skin integrity	Staff to assess feet weekly.
		Treat problems as indicated.
	Incontinence	Assess skin daily and as needed for breakdown.
		Treat as indicated.
	Impaired mobility	Evaluate range of motion (ROM). Is ROM limited because of pain?
		Consider physical therapy evaluation.
Psychological	Social skills	Ensure participation in activities within functional capacity.
	Agenda behavior	Use distraction techniques.
		Provide meaningful tasks that wanderer can successfully complete.
Environmental	Falls	Ensure proper lighting and clear pathways.
		Secure hazardous materials (cleaning supplies, medications).
	Elopement	Ensure door alarms and/or locks; camouflage exit doors.
		Prove an exit door to safe area, such as an enclosed garden.

Follow-up: Follow-up visits are scheduled as indicated by the environment in which the wanderer resides. If the patient lives at home and cannot be managed by his or her family, more intense follow-up may be indicated; patient may need placement in an environment safer than a long-term care facility.

Sequelae: The patient who wanders is at high risk for:

- Injury, such as falls and fractures, related to cognitive impairment and gait disturbance.
- Weight loss related to high expenditure of calories and inability to stay sedentary long enough to consume a meal.
- Behavior problems, such as agitation.
- Caregiver fatigue related to need for constant monitoring of wanderer.

Referral: Because wandering is often associated with negative outcomes for the patient and the caregiver, a referral for **home health** support or **long-term care (LTC) placement** may be indicated. Evidence of underlying organic or other disease state, including manifestation of a symptom not consistent with wandering, may require physician consultation.

Education: Educate the caregiver and/or the staff in the residential care facility within the contextual world of the wandering individual.

BIBLIOGRAPHY

Assessment

Abrams, WB, Beers, MH, and Berkow, R (eds): The Merck Manual of Geriatrics, ed 2. Merck, Whitehouse Station, NJ, 1995.

Brown, MM, and Hachinski, VC: Acute confusional states, amnesia, and dementia. In Isselbacher, KJ, et al (eds): Harrison's Principles of Internal Medicine, ed 13. McGraw-Hill, New York, 1994.

Buckwalter, KC: Psychosocial needs and care of the elderly. In McFarland, GK, and Thomas, MD (eds): Psychiatric Mental Health Nursing: Application of the Nursing Process. JB Lippincott, Philadelphia, 1991.

Eisendrath, SJ, and Brophy, JJ: Psychiatric disorders. In Tierney, LM Jr, McPhee, SJ, and Papadakis, MA (eds): Current Medical Diagnosis and Treatment. Appleton & Lange, Norwalk, Conn., 1995.

Gallo, JJ, Reichel, W, and Andersen, LM: Handbook of Geriatric Assessment. Aspen, Gaithersburg, 1995.

Harper, MS: Foreword. In Buckwalter, KM (ed): Geriatric Mental Health Nursing: Current and Future Challenges. Slack, Thorofare, NJ, 1992.

Plopper, M: Common psychiatric disorders. In Yoshikawa, TT, Cobbs, EL, and Brummel-Smith, K (eds): Ambulatory Geriatric Care. CV Mosby, St. Louis, 1993.

Resnick, NM: Geriatric medicine. In Isselbacher, KJ, et al (eds): Harrison's Principles of Internal Medicine, ed 13. McGraw-Hill, New York, 1994.

Wykle, ML, and Musil, CM: Mental health of older persons: Social and cultural factors. In Smyer, MA (ed): Mental Health and Aging. Springer, New York, 1993.

Alcohol Abuse

Abrams, WB, Beers, MH, and Berkow, R (eds): The Merck Manual of Geriatrics, ed 2. Merck, Whitehouse Station, NJ, 1995.

Adams, WL, Yuan, Z, Barboriak, JJ, and Rimm, AA: Alcohol-related hospitalizations of elderly people: Prevalence and geographic variation in the United States. JAMA 270:1222–1225, 1993.

Barry, R, and Burggraf, V: Elderly and alcohol: A deadly combination. In Burggraf, V, and Barry, R (eds): Gerontological Nursing: Current Practice and Research. Slack, Thorofare, NJ, 1996.

Eisendrath, SJ, and Brophy, JJ: Psychiatric disorders. In Tierney, LM Jr, McPhee, SJ, and Papadakis, MA (eds): Current Medical Diagnosis and Treatment. Appleton & Lange, Norwalk, CT, 1995.

Fankhauser, MP: Anxiolytic drugs and sedative-hypnotic agents. In Bressler, R, and Katz, MD (eds): Geriatric Pharmacology. McGraw-Hill, New York, 1993.

Gallo, JJ, Reichel, W, and Andersen, LM: Handbook of Geriatric Assessment. Aspen, Gaithersburg, 1995.

Gulanick, M, et al: Nursing Care Plans: Nursing Diagnosis and Intervention, ed 3. CV Mosby, St. Louis, 1994.

Hanna, EZ: Approach to the patient with alcohol abuse. In Goroll AH, May LA, and Mulley, AG Jr: Primary Care Medicine: Office Evaluation of the Adult Patient, ed 3. JB Lippincott, Philadelphia, 1995.

Iliffe, S, Mitchley, S, Gould, M, and Haines, A: Evaluation of the use of brief screening instruments for dementia, depression, and problem drinking among elderly people in general practice. Br J Gen Pract 44:503–507, 1994.

Plopper, M: Common psychiatric disorders. In Yoshikawa, TT, Cobbs, EL, and Brummel-Smith, K (eds): Ambulatory Geriatric Care. CV Mosby, St. Louis, 1993.

Resnick, NM: Geriatric medicine. In Isselbacher, KJ, et al (eds): Harrison's Principles of Internal Medicine, ed 13. McGraw-Hill, New York, 1994.

Welte, JW, and Mirand, AL: Lifetime drinking patterns of elders from a general population survey. Drug Alcohol Depend 35:133–140, 1994.

Williams, ME: The American Geriatrics Society's Complete Guide to Aging and Health. Harmony Books, New York, 1995.

Wykle, ML, and Musil, CM: Mental health of older persons: Social and cultural factors. In Smyer, MA (ed): Mental Health and Aging. Springer, New York, 1993.

Anxiety

Eisendrath, SJ, and Brophy, JJ: Psychiatric disorders. In Tierney, LM Jr, McPhee, SJ, and Papadakis, MA (eds): Current Medical Diagnosis and Treatment. Appleton & Lange, Norwalk, CT, 1995.

Fankhauser, MP: Anxiolytic drugs and sedative-hypnotic agents. In Bressler, R, and Katz, MD (eds): Geriatric Pharmacology. McGraw-Hill, New York, 1993.

Gulanick, M, et al: Nursing Care Plans: Nursing Diagnosis and Intervention, ed 3. CV Mosby, St. Louis, 1994.

Gurian, BS, and Miner, JH: Clinical presentation of anxiety in the elderly. In Salzman, C, and Lebowitz, BD (eds): Anxiety in the Elderly. Springer, New York, 1991.

Gurian, B, and Goisman, R: Anxiety disorders in the elderly. In Smyer, MA (ed): Mental Health and Aging. Springer, New York, 1993.

Plopper, M: Common psychiatric disorders. In Yoshikawa, TT, Cobbs, EL, and Brummel-Smith, K (eds): Ambulatory Geriatric Care. CV Mosby, St. Louis, 1993.

Rauch, SL, and Rosenbaum, JF: Psychiatric and behavioral problems. In Goroll, AH, May, LA, and Mulley, AG Jr: Primary Care Medicine: Office Evaluation of the Adult Patient, ed 3. JB Lippincott, Philadelphia, 1995.

Depression

American Psychiatric Association: Diagnostic and Statistical Manual of Mental Disorders, ed 4. American Psychiatric Association, Washington, DC, 1994.

Blazer, DG: The epidemiology of depression in late life. In Blazer DG: Depression in Late Life. CV Mosby, St. Louis, 1993.

Brooks, T, and Creary, L: Ethogeriatrics: Unique health issues of culturally diverse elderly. In Yoshikawa, L, Cobbs, EL, and Brummel-Smith, K (eds): Practical Ambulatory Geriatrics, ed 2. CV Mosby, St. Louis, 1998.

Busse, EW, and Blazer, DG (eds): Textbook of Geriatric Psychiatry, ed 3. American Psychiatric Press, Washington, DC, 1996.

Ferentz, K: The primary care setting: Managing medical comorbidity in the elderly depressed patient. Geriatrics 50(Suppl 1):S25–S31, 1995.

Fitten, LJ: Common psychiatric disorders. In Yoshikawa, T, Cobbs, EL, and Brummel-Smith, K (eds): Practical Ambulatory Geriatrics, ed 2. CV Mosby, St. Louis, 1998.

Terpstra, TL, and Terpstra, TL: Treating geriatric depression with SSRIs: What primary care practitioners need to know. Nurse Pract 22:9, 118, 1997.

US Department of Health and Human Services, Public Health Service, Agency for Health Care Policy and Research, Depression Guideline Panel: Depression in Primary Care. Vol. 2. Treatment of major depression. Clinical Practice Guideline No. 5. AHCPR Publications No. 93-0551, Rockville, Md., April 1993.

Yesavage, J, et al: Development and validation of a geriatric depression screening scale: A preliminary report. J Psychiat Res 17:215, 1983.

Elder Abuse

Abrams, WB, Beers, MH, and Berkow, R (eds): The Merck Manual of Geriatrics, ed 2. Merck, Whitehouse Station, NJ, 1995.

All, AC: A literature review: Assessment and intervention in elder abuse. Journal of Gerontological Nursing 20(7):32–35, 1994.

Brewer, and Jones, R: Reporting elder abuse: Limitations of statues. Ann Emerg Med 18:1217–1221, 1989.

Capezuti, E, Brush, BJ, and Lawson, WT: Reporting elder mistreatment. Journal of Gerontological Nursing 23(7):24–32, 1997.

Ebersole, P, and Hess, P: Toward Healthy Aging: Human Needs and Nursing Response, ed 4. CV Mosby, St. Louis, 1994.

Kaufman, SR, and Becker, G: Frailty, risk, and choice: Cultural discourses and the question of responsibility. In Smyer, M, Schaie, KW, and Kapp, MB (eds): Older Adult's Decision-Making and the Law. Springer, New York, 1996.

Lachs, MS, Berkman, L, Fulmer, T, and Horwitz, RI: A prospective community-based pilot study of risk factors for the investigation of elder mistreatment. J Am Geriatr Soc 42:169–173, 1994.

Lebowitz, B, and Light, E: Caregiver stress. In Yoshikawa, TT, Cobb, EL, and Brummel-Smith, K (eds): Ambulatory Geriatric Care. CV Mosby, St. Louis, 1993.

Regan, JJ: Commentary: Protection and empowerment of the elderly: Whose needs does the law really serve? In Smyer, M, Schaie, KW, and Kapp, MB (eds): Older Adult's Decision-Making and the Law. Springer, New York, 1996.

Williams, ME: The American Geriatric Society's Complete Guide to Aging and Health. Harmony, New York, 1995.

Grief

Abrams, WB, Beers, MH, and Berkow, R. (eds): The Merck Manual of Geriatrics, ed 2. Merck, Whitehouse Station, NJ, 1995.

Ebersole, P, and Hess, P: Toward Healthy Aging: Human Needs and Nursing Response. CV Mosby, St. Louis, 1995.

Eisendrath, SJ, and Brophy, JJ: Psychiatric disorders. In Tierney, LM Jr, McPhee, SJ, and Papadakis, MA (eds): Current Medical Diagnosis and Treatment. Appleton & Lange, Norwalk, CT, 1995.

Fankhauser, MP: Anxiolytic drugs and sedative-hypnotic agents. In Bressler, R, and Katz, MD (eds): Geriatric Pharmacology. McGraw-Hill, New York, 1993.

Gallo, JJ, Reichel, W, and Andersen, LM: Handbook of Geriatric Assessment. Aspen, Gaithersburg, 1995.

Plopper, M: Common psychiatric disorders. In Yoshikawa, TT, Cobbs, EL, and Brummel-Smith, K (eds): Ambulatory Geriatric Care. CV Mosby, St. Louis, 1993.

Rauch, SL, and Rosenbaum, JF: Psychiatric and behavioral problems. In Goroll, AH, May, LA, and Mulley, AG Jr (eds): Primary Care Medicine: Office Evaluation of the Adult Patient, ed 3. JB Lippincott, Philadelphia, 1995.

Resnick, NM: Geriatric medicine. In Isselbacher, KJ, et al (eds): Harrison's Principles of Internal Medicine, ed 13. McGraw-Hill, New York, 1994.

Zisook, S, and Shuchter, SR: Uncomplicated bereavement. J Clin Psychiatry 54:365–372, 1993.

Insomnia

Abrams, WB, Beers, MH, and Berkow, R. (eds): The Merck Manual of Geriatrics, ed 2. Merck, Whitehouse Station, NJ, 1995.

Campbell, SS, Dawson, D, and Anderson, MW: Alleviation of sleep maintenance insomnia with timed exposure to bright light. J Am Geriatr Soc 41:829–836, 1993.

Ebersole, P, and Hess, P: Toward Healthy Aging: Human Needs and Nursing Response. CV Mosby, St. Louis, 1995.

Emsellem, H: Sleep disorders. In Yoshikawa, TT, Cobbs, EL, and Brummel-Smith, K (eds): Ambulatory Geriatric Care. CV Mosby, St. Louis, 1993.

Fankhauser, MP: Anxiolytic drugs and sedative-hypnotic agent. In Bressler, R, and Katz, MD (eds): Geriatric Pharmacology. McGraw-Hill, New York, 1993.

Resnick, NM: Geriatric medicine. In Isselbacher, KJ, et al (eds): Harrison's Principles of Internal Medicine, ed 13. McGraw-Hill, New York, 1994.

Weilburg, JB: Approach to the patient with insomnia. In Goroll, AH, May, LA, and Mulley, AG Jr (eds): Primary Care Medicine: Office Evaluation of the Adult Patient, ed 3. JB Lippincott, Philadelphia, 1995.

Williams, ME: The American Geriatrics Society's Complete Guide to Aging and Health. Harmony Books, New York, 1995.

Wandering

Abrams, WB, Beers, MH, and Berkow, R. (eds): The Merck Manual of Geriatrics, ed 2. Merck, Whitehouse Station, NJ, 1995.

Algase, DL, and Struble, LM: Wandering behavior: What, why, and how? In Buckwalter, KM (ed): Geriatric Mental Health Nursing: Current and Future Challenges. Slack, Thorofare, NJ, 1992.

Ebersole, P, and Hess, P: Toward Healthy Aging: Human Needs and Nursing Response, ed 4. CV Mosby, St. Louis, 1994.

Fogel, B: Behavioral symptoms. In Morris, JN, Lipsitz, LA, Murphy, K, Belleville-Taylor, P (eds): Quality Care in the Nursing Home. Mosby–Year Book, St. Louis, 1997.

Johnson, LH, and Johnson, MA: Dementia in the elderly. In Stanley, M, and Beare, PG (eds): Gerontological Nursing. FA Davis, Philadelphia, 1995.

Matteson, MA, and Linton, A: Wandering behaviors in institutionalized persons with dementia. Journal of Gerontological Nursing 22(9):39–46, 1996.

Ouslander, JG, Osterweil, D, and Morley, J: Medical Care in the Nursing Home. McGraw-Hill, New York, 1991.

Rader, J, Doan, J, and Schwab, M: How to decrease wandering: A form of agenda behavior. Geriatric Nursing 6(4):196–199, 1985.

Scharee, DW, and Cummings, JL: Dementia. In Yoshikawa, TT, Cobbs, EL, and Brummel-Smith, K (eds): Ambulatory Geriatric Care. CV Mosby, St. Louis, 1993.

Thomas, DW: Wandering: A proposed definition. Journal of Gerontological Nursing 21(9):35–41, 1995.

Thomas, DW: Understanding the wandering patient: A continuity of personality perspective. Journal of Gerontological Nursing 23(1):16–24, 1997.

Williams, ME: The American Geriatric Society's Complete Guide to Aging and Health. Harmony, New York, 1995.

CHAPTER **17**

SYMPTOM-BASED

PROBLEMS

Assessment

Assessment of symptom-based problems in the older adult presents several challenges for the health-care practitioner. Heterogeneity increases with age, presenting the health-care provider with a great diversity of possibilities to consider in formulating diagnostic impressions. You can easily work up a patient with a single symptom or cluster of symptoms using typical symptom analysis and clinical decision-making tools. To complicate matters, however, patients may ignore symptoms initially because they do not interfere with functional activities or because they attribute the symptoms to the aging process. Conversely, patients may fear loss of independence related to a subtle decline in functional abilities and deliberately choose to conceal this until it becomes apparent to others. Acuity of symptoms may be blunted because of changes in the efficiency of certain physiologic mechanisms. New symptoms often appear in one organ system as an offshoot of preexisting disease in another organ system. Multiple symptoms may be present because of comorbidities. These factors can result in a delayed or atypical presentation.

In many cases, the first hint of illness may be a change in cognitive function or mental status. Other atypical manifestations of illness in older persons include incontinence, functional decline, falling, agitation, syncope, and/or self-neglect. These symptoms may be brought to the attention of the health-care provider by the patient or by close family members, friends, or caregivers. In the case of patients with cognitive impairment, refusal to eat or drink or a change in sleep or behavioral patterns may be symptomatic of an acute underlying process. Some patients may become agitated or hypervigilant; others may become somnolent. Because the most vulnerable organ systems are the brain, urinary tract, and cardiovascular or musculoskeletal systems, initially consider the differential diagnosis of conditions involving these systems, regardless of the predominant symptoms. Also, since many homeostatic mechanisms are affected simultaneously, evaluate the presenting picture holistically, looking for interrelated problems that may improve with minor interventions.

If the patient is new to you and is unable to give accurate information, obtain baseline data on the patient's usual state of health and functional abilities from a reputable source whenever possible.

The mnemonic OLDCARTS is helpful for symptom analysis in an older adult with intact cognition and historical reliability:

- Onset. When did you first become aware of the symptom?
- Location. Where is the symptom? Does it radiate to another location?
- Duration. How long does the symptom last? How often do you experience it?
- Character. What is the symptom like? What qualities would you use to describe it?
- Associated symptoms. Are there any other associated symptoms? What makes the symptoms worse?
- Relief. What makes the symptom better? Does it go away on its own?
- Timing. Is there a particular time when the symptom occurs?
- Setting. Is there a particular setting, place, position, activity, feeling, or circumstance in which the symptom occurs?

If the symptom or the patient's demeanor indicates a problem in function or cognition, assess these areas. Perform a thorough medication history, including the use of over-the-counter (OTC) preparations, vitamins, herbal and homeopathic remedies, and any other dietary supplements, and consider their use in formulating diagnostic possibilities. Pharmacotherapeutic or other treatment modalities can complicate or even cause illness in older patients.

Bowel Incontinence

Fecal or bowel incontinence, the inability to control evacuation of stool or flatus from the rectum, can be episodic and self-limiting or a chronic problem in the older adult. In either scenario, this socially and emotionally devastating situation interferes with quality of life and self-esteem.

Etiology: The most common cause of significant fecal incontinence, denervation of the puborectalis muscles and the external sphincters, is associated with rectal prolapse, habitual straining with defecation, childbirth (delayed onset of symptoms), diabetes mellitus, and spinal cord injuries. Fecal impaction is responsible for many of the less serious incidences of incontinence. Other contributing factors are discussed later.

Occurrence: In the community-dwelling older adult, approximately 3%–4% have a problem with bowel incontinence. In elderly persons in long-term care settings, the incidence is between 10% and 23%.

Age: Bowel incontinence is found more frequently in the older adult than in the general population.

Ethnicity: Not significant.

Gender: Bowel incontinence occurs equally in men and women.

Contributing Factors: Diarrhea from gastrointestinal (GI) disease, infectious causes, or medication side effects can contribute to acute, short-term bowel incontinence. Constipation from inadequate dietary fiber, insufficient fluid intake, or the effects of certain medications is also implicated. Fecal impaction is involved in many cases of bowel incontinence. Protracted laxative abuse can damage the myenteric plexus, leading to retention of feces and soiling. Altered cognitive functioning or depression can also contribute to inability to respond appropriately to the urge to defecate. Impaired mobility from acute musculoskeletal conditions, chronic degenerative changes, or neurologic problems is also a risk factor. Unavailability of persons to assist the dependent older adult with toileting is another risk factor.

Signs and Symptoms: Initially, patients may deny the problem or use incontinence pads because of the embarrassment associated with the problem. Family members or caregivers may notice and report fecal smearing, soiling, or "accidents." A history of abrupt onset and short course suggests an acute or self-limiting process. A more insidious and progressive course warrants a different workup. Presence or absence of associated symptoms such as pain, urinary incontinence, diarrhea, constipation, bleeding, or vomiting should be ascertained.

Has the patient recently traveled to another country?
What medications, including OTC, laxative, and herbal remedies, is the patient taking?
Has the patient recently been hospitalized or received a course of antibiotic therapy?
What is the mental status of the patient?
Is the patient depressed?
What does a diet history reveal?
What is the frequency of occurrence and timing of incontinence episodes?
What other medical conditions does the patient have?
Is the patient aware of the need to defecate?
Can the patient distinguish between the passage of flatus and the passage of solid and liquid stool?
Does the patient have any warning prior to defecating?
Does the patient have any control?

Is there a sensation of incomplete evacuation?
Has the patient recently undergone surgery of any kind?

Physical examination should include a thorough abdominal assessment, looking for rigidity, distention, hyperactive or absent bowel sounds, and pain. A rectal examination, including a digital examination to check for hemorrhoids, impaction, and sphincter control, is indicated. The patient's weight should be measured and compared with previous measurements to determine any significant change.

Diagnostic Tests: These tests are determined by the history and physical examination findings. Possible tests include abdominal ultrasound, flat plate of the abdomen, and computed tomography (CT) scan if an acute surgical abdomen or partial obstruction is suspected. Barium contrast studies, particularly a barium enema, may be helpful. Fecal hemoccult testing, sigmoidoscopy, or colonoscopy may also be indicated. If an infectious or food-borne cause is suspected, collection of stools for culture, ova, and parasites is appropriate.

Differential Diagnosis: Fecal incontinence is a symptom. Differential diagnosis includes gastroenteritis, food-borne illness, ruptured diverticulum, colon cancer, fecal impaction, anal fistula, diabetic neuropathy, or rectal prolapse; upper motor neuron lesions secondary to cerebrovascular accident (CVA), multiple sclerosis, spinal cord compression, degenerative processes, dementia, or trauma; inflammatory bowel disease, irritable bowel syndrome, or functional bowel disease; and depression with self-care deficits.

Treatment: Treatment is aimed at alleviating the cause of bowel incontinence, when possible, or at minimizing its consequences, restoring self-esteem, maintaining function, and improving quality of life. Surgery is indicated for ruptured diverticulum, rectal prolapse, some fistulas, and possibly also for colon cancer. For acute gastroenteritis and food-borne illnesses, treatment includes maintaining hydration, monitoring for life-threatening consequences, and possibly antimicrobial therapy.

For depression and functional bowel disease, treatment is individualized. Reviewing and adjusting a patient's medications is needed when the incontinence results from prescribed drugs. If chronic laxative abuse is involved, attempts to intervene and design a successful bowel management program are needed. When fecal impaction is the cause, disimpaction (manual/mechanical or pharmacologic removal of impaction) and preventive bowel hygiene measures should be instituted. Dietary modifications and the addition of a bulk-forming agent may be considered. Other treatment options include biofeedback, bowel training, and toileting. Toileting is a treatment because frail elderly persons who are dependent for activities of daily living (ADLs) need to be given the opportunity to evacuate at regular intervals. If not, they will not go, will be constipated, or will be incontinent.

Follow-up: Follow-up is indicated by cause. In any case, ongoing monitoring is needed.

Sequelae: Possible complications dependent on the cause of the symptom. Complications of bowel incontinence may include peritonitis, septic shock, dehydration, electrolyte imbalance, skin breakdown, and depression. If the patient is functionally dependent or cognitively impaired, bowel incontinence may result in placement in a long-term care facility.

Prevention/Prophylaxis: Prevention strategies depend on cause of incontinence. Eating a balanced diet with adequate fiber and fluid intake, maintaining regular physical activity, avoiding use of laxatives and cathartics, making time for bowel evacuation, and avoiding unnecessary OTC drug use are good general preventive measures. Proper food preparation and storage can prevent food-borne illness.

Referral: Refer the patient to (or consult with) appropriate specialist, as indicated by cause of incontinence symptom.

Education: Educate patient in rationale for and implementation of preventive strategies as indicated, focusing especially on the need to avoid regular laxative use and to vary the normal bowel evacuation patterns (e.g., it is not necessary to have a bowel movement every day). Explain the cause of the incontinence, the rationale for any diagnostic tests, and the appropriate treatment plan. Advise the patient when to seek medical care.

Chest Pain

Acute nontraumatic chest discomfort, perceived as pain or as a sensation of tightness, pressure, or squeezing in the chest, is associated with actual or potential tissue damage.

Etiology: The many different pathophysiologies of major chest pain syndromes may be attributed to segmental overlap of the neurons of cardiopulmonary and noncardiopulmonary origin. Chest pain may originate from organs within or outside the thorax. Visceral (organ) pain is usually characterized as vague, dull, and aching, slow in onset, and diffuse. Somatic (cutaneous and subcutaneous) pain tends to be sharp, localized, rapidly perceived, and rapidly extinguished by withdrawal of the stimulus. Deep somatic pain (bone and blood vessels) is more diffuse and difficult to localize.

Occurrence: Chest pain is one of the most common presenting symptoms, accounting for up to 7% of all visits to the emergency department or outpatient clinic.

Age: In elderly persons, the most common causes of chest pain are ischemia, gastroesophageal reflux disease (GERD), and panic disorder. The older adult is more likely to describe a symptom of chest discomfort rather than chest pain. The presentation may be different in the aged or diabetic patient with altered pain perception or altered ability to localize the discomfort. An absence of chest pain with myocardial infarction in elderly persons is not uncommon.

Ethnicity: African-Americans have a high prevalence of hypertensive heart disease, which is a cause of angina. The symptoms of coronary heart disease may differ between African-Americans and whites in that African-Americans report less typical anginal features. African-Americans are also less likely to attribute their symptoms to underlying coronary heart disease and tend to delay longer before going to the emergency department.

Gender: Coronary artery disease is more difficult to diagnose in women because of a greater prevalence of atypical symptoms, variant angina, and microvascular angina. Silent ischemia and infarction also occur more frequently in women.

Contributing Factors: Differentiating the etiology of chest pain in elderly persons is problematic owing to the more common atypical presentation and comorbidity. In elderly individuals, esophageal disease coexists with myocardial infarction in 50% of patients with coronary artery disease. Hyperventilation, a frequent symptom in patients with panic attacks, has been shown to cause coronary artery and esophageal spasm. Heartburn can reduce blood flow to the heart causing cardiac ischemia.

Signs and Symptoms: Ask the patient to describe generally the severity of the discomfort and to characterize the feeling. If there is radiation or discomfort, have the patient point to the exact location and then trace any radiation with the finger. Some of the significant parameters of symptom assessment of chest pain are listed in Table 17–1.

Focus the physical examination on the general appearance of the patient including the level of distress. For vital signs, concentrate on the regularity and symmetry of the pulse, blood pressure in both arms, and temperature. Assess the skin for moisture, color, and capillary refill. Evaluate the lower extremities for temperature, tenderness, and edema.

Conduct complete cardiac examination, assessing for extra heart sounds and checking carotid arteries for bruit, murmurs, and pericardial rubs. The pulmonary examination consists of palpation for tenderness of the chest wall and auscultation for crackles, wheezes, or pleural rubs. You might also examine the abdomen, spine, and musculoskeletal or neurologic systems, as guided by the history.

Diagnostic Tests: Order diagnostic tests based on the history and physical examination findings. These may include:

- Cardiac: blood count, thyroid function, lipids, 12-lead electrocardiogram (ECG), biochemical markers, exercise ECG, echocardiogram, perfusion studies, coronary arteriography, cardiac catheterization, chest x-ray examination.
- Pulmonary: chest x-ray examination, ECG, arterial blood gases, lung scan, pulmonary arteriography, sputum culture and/or cytology, bronchoscopy, biopsy.

TABLE 17–1 CHEST PAIN: SYMPTOM ASSESSMENT

Descriptors

Onset: Trauma relationship, predictable. **Aggravating Factors:** Emotional upset; swallowing; cold weather; sexual intercourse; deep breathing; coughing; neck, arm, or chest movement; position change. **Relieving Factors:** Food, antacid, nitroglycerine, resting, change in position, massage. **Past Treatment or Evaluation:** Electrocardiogram; upper GI, chest x-ray.

Associated Symptoms

Anxiety, depression, faintness, palpitation, numbness or tingling in hands or around mouth, fever, chills, sweating, syncope, cough, sputum production, hemoptysis, dyspnea, tenderness, trouble swallowing, nausea, vomiting, leg swelling or pain, weight change, confusion, fatigue.

Medical History

Lung disease, chest surgery, chest injury, cardiovascular disease, hypertension, diabetes, elevated cholesterol or triglyceride, angina, phlebitis, emotional problems, recent immobilization.

Medications

Hormones, diuretics, digitalis, bronchodilators, nitroglycerine, tranquilizers, sedatives, antacids.

Family History

Cardiovascular disease, diabetes, hypertension, elevated blood lipids.

Environmental History

Smoking, alcohol use, diet history, cocaine use.

- Aortic: ECG, echocardiogram, aortic angiography, CT scan, magnetic resonance imaging (MRI), transesophageal echocardiogram.
- Chest wall: chest x-ray examination.
- Gastrointestinal: esophageal manometry, acid perfusion testing, 24-hour pH monitoring.
- Psychogenic: neuropsychiatric consultation and testing, electroencephalogram (EEG), desensitization test (DST).

Differential Diagnosis: The differential diagnosis for individuals presenting with chest pain is broad, including cardiopulmonary and noncardiopulmonary possibilities.

Treatment: Therapeutic management of chest pain is always based on the specific etiology of the symptom. For cardiac pain it may include nitrates, beta-blockers, calcium channel blockers, and thrombolytics. Pulmonary embolism is treated with anticoagulation, herpes zoster with antivirals, and esophageal pain with a H2-receptor antagonist. If a psychogenic cause is determined, selected patients may benefit from antidepressants or anxiolytics.

Follow-up: Monitor patients with acute chest pain closely and appropriately as the diagnosis and response to treatment dictates. Follow regularly individuals with chronic chest pain due to known chronic disease. Instruct the patient to immediately report to the health-care professional any changes in the characteristics of the symptom.

Sequelae: The significance of an episode of chest pain is evidenced by the fact that 50% of the patients presenting with a myocardial infarction had an episode of prior angina. Silent ischemia is equally significant; 25% of all myocardial infarctions are discovered only by new ECG changes without clinically recognizable associated events. Older adults have higher frequencies of unrecognized infarcts than other groups (approximately 68%). For adults over age 70 with known infarction, the in-hospital mortality rate is 37.5% compared with 17% in individuals under age 70.

Prevention/Prophylaxis: Maintaining a healthy lifestyle including maintaining appropriate weight, eating a balanced nutritional diet, and getting adequate exercise are the best ways to prevent the development of disease. Smoking cessation and stress reduction strategies are also advantageous.

Referral: Chest pain that is acute, of recent onset, or has recently increased in frequency or severity should always be considered unstable and evaluated immediately in the hospital. Patients who have a history of coronary artery disease, who have ST-segment changes on ECG, who have rest or variant angina, or whose vital signs are unstable should also be evaluated immediately in the hospital setting. Cardiac pain may necessitate a cardiologist referral.

Education: Teach patients and families to call the emergency response system without delay when an acute new onset of chest pain or a change in chronic chest pain is experienced.

Teach patients with chronic stable etiologies for chest pain nonpharmacologic management strategies. Teach individuals with coronary artery disease and known ischemia to avoid precipitants including stress, heavy meals, and strenuous exercise. Teach patients with GERD proper weight reduction as appropriate. Prudent lifestyle changes for those with GERD include stopping smoking, avoiding alcohol and coffee, and reducing fat in the diet. Because pain often occurs after meals in a supine position, teach the patient to avoid late night feedings and to keep the head of the bed elevated.

Constipation

Constipation is subjectively defined as infrequent elimination of no more than two bowel movements per week or straining at stool 25% of the time. In true clinical constipation a large amount of stool is objectively found by the digital examination or fecal loading is revealed by x-ray examination.

Etiology: Colonic motility depends on the integrity of the nervous system impulses and circular smooth muscle tone and motor complexes stimulated by increasing intraluminal pressure generated by bulk. Any pathophysiologic process that interferes with this process can cause constipation. Common etiologies for constipation may be organic or functional (Table 17–2).

Occurrence: Constipation rates in the general public are not known, but constipation is reported more frequently among children, pregnant women, and older adults.

Age: Constipation is a frequent complaint of elderly persons; 30%–50% of individuals report taking laxatives on a regular basis.

Ethnicity: Not significant.

Gender: At all ages constipation is more frequently reported in women than in men.

Contributing Factors: The functional factors described earlier contribute to constipation if they are not the primary etiology. Additional contributing factors include anxiety, depression, and dementia. Medications that may contribute to constipation include calcium channel blockers, narcotics, iron supplements, aluminum-containing antacids, and any drug that has anticholinergic side effects. Certain types of laxatives may also be constipating such as stimulant laxatives, which may cause cathartic colon and laxative dependency, and bulk laxatives taken with insufficient fluids.

Signs and Symptoms: Patients may describe constipation as an inability to pass or difficulty in passing stool, hard or dry stool, a feeling of abdominal or rectal fullness, and less than normal frequency or less than normal amount of passing stool. Ask the patient to describe specifically the frequency, character, and amount of stool. Determine the patients fluid and fiber intake and exercise level. Conduct a through medication review to determine use of constipating drugs and laxatives. For cognitively or communication-impaired individuals who are unable to self-report bowel frequency or elimination of discomfort, encourage the caregiver to maintain a record of the frequency and character of bowel elimination. The physical examination of the constipated patient should focus on a general assessment for signs of dehydration such as inadequate skin

TABLE 17–2 ETIOLOGIES OF CONSTIPATION

Organic	Functional
Anatomic: tumors (benign or malignant), Hirschsprung's disease	Poor eating habits
Metabolic: hypothyroidism, hypercalcemia, diabetes	Inadequate fiber intake
Neurologic: multiple sclerosis, Parkinson's disease, cord lesion	Inadequate fluid intake
Gastrointestinal: idiopathic megarectum, idiopathic megacolon, diverticular disease, Chagas' disease	Lack of exercise
	Failure to respond to normal defecation impulses

turgor and/or dry mucous membranes. Perform an abdominal examination to check for distention and visible peristalsis. Auscultate bowel sounds, and check the patient for abdominal masses. Do a rectal examination, assessing for fissures and external hemorrhoids and checking for anal stricture and sensation. Do a digital examination to assess for the presence of rectal masses and stool. The absence of stool found on examination does not exclude the possibility of constipation or fecal impaction.

Diagnostic Tests: An abdominal radiograph may help to determine the extent and distribution of feces. Sigmoidoscopy and/or barium enema may be indicated in those with a recent onset of constipation when a lesion is suspected. Checking colonic transit times may be indicated in those who have a normal number of bowel movements but still complain of constipation. Colonic motility testing may be useful in identifying patterns of colonic activity.

Treatment: After the specific etiology is established and contributing factors to constipation are identified, the appropriate pharmacologic and nonpharmacologic interventions are initiated. Nonpharmacologic measures to treat constipation include encouraging fluids (1500–2000 mL/day minimum); increasing fiber intake (25–35 g/day), and prescribing exercise (20–30 min of walking daily when appropriate).

Laxatives typically prescribed and their mechanism for action are shown in Table 17–3.

If nonpharmacologic measures are unsuccessful, then consider bulk laxatives as the first line of pharmacologic laxative therapy. Start bulk laxatives slowly, increasing the dose as the patient can tolerate it. Bulk-forming laxatives are to be avoided in those who cannot take adequate fluids or those with swallowing difficulties. If these are unsuccessful or not suitable, then saline or osmotic laxatives might be added on a scheduled basis. Avoid long-term use of stimulant laxatives in the older adult, as these can cause malabsorption, electrolyte imbalance, dehydration, and cathartic colon. Mineral and castor oil are always avoided in the older adult, owing to the risk of aspiration.

TABLE 17–3 LAXATIVES AND MODE OF ACTION

Laxative	Action
Stimulant: senna, biscadyl	Stimulates myenteric plexis, increases intraluminal fluid
Bulk: bran, psyllium, methylcellulose	Increases water absorption, resists bacterial degradation
Saline: magnesium hydroxide, magnesium citrate	Osmotically draws fluid into the small bowel lumen
Hyperosmolar: sorbitol, lactolose, glycerine	Nonabsorbable dissacharrades metabolized by cecal lactobacilli

Natural laxatives, mixtures of fruits and fruit juices, have been successful in treating and preventing constipation. Fecal softeners (ducusate sodium) do not act as laxatives and are not useful in constipation, although they can reduce the strain associated with bowel elimination. Enemas work through lavage and can cause fluid and electrolyte imbalance and can increase the risk of bowel perforation, particularly if the patient is not manually disimpacted first.

Follow-up: Chronically constipated individuals often need to have combined nonpharmacologic with periodic pharmacologic intervention. When laxatives are prescribed, these individuals need regular monitoring for the side effects and the responses to treatment.

Sequelae: Constipation, though uncomfortable, is rarely life threatening. When associated with pain, distention, and/or vomiting, constipation may be a sign of a life-threatening mesenteric infarction or a partial or complete bowel obstruction. Straining in elderly persons may have serious effects on the cerebral, coronary, and peripheral arterial circulations. If stool is not eliminated from the colon and the patient becomes dehydrated, stool may harden, resulting in fecal impaction. Hardened stool may back up farther into the colon and become difficult to remove either with cathartics or enemas. Some individuals have needed surgical intervention to remove very hard stool that is obstructing the bowel.

Prevention/Prophylaxis: Adequate dietary fluid and fiber and regular exercise habits help to promote colonic mobility. Bowel elimination patterns should be monitored regularly in individuals who are unable to report bowel habits or bowel discomfort.

Referral: Constipation in elderly persons is often related to a combination of conditions and factors. When the cause is organic, the patient may need to be collaboratively managed with the appropriate physician.

Education: In addition to instruction in the dietary measures appropriate in preventing constipation, encourage older patients to maintain regular bowel habits and respond to the urge to defecate rather than suppress it. All individuals should avoid the use of laxatives and the use of over-the-counter medications known to have constipating side effects.

Dehydration

Dehydration or fluid volume depletion, which is usually accompanied by electrolyte imbalances, frequently occurs in the older patient. Often presenting as confusion, dizziness, falling, or functional decline, dehydration may initially be overlooked as a differential.

Etiology: With the aging process, total body water decreases along with protein stores. The kidneys are not efficient in concentrating urine, the antidiuretic hormone receptors do not function optimally, and the sensation of thirst decreases.

Occurrence: Dehydration is a common occurrence.

Age: Dehydration is most common in young children and older adults.

Ethnicity: Not significant.

Gender: Dehydration occurs equally in males and females.

Contributing Factors: Contributing factors include inadequate fluid intake, including unintentional or deliberate limiting of fluids because of urinary incontinence, diuretic use, decreased mobility, and unavailability of fluids to drink. Excess loss of fluids from vomiting, diarrhea, hemorrhage, or increased metabolic states (fever, infection) are also contributing factors. Frail elderly persons are particularly at risk. Depression or dementia also heightens risk, as does diabetes mellitus, neurologic disease with impaired swallowing ability, and chronic renal insufficiency. Use of diuretics, anticholinergics, or tricyclic antidepressants also increases the risk of dehydration.

Signs and Symptoms: Initially, the patient may not have any symptoms. Complaints may include dizziness, confusion, new onset of falling, or difficulty swallowing food because of inadequate saliva. Constipation or hard stools may also be associated with dehydration. Family members, neighbors, or caregivers may notice a change in the patient. A carefully elicited history may help to pinpoint the problem without an extensive workup. Caregivers of frail institutionalized elderly persons are in a key position to notice and report a decreased fluid intake or decreased urine output. If the patient is new to you as the healthcare provider, obtain baseline information whenever possible.

Objective signs may include orthostatic hypotension, tachycardia, decreased skin turgor, dry mucous membranes, a furrowed dry tongue, increased body temperature, change in mental status, or falling.

Diagnostic Tests: A complete blood count (CBC), blood urea nitrogen (BUN), creatinine, and electrolyte panel are helpful. The CBC will show an increased hematocrit; differential may indicate if infection is involved. Increased BUN and creatinine levels also signal notable volume depletion. Serum electrolyte determinations may indicate other, concurrent imbalances.

Differential Diagnosis: Anemia, dementia, delerium, gait disturbance, infectious process, or adverse drug reaction may be considered.

Treatment: Individualize treatment, depending on the underlying cause of the dehydration. Short-term parenteral fluid administration may be indicated in severe dehydration or if the patient is unable to take fluids by mouth; if the situation is permanent, enteral feeding is preferred. If the patient is already being tube-fed, it may be necessary to adjust the amount of water being given. Reevaluation of the current medication regimen may be necessary. Ensuring that the patient receives between 1500 and 1800 mL of fluid daily is important to prevent further dehydration (Tables 17–4 and 17–5).

Follow-up: See patient as indicated by cause and response to treatment.

Sequelae: Untreated dehydration can result in life-threatening electrolyte disturbances. When the patient limits fluid intake because of incontinence or diuresis, it is difficult to change this behavior on a permanent basis.

Prevention/Prophylaxis: Educate patients, families, and caregivers regarding need for daily fluid intake of 1500–1800 mL, unless medically contraindicated. Instruct the patient to avoid large amounts of caffeine and alcohol because of their diuretic effect.

Referral: Refer or consult as indicated by source of symptom. Referral for correction of urinary incontinence may help alleviate the problem if this is a causative factor.

Education: Explain causes of symptoms, measures taken to determine cause, treatment, and rationale. Emphasize the need for daily fluid intake of 1500–1800 mL, if not medically contraindicated. If the patient is incontinent, teach patient coping strategies. If use of diuretics is causing the dehydration, help patient to problem solve more acceptable lifestyle management. The patient can get up early to take the diuretic if he or she is going out for the day; or, outings can be scheduled for afternoon hours, when maximum diuresis has already occurred. Teach family members caring for patients and caregivers of institutionalized

TABLE 17–4 FORMULA FOR FREE WATER DEFICIT AND GUIDELINES FOR REPLACEMENT THERAPY

Formula for free water deficit:
(Wt [kg] × 0.45) − (140 − measured serum sodium) × (wt in kg) × (0.45)

Note: 0.45 is used instead (0.60 for the elderly to adjust for total body water decreases with age)

Guidelines
- In hemodynamic compromise (e.g., orthostatic hypotension, oliguria), replace with isotonic saline (1 to 2 liters) until stabilized.
- Calculate the free water deficit using the formula above.
- Free water deficits can be replaced orally or with 5% D5W IV.
- The approximate rate of free water initially required = {TBW/(plasma sodium)} × desired rate of decrease in plasma sodium × 1,000 (mEq/liter/hour).
- If sodium depletion is present, 0.25% or 0.5% N/S is recommended.
- Rapid correction of losses can be dangerous, especially in patients with hypernatremia. Effects include lethargy and seizures secondary to cerebral edema. Plasma sodium should be corrected at a rate not greater than 0.5 mEq/liter/hour in asymptomatic patients or 1.0 mEq/liter/hour in symptomatic patients.

Source: Adapted from Lippmann B. Fluid and electrolyte management. In: Ewald G, McKenzie C, eds. Manual of Medical Therapeutics, 28th ed. Boston: Little, Brown and Co., 1995:49–50.

TABLE 17–5 ORAL FLUID CHOICES FOR REHYDRATION

The recommended daily fluid requirement is six to eight 8-ounce glasses a day (approximately 2 quarts or 2 liters).

Water
Water makes up approximately two-thirds of the human body and remains the best choice for rehydration. Water helps prevent constipation and aids in regulating body temperature. At least half of all fluid replacement should consist of water.

Fruit/Vegetable juices
Juices are nutrient rich and make an excellent choice as a fluid source. However, caution should be taken to not overindulge in juices because they may cause diarrhea or alterations in sodium or potassium. Juices should not be used as a sole fluid source.

Milk
Milk is highly nutritious and a major source for calcium, an important vitamin for the elderly. However, it has been known to thicken sputum and promote constipation among some elderly, so judicious use based on tolerance is best.

Soft drinks/Gelatin/Sports drinks
These fluids should be taken in small amounts only because they are high in sugar and may cause further dehydration as the kidney attempts to dilute the sugar.

Caffeinated drinks (coffee, tea, and colas)
Caffeinated drinks may further compound dehydration as well as contribute to symptoms of insomnia and palpitations. It is best to eradicate caffeine from the diet or to use sparingly.

Soups
The fluid in soups is often very nutritious but can be a hidden source of high sodium in the diet. It is advised to carefully read the labels for sodium content in store-bought soups.

Alcohol
Alcohol should never be used as a fluid source for rehydration. It can exacerbate dehydration and is a major contributing factor to many medical illnesses and accidents among the elderly.

Source: Adapted from Kositzke J: A question of balance: Dehydration in the elderly. J Geront Nurs 1990; 16(5):4–1.

older patients how to encourage adequate fluid intake and monitor for inadequate intake. Advise patient or caregivers when to seek medical care.

Diarrhea

Diarrhea is an increase in the frequency, volume, or fluidity of stools. It can be acute (less than 3–5 days' duration) or chronic (more than 2 weeks' duration). Diarrhea is defined as a frequency of more than three bowel movements per day or a volume greater than 200 g/day. Regardless of its etiology, diarrhea in the frail older adult is a significant cause for concern.

Etiology: Viral infection due to rotavirus or Norwalk virus is the most common cause of acute diarrhea. Bacterial pathogens include *Escherichia coli, Shigella, Campylobacter, Salmonella,* and *Vibrio cholerae; Clostridium difficile* is a significant cause of diarrhea in the institutionalized older adult receiving antibiotic therapy. Other causes of diarrhea are travelers' diarrhea and protozoal infections with *Giardia lamblia, Cryptosporidium,* or *Entamoeba histolytica* organisms. Several drugs have significant side effect profiles for diarrhea. Inflammatory bowel disease, irritable bowel syndrome, fecal impaction, or bowel ischemia are other causes of diarrhea in the older adult.

Occurrence: Diarrhea is very common, second only to respiratory infections in frequency in the United States. Approximately 70% of deaths from diarrhea in older patients originate in nursing care facilities.

Age: Diarrhea may occur at any age; however, the most serious effects are found in the very young and very old. More than 50% of deaths from diarrheal illness occur in people over age 74.

Ethnicity: Not significant.

Gender: Diarrhea occurs equally in men and women.

Contributing Factors: Foreign travel, contaminated food and/or water, laxative abuse, immunocompromise, chronic alcohol abuse, diabetes mellitus, hyperthyroidism, infection, lactose intolerance, altered intestinal motility, malabsorption, hormone-secreting tumors, or obstructive lesions are contributing factors. The group living situation found in long-term care facilities presents an environmental factor favoring the spread of certain types of diarrhea. Medications that have the side effect of diarrhea include quinidine, digitalis, antibiotics, magnesium-based antacids, acarbose, theophylline, colchicine, levodopa, sorbitol, misoprostol, nonsteroidal anti-inflammatory drugs (NSAIDs), lactulose, fructose, chemotherapy agents, caffeine, and diuretics.

Signs and Symptoms: The history should include baseline bowel pattern data; usual dietary intake and any food intolerance; recent dining out; onset of symptom; associated symptoms; frequency, amount, and character of stools; presence of blood, mucus, or atypical color in stools; recent travel; recent hospitalization, surgery, or antibiotic therapy; exposure to others with illnesses; medications, including OTC herbal remedies and laxatives; history of neuropsychiatric problems. In the community-dwelling older adult, a history of living alone, sporadic eating patterns, and vagueness may signal a need for referral to case management or visiting nurse services for a home evaluation visit. A dietary history of the 2 days before symptom onset is helpful, with particular attention to ingestion of meat, dairy products, and seafood. Exploration of associated signs and symptoms is key in targeting the source of the problem. A history of fever, abdominal pain and distention, vomiting, myalgia, headache, and abrupt onset suggests acute diarrhea. A history of fatigue, weight loss, alternating diarrhea and constipation, incomplete evacuation, and abdominal pain indicates chronic diarrhea. The onset of travelers' diarrhea is usually 3–7 days after arrival at the new location.

Bacterial diarrhea is suspected when individuals in a group who have shared a common food source present concurrently with similar symptoms. Arthritis in conjunction with diarrhea (usually bloody or mucous) suggests inflammatory bowel disease. Pronounced weight loss in association with diarrhea implies malabsorption, cancer, or hyperthyroidism.

Physical examination should include vital signs and weight. Assess the skin for turgor, and condition of tongue and mucous membranes. Check for evidence of jaundice, rashes, or lesions. Examine the thyroid for lesions. Perform a thorough examination of the abdomen for distention, rigidity, tenderness, bowel sounds, masses, hepatomegaly, or splenomegaly. Perform a rectal examination, including hemoccult testing, to assess for bleeding, hemorrhoids, polyps, fissures, fistula, or evidence of malignancy. Also include a general inspection for arthritis or lymphadenopathy as part of the examination.

Diagnostic Tests: Diagnosis may be based on history, signs, and symptoms. In patients with diarrhea persisting for more than 3 days or with recurrent diarrhea, stool samples may need to be cultured and checked for blood, white blood cells (WBCs), *C. difficile* toxin, and ova and parasites. Blood is typically present in stool when inflammatory bowel disease, bacterial infection, or bowel ischemia occurs. WBCs are seen in *Salmonella*-, *Campylobacter*-, and *Yersinia*-associated diarrhea. Ova and parasites are present in diarrhea of protozoal origin. Concurrent use of tetracycline, sulfonamides, magnesium hydroxide, castor oil, kaolin, bismuth, antiprotozoals, or enemas with barium, soap, hypertonic saline, or tap water interferes with ova and parasite collection. Abuse of the laxative phenolphthalein also interferes with some stool testing. If you suspect laxative abuse, order a stool laxative screen.

A CBC with differential may be indicated; WBC elevation and a shift to the left may be present with infections. Decreased hemoglobin and hematocrit may signify anemia from blood loss; however, if the patient is dehydrated from the diarrhea, hemoglobin and hematocrit may actually be increased because of the fluid volume deficit. Checking serum electrolytes helps to determine imbalances caused by diarrhea and dehydration (possibly indicated by increased sodium and decreased potassium). If obstruction or ischemia is suspected, abdominal x-ray examination helps to confirm this or may point to the need for more sophisticated testing. A barium enema can reveal malignancies, polyps, or abnormalities of the mucosal pattern. Colonoscopy or sigmoidoscopy may also be desirable when bloody diarrhea is present, to explore for source of bleeding. D-xylose testing and serum iron, vitamin B_{12}, and folate levels may be needed if malabsorption is suspected in patients with chronic diarrhea. BUN and creatinine elevations may point to dehydration, but these values must be viewed in the context of the total picture (renal insufficiency, common in the older adult, affects these values). Plasma protein levels may highlight loss of protein stores in patients with chronic diarrhea.

The clinician must use careful judgment from a holistic viewpoint in determining which studies are indicated and which can be safely tolerated if the patient is severely debilitated. Also, in interpreting the laboratory results, consult reference sources for baseline values in older patients.

Differential Diagnosis: In acute diarrhea, consider inflammatory bowel disease, fecal impaction, irritable bowel syndrome, diverticulitis, antibiotic-associated pseudomembranous colitis, bowel ischemia, drug side effects, food-borne pathogens, or viral gastroenteritis. In chronic diarrhea, possibilities include malabsorption, occult neoplasm, postradiation enterocolitis, irritable bowel syndrome, and factitious and functional problems.

Treatment: Treatment depends on the cause. Frail elderly persons are at risk for dehydration and multisystem failure from diarrhea. If diarrhea is severe, refer and/or send the patient for emergent evaluation and treatment. In cases of acute-onset diarrhea in which a viral cause is likely, provide symptomatic treatment to maintain hydration and electrolyte balance. If the patient is not vomiting, encourage frequent fluids with carbohydrates and electrolytes. This can take the form of tea, juice, "flat" carbonated beverages, Gatorade, or oral rehydration products such as Pedialyte. Advance the diet to include rice, bananas, applesauce, crackers, soup, and toast. High-fiber foods, including raw fruits and cruciferous vegetables; dairy products; caffeine and alcohol; spicy or stimulant foods should be avoided until the diarrhea subsides and normal bowel function returns. If diarrhea persists for more than 3 days on this regimen, reevaluate the patient. Use of antidiarrheals is controversial owing to side effects, particularly if the patient is taking other medications. Pepto-Bismol is effective in treatment of travelers' diarrhea. *C. difficile* may be treated with metronidazole 250 mg PO qid; no alcohol is permitted with this medication. Because any antibiotic has the ability to disrupt normal bowel flora and precipitate further episodes of diarrhea, watchful waiting may be useful before prescribing.

For patients with chronic diarrhea, treat as indicated by cause. The addition of a bulk-forming agent such as psyllium may be helpful in giving stools a solid consistency; however, patients *must* take adequate fluids to prevent impaction or obstruction from use of this substance. Dietary counseling to promote adequate fiber in the diet is helpful, if this is not contraindicated.

Follow-up: Schedule follow-up visits as indicated by cause of the diarrhea. In the case of acute diarrhea, reevaluate the patient after 3 days of following the initial treatment plan. If diarrhea persists, diagnostic studies are indicated and the patient's state of hydration must be addressed.

Sequelae: Depending on the cause and extent of the diarrhea, complications may include dehydration, sepsis, shock, anemia, fluid and electrolyte imbalances, malnutrition, and peritonitis.

Prevention/Prophylaxis: Prevention depends on the cause. For community-dwelling older adults, especially those who live alone, the following guidelines are helpful:

- Careful cooking and storage of food to avoid spoilage.
- Dating leftover food and discarding after 5 days.
- Checking expiration dates on dairy and meat products before using.
- Cleansing of cutting boards and utensils.

All patients not on a medically prescribed diet should be taught about the food pyramid and the need for adequate fluid and fiber in the diet. For those contemplating travel to a foreign country, prophylactic treatment with Pepto-Bismol may be prescribed or the patient may be given a 3- to 5-day course of Floxin (antimicrobial) to take if diarrhea develops. This is particularly recommended for patients with underlying chronic disease. Caution travelers to avoid uncooked or undercooked foods, raw fruits and vegetables, buffet foods, unpasteurized dairy products, tap water, and ice. Carbonated drinks, bottled water, or boiled water are considered safe for drinking and to use for oral hygiene. Prevention of transmission of diarrhea in hospitals and long-term care facilities is extremely important. Frequent handwashing by patients and health-care workers in long-term care and hospital settings is the key to preventing transmission of infectious diarrhea. Avoidance of chronic laxative use and prudent use of antimicrobial agents are also important in preventing diarrhea.

Referral: Consult with or refer the patient to the appropriate specialist, as the cause of diarrhea indicates.

Education: Explain to patient, family, and caregivers the cause of symptoms, diagnostic and treatment measures, follow-up, and preventive strategies. Emphasize the need for early intervention to prevent dehydration.

Dizziness

Dizziness is an imprecise term commonly used to describe various subjective symptoms. The practitioner must understand the patient's personal meaning of "dizziness" in order to classify the symptom and determine its cause. The most frequently used categories of dizziness are vertigo, presyncopal lightheadedness, disequilibrium, other, and mixed (several etiologies).

Etiology: Dizziness may be caused by neurologic, systemic, psychiatric, or mixed pathologies. Causes seen most often in primary care practice are anxiety, benign positional vertigo, cerumen-impacted ears, medication, systemic or viral infections, multiple neurosensory impairments, transient vertebrobasilar ischemia, or vasovagal causes.

Occurrence: Dizziness is a common complaint in older adults. An estimated 90% of adults seen in outpatient geriatric clinics have this symptom. The frequency of dizziness increases with age.

Age: Dizziness is the most common complaint found by primary care practitioners in persons over age 75.

Ethnicity: Not significant.

Gender: Dizziness occurs equally in men and women.

Contributing Factors: Factors contributing to dizziness are related to identified causes (e.g., medications). Deficits in other body systems related to maintaining equilibrium can cause longer delays in recovery of balance for older adults than for younger adults with similar problems.

Signs and Symptoms: The patient's description of the symptom should help determine the type of dizziness experienced (Fig. 17–1).

> *Vertigo:* Patients describe the environment or self spinning; an illusion of movement, continuous or positional; the sensation of being pushed. Associated symptoms include nausea, vomiting, unsteadiness, hearing loss, visual disturbances, and tinnitus.

> *Presyncopal Lightheadedness:* Patients have the sensation one feels when about to faint. Associated symptoms include perspiration, pallor, palpitations, and syncope.

> *Disequilibrium:* Patients describe a sense of imbalance. It may be sensation localized to the body and relieved by bracing oneself, sitting, or lying down. Associated symptoms are numbness, poor coordination, and general weakness.

> *Other:* Patients may give a vague description of dizziness. Coexistence of psychiatric or organic disease is possible.

> *Mixed:* More than one type of dizziness may exist in 40% of patients.

Diagnostic Tests

> *General:* Observe how the patient moves around in the physician's office. Does he or she hold onto the furniture or walls?
>
> Check vital signs, especially postural blood pressure (BP). A drop in systolic BP of 20 mmHg or more without normalization after 2 minutes is significant. In older adults, an initial drop is also significant in patients who normally have low blood pressure. Causes of postural hypotension include decreased cardiac output, hypovolemia, impaired venous return, and medication side effects. It is important to determine whether the test of abruptly going from a lying to a sitting or standing position reproduces the patient's sensation.
>
> Test for extraocular movement (EOM), watching for nystagmus. Rotatory nystagmus suggests a peripheral cause of dizziness; vertical nystagmus suggests a central lesion.

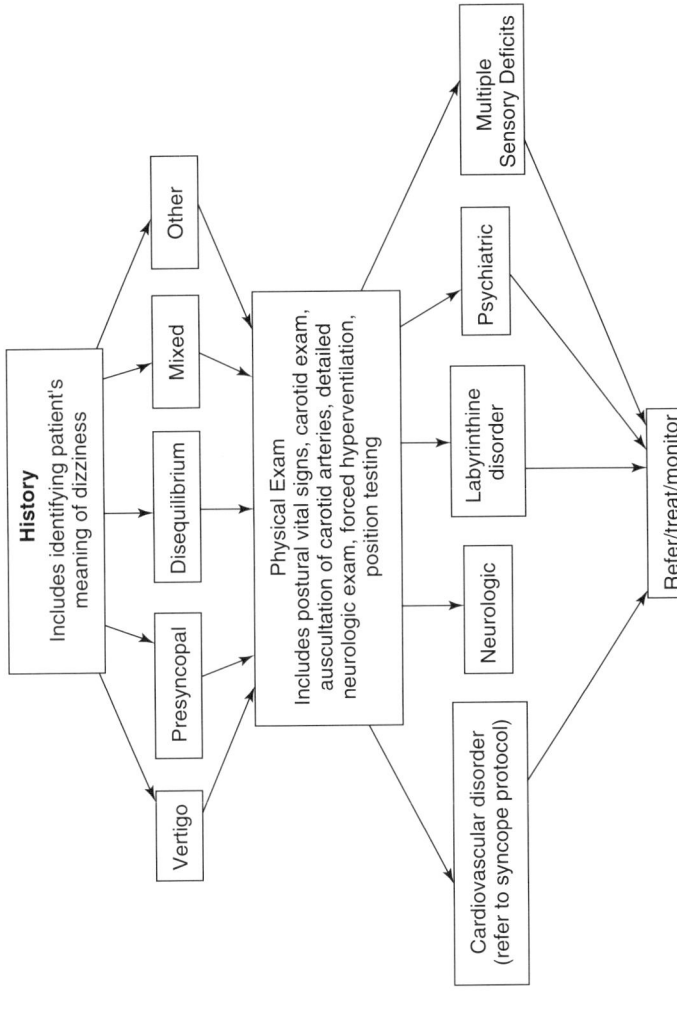

FIGURE 17–1 Dizziness. (Adapted from Jonsson, PV, and Lipsitz, LA: Dizziness and syncope. In Hazzard, W, et al: Principles of Geriatric Medicine and Gerontology, ed. 3. McGraw-Hill, New York, 1994.)

Check the patient's visual acuity and corneal reflexes. Perform a fundoscopic examination, looking for papilledema.

Inspect the ears for accumulation of fluid, bulging tympanic membrane (TM), inflamed TM, presence of cerumen impaction or pus accumulation and discharge. Perform Weber's and Rinne's hearing tests if gross hearing is diminished. Hearing loss in Menière's disease is initially of low intensity and noted only during attacks of dizziness; in later stages of the disease, hearing loss becomes fixed. Hearing tests at this time can provide baseline data for follow-up testing.

Auscultate the carotid artery, checking for bruits.

Neurologic Function

- Cerebellar testing: If the patient points past the examiner's finger, suspect a vestibular lesion. Intentional tremor or abnormal alternating movements suggest cerebellar dysfunction (point-to-point).
- Sensory testing.
- Position sense.
- Romberg's test: Patients with cerebellar disease will have difficulty standing with their feet together. Patients with decreased position sense will be able to compensate with eyes open, but sway with eyes closed.
- Gait assessment: Patients with cerebellar disease will perform this maneuver poorly.

Special Diagnostic and Screening Tests

Have the patient breathe 20–30 times a minute for 2–3 minutes (forced hyperventilation). This normally causes dizziness and finger and perioral numbness. Determine whether these are the same sensations the patient has been feeling; if so, the dizziness may be related to anxiety.

Have the patient march in place for 30 seconds with the eyes closed and arms extended in front. Be careful not to orient the patient with any sounds (e.g., your voice or a ticking clock). Patients with absent or reduced vestibular function (from prior vestibular damage) will rotate more than 30–45 degrees while marching.

For the Hallpike maneuver (also called the Bereny's positional test), have the patient sit on the examination table. The examiner quickly but gently helps the patient lie down with the head hanging over the back of the table at about a 30-degree angle and the face turned 45 degrees to the right (the head-hanging part of the maneuver can be omitted for frail patients). While holding the patient's head in place for 1 minute, observe the patient for nystagmus and ask whether this reproduces the dizziness (vertigo) symptoms. Bring the patient back to a sitting position and observe for 1 minute. Repeat the test with the head turned 45 degrees to the left. If vertigo is reproduced, the test should be repeated two or three times on the side that caused the most severe symptoms to determine if the nystagmus and symptoms begin to disappear. Patients with benign postural vertigo experience severe vertigo 5–15 seconds after the head is turned; the sign fades in less than a minute. Repeated testing will cause the symptoms to disappear. Suspect a central lesion if vertigo is dissociated from nystagmus or occurs just after positioning, is primarily vertical or horizontal, lasts longer than a minute, or does not disappear with repeated testing.

Perform the minicalorie test to screen for vestibular dysfunction. Position the patient supine with the head turned 30 degrees. Instill 0.2 mL of ice water from a tuberculin (TB) syringe into the ear canal. Then turn the patient's head to midline and observe the eyes for nystagmus. With repetition, failure to induce nystagmus indicates peripheral disease on that side.

More Diagnostic Tests: If indicated by history, perform the following:

ECG.
Audiometric examination.
Hematologic testing (CBC).
Serum glucose test (for hypoglycemia).
Thyroid function test.
Serology/Venereal disease research laboratory (VDRL) test (for syphilis): Neurosyphilis is a rare but treatable condition; hearing loss is usually bilateral with less dizziness.

> *Ill-Defined:* Evaluate drug and carbon monoxide levels, if appropriate with history (i.e., patient is indoors during winter months and complains of headaches).

Differential Diagnosis

Neurologic Disorders

Benign positional vertigo.
Vestibulopathy.
Ménière's disease.
Medication toxicity.
Acoustic neuroma.
Transient ischemic attack.
Cerebellar stroke.
Parkinson's disease.

Systemic Causes

Hypotension.
Transient arrhythmias.
Lead or arsenic poisoning.
Metabolic disorders.

Psychiatric

Anxiety.

Psychosis.

Affective disorders.

Mixed/Other

Combination of vestibular, visual, and proprioception deficits.

Treatment: Patients are treated according to the cause of the dizziness. For acoustic neuroma, surgery may be indicated. Patients with benign positional vertigo should perform the following therapeutic exercise. While lying in bed, the patient rolls over to the left, reproducing the dizziness. The patient holds that position until the dizziness subsides, then repeats this exercise five times (this will fatigue the vertigo response). This exercise should be done every 3 hours, until the patient is symptom-free for several days.

Medication will not help symptoms of vertigo and may cause a state of heightened alertness.

If dizziness is caused by toxicity from medication side effects, discontinue use of the offending drug, if possible.

Symptomatic treatment with antihistamines and sedatives may be marginally effective but may increase falls in older adults.

Follow-up: Patients should return for follow-up visits if symptoms worsen, change from one type of dizziness to another, or do not resolve within 2 weeks.

Sequelae: This depends on the underlying cause of the dizziness.

Prevention/Prophylaxis: Teach older adults to move extremities before rising from positions held for any length of time to compensate for age-related changes in vascularity. Try to determine if dizziness is from medication side effects before adding additional medications to combat the dizziness.

Referral: If etiology remains unclear, refer the patient to a specialist. For suspected peripheral nervous system disorders, dynamic testing of the patient's vestibular function such as audiograms, otoneurology examination, electronystagmography, and caloric testing is indicated.

For cardiac etiology, refer the patient to a cardiologist for possible echocardiography, Holter monitoring, and an exercise stress test.

Patients with central nervous system involvement are referred to a neurologist for CT, MRI, and EEG.

For psychiatric conditions, refer the patient to Psych-Mental Health CNS/NP, psychologist, or psychiatrist.

Education

- Explain the underlying cause, rationale for treatment, and importance of exercises.
- Teach the patient the exercises and ask him or her to demonstrate.
- Explain that this condition may return intermittently for several years.

- Encourage the use of assistive devices for safety until the condition resolves. Placement of handrails in the bathroom and halls may assist with safe ambulation.
- If the condition worsens (e.g., the patient develops a fever, increased dizziness, or tinnitus, advise the patient to seek medical attention.

Dysphagia

Dysphagia, the sensation of a food bolus lodged in the esophagus, is a disorder of esophageal transport and a symptom of an underlying process. The problem is commonly divided into oropharyngeal (transfer dysphagia, the inability to initiate deglutition successfully) and esophageal (the sensation of impeded transit through the esophagus). The feeling of a reduced ability to transport food or beverage from the upper esophagus to the stomach may resemble that of an obstruction in the chest.

Etiology: Aging itself does not cause clinical dysphagia; however, some normal changes of aging can aggravate any preexisting swallowing problems. A lack of movement of the contents of the esophagus indicates the presence of a motility disorder or an obstruction from either an intrinsic or an extrinsic source. Motor or motility disorders of the esophagus may be due to primary muscle disease (myopathy) or to neurologic disease (neuropathy). Muscle diseases that may result in motor disorders of the esophagus include muscular dystrophy, myasthenia gravis, and scleroderma. Neurologic disorders that may result in motor disorders of the esophagus include achalasia, multiple sclerosis, and amyotrophic lateral sclerosis. All dysphagia is caused by motor impairment or physical narrowing of the esophagus, either intrinsically (carcinoma, stricture, and web) or extrinsically (mediastinal tumors and vascular anomalies).

Occurrence: The occurrence rate of dysphagia is unknown.

Age: Dysphagia occurs at any age.

Ethnicity: Not significant.

Gender: Dysphagia occurs equally in males and females.

Contributing Factors: Factors that contribute to dysphagia include increasing age when cancer of the esophagus is more likely; smoking; long history of gastroesophageal reflux; medications (antidepressants, sedatives, neuroleptic agents, such as anticholinergics, antihistamines, antihypertensives, and diuretics: these may produce slowing or disruption of the oral phase of swallowing and affect salivation). Tetracycline, doxycycline, potassium, ferrous sulfate, calcium channel blockers, beta-adrenergic agents, quinidine, aspirin, theophylline, and nitrates may cause a decrease in lower esophageal sphincter pressure, causing increased reflux disease. Vitamin C, NSAIDs, and several other agents also increase reflux if the patient has inadequate fluid intake. Inadequate fluid intake with medication and/or meals, decreased mental status, functional limitations are all prevalent conditions in the older adult that may lead to dysphagia.

Signs and Symptoms: Patients complain of food "stuck" in the esophagus. They may localize the sensation to a specific area, usually behind the sternum or in the suprasternal area (if localized behind the sternum, good correlation with anatomic site exists). Patients report choking and feeling a pressure sensation in the mid-chest. If total obstruction occurs, salivation increases, and vomiting and choking occur. Patients should distinguish between difficulty swallowing solids, liquids, or both. Associated pneumonia, weight loss, and symptoms of gastroesophageal reflux may occur. The time of the presentation of signs and symptoms is important, as a rapid onset may indicate infection, irritation, a food impaction, or a tumor, whereas a slower progressive illness suggests a motor disorder. Patients should be examined for pallor and signs of scleroderma. The mouth should be assessed for signs of irritation, ill-fitting dentures, and any pharyngeal masses. Check for lymph node enlargement and goiter. Examine the abdomen for evidence of any masses or tenderness (Fig. 17–2).

Diagnostic Tests: Test stool for occult blood if associated esophagitis is suspected. Endoscopy with biopsy, esophageal manometry, barium cine/video esophagram, and modified cine-esophagram (cookie swallow) are all valuable tests to determine a structural impediment and/or obstructing lesion. Ambulatory 24-hour pH testing of intraesophageal pH and pressures has found to be useful when evaluating noncardiac chest pain. If malnutrition is suspected, a serum albumin level and a CBC with indices should be ordered.

Differential Diagnosis: Motor diseases that need to be ruled out in a patient complaining of dysphagia include pseudobulbar palsy, myasthenia gravis, multiple sclerosis, amyotrophic lateral sclerosis, and Parkinson's disease. If an obstruction is suspected, then consider tumor, goiter, enlarged lymph nodes, cervical spine osteophytes, sideropenic webs (Plummer-Vinson syndrome), Zenker's diverticulum, pervasive carcinoma, foreign bodies, food impaction, and aortic aneurysm as the underlying cause of this symptom. For the patient complaining of burning associated with swallowing, reflux esophagitis, esophageal infection, and tablet-induced esophagitis need to be explored. Patients with noncardiac chest pain and globus hystericus may also experience dysphagia.

Treatment: Stable patients can be treated as outpatients. Hospitalization may be required when dysphagia is associated with total or near-total obstruction of the esophageal lumen. Esophageal dilatation (pneumatic or bougie), surgical intervention for an esophageal stent, or laser therapy for late cancer may also be part of the treatment plan, depending on the etiology of the dysphagia. Some general measures recommended in the treatment of dysphagia include determining esophageal patency, ensuring airway and pulmonary function, excluding cardiac disease, and assessing nutritional status. Patients with suspected obstructions may need to be given nothing by mouth (NPO); in general, liquids

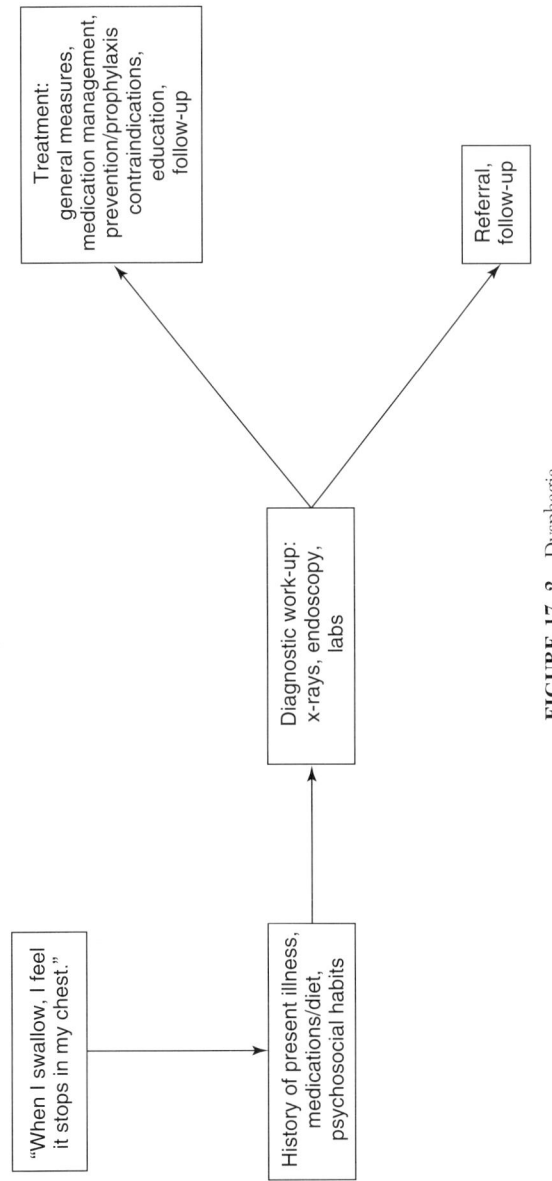

FIGURE 17–2 Dysphagia.

and soft foods only are recommended, until evaluation is completed. Patients with esophageal spasms can be given calcium channel blockers (nifedipine 10–30 mg tid). Patients with associated esophagitis may receive antacids; H2 blockers, adjusting the dosage for the creatinine clearance (ranitidine 150 mg PO bid, nizatidine 150 mg bid, or famotidine 20 mg bid); or, in cases of severe esophagitis, omeprazole 20 mg once a day for 4–8 weeks.

Follow-up: Patient monitoring depends on the specific etiology of the dysphagia.

Sequelae: Complications from dysphagia depend on its cause. An esophageal stricture that responds to dilatation or esophagitis that is resolved with medication has a good prognosis, whereas an obstruction from carcinoma has a poor prognosis.

Prevention/Prophylaxis: Extremely hot or cold foods may worsen symptoms of dysphagia. Observe for aspiration. Assess and advise patients in regard to properly fitting dentures. Monitor for oversedation from medications. Patients should remain upright while eating or drinking.

Referral: A gastroenterologist should be consulted for the endoscopy and for possible hospitalization of patients with severe dysphagia. Other referrals to consider may include speech therapist, radiologist, and dentist (in case of ill-fitting dentures).

Education: Patients should be encouraged to drink fluids with their meals if they are having difficulty swallowing solids. All foods, especially meat products, should be chewed thoroughly. Patients should also be informed that it is important to swallow all medications with plenty of fluid while in an upright position.

Fatigue

Fatigue is a feeling of tiredness or weariness; patients usually refer to it as exhaustion, lack of energy, or weakness.

Etiology: Patients seldom seek medical advice for fatigue that is related to normal physical and/or mental activity. Continuation of fatigue interrupting the patient's activities of daily living (ADLs) may have a physical or psychological cause (Table 17–6).

Fatigue lasting longer than 6 months should be considered chronic.

Occurrence: Fatigue is common among the elderly population. It is problematic for 70% of elderly persons; 59% report experiencing it often.

Age: Not significant.

Ethnicity: Not significant.

Gender: Fatigue occurs equally in males and females.

TABLE 17-6 PHYSICAL AND PSYCHOLOGICAL
CAUSES OF CHRONIC FATIGUE

Physical	Psychological
Infections	Depression
Anemia	Anxiety
Lymphoma	Drug or alcohol abuse
Leukemia	
Acute or chronic hepatitis	
Endocarditis	
Tuberculosis	
Diabetes mellitus	
Hypothyroidism	
Hypoparathyroidism	
Acute or chronic renal failure	
Hepatocellular failure	
Malignancies	
Congestive heart failure	
Drug interactions or misuse	
Inflammatory disease	
Neuromuscular disorders	
Chronic obstructive pulmonary disease	

Contributing Factors: Poor dietary habits, alcohol abuse, smoking, stressful situations (e.g., loss of a loved one or change in environment), chronic illness, drug interactions, misuse of drugs, and sleep apnea may contribute to fatigue.

Signs and Symptoms: Obtain a complete medical history and perform a physical examination, as fatigue may indicate various psychological or physiologic illnesses. Each cause has specific signs and symptoms. Try to distinguish between generalized fatigue and actual weakness by testing for muscle strength and presence of localized tenderness. A mental status examination should be included as part of the physical examination to screen for dementia. Using a geriatric depression scale, establish a baseline diagnosis (Fig. 17-3).

Diagnostic Tests: Consider the following diagnostic tests when a patient complains of persistent, unresolved fatigue. To rule out anemia, order a CBC with indices. Table 17-7 shows the CBC components, the range of normal values for each, and possible causes for abnormal laboratory findings.

Peripheral blood smear red blood cells (RBCs) should be round and equal in size. Central pallor should occupy approximately one-third to one-half the cell's diameter; pallor covering a greater area indicates hypochromia.

Reticulocyte count (25,000–75,000) enables kinetic classification of the anemia, prompted by the question "Is the marrow failing to make blood, or is blood loss occurring?"

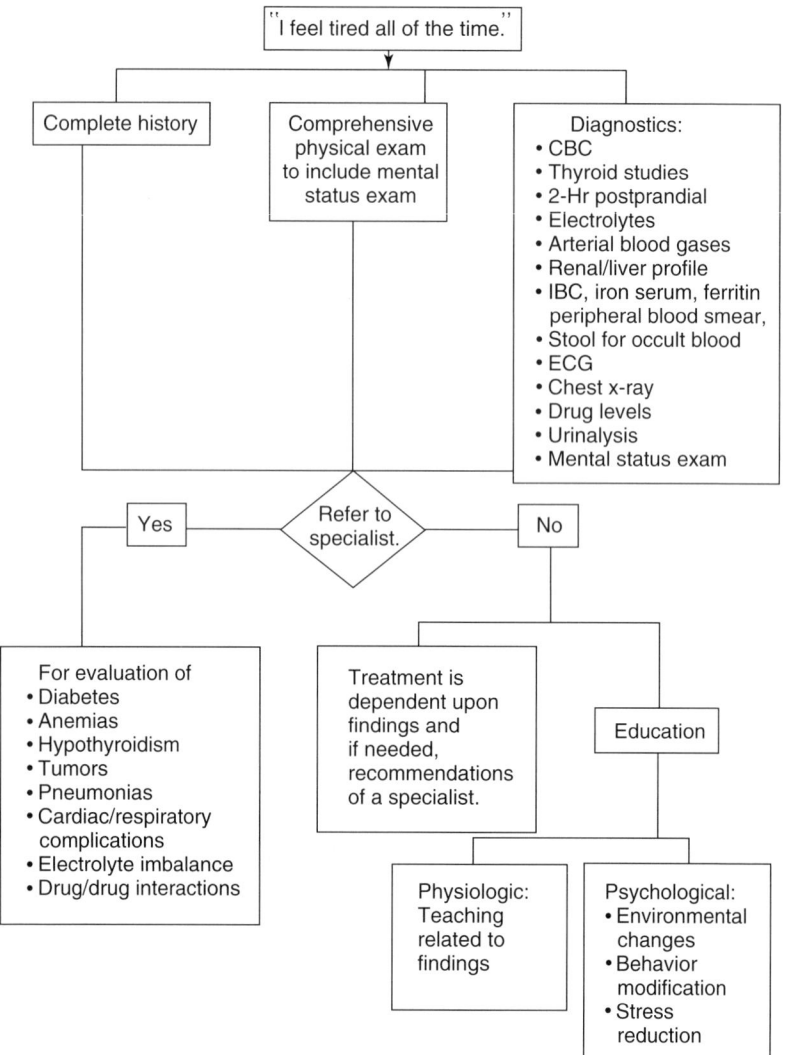

FIGURE 17–3 Fatigue.

Bone marrow aspiration sampling, a means of testing for anemia, is somewhat limited; this evaluation is done when other test results are found to be normal in patients with normocytic, hypoproliferative, normochromic anemia.

Stool should be tested for occult blood to determine hidden blood loss.

Because fatigue may be a presenting symptom of hypothyroid disease, investigation of thyroid functioning is warranted. Low levels of triiodothyronine (T_3) and thyroxine (T_4) indicate primary or secondary hypothyroidism. Only T_3

TABLE 17–7 DIAGNOSTIC TESTS FOR FATIGUE TO RULE OUT ANEMIA

Laboratory Study (Normal Values)	Causes for Abnormal Findings
Red blood cells (RBCs) (4.0–5.0)	
Mean corpuscular volume (MCV) (80–98)	If MCV is less than 80, suspect microcytic anemia.
Mean corpuscular hemoglobin (MCH) (27–31)	If MCH is less than 27%, suspect hypochromic anemia.
Mean corpuscular hemoglobin concentration (MCHC) (32–36)	If MCHC is less than 32%, suspect hypochromic anemia.
Hemoglobin (elderly man 12.4–14.9; elderly woman 11.7–13.8)	If hemoglobin is abnormal, suspect anemia.
Hematocrit (elderly man 42%–54%; elderly woman 38%–46%)	If hemoglobin is abnormal, suspect anemia.
Iron-binding capacity (IBC) (two to three times greater than the serum iron level)	When serum iron is decreased, the IBC is increased. If IBC is increased, suspect iron-deficiency anemia.
Total iron-binding capacity (TIBC) (250–450 mg/dL)	If TIBC is decreased, suspect hemochromatosis (excess iron deposits in organs and tissues) and anemia.
Serum iron (50–150 mg/mL)	If serum iron is decreased, suspect iron-deficiency anemia.
Serum ferritin (men 20–300 ng/mL; women 20–120 ng/mL)	If serum ferritin is decreased, suspect iron-deficiency anemia.

rises in toxicosis; free T_4 remains within normal limits. Thyroid-stimulating hormone (TSH) levels greater than 20 mIU/mL suggest primary hypothyroidism.

To rule out new-onset diabetes, common in older adults, check fasting (FBS) and postprandial (PP) blood sugar levels; an FBS level greater than or equal to 140 mg/dL or a 2-hr PP blood sugar level greater than or equal to 200 mg/dL indicates diabetes.

An electrolyte panel, particularly to check the potassium level, is warranted. Patients taking a potassium-wasting diuretic can become hypokalemic (K^+ less than 3.5 mEq/L) and may experience resultant vertigo, hypotension, nausea and vomiting, and muscle weakness. Elevated levels of BUN (greater than 25 mg) and creatinine (greater than 1.2 mg/dL) may indicate renal disease. Order a urinalysis to assess for renal disorders and other systemic abnormalities.

Lactate dehydrogenase (LDH) is usually 55–102 U/L for adults over age 60. Elevations may indicate lung, liver, or renal disease.

For patients with dyspnea accompanying fatigue, evaluate arterial blood gases (ABGs) and order a chest x-ray examination to rule out congestive heart failure and chronic obstructive pulmonary disease (COPD).

ECG reveals any cardiac arrhythmias, enlargement of the heart, myocardial infarct, and any abnormalities in the conduction system.

Monitor drug levels carefully in older persons, keeping in mind the age-related decrease body fluid levels, increased body fat, decreased glomerular filtration rate, and decreased hepatic blood flow. The effects of digoxin toxicity, which is especially common in older adults, are similar to the signs and symptoms of anemia.

Differential Diagnosis: Fatigue can be related to a number of psychological and physiologic etiologies.

Treatment: Treatment depends on the findings during a comprehensive workup.

Follow-up: Follow-up depends on the findings. Monitor the patient periodically as indicated by diagnosis or symptoms. Additional signs and symptoms may occur if the etiology is physiologic.

Sequelae: The condition relates to the etiology of fatigue.

Prevention/Prophylaxis: Optimal health maintenance and knowledge of prescription and over-the-counter medications may prevent, or enable early recognition of, signs and symptoms of systemic or psychological illness.

Referral: Referral to a specialist is indicated pending results of the workup.

Education: If the fatigue has a physiologic cause, teaching should be related to the findings; psychological, changes in the environment, behavior modification, and stress reduction may be needed.

Headache

Headache describes many entities in which the primary symptom is pain in the head, neck, or face. Headache is one of the most commonly encountered problems in primary care of older adults. Many types and causes of headache exist. Although many causes are benign, some are life threatening. In any case, the symptoms of headache interfere with optimal functioning and quality of life.

Etiology: The most common type of headache, the tension headache, is caused by stress and muscle contraction. Migraine and cluster headaches are also common, although less so in older persons than the general population. In older patients with migraine or cluster headaches, the initial onset occurs in early to mid-adulthood. Many people with chronic or recurrent headaches have a combination of these (tension and migraine or cluster) (Table 17–8).

Occurrence: Headache is one of the 10 most common symptoms seen in primary care. Up to 90% of the population have had headaches, with 45 million individuals reporting recurring headache.

TABLE 17–8 LESS COMMON CAUSES OF
HEADACHES IN ELDERLY PERSONS

Acute/Emergent	Other
Subarachnoid hemorrhage	Sleep apnea
Giant cell arteritis	Sinus headache
Bacterial meningitis	Temporomandibular joint syndrome
Herpes zoster	Parkinson's disease
Ischemic or thrombotic stroke	Drug-related/polypharmacy
Trigeminal neuralgia (may become chronic)	Psychogenic
Acute narrow-angle glaucoma	Chronic open-angle glaucoma
Intracranial tumors	Cervical radiculopathy
Unstable hypertension	Thyroid disorders

Age: Prevalence of headache in patients over age 65 may be as low as 8% or as high as 50%, depending on defining factors. Tension headaches often increase in frequency with age. New or sudden onset of headache after age 50 must be investigated, as it may indicate new disease.

Ethnicity: Not significant.

Gender: Women are affected more often than men; 76% of women and 57% of men report one headache per month. Migraine headaches are more common in women than in men, tending to begin in early adulthood. Cluster headaches are more common in men than in women, with a mean age of onset at 30 years.

Contributing Factors: In older adults, poor posture, cervical osteoarthritis, use of eyeglasses, depression, bereavement, ill-fitting dentures, sleep disorders, and joint pain may contribute to or complicate the symptoms of headaches.

Signs and Symptoms: Diagnosis is frequently made on the basis of history, particularly for the most common types of headaches, by characterizing the symptom and associated manifestations including onset, location, duration, frequency, character, triggering or aggravating factors, alleviating factors, prior history and initial onset of problem, prodromal symptoms, severity rating, sleep problems, use of prescribed or OTC medications and herbal remedies, use of caffeine, use of alcohol, and history of allergies. If the patient is physically and mentally able to participate, having him or her keep a headache diary is very helpful in identifying patterns. Problems associated with history taking in older patients may include an inability to localize or accurately describe symptoms or the underreporting of symptoms. Table 17–9 provides further guidance in establishing the cause of the headache.

The physical examination should include observation of general appearance, including facies, and evaluation of mental status. Assess vital signs for extremes in blood pressure, suggesting a neurologic event. Examine the head and palpate for tenderness, signs of trauma, pain over the temporal artery, and strength of

TABLE 17–9 CLINICAL FEATURES OF VARIOUS TYPES AND CAUSES OF HEADACHES IN OLDER PERSONS

Type/Cause of Headache	Characteristics of Headache	Other Features
	Acute/Subacute	
Accelerated hypertension	Generalized; throbbing	Rapid rise in blood pressure; chronic type is often occipital
Giant cell arteritis	Variable location (often temples, scalp, post cervical); variable quality	Tenderness over arteries; jaw pain with chewing; systemic symptoms may be present; more common in women
Ischemic or thrombotic stroke	Variable quality; moderate to severe intensity	More common with history of headache; neurologic deficits
Subarachnoid hemorrhage	Sudden onset; moderate to severe intensity	Associated with hypertension, trauma, aneurysm; high mortality; meningeal irritation; blood in cerebrospinal fluid; necessitates neuroimaging scan (CT; more sensitive to blood)
Intracranial tumors	Recent onset; increasing frequency and intensity; present when patient awakens, worse with head movement	Headache often absent with primary or metastatic brain tumors
Intracranial infection	Variable quality; variable location	Other signs more important (e.g., fever, meningeal signs, confusion)
Herpes zoster	Cranial nerve involvement; unilateral	Dysesthesia along cranial nerve distribution; vesicular lesions; malaise; low-grade fever

Recurrent

Trigeminal neuralgia (tic douloureux)	Unilateral; lightning-like stabbing along trigeminal nerve distribution; during waking hours	May see motor or sensory changes in face owing to brain stem or gasserian lesion; also may be idiopathic
Cluster	Episodic; unilateral; excruciating; around the eye	80% are men; severity makes patient consider suicide; patient should avoid alcohol and smoking; may be familial

Chronic

Migraine	Unilateral; pulsating moderate to severe; lasts hours to days	Nausea, photophobia, intolerant to noise; aura or prodrome; family history in 50%–70%; more common in women; greatest prevalence in fourth or fifth decades
Muscle contraction (tension)	Begins in muscle units of head or neck and spreads over entire head; trigger point of tenderness over muscle involved	Caused by physical and psychologic stress that makes muscle units contract
Cervical radiculopathy	Begins as cervical spine pain; spreads to occipital area and becomes generalized; worse with neck movement	Caused by osteoarthritis; neck radiographs show characteristic changes; increases in prevalence with age
Sleep apnea syndrome	Variable intensity and quality; nocturnal or morning common	Improves greatly after treatment for sleep apnea
Medication related	Generalized; variable intensity and quality, depending on medication	Establish temporal relationship when patient takes medication; any medication may be a potential cause; polypharmacy related
Sinus	Begins early in day, but improves during day with sinus drainage; pressure or aching may be over sinus areas or generalized	History of chronic sinusitis; possible allergies must be excluded; may have tenderness over sinus area; associated with chronic cough

Source: From Yoshikawa, TT, Cobbs, EL, and Brummel-Smith, K: Practical Ambulatory Geriatrics, ed 2. CV Mosby, St. Louis, 1998, with permission.

the temporal arterial pulse. Test the cranial nerves. Perform a fundoscopic examination to assess for papilledema, hemorrhages, exudates, and venous pulsations. Evaluate gross and fine motor and sensory functions including gait, balance, and tactile sense. Test deep tendon reflexes for presence and symmetry; measure muscle strength for grading and equality.

Conduct an examination of the head and neck for lymphadenopathy, thyroid enlargement, carotid bruits, trigger points, meningeal irritation, or limitation in normal range of motion. Check the temporomandibular joint for alignment, mobility, and clicking. Examine the ears, nose, and throat, including the teeth for contributing problems.

Evaluate the patient for postural alignment problems, muscle spasms, or trigger points in the back or shoulders. Investigate in depth the presence of any new-onset headache in patients over age 50 or any acute-onset headache with positive neurologic findings.

Diagnostic Tests: Individualize diagnostic tests according to the suspected cause of the symptom. If you suspect anemia, infection, or electrolyte imbalance, obtain a CBC with differential, glucose level, and chemistry profile. An erythrocyte sedimentation rate (ESR) helps if you suspect inflammatory conditions such as giant cell arteritis. An elevated ESR warrants referral of the patient for temporal artery biopsy to confirm diagnosis. If thyroid abnormalities are a possibility, perform thyroid function studies. Do a lumbar puncture for cerebrospinal fluid analysis if a diagnosis of subarachnoid hemorrhage or meningeal infection is being considered. CT scanning or MRI is indicated for emergency evaluation of subarachnoid hemorrhage, arteriovenous (AV) malformation with cerebral aneurysm, possible CVA or intracranial neoplasm; arteriography may also be necessary. Sinus x-ray examination with a Water's view helps when recurrent or chronic symptoms suggest the sinus as a possible origin of headache. Cervical spine x-ray examination may reveal a musculoskeletal source of pain.

Differential Diagnosis: Symptoms of headaches of various types and etiologies can mimic each other. CVA can mimic some types of headache. See also Etiology and Contributing Factors sections.

Treatment: Treatment of headache depends on its cause. Because of the potential for drug-related problems in older adults, nonpharmacologic treatment including biofeedback, imagery, progressive relaxation techniques, and other stress management strategies should be tried initially for muscle tension, migraine, and mixed (tension and migraine) headaches. Other nonpharmacologic treatments that may be effective include acupuncture, acupressure, transcutaneous electrical nerve stimulation (TENS), massage, intermittent use of a cervical collar, heat or cold application, and resting in a darkened room.

Before instituting drug therapy, evaluate renal function, and in selected cases, liver function also. The use of analgesics such as acetaminophen, aspirin or other NSAIDs, along with any of the nonpharmacologic modalities described earlier, is often effective for pain relief. The availability and use of the medication at the onset of symptoms is essential for maximal benefit. Use caution in prescribing these medications. Patients who are receiving anticoagulant therapy, have a history of sensitivity to salicylates or of GI bleeding or peptic ulcer disease, should not use aspirin. Similarly, NSAIDs should not be used if these conditions or compromised renal function exist.

The NSAID naproxen sodium 500 mg PO bid, ibuprofen 400 mg PO tid, or Orudis 50 mg PO tid is frequently used to treat headache. These should be taken with food to minimize GI effects. Acetaminophen can cause liver failure in toxic doses; if not contraindicated, dosages of 500–650 mg PO qid should be used. These medications are mainly used abortively to alleviate or minimize the severity of headache symptoms.

For frequent headaches, prophylactic therapy may be instituted to prevent development of symptoms. Medication is taken daily for a trial period (usually 1–2 months) to evaluate the effect on headache frequency. Although beta-blockers have been used prophylactically for migraine and cluster headaches, they are contraindicated in patients with a history of bronchospastic disease, asthma, diabetes, or congestive heart failure (CHF). Beta-blocker Inderal LA 80 mg PO daily, Tenormin, 50–100 mg PO daily, or Corgard 40 mg PO daily may be used.

Calcium channel blockers such as verapamil 240 mg PO daily or nifedipine 30–180 mg PO daily have also been used prophylactically to prevent migraines. Contraindications include CHF, heart block, hypotension, sick sinus syndrome, and atrial fibrillation. Low-doses of tricyclic antidepressants (e.g., Elavil 50 mg PO daily or Norpramin 50 mg PO daily) have been prescribed to take at bedtime. Selection of the agent should be based on patient profile; many are contraindicated because of adverse effects on the cardiovascular system or anticholinergic effects.

For abortive treatment of migraine or cluster headache, if nonprescription analgesics such as aspirin and acetaminophen are ineffective, ergotrate preparations such as Midrin and Cafergot have been used with some success in adults. These drugs are contraindicated in patients with coronary artery disease (CAD) or peripheral vascular disease, limiting their use in older patients. Imitrex has also been prescribed, although it is contraindicated in the presence of ischemic heart disease, CAD, coronary artery vasospasm (including Prinzmetal's angina), uncontrolled hypertension, potential for cerebrovascular event, basilar or hemiplegic migraine, use of monoamine oxidase (MAO) inhibitors within 2 weeks, or use of ergot-based drugs within 24 hours. Low-range doses are 5 mg as a nasal spray, 6 mg subcutaneously, or 25 mg PO.

For patients with cluster headaches, 100% oxygen, 7 L by mask for 15 minutes, may be used in the absence of COPD or other respiratory complications. If not contraindicated, prednisone, 40–60 mg PO daily for 1 week, then tapered off for another week, may also be prescribed for cluster headaches. Intranasal lidocaine 4% topical solution, 1 mL in the nostril corresponding to the location of the headache has also been effective in relieving migraine or cluster headaches. Cluster headaches may also be treated with medications used for migraine.

For giant cell arteritis, patients may take prednisone, 40–60 mg daily for several weeks, then tapered gradually to 10–20 mg daily and continued for 18 months. Long-term steroid therapy of this nature has important implications related to immune system function, GI bleeding, and bone deterioration.

Follow-up: Monitoring depends on cause and treatment strategies. Patients should be monitored for effectiveness of treatment.

Sequelae: Depends on cause. Missed diagnosis of acute, life-threatening symptoms can prove fatal. Most common causes have recurrence or chronicity, which affects quality of life.

Prevention/Prophylaxis: Avoidance of triggers, early intervention with medication as soon as symptoms present, stress reduction techniques as appropriate.

Referral: Refer patients to collaborating physician or neurologist whenever "red flags" are noted present (Table 17–10).

Education: Teach patients how to live with a chronic or recurrent problem, to avoid triggers to reduce stress reduction, and to promote self-care.

TABLE 17–10 "RED FLAGS" IN THE DIAGNOSIS OF HEADACHE

1. Onset of headache after age 50
2. Onset of new or different headache
3. "Worst" headache ever experienced
4. Onset of subacute headache that progressively worsens
5. Onset of headache with exertion, sexual activity, coughing, or sneezing
6. Headache associated with any of the following changes in neurologic evaluation
   a. Drowsiness, confusion, memory impairment
   b. Weakness, ataxia, loss of coordination
   c. Numbness and/or tingling in extremities
   d. Paralysis
   e. Sensory loss associated with headache
   f. Asymmetry of pupillary response, deep tendon reflexes, or Babinski response
   g. Signs of meningeal irritation
   h. Progressive visual or neurologic changes
   i. Other evidence to suggest an underlying neurologic disorder such as persistent tinnitus, loss of sense of smell, loss of sensation over the face, dysphagia
7. Abnormal medical evaluation
   a. Fever
   b. Stiff neck
   c. Hypertension
   d. Weight loss
   e. Tender, poorly pulsatile temporal arteries
   f. Papilledema
   g. Chronic cough, lymphadenopathy, recurrent nasal drainage or discharge, or other evidence to suggest a systemic illness

Hematuria

Hematuria is abnormal presence of blood (erythrocytes) in the urine. Regardless of age, this can be defined as two to four RBCs per high-power field (HPF).

Etiology: Hematuria usually signifies structural genitourinary abnormalities. Other causes include a urinary tract infection (UTI), renal stones, coagulation defects, glomerular disease, trauma to the genitourinary (GU) tract, tumors or neoplasms, vascular disease, opiate abuse, or benign familial hematuria. Blood seen upon starting to void is usually from the prostate, urethra, or penis. Blood seen at the end of voiding is most likely from the bladder neck or prostatic urethra. Total hematuria or blood during the entire void is from typically the bladder, kidney, or ureters.

The etiology of hematuria can vary depending on the location of disease in the GU tract. Infection and trauma can cause bleeding from the urethra. Kidney stones, infection, benign prostatic hyperplasia (BPH) involving the bladder neck, and cancer can cause hematuria from the bladder region. Hematuria from the kidney can result from trauma, infection, stones, structural anatomic anomalies, cancer, or glomerular disease. In addition, patients with infections, tumors, or stones in the ureters can present with hematuria. Other causes include sickle cell disease, anticoagulant therapy, bleeding disorders (disseminated intravascular coagulation [DIC], thrombocytopenia, hemophilia), cocaine abuse, and hemolytic uremic syndrome. In male and female patients under age 20, suspect congenital urinary tract anomaly, acute UTI, or acute glomerulonephritis. In men and women between ages 20 and 40 the cause is usually UTI, kidney stones, trauma, or bladder tumor. In men ages 40–60, suspect bladder tumor, renal stones, UTI, or renal neoplasm. In women ages 40–60, suspect acute UTI, kidney stone, or bladder tumor. In elderly men over age 60, initially suspect prostate disease, then bladder tumor and acute UTI. For women, age 60 and older, rule out bladder tumor and acute UTI.

Ethnicity: Those prone to sickle cell disease (almost exclusively African-Americans) or those who carry the sickle cell trait (10% of African-Americans) should have this factor assessed in the workup of asymptomatic hematuria.

Contributing Factors: Transient macroscopic or microscopic hematuria may be triggered by recent strenuous activity, indwelling or straight catheterization, or food or pollen allergies.

Signs and Symptoms: Patients may present with painless hematuria or dysuria and urgency with hematuria. Patients may describe the hematuria as occurring just at the onset of urination, at the end of urination, or throughout the entire void. Clots may be present. Other complaints may include vaginal discharge, urgency or frequency of urination, nocturia, polyuria, incontinence, dribbling, reduced or slow urinary stream, abdominal or flank pain, fever, anorexia, nausea, weight loss, scrotal pain, and urinary hesitancy.

The history should include any significant medical history, surgery, family history, and medications (OTC and prescription). Any history of urinary calculi (nephrolithiasis or urolithiasis), frequent UTIs, congenital kidney malformation, or prostate disease. Inquire about the use of hormonal replacement therapy and the last incident of vaginal bleeding. Take a complete sex history and inquire about the presence of penile lesions, discharge, or hematospermia. Assess the onset, duration, frequency, and severity of the hematuria. Ask about any recent alteration in the volume of urine produced in a day.

During the physical examination, assess blood pressure, temperature, skin (for jaundice), and eyes (for pallor). Palpate the abdomen for any mass, suprapubic tenderness, or rigidity. Assess for any costovertebral tenderness. Auscultate for any renal artery bruits. Thoroughly inspect the female and male genitalia for any abnormalities. In women, inspect the urethral meatus and vaginal wall (checking for atrophy, tears, cystocele), and note any signs of infection (discharge or lesions). In men, carefully examine the external shaft of the penis and the position of the urethra, noting any discharge, lesions, or inflammation. Palpate the spermatic cord, testes, epidiymus, and prostate, unless you suspect acute prostatitis. Assess the patient for any signs of hemolytic disease and for any systemic signs of renal failure.

Objective findings associated with hematuria include:

Bruit over the flank region (renal arteriovenous fistula).

Bruit over the epigastric region in a hypertensive patient (could be related to renal artery stenosis).

Costovertebral angle tenderness with renal stones or acute UTI.

Suprapubic or abdominal tenderness with UTI.

Inguinal lymphadenopathy with inflammation, infection, or malignancy of the penis, urethra (male or female), scrotum, or vulva.

Urethral discharge in men, indicating urethritis.

Abdominal or pelvic mass that may be associated with a malignancy in the bladder.

Fever with acute UTI.

Glomerular nephritis.

Proteinuria with kidney disease.

Diagnostic Testing: The clinical tests ordered are based on the patient presentation, history of present illness, and physical examination findings. For diagnosis of hematuria, a freshly voided urine specimen should be obtained and examined within 30 minutes. Microscopic examination after centrifugal sedimentation is the most sensitive way to identify formed elements such as cells, casts, crystals, and microorganisms. A urine dipstick test can be done in the office to detect the presence and quantity of blood (normal is negative or 0–1 RBCs/HPF), bacteria (normal is 0–4 WBCs/HPF), protein, ketones, and general appearance of the urine. Note the presence of clots or frank blood. Send a urinalysis for a culture and sensitivity (C&S) testing if you suspect an infection. This will allow you to quantify the amount of blood present in the urine (hematuria is generally defined as 2–4 RBC/HPF). Results of the culture will determine the specific bacteria present; results of the sensitivity test will help determine the antibiotic to use for treatment.

Serum BUN and creatinine levels should be sent for evaluation of actual kidney function. Elevated BUN is most common with inadequate excretion secondary to urinary obstruction, prostate enlargement, or kidney disease. An increase of 50–150 mg/100 mL indicates serious kidney problems. Increased serum creatinine levels can be seen with chronic nephritis, altered renal function, and urinary tract obstruction. Patients with known kidney disease or proteinuria with hematuria may need a 24-hour urine collection to assess total urine protein, as well as creatinine clearance testing. A recent BUN and creatinine level will be required before intravenous pyelography (IVP) is ordered.

If the patient is receiving anticoagulant therapy, obtain a CBC, checking the total platelet count, and a coagulation panel to check clotting times, including a prothrombin time (PT), partial thromboplastin time (PTT), and international normalized ratio (INR).

If the clinical presentation of hematuria suggests kidney stones and the pain is tolerable, outpatient treatment includes an abdominal x-ray of kidney ureter and bladder (KUB) film to assess for the presence of stones. Pushing liquids and straining the urine is also necessary. Consider the need for pain management; if pain persists, an ultrasound or IVP to determine the actual position of the stone, and stone removal by a urologist, may be necessary.

Differential Diagnosis: The following should be considered in the differential diagnosis:

- Uncomplicated or complicated cystitis.
- UTI.
- Pyelonephritis.
- Glomerular nephritis.
- Kidney stones.
- Renal calculi.
- IgA nephropathy.
- March hemoglobinuria (exercise related).
- BPH.
- Prostatitis.
- Trauma.
- Urologic cancer.
- Hemolytic and clotting disorders.
- Medication-related papillary necrosis, nephritis, or cystitis.
- Benign familial hematuria.
- Pseudohematuria secondary to excessive ingestion of beets, laxatives and tea containing phenolphthalein, vegetable dyes, pyridium, concentrated urine.

Treatment: Therapy depends completely on the suspected or known cause of the hematuria.

For UTI and nongonococcal urethritis: Empirical treatment or specific antibiotic treatment as determined from C&S report
Consult with physician regarding the clinical presentation of patients with acute prostatitis, as many require hospitalization and intravenous (IV) antibiotic therapy.

For chronic prostatitis, long-term antibiotic therapy is often indicated.
Dosage adjustments should be made for reduced kidney function.
For kidney stones and renal calculi: Outpatient management, depending on pain management, passage of the stone, and position of the calculi
Patients treated as outpatients should increase their fluid intake to 1–3 L/day and strain their urine. Pain medications are usually required.
See "Referral" section for specialized management.

Follow-up: Protocol for follow-up depends on the workup and clinical findings. Patients need routine follow-up to determine the exact cause of the hematuria. Any patients treated as outpatients for UTIs, prostatitis, BPH, kidney stones, or idiopathic hematuria should be reevaluated 24–72 hr after treatment initiation. Patients with any acute problems or changes in symptom status should be referred for emergency evaluation. Depending on the nature of the hematuria, urologic consultation and further diagnostic testing may be required.

Sequelae: Complications of hematuria are directly related to the underlying condition or the cause of the hematuria.

Prevention/Prophylaxis: Patients with chronic UTIs, chronic prostatitis, or recurrent renal stones should seek medical intervention at the appropriate time (see also "Education"). Patients with a history of calcium oxalate stones should follow low-purine dietary recommendations.

Referral: Depending on the complexity and nature of the hematuria, physician consultation may be required. Refer patients to urology if:
- Stone removal is needed.
- Acute or chronic prostatitis, UTI, or BPH accompanies hematuria, for cystoscopy or other cytologic testing (in men).
- Persistent hematuria, without infection or obstruction, is present, for further workup.
- Persistent hematuria is present, to rule out tumors and bladder carcinoma and possibly for cystoscopy.
- Pseudohematuria (caused by pigments other than blood) needs confirmation.

Emergency care or hospitalization may be necessary for patients with acute disease or hemorrhage. Hospitalization may also be needed for older adults with complicated UTIs, glomerular nephritis, or acute pyelonephritis.

Education: Teach patients with chronic UTIs, pancreatitis, or renal stones the appropriate time to seek medical attention. Teach low-purine diet recommendations to those with a history of calcium oxalate stones. Teach the importance of treatment compliance in patients taking medications for chronic prostatitis and BPH. Discuss routine health maintenance with patients including personal hygiene and safe sex practices. All medications should be reviewed by the health-care provider.

Hemoptysis

Hemoptysis is defined as coughing up blood from the respiratory tract. This may be in the form of blood-tinged sputum or actual clots of blood.

Etiology: To determine the etiology of the hemoptysis, it is crucial to decide whether the source of bleeding is from the respiratory tract, GI tract, or nasopharynx. Most cases of hemoptysis are caused by lung diseases, including:

Acute or chronic bronchitis.
Inflammation or disease or the larynx, trachea, or pharynx.
Pneumonia.
Lung abscess.
Tumors.
Bronchogenic carcinomas.
Tuberculosis.

There are also cardiovascular causes of hemoptysis. Pulmonary infarct with thromboembolus or left-sided heart failure with mitral stenosis can cause lung irritation, leading to hemoptysis. Less commonly, bloody respiratory secretions are seen in patients with fungal infections, parasites, chest trauma, or metastatic neoplasms. Persons with clotting defects (thrombocytopenia, vitamin K deficiency, DIC) and those taking anticoagulants may present with hemoptysis. In the case of gross hemoptysis, determining the etiology is secondary to emergency intervention to control the hemorrhage.

Occurrence: Blood-streaked sputum is seen in 30%–60% of patients with inflammatory factors (bronchitis or bronchiectasis) and in only 20%–30% of those with pneumonia or hemoptysis caused by other severe diseases. Older patients with chronic lung disease, immunosuppression, or other coexisting chronic diseases, and those who smoke cigarettes, are more likely to develop this problem.

Age: Hemoptysis can occur at any age. However, elderly persons presenting with hemoptysis more commonly have chronic disease, cardiovascular problems (e.g., mitral stenosis), and clotting deficits should be assessed thoroughly.

Ethnicity: No documentation found.

Gender: No documentation found.

Contributing Factors: The following factors contribute to the development of hemoptysis:

Smoking history.

Chronic bronchitis or lung disease.

Recent viral or bacterial lung infections.

Immunocompromised status.

Recent surgery placing patient at risk for DVT with pulmonary emboli or infarct. Patients with a

    History of mitral stenosis (related to earlier history of rheumatic fever).

    History of atrial fibrillation (with embolic phenomena).

    Tuberculosis.

    Anticoagulant therapy.

Signs and Symptoms: It is critical to determine the source of the bleeding. Patients with hemoptysis generally have respiratory symptoms and complain of irritation or burning in the throat or chest, usually accompanied with a cough or the urge to cough. Blood is present with the sputum and is usually bright red or frothy with an alkaline pH. Patients with bleeding from the GI tract or hematemesis (bloody vomit) often present complaining of GI symptoms associated with nausea or vomiting, dyspepsia, heartburn, or difficulty swallowing. The blood is usually dark red, has a coffee-grounds appearance, or may contain food particles. Blood from the GI tract has an acidic pH.

    Have the patient clarify the symptoms.

Did they occur suddenly?

Was there a cough or other upper respiratory sign?

Is it blood-tinged sputum or actual clots?

Does the patient have any associated symptoms such as vomiting, fever, chest pain, shortness of breath, palpitations, leg pain or cramps, weight loss, or night sweats?

Is there throat, mouth, or tongue pain or hoarseness?

Has the patient ever been diagnosed with tuberculosis?

Does the patient have a history of frequent nosebleeds?

Does the patient take Coumadin or have an irregular heartbeat?

    Patients' complaints may vary, but the subjective data are critical to the differential diagnosis.

    Perform a physical examination thoroughly examining the nasal passages, turbinates, and sinuses and assessing completely the mouth, throat, and neck. Assess the presence of cervical and supraclavicular adenopathy and fever. Auscultate the lungs for rales, wheezing, or friction rubs. Inspect cardiac and thorax regions for physical evidence of chronic lung disease (increased anteroposterior diameter), respiratory distress, or asymmetric chest excursion or movement. Auscultate the heart for murmurs, S_3, S_4, or rubs. Measure the respiratory and pulse rates. If it is unclear if the bleeding is related to the GI tract, also carefully inspect and assess the abdomen and check the stool for blood. Evidence of deep vein disease in the legs should be assessed.

Diagnostic Tests: The cause of the hemoptysis determines what diagnostic tests should be performed. Generally, the tests are done to support the diagnosis and guide the treatment. To assess possible infection or any significant blood loss, obtain a CBC with indices. Assess the WBC for any increase in the presence of infection or decrease in the presence of immunosuppression from liver disease, neoplasms, or medications. Be careful not to rely on an elevated WBC count to diagnose pneumonia or infection in elderly individuals, as the count is often normal and fever absent in those with these conditions. Evaluate RBCs, hemoglobin, and hematocrit to assess for blood or volume loss. A tuberculin (0.1 mL Mantoux) test may be needed to screen for tuberculosis. Carefully assess the need for anergy testing in the patient. Check platelets (PLT) for any evidence of thrombocytopenia. In the differential the monocytes may be increased in the presence of infection. PT and partial thromboplastin time (normal ranges vary among laboratories) and INR should be measured if the patient is taking anticoagulants, to assess for alterations in clotting times. Conduct serum electrolyte and liver function tests to rule out other disease processes in the differential diagnosis. An elevated LDH may indicate liver, lung, or renal disease. Check aspartate aminotransferase (AST) and alanine aminotransferase (ALT) levels for assessment of inflammatory or chronic liver disease resulting in low platelet levels that could cause bleeding. If systemic liver disease is considered, do complete screening for hepatitis.

Sputum may be cultured and tested for acid-fast bacilli (AFB) and sent for evaluation to determine the bacterial source of infection and rule out tuberculosis. If any exudate of symptoms of *Candida* infection are visualized during the physical examination, a throat culture should be done. A chest x-ray examination can be helpful in evaluating presence of infiltrates, inflammatory disease, tuberculosis, apical scarring, effusions, or neoplastic disease.

If the hemoptysis does not resolve or worsens, a referral and indirect laryngoscopy or fiberoptic bronchscopy may be needed. Cytologic or tissue samples are necessary to establish a diagnosis of lung cancer. If the results of the chest x-ray examination are not conclusive, CT scan of the chest may be required for further evaluation of abnormalities. Patients with a history of mitral stenosis or atrial fibrillation, or cardiac abnormality on examination should have an ECG to assess for cardiac arrhythmias, left-ventricular hypertrophy (LVH), or conduction anomalies.

In the presence of lung hemorrhage, suspect DVT with pulmonary embolism and refer patient for emergency intervention.

Differential Diagnosis: Careful history taking and evaluation are necessary to rule out hematemesis. The differential diagnosis includes sinus infection, inflammation or disease of the pharynx or larynx, bronchitis; pneumonia, tumors, carcinomas, pulmonary infarct associated with thromboembolism; left-sided heart failure with mitral stenosis, clotting disorders, tuberculosis (TB), fungal or parasitic infections, and rarely, blunt chest trauma. Neoplasms (bronchogenic carcinomas) in elderly persons with a history of smoking need to be ruled out.

Treatment: The decision to treat hemoptysis is based on the clinical presentation, diagnostic evaluation, and clinical evidence of disease. Acute and chronic bronchitis are the most common causes of hemoptysis. In patients with chronic bronchitis who smoke, the agents vary (viral *Streptococcus pneumoniae, Haemophilus influenzae,* or *M. catarrhalis*) and are treated with appropriate antibiotics, antitussives, and bedrest. The following medications can be used dependent of liver, renal function, and allergies:

Patients over age 65 with chronic disease and immunosuppression with WBCs less than 4000 or greater than 30,000/mm^3 may require hospitalization. Others who may need hospitalization are patients with persistent hemoptysis, suspected or active tuberculosis, clotting disorders, cardiac disease, or suspected neoplasm. Carefully evaluate persons with clotting defects (e.g., thrombocytopenia, vitamin K deficiency, DIC) and those taking anticoagulants, if hemoptysis is their presenting symptom. If bleeding is secondary to lung cancer, external-beam radiotherapy for palliation is used most often.

Follow-up: Monitor patient for full resolution of the hemoptysis. Reevaluate patients taking antibiotics when the medication is finished. The hemoptysis should resolve in 2–3 days. Ask patients to seek medical attention if symptoms persist or worsen. Patients with documented infiltrates or abnormalities on chest x-ray examination should have another film done 2–3 weeks after treatment. Have patients report any lingering systemic symptoms (fever, weight loss, fatigue). Persistent or recurring hemoptysis in smokers, or in any elderly person, probably requires assessment of GI or nasopharynx tract bronchoscopy, and testing to reveal source of blood. Repeat blood studies as indicated.

Sequelae: Complications of hemoptysis depend on the etiology of the blood production and the amount of blood lost. Hemoptysis becomes life threatening by causing cardiovascular collapse or acute respiratory insufficiency.

Prevention/Prophylaxis: Teach all patients about smoking cessation. Instruct patients who are being medically managed for bronchitis or pneumonia to complete all medications and report any persistent or systemic symptoms. Encourage patients with chronic sinusitis to humidify the air and avoid overuse of nasal sprays or oral decongestants. Older patients should receive a flu shot annually and all patients over 65 should have a pneumococcal vaccine. Patients taking Coumadin should be seen regularly for blood studies (PT/PTT, INR, CBC).

Referral: Consultation with a physician may be necessary, depending on the clarity of the patient's clinical presentation. Discussion may be needed to further assess the diagnostic findings and plan the appropriate treatment. Gross hemoptysis or hemorrhage will require emergency intervention. Patients with persistent hemoptysis should be referred to a pulmonary specialist for a bronchoscopy.

If TB or a fungal infection is isolated, you may have to consult with an infectious disease specialist to construct the best treatment plan.

Education: Appropriate instruction and education depends on the diagnosis and treatment plan. Patients receiving anticoagulant therapy should be taught the symptoms that need to be reported to their provider. Finally, all patients must be instructed about the need for follow-up care.

Hoarseness

Hoarseness describes a voice with a harsh quality and low pitch, or one that sounds weak or raspy. Hoarseness can simply indicate any change from the individual's usual voice quality.

Etiology: This symptom is caused by an abnormality somewhere along the vocal tract. An abnormal flow of air past the vocal cords causes hoarseness. An abnormally harsh quality to the voice is caused by a turbulence created by irregularity in the vocal cords. Hoarseness can be acute, arising from an infectious or inflammatory process in the larynx, or chronic, usually developing from more serious problems such as compression or disruption of the vocal cords from malignant and benign polyps, nodules, or tumors or from vocal cord paralysis, systemic disorders such as rheumatoid arthritis, Sjögren's disease, myxedema, lupus, retrosternal goiter, myasthenia gravis, and the laryngeal muscle atrophy seen with aging. Gastroesophageal reflux can also cause laryngeal irritation that can cause hoarseness.

Occurrence: Hoarseness is a common occurrence.

Age: Hoarseness occurs at any age.

Ethnicity: Not significant.

Gender: Hoarseness occurs equally in men and women.

Contributing Factors: Trauma to the larynx may be caused by:
- Excessive alcohol intake.
- Inhalation of noxious fumes and cigarettes.
- Excessive talking and shouting.

Signs and Symptoms: Note the duration of symptoms. Acute onset is more likely to be from infection or trauma, whereas a complaint of progressively increasing hoarseness is more likely to be from cancer or other serious disease. If the hoarseness becomes progressively worse during the day, suspect myasthenia gravis. Review voice use and lifestyle. A professional singer or weekend football fan can suffer voice overuse and abuse. A cigarette smoker of 2 packs per day for 45 years may have irritation or malignancy. A scratchy throat the morning after eating spicy foods late in the evening suggests gastroesophageal reflux.

Sore throat and otalgia accompanying hoarseness is frequently seen in patients with malignant tumors of the larynx or pharynx. Dysphagia or odynophagia with hoarseness may indicate a disease affecting the pharynx or esophagus. Cough and hoarseness suggests irritation of the endolarynx and/or pulmonary disease. Hemoptysis along with hoarseness may indicate a malignant process of the pharyngeal, laryngeal, or pulmonary areas. Fever and oral, nasal, or otalgic discharge with hoarseness suggests an infectious process.

The physical examination may reveal infection or masses.

Diagnostic Tests: Laboratory testing should include:

- CBC.
- Elevated WBCs seen with infection.
- Culture and sensitivity of oral, nasal, or otalgic discharge: reveals responsible organism; guides antibiotic therapy.

If hoarseness is not clearly the result of a short-duration, self-limited process such as URI, then refer the patient for laryngoscopy. Laryngoscopy with or without biopsy is mandatory if hoarseness has persisted more than 2 weeks. Stroboscopy improves detection of small lesions: If the patient has vocal cord paralysis, CT scans from the skull base to the aortic arch, are needed, to assess compression of the vagus and/or laryngeal nerves.

Differential Diagnosis: The following should be considered when diagnosing hoarseness:

- Viral or bacterial laryngitis.
- Papillomatosis.
- Traumatic hoarseness.
- Compressed laryngeal nerves.
- Bilateral or unilateral vocal cord paralysis.
- Emotional or psychiatric disorders.

Treatment: Treat cause or refer as appropriate. Laryngeal papillomatosis, vocal polyps, and tumors require surgical removal. Smoking cessation, voice rest, and humidification may relieve symptoms of irritation.

Follow-up: See patient as indicated by cause of symptom, until problem resolves.

Sequelae: Possible complications depend on the cause of the hoarseness. Airway obstruction may occur if patient has inflammation and/or lesions.

Prevention/Prophylaxis: Prevention strategies depend on the cause of the symptom. Advise patients to maintain a healthy lifestyle and to avoid noxious inhalants, alcohol, and overuse of the voice.

Referral: Refer to or consult with appropriate specialist, as indicated by the cause of the symptom. Referral to a speech therapist may also be indicated.

Education: Explain causes of symptoms, measures taken to determine the cause, and any symptomatic treatment given. Advise patient when to seek medical care.

Involuntary Weight Loss

Involuntary weight loss is the process by which the number of calories available is less than the patient's daily needs. Recent, marked weight loss is a more ominous sign than gradual loss over an extended period of many months or years; the rapidity of weight loss is an important clue. Recent loss is usually defined as a substantial loss of 10 lb or more occurring over the past 3–6 months. In the older adult, a loss of at least 10% of body weight over 2 months is cause for concern.

Etiology: Involuntary weight loss can be classified into three groups:

- Inadequate nutrient intake.
- Excessive energy expenditure that occurs in catabolism.
- A combination of inadequate intake and excessive energy expenditure.

Organic causes of inadequate nutrient intake include alcoholism, mechanical causes such as poor dentition, and dysphagia. Psychogenic causes of unexplainable weight loss can be depression, anxiety, and/or a form of dementia. Patients who have hyperthyroidism, diabetes mellitus, pheochromocytoma, malignancy, or fever lose weight via excessive energy expenditure. For patients with neoplasms, infection, liver disease, renal disease, endocrine disorder, and GI disease, weight loss results from the anorexia that often occurs with these diseases and the excessive energy that is expended.

Occurrence: The occurrence of involuntary weight loss completely depends on the etiology and underlying disease. For example, in COPD, weight loss is as common as 71%. A high incidence of involuntary weight loss occurs with metastatic disease, alcoholism, dementia, depression, and acquired immunodeficiency syndrome (AIDS).

Age: No documented significance; however, age-related changes (e.g., in smell, taste, dentition) and chronic diseases more common in the elderly predispose this age group to weight loss. About one-half of Americans over age 65 have lost all their teeth.

Ethnicity: Not significant.

Gender: No documented significance; however, gender data are affected if the specific underlying disease causing the weight loss is more common in men or in women.

Contributing Factors: Pulmonary and cardiac diseases, cancer, dementia, alcoholism, depression, medications, GI tract dysmotility, sensory changes, decreased functional status, lack of transportation, financial problems, malnutrition, hyperthyroidism, chronic infection, dentition, smoking, family history of involuntary weight loss, and history of exposure to hepatitis have been known to contribute to involuntary weight loss.

Signs and Symptoms: Patients may report depression, poor dentition, dysphagia, alcohol and drug use, persistent localized pain, sore tongue, paresthesia, anorexia, nausea, vomiting, change in stools, and diarrhea. Patients with accelerated metabolism may describe episodes of fatigue, fever, melena, heat intolerance, polydipsia, polyphagia, and polyuria. On physical examination, patients appear pale, cachectic, with a malnourished appearance (hair loss, muscle wasting, loss of subcutaneous fat, especially around face). Look for evidence of loose skin, petechiae, cyanosis, clubbing of the fingers, and edema. There may be temporal wasting, icterus, dry mucous membranes, poor-fitting dentures, stomatitis, candidiasis, and flattened lingual papillae. Examination of the cardiorespiratory system may reveal loud or palpable murmurs and diminished breath sounds. Liver or spleen may be palpable. Check for masses in the abdomen, breasts, and rectum. Muscle wasting may be apparent on the extremities and deep tendon reflexes may have a prolonged relaxation phase. Patients may have diminished position and vibratory sense. Check women for ovarian masses, cervical lesions, and any obvious neoplasia. Examine men's prostate gland for enlargement.

Diagnostic Tests: Physical findings indicate most organic causes of weight loss and guide the choice of diagnostic tests. Standard tests include CBC with differential; electrolyte values; renal and liver function; serum levels of albumin, calcium, phosphorus, and glucose; ESR, TSH level; urinalysis; chest x-ray examination; and nutritional or diet history. Add human immunodeficiency virus (HIV) testing if indicated and a complete review of medications. In the absence of localized symptoms, routine cancer screening is indicated in certain patients. Consider a neoplastic origin when benign causes of weight loss appear unlikely: cancers of the lung, stomach, and pancreas; lymphoma; or leukemia (Fig. 17–4).

If the cause of weight loss is not clear from these results, watchful waiting is recommended; watch for further weight loss or specific symptoms and reconsider a functional cause of weight loss. If no abnormalities are detected from the standard tests, history, and physical examination, an organic cause is unlikely (less than 5%). When the findings from the initial workup are negative, psychological problems, particularly depression and anxiety, are among the most common reasons for weight loss.

Evidence of blood loss anemia on the CBC or one positive fecal occult blood result is reason to perform GI imaging. In general, imaging studies performed in the hope that they "will turn up something" are expensive, are as likely to yield false-positive results as true-positive results, and are overused for general screenings. These methods do have a higher diagnostic yield if directed at a specific organ, system, or region of the body.

For gradual weight loss, the workup can take as long as six months.

Differential Diagnosis: For weight loss that occurs with increased food intake, consider diabetes, thyrotoxicosis, malabsorption, leukemia, lymphoma, and adrenal insufficiency. For weight loss that occurs with normal or decreased food intake, consider alcoholism; malignancy; infection; gastrointestinal, hepatic, renal, dental, endocrine, respiratory, cardiac, or psychological etiology; anorexia nervosa; malnutrition; and functional origin.

Treatment: Watchful waiting is recommended if no organic cause is determined immediately. Otherwise, treat or manage the identified underlying cause.

Follow-up: If results of the standard tests listed earlier are negative, and the history and physical examination are negative, the recommended approach is to watch for further weight loss and to reconsider functional causes. Have patient or caregiver keep a daily record of food intake, activity levels and symptoms, and schedule return visit in 2–4 weeks.

Sequelae: Malnutrition is the first complication to consider in involuntary weight loss. Long-term unexplained weight loss may be indicative of failure to thrive.

Prevention/Prophylaxis: Discuss proper nutrition and the need for dental care, if appropriate.

Referral: Refer to a specialist for rapid or acute decline; for positive diagnostic test results indicating malignancy, thyrotoxicosis, or other acute organic illnesses requiring sophisticated diagnostic workup and/or management; or for a patient condition beyond your current scope of practice. Refer patients for assistance if social issues may be contributing to weight loss. Refer to appropriate specialist or perform additional assessments, to confirm patient's denial of problems (e.g., nutritional, psychologic, in-home, functional).

Education: Instruct patients about proper nutrition. Encourage exercise to improve strength or function. Teach patients about proper medication use and about signs or symptoms of overmedication or undermedication.

Joint Pain

Joint pain is discomfort or pain arising from one of the various joints in the body (neck, spine, shoulder, hand, wrist, distal interphalangeal, proximal interphalangeal, elbow, hip, knee, ankle, or metatarsophalangeal). Joint pain can arise from muscular, bone, or systemic disease.

Etiology The description, location, onset, and associated symptoms are critical to diagnosing the etiology of joint pain. The cause can be as varied as the type of pain the patient presents with. Narrowing down or clarifying the etiology of the pain depends on the clinical presentation, complete history, and findings from physical examination and appropriate diagnostic testing. The pain can be mild (from strained muscles or ligaments that support the joint), chronic (lasting more than 6 months, from degenerative joint disease [DJD] arthritis, osteoarthritis [OA]), inflammatory (from joint effusion, rheumatoid arthritis [RA]), or severe and acute (from fracture, cartilage injury, avascular septic necrosis). The following should be considered as causes of joint pain:

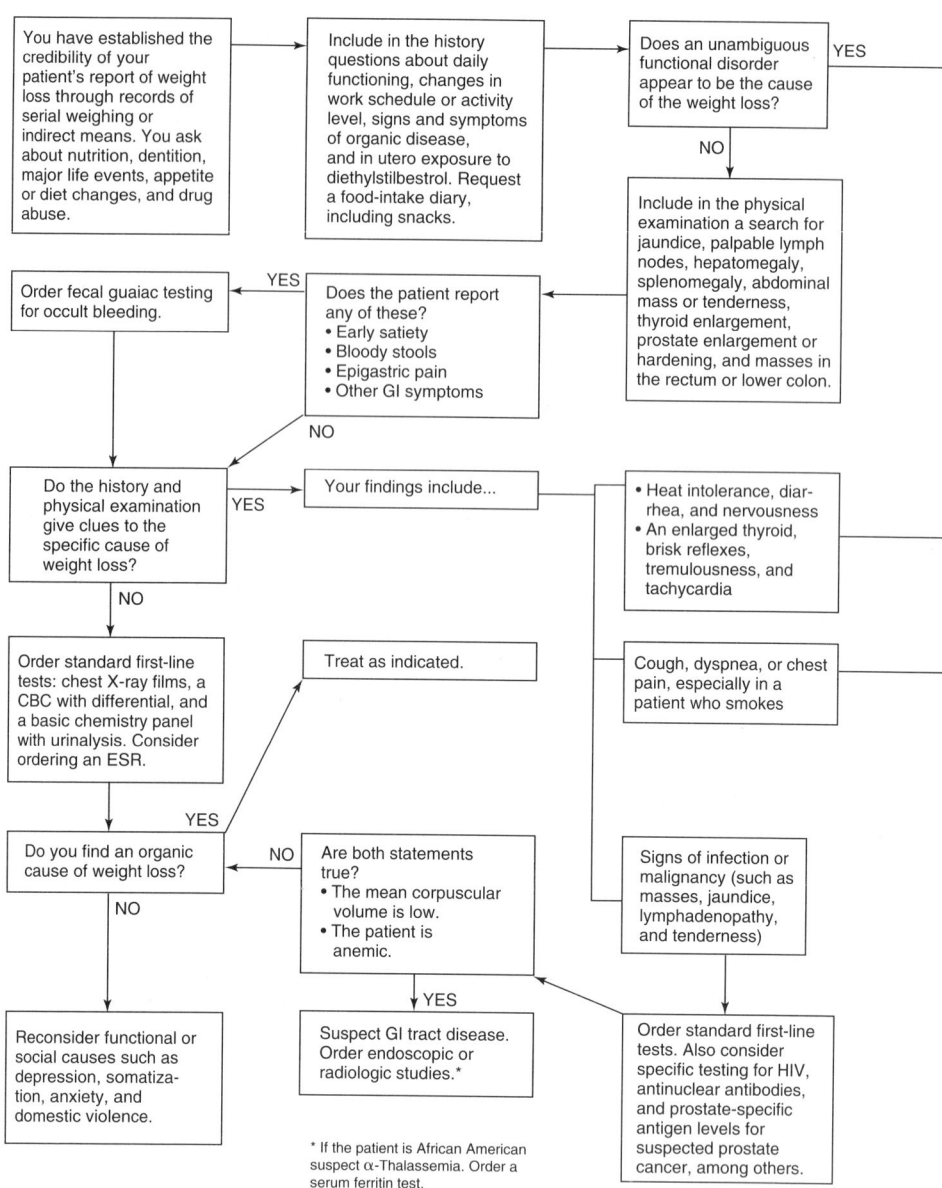

FIGURE 17–4 Involuntary weight loss.

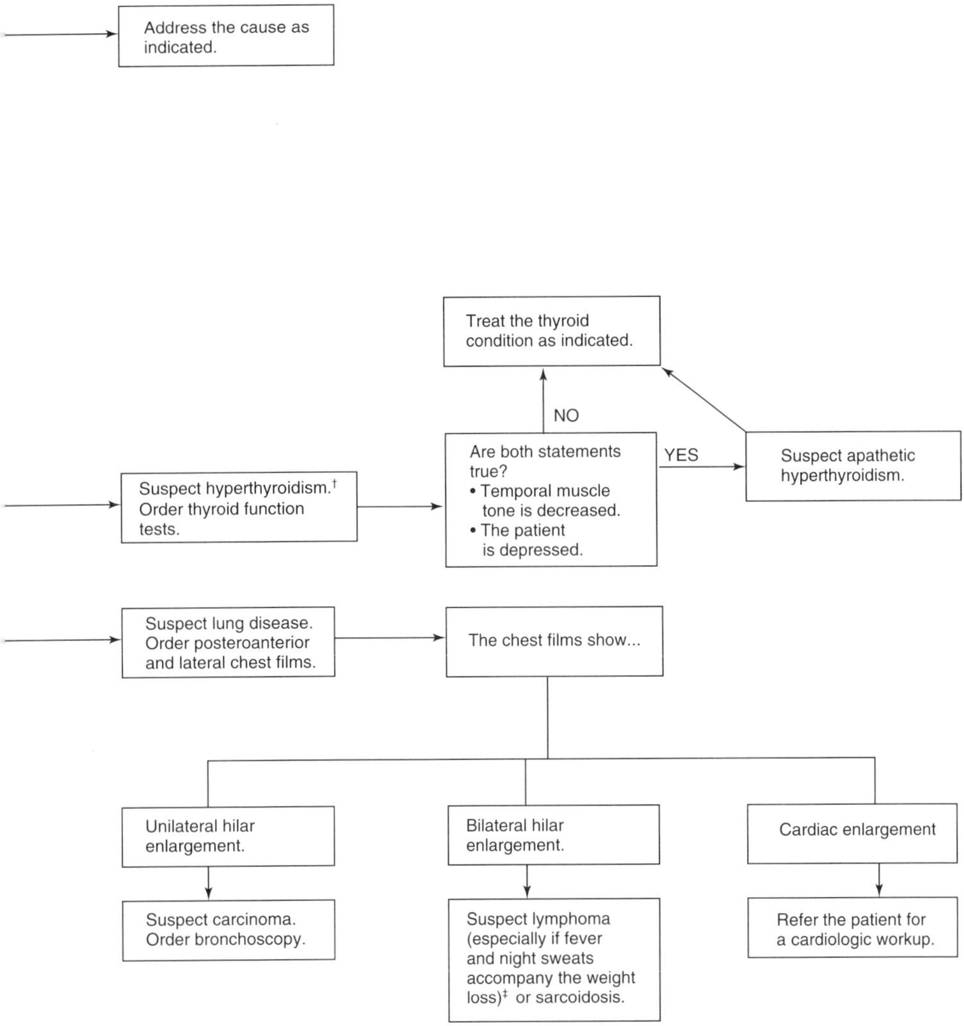

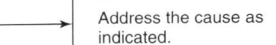

Address the cause as indicated.

Treat the thyroid condition as indicated.

NO

Are both statements true?
• Temporal muscle tone is decreased.
• The patient is depressed.

YES → Suspect apathetic hyperthyroidism.

Suspect hyperthyroidism.[†]
Order thyroid function tests.

Suspect lung disease. Order posteroanterior and lateral chest films.

The chest films show...

Unilateral hilar enlargement.

Bilateral hilar enlargement.

Cardiac enlargement

Suspect carcinoma. Order bronchoscopy.

Suspect lymphoma (especially if fever and night sweats accompany the weight loss)[‡] or sarcoidosis.

Refer the patient for a cardiologic workup.

† Hypothyroidism, often accompanied by depression, may also cause weight loss and requires similar testing.

‡ Fever and night sweats may also signal tuberculosis (TB). If chest films suggest TB, arrange for tuberculin purified protein derivative (Mantoux) testing.

Chronic infection (TB, fungal).

Gout.

Arthritis (OA, RA, gonococcal, septic).

Bursitis.

Tendinitis.

Ankylosing spondylitis.

Fracture (stress or traumatic).

Peripheral entrapment syndromes (carpal tunnel, thoracic outlet).

Neuropathies.

DJD.

Disc problems.

Systemic causes (systemic lupus erythematosus [SLE], sarcoidosis, Lyme disease, hemophilia, Raynaud's disease, Paget's disease, hemochromatosis).

If the patient presents with an atypical case of joint pain, systemic disease may be the underlying cause.

Occurrence: Joint pain is a common complaint among elderly patients.

Age: No age is specified; however, joint pain is found more frequently in the elderly patient as a result of age-related muscle atrophy, demineralization of trabecular bone, atrophy of cortical bone, chronic disease, and loss of bone density.

Ethnicity: No documentation is found specifically for joint pain; however, the prevalence of certain types of inflammatory joint disease and systemic disorders is higher in various ethnic groups.

Gender: Joint pain occurs equally in males and females.

Contributing Factors: Factors that may lead to joint pain include overuse or strain, previous injury or trauma to the joint, alterations in gait or balance, past surgery or joint replacement, known history of arthritis or joint disease and postmenopausal women with no hormonal replacement therapy. Weight, physical stature, smoking and family history should be assessed in reviewing the risk factors for osteoporosis. Other contributing factors include obesity, poor nutritional habits, low calcium intake, alcohol consumption, medications, and exercise habits. Note any balance or gait disorders, as well as the use of any equipment for ambulation.

Signs and Symptoms: The inability to maintain normal physical activity or alteration in mobility because of pain in a joint often leads patients to seek medical care for this complaint. Joint pain may be the presenting sign in joint, bone, muscle, or systemic disease. A complete medical history and physical examination are necessary. Symptoms associated with joint pain may include general weakness, stiffness, decreased range of motion, and inflammation.

The history should include the onset of the pain (sudden, insidious); character of the pain (dull sharp); and the pain's duration and location (including radiation). Inquire about any associated symptoms, any alleviating or aggravating factors, and timing (e.g., worse in morning, better late in the day). Discuss normal activity levels and the possibility of overuse or strain. Has there been any old or recent trauma to the joint? If there was an injury, did the patient hear any popping or clicking? Discuss the limitation in joint mobility, and note the presence of any edema, redness, or fever. Review if there is any associated muscle fatigue, joint deformity, or inability to perform certain movements.

The physical examination includes a complete assessment of the patient, paying specific attention to any joint pain complaints. Inspect, palpate, and percuss (if needed) each joint, and assess the appropriate range of motion, noting any pain or limitations in movement. Note the patient's gait, balance, and posture. Inspect each joint, noting the musculature, any atrophy, contractures, nodules (Heberden's or Bouchard's nodes), asymmetry, or gross deformity. Note any erythema, inflammation, or soft tissue swelling on or near the joint. Palpate for any tenderness on or around the joint. Palpate any areas of effusion. Assess for any lymphadenopathy. Check for crepitus, clicking, or popping in or around the joint.

Diagnostic Tests: This depends on the suspected or differential diagnosis. Problem-specific complaints and physical examination findings dictate which tests are required. A CBC with differential is needed to rule out infection (elevated WBCs). Normocytic, normochromia anemia is seen with RA. ESR helps determine inflammatory disease (normal values depending on the method and laboratory parameters). An elevated ESR is seen in persons with collagen vascular disease, infection, inflammatory disease, and RA. Marked elevations in alkaline phosphatase level (20–90 IU/L) are seen in those with bone disease (e.g., Paget's disease, metastatic bone disease). Hypercalcemia with marked alkaline phosphatase is seen in patients with hyperparathyroidism or carcinoma of the bone. Serum creatine kinase (CK) isoenzymes are elevated in persons with muscle trauma and progressive muscular disease.

Obtain a complete electrolyte panel and urinalysis, checking BUN and creatinine, to assess renal function. Many causes of joint pain are treated with NSAIDs, which can potentially alter renal function. Because kidney function decreases with aging, routine testing is necessary. Other, more problem-specific, tests include:

Hepatitis B profile with liver function tests (patients with recent infection can present with arthritic joint pain).

Uric acid levels in patients with suspected gout.

Antinuclear antibody (ANA) testing, results positive in those with SLE and in 25% of persons with RA.

RA latex fixation test revealing high titers with severe joint disease.

Rheumatoid factor, which may or may not be present with RA, but is elevated in chronic infection, TB, and sarcoidosis.

X-ray examination of the joint can be useful to detect any fracture, joint space destruction or narrowing, erosion, arthritic changes, and degeneration.

Joint effusions may require aspiration and culture of the aspirate to assess for sepsis. Further evaluation with CT scans or MRI may also be necessary.

Differential Diagnosis: The disease processes associated with joint pain are considered in the differential diagnosis. Some others to rule out include psoriatic arthritis, connective tissue disease, Reiter's disease, multiple myeloma, and scleroderma.

Treatment: Medical management of joint pain depends on the findings of the comprehensive assessment. The goal to decrease pain may include physical therapy, analgesic and anti-inflammatory medications, moist heat, intra-articular steroid injections, assistive devices, and/or surgery. Emergency intervention is required if you suspect a fracture, avascular necrosis, or sepsis.

Follow-up: Monitoring of patients depends on findings. Patients with acute or severe joint pain may need emergency care and intervention. Monitor patients with chronic pain frequently until the clinical workup is completed. Management of chronic joint pain or disease requires routine visits to monitor medications and laboratory and diagnostic test results.

Sequelae: The condition and prognosis relates to the etiology of the joint pain.

Prevention/Prophylaxis: Prevention methods depend on the etiology of the joint pain. When applicable, use weight reduction to decrease stress on the joint, physical therapy and exercise for strengthening; moist heat, topical medications, and steroid injections to reduce pain and spasms. Explore alternative methods of pain control (accupuncture, yoga, medication, or massage therapy). Address fall prevention for patients using assistive devices (canes, crutches, or walkers). Instruct the patient concerning joint protection and preservation. Discuss proper nutrition, calcium supplements, and smoking cessation.

Referral: Refer patients to a specialist pending the results of the workup. Refer patients to the appropriate emergency service if you suspect sepsis, fracture, or avascular necrosis.

Education: Teach patients about the appropriate dose of medications and the potential side effects that need to be reported. Instruct patients about appropriate follow-up and referrals. Tell the patient to report any persisting or worsening joint pain as well as any systemic involvement. Instruct patients on the appropriate methods for pain control. Review the use of any adaptive equipment.

Nausea and Vomiting

Nausea is a subjective, unpleasant sensation that usually precedes vomiting and is often accompanied by increased parasympathetic activity such as pallor, diaphoresis, salivation, and other vasovagal signs such as hypotension and bradycardia.

Vomiting is a reflex causing the forceful ejection, as opposed to passive reflux, of gastric contents. Nausea and vomiting often occur together.

Etiology: Nausea is caused by alterations in the motility of the stomach and small intestine. The vomiting reflex involves visceral and somatic components, and is integrated in the vomiting center and the chemoreceptor trigger zone (CTZ) of the medulla oblongata. The vomiting reflex begins in the stimulation of receptor sites in the mucosa of the upper GI tract, the labyrinth apparatus (inner ear), higher cortical centers (such as emotional stimuli), or the CTZ (dopamine receptors), which is stimulated by specific mediators in the blood. The afferent nerves carry the impulses to the vomiting center, then the efferent pathways (including the phrenic nerves to the diaphragm, spinal nerves to the abdominal musculature, and visceral nerves to the stomach and esophagus) carry the impulses to the effector muscles, resulting in relaxation of the gastric fundus and gastroesophageal sphincter, contraction of the gastric pylorus, and reverse peristalsis in the esophagus. The glottis closes, preventing aspiration and increasing intrathoracic pressure; the abdominal wall muscles and the diaphragm contract, causing an increase in intra-abdominal pressure, resulting in the forcing of the stomach contents through the mouth.

Occurrence: Nausea and vomiting are common.

Age: Nausea and vomiting occurs at all ages.

Ethnicity: Not significant.

Gender: Nausea and vomiting occur more often in women than in men, primarily because of female hormonal fluctuations.

Contributing Factors: The following can contribute to the development of nausea and vomiting:

Structural malformations such as hiatal hernia.
GI disorders such as gastroenteritis or obstruction.
Abdominal surgery.
Central nervous system (CNS) disorders and dysfunction such as migraine headache or tumor.
Pancreatic and biliary disturbances.
Underlying chronic conditions such as diabetes, heart disease, or renal insufficiency.
Vestibular disturbances.
Psychological disorders.
Sight or odor of noxious and/or emotionally upsetting stimuli.
Hormone imbalances and pregnancy.
Motion sickness.
Toxins.
Drug ingestion.
Fever and infection.

Signs and Symptoms: Obtain information about the timing, frequency, and duration of the nausea and/or vomiting. A 1–2 day history of nausea and vomiting in an otherwise healthy patient suggests acute gastroenteritis, which is usually self-limiting. Nausea and vomiting in the morning is often associated with pregnancy, uremia, and alcoholic gastritis. If nausea and vomiting occur shortly after eating, suspect pylorospasm, gastritis, or a psychogenic cause. Vomiting 4–6 hours after eating and composed of undigested food suggests gastric distention.

If the patient complains of vomiting without nausea and muscular contraction of the diaphragm and/or abdominal wall, suspect hiatal hernia or GERD. Projectile vomiting without nausea is an ominous symptom suggesting a CNS disturbance such as a lesion. Blood in the vomitus warrants further assessment, as the cause may be minor (e.g., swallowed blood from a nose bleed) or major (e.g., GI bleeding). A putrid odor associated with the vomitus occurs with lower intestinal obstruction or gastrocolic fistula. Bile will be present from prolonged vomiting of any cause.

The physical exam should identify patients with dry mucous membranes, orthostatic hypotension, weight loss, excessive thirst, and decreased urination; these patients may be dehydrated. The presence of jaundice suggests hepatitis or cholestasis. Abdominal distention suggests ileus, obstruction, or ascites. The absence of bowel sounds suggests ielus; high-pitched, tinkling sounds suggest intestinal obstruction; hyperactive bowel sounds may indicate acute gastroenteritis. If the patient has tenderness with guarding (muscular rigidity) and/or rebound tenderness, suspect peritoneal or visceral inflammation. The location of these signs may help pinpoint the underlying cause of the nausea and vomiting. A neurologic, cardiovascular, or pelvic examination may also be indicated by patient history and complaint.

Diagnostic Tests: To determine the cause, tests that may be performed include:

- Urine for specific gravity (increased specific gravity may indicate dehydration; WBCs may indicate infection such as pyelonephritis).
- Serum or urine pregnancy test or human chorionic gonadotropin (hCG) level (to detect pregnancy).
- Liver function tests (screen for hepatitis, cholestasis, or other hepatic involvement).
- BUN level for renal impairment.
- Creatinine level (to screen for dehydration and underlying renal disease); glucose and electrolytes (to rule out diabetic ketoacidosis and/or diabetic gastroparesis; to evaluate degree of dehydration).
- CBC (WBCs may be elevated in acute infections and appendicitis).
- Drug levels and/or screens (to check for toxicity and presence of drugs).
- Abdominal flat plate and upright x-ray examinations (to diagnose obstruction or ileus).
- Upper GI series or endoscopy (to diagnose gastritis or peptic ulcer).

- Abdominal ultrasound (to help diagnose cholelithiasis).
- ECG (to rule out myocardial infarction and other cardiac problems).

Differential Diagnosis: Self-limiting nausea and vomiting should be differentiated from acute (serious) nausea and vomiting.

Treatment: Projectile vomiting may indicate a CNS problem; evaluate and/or refer these patients immediately. Treat cause or refer as appropriate.

General measures include having the patient follow a clear-liquid diet to replace fluids and electrolytes and to prevent dehydration when the acute episode has subsided. During the acute episode, encourage small sips of clear fluids and/or ice chips. Examples of recommended liquids include Gatorade (or other sports or electrolyte-replacement drink), tea, clear broth, and clear caffeine-free carbonated beverages such as ginger ale. After the nausea and vomiting has decreased for 12 hours, advise the patient to try foods such as salted crackers or dry toast, then gradually to add foods such as rice, baked potato, and chicken soup with noodles. Continue to add foods to the diet as tolerated, gradually returning to a full normal diet. Patients must avoid caffeine-containing foods and fluids, alcohol, dairy products, most fruits and vegetables, red meats, and spicy and/or heavily seasoned foods until they have fully recovered. Have all patients rest as much as possible; provide reassurance.

Pharmacologic

Adjusting the timing, dosage, and/or preparation of medications may help relieve nausea and/or vomiting associated with medication use. Antiemetic medications may provide symptomatic relief; many have combined anticholinergic, antihistamine, and/or CNS-depressant actions and should be used judiciously in elderly patients. Examples include metoclopramide (for diabetic gastroparesis or postoperatively) 5 mg PO 30 minutes before meals and at bedtime for 2–8 weeks, increasing to 10 mg qid only if the initial dosage brings no response; and antihistamines such as dimenhydrinate or hydroxyzine (for motion sickness, postoperative nausea, or drug-induced nausea).

Follow-up: See the patient for follow-up as indicated by the cause of the symptom(s). See the patient in 3 days to assess whether or not nausea and vomiting have stopped and/or for reevaluation.

Sequelae: Possible complications depend on the cause of the symptom(s) and may include dehydration, metabolic acidosis, electrolyte imbalances, aspiration, and aspiration pneumonia.

Prevention/Prophylaxis: Prevention strategies depend on the cause of the symptom(s). Advise patient of dietary precautions such as:

- Avoiding fatty or spicy foods.
- Proper handling of food.
- Proper handwashing techniques.
- Precautions for traveling outside of the United States.

Monitor and prevent dehydration during acute episode.

Referral: Refer patients to, or consult with, specialist appropriate for the cause of the symptom(s).

Education: Explain causes of symptoms, measures taken to determine the cause, and symptomatic treatment if any. Advise patient when to seek medical care.

Peripheral Edema

Peripheral edema is an increase in the interstitial fluid component as a result of an expansion of the extracellular fluid volume. When an accumulation of lymph in the extremities causes an increase in hydrostatic pressure, the term "lymphedema" is used.

Etiology: Normally the distribution of water between the blood and interstitial tissues is maintained by an equilibrium. Remembering Starling's concept that the osmotic pressure of the plasma proteins balances the hydrostatic pressure in the capillaries helps in the understanding of fluid dynamics. Fluid flows from the vessels to the interstitial area in response to intravascular hydrostatic pressure and the colloid osmotic pressure of the interstitial fluid. In the opposite direction fluid enters the blood because of the interstitial tissue tension and the oncotic pressure of the plasma proteins. Interstitial fluid is also returned to the blood as lymph. Under steady-state conditions, net fluid flux out of the capillary is balanced by lymph flow back into circulation. Alteration in any of these components upsets the equilibrium and leg edema occurs. Two basic steps occur in edema formation: sodium and water are retained, and capillary hemodynamics are altered.

Leg edema, common in elderly persons, often has diverse etiologies (Table 17–11). In a study of elderly patients with leg edema, the most common causes were venous insufficiency (63.2%), congestive heart failure (15.1%), drug-induced edema (13.8%), and other conditions (11.1%) including lymphedema, ovarian and prostate cancers, and postphlebitic syndrome (Ciocon, 1995).

Occurrence: The frequency of occurrence completely depends on the underlying etiology and combined etiologies.

Age: Peripheral edema occurs frequently in older adults.

Ethnicity: Not significant.

Gender: No documented significance is found, but gender statistics vary according to the specific etiology (e.g., idiopathic edema is more common in woman, heart failure edema more common in men).

Contributing Factors: Physiologic age-related changes increase the vulnerability to fluid retention. The older individual has a smaller amount of total body water overall (80% of body weight for a newborn; 60% for a young adult; 50% for

TABLE 17–11 CAUSES OF LEG EDEMA

Bilateral	Unilateral
Cardiovascular disease (heart failure, pulmonary hypertension, valvular disease, chronic venous insufficiency)	Impaired lymphatic flow
	Venous obstruction
	Inflammation
Renal insufficiency	Infection
Hyperthyroidism, hypothyroidism	Tumor
Liver disease	Trauma
Obesity	Compartment syndrome
Adverse drug reaction	Ruptured cyst, tendon, or muscle
Sodium-retaining drug	Reflex sympathetic dystrophy
Hypoproteinemia	
Allergic	
Idiopathic edema	

an older adult). As more intercellular fluid is lost over time, extracellular fluid volume starts to comprise the greater composition. Risk factors for leg edema from age-related changes include a decrease in:

Serum albumin.
Glomerular filtration rate (GFR).
Hepatic blood flow.
Sodium concentrating ability of the kidney.
Myocardial contractility and cardiac output.
Baroreceptor sensitivity.

Additional contributing factors include dependent positioning of the lower extremities, excessive intake of sodium, hot weather, and use of medicines that contribute to sodium retention.

Signs and Symptoms: The patient may complain of fullness, discomfort, aching pain, shoes that are too tight, or weight gain. The history should elicit the seven dimensions of the signs and symptoms of edema, emphasizing location (unilateral or bilateral) and chronologic evolution (acute or chronic progression). The presence or absence of pain is helpful in determining the differential diagnosis.

The physical examination begins with weight. Assess skin changes, including lesions, discoloration, texture, and induration. Evaluate the venous and arterial circulation, checking pulses throughout, capillary refill, and dependent rubor. Varicose veins are usually readily apparent with the inspection of the legs while the patient stands.

Assess the extremity for local or diffuse tenderness and for pitting or nonpitting edema. Measure and compare the circumference bilaterally at a designated point (e.g., patella, calf, mid-calf). Assess any localized enlargement.

Examine body systems indicated by the history (e.g., cardiac, renal, endocrine, pulmonary).

Diagnostic Tests: Diagnostic tests depend on the probable etiology of leg edema. Cardiac etiologies may warrant a chest x-ray examination, ECG, or echocardiogram. Thyroid panel evaluates TSH and free thyroxine (T_4). CBC with differential, serum protein albumin level, and electrolyte values should be obtained. Renal and liver panels are generally usually done as part of an automated chemistry test. Additional studies may include ultrasound, venogram, venous Doppler studies, and lymphangiography. CT scans for pelvic masses and lymphoma may be indicated.

Differential Diagnosis: Leg edema is an important clinical sign, and its causes are diverse. The difference is facilitated in part by noting if edema is unilateral or bilateral (see Table 17–11).

Treatment: Always direct treatment at the cause of leg edema: diuretics for heart failure, a high-protein diet for hypoalbuminemia, angiotensin-converting enzyme (ACE) inhibitors for proteinurea, and thrombolytics for acute deep venous thrombosis.

Follow-Up: Closely monitor patients for effectiveness of therapy and adverse events. Monitor the weight and limb circumference measurements.

Sequelae: When administering diuretics the health-care professional must be alert to potential volume depletion (such as dizziness and metabolic abnormalities). Patients with edema as a result of deep venous insufficiency are prone to recurrent ulceration.

Prevention/Prophylaxis: With recurrent lymphangitis and cellulitis, prescribe intermittent long-term antibiotic prophylaxis. For those with leg swelling secondary to deep venous thrombosis, thrombolytics may limit the tissue loss, pulmonary embolus, and more extensive thrombosis of the deep venous system.

Referral: Regardless of the cause of leg swelling, you can achieve the best fluid removal while the patient is hospitalized. This is particularly true when the process is an acute one such as deep venous thrombophlebitis or cellulitis. When thrombolytic therapy is indicated, consult a vascular specialist.

Education: Patients need specific information related to the edema and the management of symptoms. Typically the patient with edema is instructed to avoid highly salted foods. If compression stockings are recommended, emphasize the importance of proper application technique to avoid excessive pressure. Instruct patients to elevate the legs to decrease peripheral vascular pressure. Periodic active muscle contraction exercises are important for those persons who must sit for long periods. Teach patients with peripheral vascular disorders to avoid excessive heat and to reduce weight if indicated. Special care of the skin, including proper shoes and prevention of trauma, is important.

Syncope

Syncope is defined as a transient loss of consciousness and postural tone.

Etiologies: In most instances the loss of consciousness reflects a transient decrease in cerebral blood flow that is usually secondary to a fall in the systemic arterial blood pressure. Interruption of cerebral blood flow for 8–10 seconds or less than 30 mL of blood flow/100 g of brain tissue per minute results in syncope. Most etiologies of syncope can be separated into cardiovascular and noncardiovascular causes (see table under differential diagnosis).

Occurrence: The Framingham study showed that 3% of men and 3.5% of women had experienced at least one syncopal episode. Syncope accounts for about 3% of all emergency department visits and 6% of all hospital admissions.

Age: Syncope occurs annually in 6% of individuals age 65 and older, with a recurrence rate of 17%–63% in this age group. Some forms of syncope (i.e., vasovagal, carotid sinus hypersensitivity) are more common in younger persons than in older persons; other forms of syncope (i.e., cardiac, orthostatic, micturation-related) occur more often in older than in younger individuals.

Ethnicity: Not significant.

Gender: Among younger adults, women have nearly twice the rate of syncope as men; but among elderly adults, men have the greater incidence. This likely reflects the most common etiologies in the different age groups.

Contributing Factors: Cerebral blood flow has been reported to decline as much as 25% with physiologic aging. Hormonal regulation of extracellular volume may become impaired with age. Cardiac reflexes and baroreceptor sensitivity may also become impaired. The kidneys' ability to conserve sodium and water declines. Hypertension, diabetes, and alcoholic peripheral neuropathy are predisposing diseases. Diuretic-induced volume depletion and electrolyte imbalances cause a reduction in systolic blood pressure in response to postural stress. Alcohol is a contributing factor in vasovagal syncope. An emotional response can cause a neurally mediated syncope in susceptible individuals in stressful circumstances. Situational syncope can occur with micturation, defecation, or cough or after meals.

Signs and Symptoms: Because the patient may not be able to recall the event precisely, gather corroborating historic information from others. Obtain the patient's description of symptoms preceding the event and of activities that may have precipitated the event. Cardiac-related syncope may be sudden and without warning. A brief prodrome of symptoms such as nausea, pallor, or diaphoresis may suggest a vasovagal episode. Determine if any focal neurologic symptoms were present (i.e., dysphagia, diplopia, motor and sensory symptoms). Review significant past medical history, all medications being used, and alcohol intake. The history is very important in distinguishing actual syncope from dizziness, vertigo, seizure, pseudovertigo, and disequilibrium.

Focus the physical examination on the cardiovascular and neurologic components. Check blood pressure in both arms and positionally. Determine the compensatory pulse rate. Check the carotids for bruits. Examine the heart, assessing for signs of arrhythmia, vascular disease, and left ventricular dysfunction. Perform a thorough neurologic examination, paying particular attention to focal abnormalities that may suggest neurologic syncope. Generalized anxiety disorders can cause hyperventilation and trigger a vasodepressor reaction; this should be evaluated during the physical examination.

Diagnostic Tests: An ECG is indicated in all patients with syncope looking for rhythm disturbance, QRS pathology, and structural heart disease. Additional cardiac diagnostics may include echocardiogram, ambulatory ECG monitoring, and electrophysiological studies. Carotid sinus compression is sometimes used to provoke symptoms, but this should be done cautiously and selectively. A chest x-ray which may reveal cardiomyopathy, is indicated in patients with new abnormal findings, dyspnea, and those without a recorded baseline.

Tilt table testing is useful in patients with syncope of unknown etiology or those with recurrent syncope. Vasovagal syncope may be induced with this procedure; this may be done with or without isoproterenol. Laboratory evaluation should include a CBC with differential, creatinine, and BUN. Electrolytes may also be indicated.

Differential Diagnosis: Once a true syncopal event has been determined, the differential is primarily cardiac and noncardiac etiologies (Table 17–12).

Treatment: Once you identify the specific cause of syncope, you can initiate the appropriate treatment. This may include beta-adrenergic blockade, scopolamine, or theophylline for vasovagal syncope. Antiarrhythmic therapy is initiated, if indicated, and drug-induced or idiopathic orthostatic hypotension treated appropriately. Cardiac surgery is the treatment of choice for obstructive heart

TABLE 17–12 DIFFERENTIAL DIAGNOSIS: SYNCOPE IN OLDER ADULTS

Cardiovascular	Noncardiovascular
Dysrhythmias	Hypoxemia
Carotid sinus hypersensitivity	Vasovagal attack
Aortic stenosis	Vagal glossopharyngeal neuralgia
Aortic arch syndrome	Situational syncope (micturation, cough,
Orthostatic hypertension	postprandial defecation)
Transient ischemic attacks	
Aortic dissection	
Myocardial infarction	
Pulmonary embolism	

disease. Always correct underlying anemia and metabolic imbalance and optimize cardiac and pulmonary status in the elderly patient.

Follow-up: Unknown causes precipitate a high incidence (38%–47%) of syncopal events. Although the syncope may be isolated, in up to one-third of patients it is a recurring event. Because recurrences may reflect lack of effective therapy or a failure to diagnose correctly, close monitoring is indicated.

Sequelae: Morbidity from syncope varies from 5%–53% in elderly patients. Syncope from cardiovascular causes tends to be more dangerous, having a 1-year mortality of 20%–30% compared with 5% for noncardiovascular or unknown causes. Sudden death with syncope has been attributed to arrhythmia. Patients with syncope are at risk for fall-related injury (fracture, subdural) and reduced functional capacity.

Prevention/Prophylaxis: Patients with vasovagal syncope are taught to avoid triggers and, if premonitory symptoms occur, to lie down immediately and elevate the feet higher than the chest. Adequate fluid intake is a precaution, and for selected individuals with vasovagal syncope a higher salt intake may be advised. Support hose may help prevent reduction in central plasma volume. Patients are encouraged to avoid a sudden change in position. For syncope caused by atrial fibrillation, low-dose warfarin or aspirin therapy may be prescribed.

Referral: Hospitalization is necessary for patients in whom you suspect an arrhythmia or myocardial infarction as the cause of the syncope and for those who sustain significant injury during the syncopal event. Consultation with a cardiologist may be appropriate for managing cardiac syncope, and with a neurologist for neurally mediated syncope.

Education: In addition to teaching preventive strategies, teach individuals with recurrent syncope safety precautions related to driving or the use of dangerous machinery.

Tremor

Tremor is an involuntary movement characterized by rhythmic oscillation of a body part.

Etiology: Tremor results from regular oscillatory contractions of agonistic and antagonistic muscles. It may be associated with overactivity of a common circuit involving cerebellothalamic connections.

    Action tremor, a fine tremor, is present when the limbs and trunk are held in certain positions or engaged in active movements; this type of tremor may be classified as physiologic, essential, primary writing, and rubral. *Physiologic* tremor is aggravated by stress, endocrine disorders (hyperthyroidism, hypoglycemia, and pheochromocytoma), or drugs (such as lithium, tricyclics, phenothiazines, epinephrine, theophylline, amphetamines, thyroid hormones, isoproterenol, corticosteroids, valproate, levodopa, and butyrophenones) toxins (such as mercury, lead, arsenic, bismuth, and carbon monoxide), and dietary factors (e.g., caffeine and monosodium glutamate intake and ethanol withdrawal). *Essential* tremor may be familial (autosomal dominant inheritant), sporadic, or associated with other movement disorders (Parkinson's disease, torsion dystonia, or torticollis). *Primary writing* tremor is a form of dystonia that occurs only during writing. *Rubral* tremor, a coarse tremor that may be present at rest, increases with postural maintenance and movement and may indicate an ipsilateral cerebellar outflow lesion.

Intention tremor, a tremor that increases with precise movements, may be caused by lesions of cerebellar pathways, cerebellar degeneration, Wilson's disease, and drugs or toxins (such as phenytoin, barbiturates, lithium, ethanol, mercury, and fluorouracil). Neuropathologic studies of autopsy cases have found no significant pathology of essential tremor. However, results using positron emission tomography (PET) scanning show alteration of glucose metabolism in the thalamus and inferior olives of patients with essential tremor.

Rest tremor, a tremor present at rest that often disappears with movement, is associated with lesions in the extrapyramidal pathways (as found in Parkinson's and cerebellar diseases). Rest tremor originates in the basal ganglia or cerebellum areas, which influence lower motor neurons responsible for coordinated muscle control.

Occurrence: Everyone has a very low amplitude physiologic tremor that can be observed when the arms are extended. Present in all muscle groups, it persists throughout the waking state. Estimates suggest that 3–4 million people in the United States have an essential tremor; in 50% of cases the disease is familial (autosomal dominant, meaning 50% of an affected individual's children have it). The incidence of familial tremor is estimated at 415 in 100,000.

Age: Occasionally familial tremor may begin in childhood; however, the mean age of onset is age 45. Essential tremor begins in young to middle-aged people and gradually intensifies with age. Most studies report a significant age-associated increase in the prevalence of essential tremor. Aging is also associated with a decrease in rate of the tremor and an increase in amplitude.

Ethnicity: Tremor is more prevalent in whites than in blacks and is of intermediate prevalence in Hispanics.

Gender: Tremor afflicts both genders nearly equally, with slightly more frequency in men than in women.

Contributing Factors: During times of stress, the amplitude of a physiologic tremor increases. Fatigue, anxiety, hyperthyroidism, systemic illness, use of medications, drug withdrawal (especially from alcohol), use of methylxanthines, and excess caffeine intake exaggerate this symptom. Alcohol in small quantities often decreases an essential tremor.

Anxiety and stress accentuate the tremor; frequently the symptoms are reported as being worse in public situations.

Signs and Symptoms: History of the onset and duration of the tremor, including posture, behavioral context, motor performance and body part(s) involved, aids in categorizing the symptom. Tremor is assessed clinically on the basis of distribution, amplitude, posture, and motor performances that elicit it. History, physical examination with attention to neurologic and musculoskeletal systems, and observation of gait are required for diagnosis. The history may include trembling, nervousness, jitters, twitching, anxiety, tenseness, spasms, inability to relax, achiness, shakes, and fatigue in an extremity. In some cases, a family member or friend first observes the tremor, becoming noticeable to the patient later. Tremor may occur in various body parts such as the hands, head, facial structures (chin, tongue, lips, and ears), vocal cords, trunk, and legs. Ninety-four percent of all tremors occur in the hands, either unilaterally or bilaterally.

In evaluation of tremor, first establish if the tremor is present at rest or with action.

Physiologic tremor occurs normally when attempting to maintain a posture, such as holding hands extended or standing still, and can increase and become symptomatic under circumstances involving stress, exercise, and drugs. The frequency decreases with age, especially after the fifth decade. Test for a postural tremor by having the patient hold the arms stretched out in front. Placing a sheet of paper over the outstretched hands may enhance the tremor further. Essential or familial tremor may be limited to the upper limbs or a side-to-side nodding movement of the head. Tremor of the head may precede tremor of the hands, but more often head tremor follows hand tremor. Head tremor, which is also postural, disappears when the head is supported. Listening to the patient speak or having the patient hold a note as long as possible may reveal a quivering intonation.

Action and intention tremors both occur during purposeful movement. Carrying a cup of liquid, pouring liquids, or eating with a spoon often brings out the tremor. Writing may be tremulous and sloppy. The individual may report giving up tasks or using the lesser-affected hand for tasks. Action or intention tremor is tested by the finger-to-nose maneuver or heel-to-shin testing.

Orthostatic tremor, a tremor of the legs, is present only during standing, decreasing or disappearing with walking, sitting, or reclining. This tremor can be evoked by strong contraction of the leg muscles against resistance. Also, have patient stand with feet together and observe for rapid rhythmic contractions of leg muscles that cause the kneecaps to bob up and down (Fig. 17–5).

Patients with hysterical tremor, a possible symptom of conversion disorder, may present with a complex combination of resting, postural, and kinetic tremors. History reveals an abrupt onset with variable course, absence of other neurologic symptoms, selective ability to perform some functions with severe tremors and unusual handwriting. Restraining the affected limb may induce

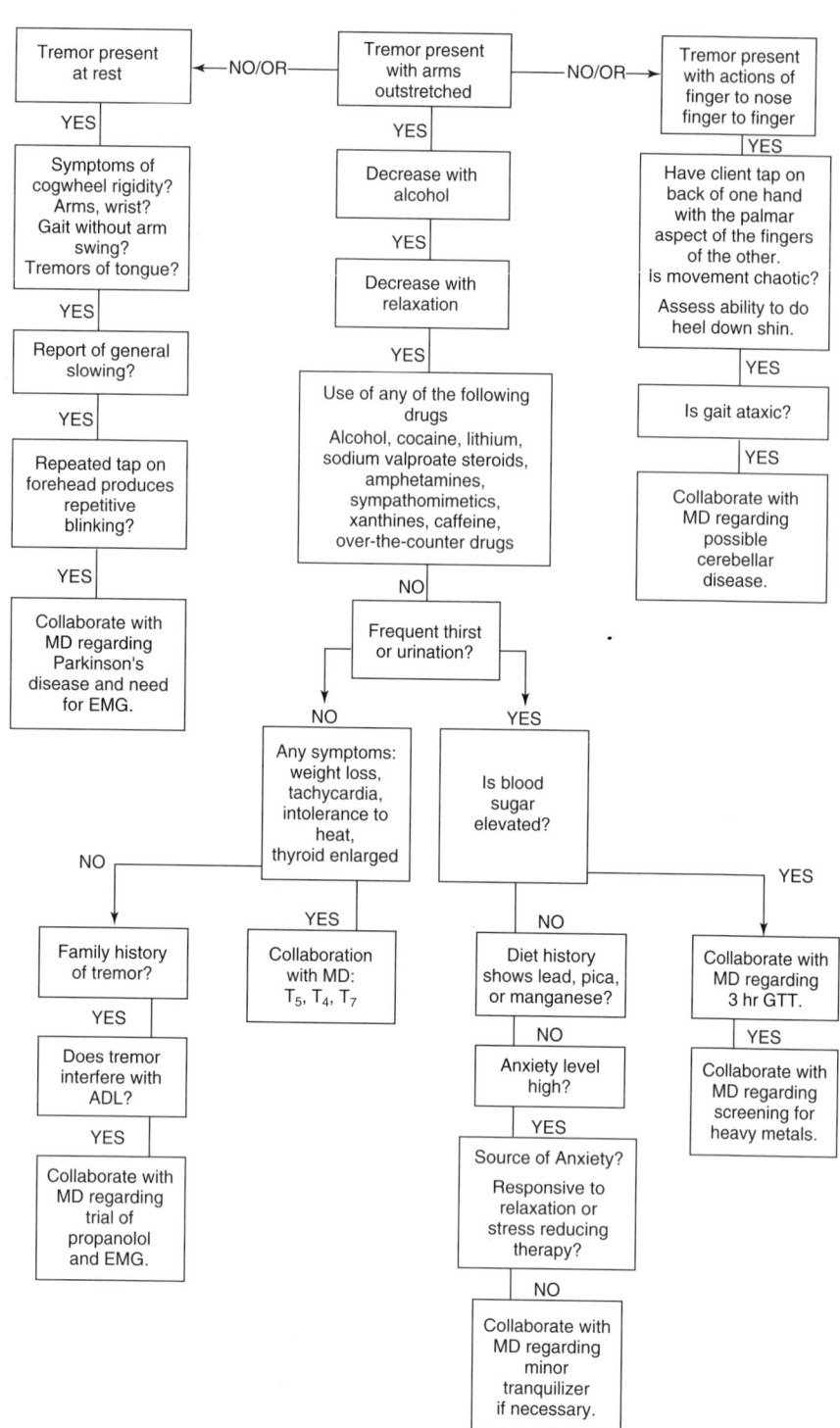

FIGURE 17–5 Tremor.

the tremor to move to another body part. An important clue to diagnosis is that it disappears when the patient's attention is distracted.

Rest tremor, most frequently seen in Parkinson's disease, occurs at rest and disappears during sleep. A resting or static tremor is observed when the muscle is at rest, such as when the hands are on the lap and the "pill-rolling" motion of the distal fingers is observed.

Finger-to-nose testing usually causes the tremor to decrease or to cease completely. Cerebellar tremor presents as both postural and kinetic. The most common type consists of oscillations of the arms about the shoulder or of the legs about the hips. When it affects the trunk and head, it is referred to as titubation. Finger-to-nose testing reveals an increased intensity of the tremor as the target is approached. This kind of tremor can resemble flapping or wing beating, similar to a bird flapping its wings. Ophthalmologic examination should be considered, as it may aid in diagnosis of multiple sclerosis or the Kayser-Fleischer ring seen in Wilson's disease.

Diagnostic Tests: Serum chemistries and metabolic studies, particularly thyroid function tests, should be done routinely. Electromyography (EMG) is used to subdivide tremors according to their rate and their relationship to posture of the limbs and volitional movement. Approximate frequency ranges include:

Cerebellar tremor 3–5 Hz (very coarse).
Parkinsonian 4–6 Hz.
Essential tremor 4–9 Hz.
Physiologic tremor 8–12 Hz.
Primary orthostatic tremor 14–16 Hz.
Postural or action tremor 10–12 Hz (generally invisible but can be enhanced).

Brain imaging is indicated when the tremor is cerebellar or when associated with other neurological symptoms or signs.

Differential Diagnosis: Fasciculations, sensory ataxia, myoclonus, asterixis, clonus, shivering, peripheral neuropathy, and focal dystonia can mimic tremor. Tremor has a wide range of etiologies.

Treatment: Physiologic tremor treatment is aimed at decreasing factors that exacerbate the tremor and any underlying disorder. Identify and remove the precipitating cause if possible. Offer reassurance tremor may be a normal response. Stress reduction may be helpful. Remove all caffeine products from diet. A small dose of propranolol taken prior to the anxiety-provoking event, such as public speaking, may be effective. Essential or familial tremor is treated with propranolol (Inderal) 20 mg tid, or 60 mg/day in a long-acting capsule, and increasing the dosage to 240–300 mg/day before the patient is considered to be a nonresponder. This drug is contraindicated in those with pulmonary or cardiac disease and diabetes; it may cause depression or impotence. Primidone (Mysoline), an anticonvulsant, is just as effective as propranolol. Initially a 50-mg dose is taken at bedtime, increasing to 250–300 mg, until a therapeutic response is achieved. Approximately 20% of patients report dizziness, headache, ataxia, nausea, and vomiting. Metoprolol (Lopressor), a selective beta-blocker, has been useful when asthma is present, at dosage of 50 mg bid. Nadolol (Corgard) 40 mg qid is also effective, and has fewer CNS side effects. Minor tranquilizers such as diazepam and alprazolam are occasionally helpful when given in conjunction with propranolol. Nimodipine has recently been found effective in clinical study.

For orthostatic tremor treatment is initiated at a low dose, but clonazepam 4–6 mg/day may be given. Cerebellar and rubral tremor has not shown significant improvement with any drug treatment. Stereotactic thalamotomy may improve this type of tremor but not overall function.

Follow-up: Patients should be evaluated for therapeutic effects and side effects of medications within 1 week of starting treatment. If primidone is started, begin on a Friday night so the patient can identify any side effects over the weekend. Warn patients of the possibility of side effects and reassure them that these effects should last no longer than a few days. Annual monitoring for weight loss, depression, and decline in functional status is necessary.

Sequelae: Functional disabilities may occur in ADLs, including compromised eating, drinking, and preparing food. Decreased caloric intake and weight loss may be observed. Ambulation, especially on stairs, may be hazardous if the patient has tremor of the head, lower extremity, or even upper extremity, which makes holding onto handrails difficult. Withdrawal from social situations may occur. Depression is common.

Prevention/Prophylaxis: Reduce factors that can exacerbate the tremor. Continue medication regimen.

Referral: A neurologist should be consulted for cerebellar tremors, mixed tremors, parkinsonian tremor, or when a focal neurologic deficit is identified. An ophthalmologist should be consulted when Wilson's disease is suspected. A mental health provider or psychiatrist should be consulted when a hysterical tremor is suspected. A physical or occupational therapy consult may be helpful in advanced or disabling cases. A nutritional consult should be considered when weight loss is identified and food supplements are required.

Education: Include information related to the illness and medications, and practical information on disabling effects. Practical solutions include Velcro closure on clothes, use of special eating utensils, and increased use of finger foods and straws. Use of a signature stamp may be helpful for patients who can no longer write their names; many banks now approve this. Medication information for beta-blockers should include monitoring of pulse and orthostatic blood pressures. The patient should be taught to not abruptly stop taking the medications because of possible rebound cardiac effects. Patients receiving primidone should be taught about its adverse effects and to avoid abrupt discontinuation, as this may cause a rebound tremor phenomenon. Information on the International Tremor Foundation, 360 West Superior Street, Chicago, IL 60610 (312-664-2344), which publishes a quarterly newsletter, may be helpful to patients.

Urinary Incontinence

Urinary incontinence is the involuntary loss of urine sufficient enough to be a problem. Types of incontinence include acute/transient and persistent. Subtypes of persistent incontinence include urge, stress, mixed, overflow, functional, and reflex. Acute urinary incontinence usually is of sudden onset and is related to an illness, treatment, or medication. When the illness is over or the identified cause is addressed, this condition usually resolves.

Persistent urinary incontinence definitions include:

Urge incontinence is the involuntary loss of urine in association with a strong sensation of urinary urgency. The pressure in the bladder (detrusor) exceeds the pressure in the urethra.

Stress incontinence occurs when intra-abdominal pressure is increased by coughing or sneezing, and the pelvic floor and urethral muscles are weak. Stress incontinence is the most common type of incontinence in women.

Mixed incontinence, a combination of stress and urge incontinence, is especially common in elderly women.

Overflow incontinence is the failure to empty the bladder completely, resulting in overdistention.

Functional incontinence, a result of chronic cognitive or physical impairments, interferes with the ability of patients to toilet.

Reflex, or unconscious, incontinence occurs in patients with neurologic problems, including spinal cord lesions.

Etiology: Urinary incontinence can be caused by several factors affecting the anatomy and/or physiology of the lower urinary tract or by other factors including changes in cognition and/or mobility.

Occurrence: Approximately 13 million people in the United States, or 10%–35% of adults and at least 50% of nursing home residents, have urinary incontinence.

Age: In the community-dwelling older population, the prevalence of urinary incontinence is 15%–35%. Caregivers of homebound elderly persons report that 53% are incontinent of urine. At least half of the 1.5 million nursing home residents are incontinent.

Ethnicity: Not significant.

Gender: Urinary incontinence is twice as prevalent in women as in men; however, overflow incontinence is more prevalent in men.

Contributing Factors: Many contributing factors for urinary incontinence include pelvic muscle weakness, multiparity, estrogen depletion (menopause), diabetes, stroke, multiple sclerosis, spinal cord injury, benign prostatic hypertrophy, urinary tract infection, fecal impaction, poor fluid intake, excessive fluid intake, smoking, pregnancy, vaginal delivery, episiotomy, lack of postpartum exercise, age, female gender, delirium, cognitive impairment, immobility or impaired mobility commonly associated with chronic degenerative disease, environmental barriers, and high-impact physical activities.

The side effects of many medications can also contribute to urinary incontinence (Table 17–13).

Signs and Symptoms: Because urinary incontinence is not life threatening and may be a source of embarrassment, the patient may not seek evaluation and treatment unless the health-care provider broaches the question. Asking "Do you ever have difficulty getting to the bathroom in time?" or "Do you ever have a problem with leaking urine when you cough, sneeze, or laugh?" will yield more results than asking directly about "incontinence." Other helpful questions include:

How frequently do you get up at night to use the bathroom?
Do you have any problems with constipation?
Do you visit the bathroom frequently during the day?
Do you feel like you are not emptying your bladder completely?
Do you wear a pad to prevent wetness?

Urge incontinence manifests as a sudden, strong urge to void, as a loss of urine on the way to the bathroom or as a loss of urine without any symptoms. The history with stress incontinence includes that of leakage of small amounts of urine with a cough, sneeze, laugh, or other physical exertion; in some cases, urine is lost with postural changes. Mixed incontinence presents with a blend of urge and stress symptoms, with one troubling the patient more than the other. Patients with overflow incontinence may report several symptoms, including urgency, frequency, dribbling, or urge or stress incontinence symptoms; men often talk about hesitancy or slow stream.

Functional incontinence may present as urgency or the functional limitations may be obvious, such as in patients with arthritis, Parkinson's disease, or post-CVA residual. Patients with cognitive impairment or depression may not have the

TABLE 17–13 DRUG CLASSIFICATIONS THAT CONTRIBUTE TO URINARY INCONTINENCE

Diuretics	Caffeine
Anticholinergic agents	Psychotropics
Tricyclic antidepressants	Phenothiazines
Antispasmodics	Antiparkinsonian agents
Narcotic analgesics	Sedative/hypnotics
CNS depressants, including alcohol	Angiotensin-converting enzyme (ACE) inhibitors
Beta-agonists	
Alpha-adrenergic agents, including antihistamines, sympathomimetics, sympatholytics	
Calcium channel blockers	

ability to describe their symptoms; the history of the problem in these patients may come from a family member or caregiver.

Patients with unconscious or reflex incontinence may experience postvoiding or continual incontinence; some may have urgency and bladder irritability. A history of the problem should include onset, duration, aggravating and relieving factors, associated symptoms, and current self-management. Obtain a thorough drug history, including prescribed and OTC medications, herbal remedies, homeopathics, caffeine and alcohol use. A surgical history including any gynecologic, colorectal, urologic, and neurosurgical procedures should be explored. Ask about a past history of urethral structure with dilation. A history of any concurrent chronic diseases such as diabetes mellitus, multiple sclerosis, stroke, spinal stenosis, parkinsonism, congestive heart failure, hypertension, or cancer (particularly with past radiation therapy) is essential. Note if the patient has recently been hospitalized or had an indwelling catheter. Investigation of nutritional status and fluid intake, as well as recent changes in functional status, is also helpful.

The mnemonics DRIP and DIAPERS (see Differential Diagnosis) may help you differentiate between transient and persistent incontinence. Having the patient keep a bladder diary, including voiding patterns, frequency, amount, episodes of incontinence, activity, and fluid intake is also helpful in differentiating symptoms. A visit to the patient's residence helps to assess for environmental barriers to continence.

Physical examination should include functional assessment, with special attention to mobility, to the person's ability to remove necessary clothing in time to use the toilet, and to toileting hygiene. Mental status, including cognition and evidence of depression, should be assessed. The abdomen should be examined for clues such as bladder distention, pelvic masses, or tenderness in the suprapubic region. Distention can be found in overflow incontinence due to some type of obstruction. A malignancy, benign myoma, or prolapse in the pelvic region creates pressure on the bladder seen in urge, stress, or mixed incontinence. A vaginal examination may reveal poor perineal hygiene, skin breakdown from urine soaking, or redness and thinning of tissue typical of atrophic changes. Prolapse of genitourinary structures or rectum may also be seen. To assess for pelvic floor muscle strength and relaxation, instruct the patient to bear down as though having a bowel movement, then tighten or squeeze by pulling up on pelvic floor muscles; in patients with pelvic floor relaxation, you will see the inability to contract or weak contractions. Positive neurologic findings in the perineal area include hypersensation, hyposensation, or absence of the bulbocavernosus ("anal wink") reflex. A rectal examination may uncover fecal impaction, rectal prolapse, hemorrhoids, masses, or, in men, prostatic enlargement. Whenever possible, the examiner should observe the patient voiding, having the patient void into a measurable receptacle. This should be followed by evaluation of a postvoiding residual (PVR). Studies are inconclusive with respect to the amount of PVR that is significant, with values ranging from greater than 50 mL to greater than 200 mL (Fig. 17–6).

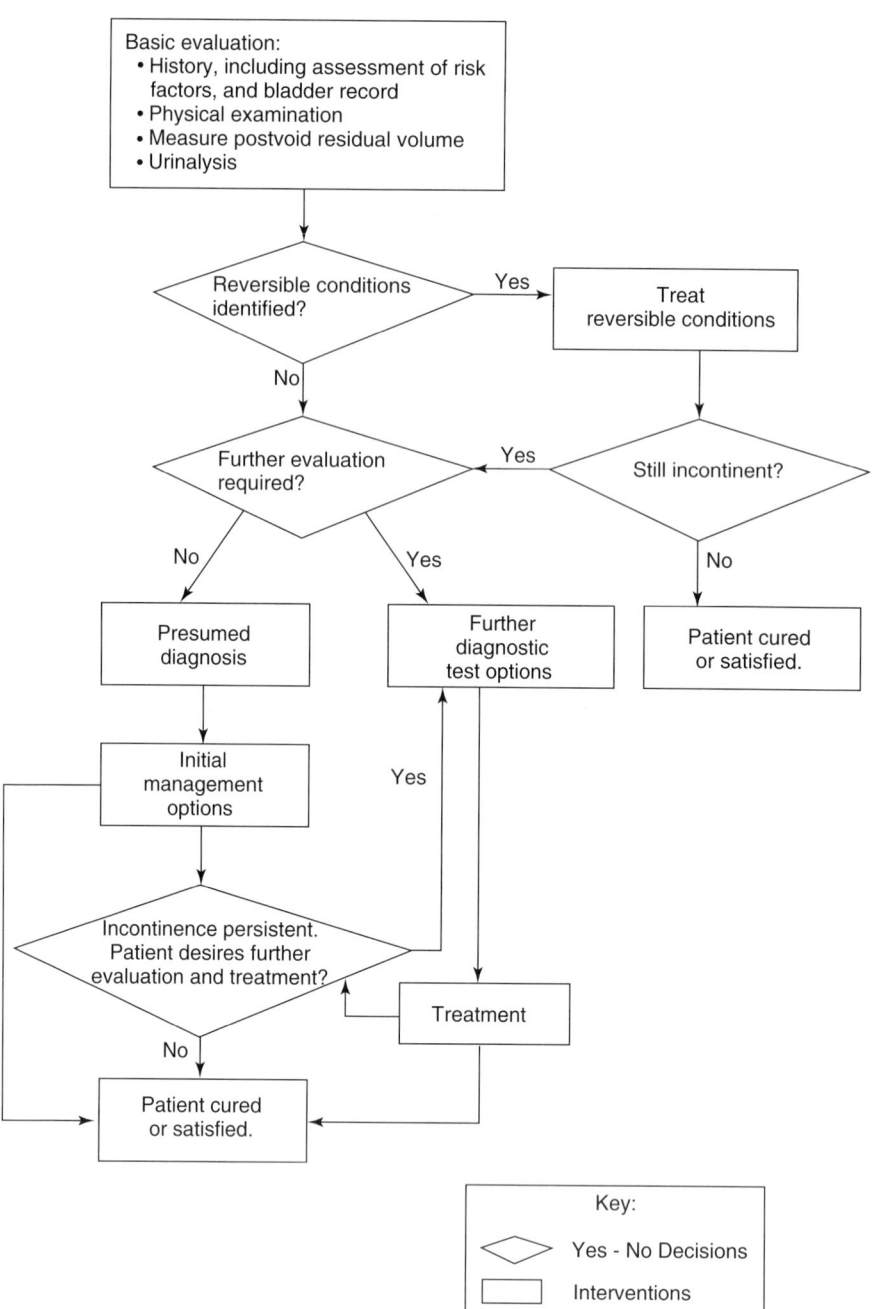

FIGURE 17–6   Urinary incontinence.

Diagnostic Tests: Perform a provocative stress test if possible, if you suspect stress or urge incontinence. Immediate leakage with the stress maneuver indicates stress incontinence. Delayed leakage suggests other causes of incontinence.

A urinalysis is also indicated. Positive findings include the presence of leukocytes or nitrites, suggestive of infection; the presence of occult blood, suggestive of infection or obstruction (including malignancy); proteinuria, suggestive of a problem with the renal filtration system.

These findings, in turn, will necessitate other studies to get to the source of the problem. For suspected infections, a urine culture and sensitivity is indicated to identify the causative organism and the appropriate antibiotic treatment. If renal problems are likely, a creatinine clearance test will yield further information. If diabetes is a consideration, order a fasting glucose test. Further diagnostic studies are considered individually in patients who are unsuitable for presumptive diagnosis and treatment, who do not respond to trial management following the basic evaluation, who have comorbid conditions, or who are candidates for surgical intervention. Specialized testing includes urodynamic testing, ultrasound, and cystoscopic procedures designed to identify the cause of urinary incontinence.

Differential Diagnosis: Urinary incontinence is a symptom, not a diagnosis in itself. Differential diagnosis includes vaginal or urethral discharge, urinary tract infection, and medication side effect. The two mneumonics DRIP and DIAPERS are often used to differentiate transient (acute) from persistent urinary incontinence:

DRIP		DIAPERS	
D	Delirium	D	Delirium
R	Restricted mobility	I	Infection
I	Infection, impaction, inflammation	A	Atrophic vaginitis
P	Pharmaceuticals, polyuria	P	Psychological, pharmaceuticals, psychotropics
		E	Endocrine problem
		R	Restricted mobility
		S	Stool impaction

Treatment: The treatment depends on the cause of the incontinence. For transient or acute urinary incontinence, treating, eliminating, or modifying the cause usually alleviates the symptom. Guidelines from the Agency for Health Care Policy and Research (AHCPR) address this area comprehensively. For persistent incontinence, treatment is categorized as behavioral, pharmacologic, or surgical. AHCPR guidelines advise going from least-invasive treatment to most-invasive treatment, as indicated (Fig. 17–6). Frequently used behavioral interventions include pelvic muscle exercises (PMEs) or Kegel exercises, performed alone or in combination with biofeedback, to help stregthen periurethral muscles, and toileting programs such as timed voiding, prompted voiding, and bladder training. The degree of independent participation by the patient in these programs depends on cognition and mobility. Electrical stimulation using intravaginal and/or intra-anal electrodes to inhibit bladder instability and improve sphincter and levator ani contractility is also useful as an adjunct therapy. If nocturia is a problem, limiting fluids before bedtime is helpful. Physical devices such as a pessary may be indicated for women with organ prolapse for whom surgery is not recommended or desired. Requirements for pessary use include intact cognition, manual dexterity, and the ability to follow instructions.

Always approach pharmacologic therapy cautiously in older patients. Consider comorbidities and potential interactions with other prescribed medications before deciding on a pharmaceutic agent. Treat stress or mixed incontinence associated with atrophic vaginitis with estrogen preparations, applied topically or taken orally. Various estrogen preparations are available, with new developments constantly in progress. Topical estrogen preparations are preferred because of the decreased incidence of side effects. Vaginal estrogen cream 2 g contains 1.25 mg conjugated estrogens per applicatorful. Dosage is one applicator daily, which may be reduced in frequency or given in a 3-weeks on, 1-week-off regimen. Oral estrogen dosage is 0.3–0.625 mg daily. Progesterone must be given to women with an intact uterus, to prevent endometrial hyperplasia and malignancy; medroxyprogesterone 2.5 mg daily, continuously or intermittently, may be prescribed.

Estrogen is contraindicated in patients with suspected or confirmed uterine or breast cancer, undiagnosed vaginal bleeding, or a history of thrombophlebitis. Patients receiving estrogen therapy should have annual Pap tests and mammograms.

Phenylpropanolamine (PPA) and pseudoephedrine are sympathomimetic drugs with alpha-adrenergic agonist properties; these drugs are thought to increase bladder outlet resistance, which is desirable in stress incontinence. The dosage of PPA is 25–100 mg PO bid in a sustained-release form. Pseudoephedrine dosage is 15–30 mg PO tid. This class of medications has many significant side effects, including tachycardia, elevated blood pressure, anxiety, insomnia, agitation, cardioarrhythmia, sweating, and respiratory difficulty, and should not be used by patients with cardiac problems, hypertension, or any type of obstructive syndromes. Imipramine, discussed farther on, can be used as a second-line agent for stress incontinence when other drugs are ineffective.

Urge incontinence and detrusor hyperreflexia have both been treated successfully with pharmacologic therapy. Anticholinergic agents and tricyclic antidepressants (with anticholinergic properties) are the agents of choice. These drugs are contraindicated in patients with glaucoma or prostatic hypertrophy. Tricyclics, which cannot be taken concomitantly with MAO inhibitors, should be used selectively in patients with heart disease. Common side effects include dry mouth, blurred vision, constipation, dry skin, confusion, and postural hypotension. Oxybutynin (Ditropan) 2.5 mg PO bid, which is recommended for older patients, has an antispasmodic effect on bladder smooth muscle, delaying the urge to void. Propantheline (Pro-Banthīne) is also used, in dosages of 7.5–30 mg PO tid, but it has an undesirable side effect profile; monitor PVR to prevent urine retention. Flavoxate (Urispas) 100–200 mg tid or dicyclomine (Bentyl) 10–20 mg tid are other anticholinergic choices.

Imipramine (Tofranil) 10–25 mg PO taken one to three times daily is the prototype tricyclic; it exerts a twofold action, decreasing bladder contractions and increasing outflow resistance. Doxepin, desipramine, or nortriptyline can also be used.

For overflow incontinence unrelated to obstructive uropathy (e.g., atonic bladder), bethanechol (Urecholine) 10–30 mg PO tid can be prescribed. Its cholinergic effects include stimulation of the detrusor muscle. Because this drug has a high profile of undesirable side effects and is contraindicated in patients with asthma, Parkinson's disease, peptic ulcer, hypertension, cardiac disease, hyperthyroidism, or epilepsy, it is of limited usefulness in the older patient.

For patients with overflow incontinence due to prostatic hypertrophy, surgery was previously the only available option. Now, however, several drugs are being used in selected patients. Urologic consultation and workup is advised prior to prescribing these medications. Finasteride (Proscar) 5 mg PO daily inhibits the enzyme that converts testosterone into its active form; this results in a regression of prostate tissue. Not all patients show an increase in urine outflow; in fact, some patients must take this drug for 6–12 months to determine its effectiveness. Use Proscar cautiously in those with impaired liver function. Side effects include decreased libido and impotence. Measure prostate size and monitor for reduction through digital rectal examinations. Patients should also be monitored for changes in urine output and PVR volume, indicative of obstructive uropathy. The drug should not be prescribed to sexually active patients with partners of childbearing age because of potentially harmful effects on the male fetus; for this reason, also, it should not be crushed and handled by pregnant women or by women capable of becoming pregnant. Other drugs currently being used for treatment of prostatic hypertrophy include α_1-adrenergic blockers terazosin (Hytrin) and prazosin (Minipress), antihypertensive agents that also relax the smooth muscle of the prostate and bladder neck, alleviating pressure on the urethra. Dosages for each of these are individualized, starting with 1 mg PO daily for terazosin and 1 mg PO bid for Minipress. Because older patients are very sensitive to the hypotensive effects of these drugs, monitor carefully for safety and adverse events. Although not an approved usage, many older men are using saw palmetto, an herbal product, for reduction of prostatic enlargement.

Other treatments for urinary incontinence include surgical interventions for stress incontinence in women or prostatic hypertrophy in men. Nonsurgical management of persistent urinary incontinence includes intermittent catheterization, use of pelvic organ support devices such as pessaries in women, physical and environmental modifications to improve access to the toilet, or use of absorptive products.

Follow-up: To evaluate the efficacy of the prescribed treatment, schedule follow-up visits biweekly initially, and on an individualized basis thereafter. Patients following PME routines may need extra support to establish and maintain the program.

Patients taking replacement estrogen should have annual Pap smears. Medication therapy should be monitored for effectiveness, side effects, and drug interactions. Behavioral therapy requires patient or caregiver support and reinforcement to establish a desired habit or pattern.

Sequelae: Possible complications include UTI, hydronephrosis (with overflow or obstruction), renal failure secondary to hydronephrosis, adverse drug events, or failure of behavioral therapy. Skin breakdown is a significant complication with persistent urinary incontinence. Urosepsis can occur with unrecognized UTIs. Falls can occur after episodes of urinary incontinence, particularly with persons in a group residence or living alone.

Prevention/Prophylaxis: Ways to help prevent incontinence include:

- Early identification and remediation of causes of acute or transient urinary incontinence.
- Routine instruction of women in Kegel exercises after childbirth and in the early postmenopausal stage.
- Teaching patient and family that urinary incontinence is not a normal aging change and is treatable.
- Regular gynecologic examinations for women to detect pelvic pathology.
- Regular rectal examination in men to detect and treat early prostatic hypertrophy.
- Careful attention to prescribing only essential drugs in the older population.

Referral: Refer men with overflow incontinence for urologic evaluation. If management is conservative (i.e., prescribing medications), it can be collaborative. If you have not studied the use of biofeedback or electrical stimulation, refer the patient to a knowledgeable nurse practitioner or to a health-care continence specialty group. In many long-term care settings, consultations with and patient referrals to such groups for evaluation and management suggestions are routine. Refer for further evaluation patients with an uncertain diagnosis, for whom you are unable to develop a management plan from the basic diagnostic evaluation, and those with a lack of correlation between symptoms and clinical findings. Refer patients for whom surgical intervention is considered, patients with hematuria without infection, patients who fail a therapeutic trial and desire further intervention, and those with other comorbidities, including:

History of prior surgery for incontinence or radical pelvic surgery.
Suspicion of prostate cancer.
Abnormal PVR urine.
Neurologic condition such as multiple sclerosis; spinal cord injury or lesions.
Persistent symptoms of difficulty emptying bladder.
Incontinence in conjunction with recurrent symptomatic UTIs.

Education: Teach patients, family, caregivers, health-care providers, and the public that urinary incontinence is *not* a normal consequence of aging and *is* treatable. Teach the patient, family, and caregivers behavioral therapy techniques. Teach Kegel exercises, pessary use (when necessary), intermittent catherization, medication actions, and medication side effects. Teach patients how to use a bladder record or incontinence monitoring record. Teach signs and symptoms of UTI, the role of diet in the prevention of constipation, avoidance of irritant and diuretic beverages, and good perineal hygiene to avoid infection.

REFERENCES

Assessment

Abrams, WB, Beers, MH, and Berkow, R: The Merck Manual of Geriatrics, ed 2. Merck Research Laboratories, Whitehouse Station, NJ, 1995.
Merck Research Laboratories, Whitehouse Station, NJ, 1995.
Bates, B, Bickley, LS, and Hoekelman, RA: Physical Examination and History Taking, ed 6. JB Lippincott, Philadelphia, 1995.
Finucane, TE, and Burton, JR: Geriatric medicine. In Barker, LR, Burton, JR, and Zieve, PD (eds): Principles of Ambulatory Medicine, ed 4. Williams & Wilkins, Baltimore, 1995.
Hamm, JR, and Sloane, PD: Primary care geriatrics, ed 3. CV Mosby, St. Louis, 1997.
Lonergan, ET: Clinical evaluation. In Lonergan, ET (ed): Geriatrics. Appleton & Lange, Stamford, CT, 1996.
Tierney, LM, McPhee, SJ, and Papadakis, MA (eds): Current Medical Diagnosis and Treatment, ed 36. Appleton & Lange, Stamford, CT, 1997.
Yoshikawa, TT, Cobbs, EL, and Brummel-Smith, K: Practical Ambulatory Geriatrics, ed 2. CV Mosby, St. Louis, 1998.

Bowel Incontinence

Abrams, WB, Beers, MH, and Berkow, R: The Merck Manual of Geriatrics, ed 2. Merck Research Laboratories, Whitehouse Station, NJ, 1995.
Ebersole, P, and Hess, P: Toward Healthy Aging, ed 4. CV Mosby, St. Louis, 1994.
Hamm, RJ, and Sloane, PD: Primary Care Geriatrics, ed 3. CV Mosby, St. Louis, 1997.
Lueckenotte, AG: Gerontologic Nursing, CV Mosby, St. Louis, 1996.
Matteson, MA, McConnell, ES, and Linton, AD: Gerontologic Nursing, ed 2. WB Saunders, Philadelphia, 1997.
Schrock, TR: Fecal incontinence. In Lonergan, ET (ed): Geriatrics. Appleton & Lange, Stamford, CT, 1996.

Chest Pain

Aisenberg, J, and Castell, D: Approach to the patient with unexplained chest pain. Mt Sinai J Med 61:481, 1994.
American College of Emergency Physicians: Clinical policy for the initial approach to adults presenting with a chief complaint of chest pain with no history of trauma. Ann Emerg Med 25:274–299, 1995.
Bittner, V, and Clark, D: Chest pain of unknown origin: The differential diagnosis. Hospital Medicine 31:12–19, July 1995.
Bittner, V, and Clark, D: Chest pain of unknown origin: Initial evaluation and management. Hospital Medicine 31:30–34, August 1995.
Fowler, N: Chest pain: A practical method of evaluation. Hospital Medicine 20:38–82, September 1984.
Limacher, M: Clinical features of coronary heart disease in the elderly. In Lowenthal, D (ed): Geriatric Cardiology. Cardiovascular Clinics, 22, FA Davis, Philadelphia, 1992.

Williams, B: Chest pain. In Martin, A, and Camm, AJ (eds): Geriatric Cardiology: Principles and practice. John Wiley, New York, 1994.

Constipation

Allison, OC, Porter, ME, and Briggs, GC: Chronic constipation: assessment and management in the elderly. Journal of the American Academy of Nurse Practitioners 6:7, 311–317, July 1994.

Beverley, L, and Travis, I: Constipation: Proposed natural laxative mixtures. Journal of Gerontological Nursing 18:10, 5–12, October 1992.

Harari, D, Gurwitz, J, and Minaker, K: Constipation in the elderly. JAGS 41:1130–1140, 1993.

Sandler, RS, Jordan, MC, and Shelton, BJ: Demography and dietary determinants of constipation in the US population. Journal of Public Health 80:185–189, 1990.

Dehydration

Abrams, WB, Beers, MH, and Berkow, R: The Merck Manual of Geriatrics, ed 2. Merck Research Laboratories, Whitehouse Station, NJ, 1995.

Chernoff, R: Nutrition. In Jahnigen, DW, and Schrier, RW: Geriatric Medicine, ed 2. Blackwell Scientific, Cambridge, MA, 1997.

Ebersole, P, and Hess, P: Toward Healthy Aging, ed 4. CV Mosby, St. Louis, 1994.

Kayser-Jones, J: Mealtime in nursing homes: The importance of individualized care. Journal of Gerontologic Nursing 22:26–32, 1996.

Matteson, MA, McConnell, ES, and Linton, AD: Gerontologic Nursing, ed 2. WB Saunders, Philadelphia, 1997.

Yoshikawa, TT, Cobbs, EL, and Brummel-Smith, K: Practical Ambulatory Geriatrics, ed 2. CV Mosby, St. Louis, 1998.

Zembrzuski, CD: A three-dimensional approach to hydration of elders: Administration, clinical staff and in-service education. Geriatric Nursing 18:20–26, 1997.

Diarrhea

Bennett, RG, and Greenough, WB: Diarrhea. In Hazzard, WR, et al: Principles of Geriatric Medicine and Gerontology, ed 3. McGraw-Hill, New York, 1994.

Chernecky, CC, and Bergey, BJ: Laboratory Tests and Diagnostic Procedures, ed 2. WB Saunders, Philadelphia, 1997.

Cole, MC: Chronic and acute diarrhea. In Rakel, RE: Saunders Manual of Medical Practice. WB Saunders, Philadelphia, 1996.

LaForce, FM: Infections. In Jahnigen, DW, and Schrier, RW: Geriatric Medicine, ed 2. Blackwell Scientific, Cambridge, MA, 1997.

Seller, RH: Differential Diagnosis of Common Complaints, ed 3. WB Saunders, Philadelphia, 1996.

Dizziness

Abrams, WB, and Berkow, R (eds): The Merck Manual of Geriatrics. Merck Sharp & Dohme Research Laboratories, Rahway, NJ, 1990.

Basmajian, JV, et al: Stedman's Medical Dictionary, ed 24. Williams & Wilkins, Baltimore, 1982.

Bates, B: A Guide to Physical Examination and History Taking, ed 5. JB Lippincott, Philadelphia, 1991.

Brocklehurst, JC, Tallis, RC, and Fillit, HM (eds): Textbook of Geriatric Medicine and Gerontology. Churchill Livingstone, Edinburgh, 1992, p. 318.

Burnside, IM: Nursing and the Aged, ed 3. McGraw-Hill, New York, 1988, pp. 394–395.

Carnevali, DL, and Patrick, M (eds): Nursing Management for the Elderly. JB Lippincott, Philadelphia, 1979.

Carpenito, LJ: Nursing Diagnosis: Application to Clinical Practice, ed 5. JB Lippincott, Philadelphia, 1993.

Chenitz, WC, Stone, JT, and Salisbury, SA: Clinical Gerontological Nursing: A guide to advanced practice. WB Saunders, Philadelphia, 1991, pp. 304–305.

Jonsson, PV, and Lipsitz, LA: Dizziness and syncope. In Hazzard, WR, et al: Principles of Geriatric Medicine and Gerontology, ed 3. McGraw-Hill, New York, 1994, pp. 1165–1171.

Kane, RL, Ouslander, JG, and Abrass, IB: Essentials of Clinical Geriatrics, ed 3. McGraw-Hill, New York, 1994.

Pearson, LB: Protocols: How to develop and implement within the nurse practitioner setting. Nurse Practitioner 2(1):9–12, September-October 1976.

Sloane, PD: Dizziness. In Ham, RJ, and Sloane, PD: Primary Care Geriatrics, ed 2. CV Mosby, St. Louis, 1992, pp. 336–342.

Thompson, C, Cox, A, and Jones, JM: Protocols: Guidelines for practice in occupational health care setting. Occupational Health Nursing 33(10):516–521, October 1984.

U.S. Prevention Services Task Force: Guide to Clinical Preventative Services: An Assessment of 169 Interventions. Williams and Wilkins, Baltimore, 1989.

Yoshikawa, TT, Cobbs, EL, and Brummel-Smith, K: Ambulatory Geriatric Care. CV Mosby, St. Louis, 1993, pp. 305–310.

Dysphagia

Bates, B: A Pocket Guide to Physical Examination and History Taking. JB Lippincott, Philadelphia, 1995.

Carpenito, LJ: Handbook of Nursing Diagnosis, ed 5. JB Lippincott, Philadelphia, 1993.

Cole-Arvin, C, Notich, L, and Underhill, A: Identifying and managing dysphagia. Nursing 94, 7:48, 1994.

Ergun, GA, and Miskovitz, PF: Aging and the esophagus: Common pathologic conditions and their effect upon swallowing in the geriatric population. Dysphagia 7:58, 1992.

Gustafsson, B, and Tibbling, L: Dysphagia, an unrecognized handicap. Dysphagia 6:193, 1991.

Hendrix, TR: Art and science of history taking in the patient with difficulty swallowing. Dysphagia 8:69, 1993.

Lorenze, R, Jorysz, G, Tornieporth, N, and Classen, M: The gastroenterologist's approach to dysphagia. Dysphagia 8:79, 1993.

Roe, D: Dysphagia. In Griffith, HW, Dambro, MR: The Five Minute Clinical Consultant. Lea & Febiger, Philadelphia, 1994.

Veldee, MS, and Peth, LD: Can protein-calorie malnutrition cause dysphagia? Dysphagia 7:86, 1992.

Fatigue

Abrams, W, Beers, MH, and Berkow, R: The Merck Manual of Geriatrics, ed 2. Merck Research Laboratories, Whitehouse Station, NJ, 1995.

Ahronheim, J: Case studies in geriatrics for the house officer. Williams and Wilkins, Baltimore, 1990.

Ahronheim, J: Handbook of prescribing medications for geriatric patients. Little, Brown, Boston, 1992.

Bates, B: A Guide to Physical Examination. JB Lippincott, Philadelphia, 1994.

Beland, I, and Passos, J: Clinical Nursing: Pathophysiological and Psychological Approaches. MacMillan, New York, 1981.

Friedman, H: Problem-Oriented Medical Diagnosis, ed 5. Little, Brown, Boston/Toronto/London, 1991.

Gorman, RS: Fatigue. Decision making in medicine. In Greene, HL, Johnson, WP, and Maricic, MJ (eds): Decision Making in Medicine. Mosby Year Books, St. Louis, 1993.

Girl, AH: Management of diverticular disease. In Goroll, AH, May, LA, and Mulley, AG (eds): Primary care medicine: Office Evaluation of the Adult Patient, ed 3. JB Lippincott, Philadelphia, 1995.

Lipschitz, D: The anemia of chronic disease. Journal of American Geriatrics Society 38:1238–1263, 1990.

Rice, L: Anemia: Using a rational approach to diagnosis. Consultant 30:39–40, 43–44, 47–49, 1990.

Stabb, A, and Lyles, M: Manual of Geriatric Nursing. Scott, Foresman/Little, Brown Higher Education, Glenview, IL, 1990.

Headache

Allen, TG: Evaluating and treating headaches. In AJN 94(4):16B–16H, April 1994.

Cargill, J: Headaches in the Older Adult. ADVANCE for Nurse Practitioners 2(4):8–10, 32, 1994.

Coutin, IB, and Glass, SF: Recognizing uncommon headache syndromes. Am Fam Physician 54(7):2247–2252, 1994.

Dambro, M: Griffith's 5 Minute Clinical Consult. Williams & Wilkins, Baltimore, 1997.

Peroutka, SJ: Drugs effective in the therapy of migraine. In Goodman & Gilman's The Pharmacological Basis of Therapeutics, ed 9. McGraw-Hill, New York, 1996.

Pfeiffer, GM: Easing the pain of tension headaches. ADVANCE for Nurse Practitioners (5)5:25–31, 1997.

Seller, RH: Differential Diagnosis of Common Complaints, ed 3. WB Saunders, Philadelphia, 1996.

Weiss, J: Assessment and management of the client with headaches. Nurse Practitioner 18(4):44–57, 1993.

Yoshikawa, TT, Cobbs, EL, and Brummel-Smith, K: Practical Ambulatory Geriatrics, ed 2. CV Mosby, St. Louis, 1998.

Hematuria

Barker, LR, Burton, JR, and Zieve, PD: Principles of Ambulatory Medicine, ed 3. Williams & Wilkins, Baltimore, 1991, pp. 490–494.

Doenges, ME, Moorhouse, M, and Geissler, AC: Nursing Care Plans: Guidelines for Individualizing Patient Care, ed 4. FA Davis, Philadelphia, 1997.

Isselbacher, KJ, et al: Harrison's Principles of Internal Medicine, ed 13. McGraw-Hill, New York, 1994, pp. 237, 1305–1306.

Fishbach, F: A Manual of Laboratory Diagnostic Tests, ed 2. JB Lippincott, Philadelphia, 1984.

McCarthy, JJ: Outpatient evaluation of hematuria. Postgrad Med 101(2):125–131, 1997.

Restrepo, N, et al. Evaluating hematuria in adults. Am Fam Physician 40(2):149–155, 1989.

Sanford, JP, Gilbert, DN, Sande, MA: Guide to Antimicrobial Therapy, Inc., Dallas, TX, 1996.

Schwartz, MH: Textbook of Physical Diagnosis, ed 2. WB Saunders, Philadelphia, pp. 345–346, 1994.

Hemoptysis

Barker, LR, Burton, JR, and Zieve, PD: Principles of Ambulatory Medicine, ed 3. Williams & Wilkins, Baltimore, 1991, pp. 589–591.

Bartlett, JG: Pocket Book of Infectious Disease Therapy. Williams & Wilkins, Baltimore, 1997.

Colice, GL: Hemoptysis: Three questions that can direct management. Postgrad Med 100(1):227–236, 1996.

Doenges, ME, Moorhouse, M, and Geissler, AC: Nursing Care Plans: Guidelines for Individualizing Patient Care, ed 4. Philadelphia, FA Davis, 1997.

Fischbach, F: A Manual of Laboratory Diagnostic Tests, ed 2. JB Lippincott, Philadelphia, 1984.

Isselbacher, KJ, et al: Harrison's Principles of Internal Medicine, ed 13. McGraw-Hill, New York, 1994, pp. 172–174.

Merck Manual of Diagnosis and Therapy, ed 17. Merck & Co., Rahway, NJ, 1997, pp. 603–605.

Nurse Practitioner's Drug Handbook. Springhouse, PA, Springhouse Corporation, 1996.

Hoarseness

Dettelbach, M, Eibling, D, and Johnson, J: Hoarseness: From viral laryngitis to glottic cancer. Postgrad Med 5:143, 1994.

Involuntary Weight Loss

Mansouri, A, Morton, KI, and Verdery, RB: Pinpointing the causes of unexplained weight loss. Patient Care 28:46, 1994.

Marton, KI, Sox, HC, and Krupp, JR: Involuntary weight loss: Diagnostic and prognostic significance. Ann Intern Med 95:568, 1981.

Robbins, LJ: Evaluation of weight loss in the elderly. Geriatrics 44:31, 1984.

Uphold, CR, and Graham, MV: Weight Loss. Clinical Guidelines in Adult Health. Barmarrae Books, Gainesville, FL, 1993, pp. 39–44.

Vandenbergh, E, Vandewwoestijne, KP, and Gyselen, A: Weight changes in the terminal stages of chronic obstructive pulmonary disease: Relation to respiratory function and prognosis. Am Rev Respir Dis 95:556, 1967.
Wise, GR, and CD: Evaluation of involuntary weight loss: Where do you start? Postgrad Med 95:143, 1994.

Joint Pain

Abrams, WB, Beers, MH, and Berkow, R (eds): Merck Manual of Diagnosis and Therapy, ed 17. Merck & Co., Rahway, NJ, 1997, pp. 1297–1304.
Bates, B: A Guide to Physical Examination and History Taking, ed 5. JB Lippincott, Philadelphia, 1991.
Barker, LR, Burton, JR, and Zieve, PD: Principles of Ambulatory Medicine, ed 3. Williams & Wilkins, Baltimore, 1991.
Berg, D: Handbook of Primary Care Medicine. JB Lippincott, Philadelphia, 1993.
Doenges, ME, Moorhouse, M, and Geissler, AC: Nursing Care Plans: Guidelines for Individualizing Patient Care, ed 4. FA Davis, Philadelphia, 1997.
Fischbach, F: A Manual of Laboratory Diagnostic Tests, ed 2. JB Lippincott, Philadelphia, 1984.
Schwartz, M: Textbook of Physical Diagnosis, ed 2. WB Saunders, Philadelphia, 1994, p. 408.

Peripheral Edema

Ciocon, J, Fernandez, B, and Ciocon, DG: Leg edema: Clinical clues to the differential diagnosis. Geriatrics 48(5):34–45, May 1993.
Ciocon, J, Galindo-Ciocon, D, and Galindo, D: Raised leg exercises for leg edema in the elderly. Angiology 46(1):19–24, 1995.
Galindo-Ciocon, D: Nursing care of elders with leg edema. J Gerontol Nurs 22(7):7, July 1995.
Merli, G, and Spandorfer, J: The outpatient with unilateral leg swelling. Med Clin North Am 79(2):435–441, March 1995.

Syncope

Bonema, JD, and Maddens, ME: Syncope in elderly patients: Why their risk is higher. Postgrad Med 91(1):129–144, January 1992.
Farreh, PM, Santnga, JT, and Eagle, KA: Syncope: Diagnosis of cardiac and noncardiac causes. Geriatrics 50:24–30, 1995.
Hart, G: Evaluation of syncope. Am Fam Physician 51(8):1914–1948, June 1995.
Hayes, O: The evaluation of syncope in the emergency department. Emergency Clinics of North America (16)3:601–615, 1998.
Schaal, S, et al: Syncope. Curr Prob Cardiol 207–264, April 1992.
Schraeder, P, Lathers, C, and Charles, J: The spectrum of syncope. J Clin Pharmacol 34:454, 1994.

Tremor

Adams, RD, and Victor, M: Tremor, myoclonus, spasms, and tics. In Principles of Neurology, ed 5. McGraw-Hill, New York, 1993.
Anouti, A, and Koller, WC: Tremor disorders: Diagnosis and management. West J Med 162:510, 1995.
Bain, PG, et al: Tremor associated with benign IgM paraproteinaemic neuropathy. Brain 119:789, 1996.
Biary, N, et al: The effect of nimodipine on essential tremor. Neurology 45:8, 1995.
Bradley, WG, Daroff, RB, Fenichel, GM, Marsden, CD (eds): ed 2. Vol I. Butterworth-Heinemann, Boston, 1996.
Branch, WT: Office Practice of Medicine, ed 3. WB Saunders, Philadelphia, 1994.
Gillespie, MM: Tremor. J Neurosci Nurs 23:3, 1991.
Koller, WC: Evaluation of tremor disorders. Hosp Pract 5:23, 1990.
Louis, ED, et al: Differences in prevalence of essential tremor among elderly African-Americans, whites, and Hispanics in Northern Manhattan, NY. Arch Neurol 52:1201, 1995.
Samuels, MA: Making sense of movement disorders. Emerg Med 11:21, 1989.
Sweeney, PJ: Understanding tremor. Emerg Med 1:88, 1993.

Wills, AJ, Thompson, PD, Findley, LJ, Brooks, DJ. A positron emission tomography study of primary orthostatic tremor. Neurology 46:3, 1996.

Urinary Incontinence

ACOG Technical Bulletin #213—October 1995: Urinary Incontinence.

Augspurger, RR: Urinary incontinence and catheters in the elderly male and female. In Jahnigen, DW, and Schrier, RW: Geriatric Medicine, ed 2. Blackwell Scientific, Cambridge, MA, 1997.

Chernecky, CC, and Bergey, BJ: Laboratory Tests and Diagnostic Procedures, ed 2. WB Saunders, Philadelphia, 1997.

Dambro, M: Griffith's 5 Minute Clinical Consult., Williams & Wilkins, Baltimore, 1997.

Newman, DK, Steidle, C, and Wallace, D: Urinary incontinence: An overview of the diagnosis and management. American Journal of Managed Care, 68–74, Sept. 1995.

Spratto, GR, and Woods, AL: PDR Nurse's Handbook, ed 2, Medical Economics, Montvale, NJ, 1997.

US Department of Health and Human Services, Public Health Service, Agency for Health Care Policy and Research: Clinical Practice Guideline Number 2—1996 Update. Urinary Incontinence in Adults: Acute and Chronic Management. AHCPR Pub No 96-0682, Rockville, MD, 1996.

Yoshikawa, TT, Cobbs, EL, and Brummel-Smith, K: Practical Ambulatory Geriatrics, ed 2. CV Mosby, St. Louis, 1998.

APPENDIX **A**

PHYSIOLOGIC

INFLUENCES OF

THE AGING PROCESS

Integumentary System

Age-Related Change	Appearance or Functional Change	Implication
Loss of dermal and epidermal thickness	Paper-thin skin	Prone to skin breakdown and injury
Flattening of papillae	Shearing and friction force more readily peels off the epidermis	
	Diminished cell-mediated immunity in the skin	
Atrophy of the sweat glands	Decreased sweating	Frequent pruritus
Decreased vascularity	Slower recruitment of sweat glands by thermal stimulation	Alteration in thermoregularity response
	Decreased body odor	Fluid requirements may change seasonally
	Decreased heat loss	Loss of skin water
	Dryness	Increased risk of heat stroke
Collagen cross-linking	Increased wrinkling	Potential effect on one's morale and feeling of self-worth
Elastin regression	Laxity of skin	
Loss of subcutaneous fat	Intraosseous atrophy, especially to back of hands and face	Loss of fat tissue on soles of feet—trauma of walking increases foot problems
Decreased elasticity	Purpuric patches after minor surgery	Reduced insulation against cold temperatures; *prone to hypothermia*
Loss of subcutaneous tissue		Check why injury is occurring; be alert—potential abuse or falls
Decreased number of melanocytes	Loss of pigment	Teach importance of using sun block creams; refer to dermatologist as needed
Decline in fibroblast proliferation	Pigment plaque appears	Decreased tissue repair response
	Decreased epidermal growth rate	
	Slower reepithelialization	
	Decreased vitamin D production and synthesis	
Decreased hair follicle density	Loss of body hair	
Decreased growth phase of individual fibers	Thin, short villus hairs predominate	
	Slower hair growth	
Loss of melanocytes from the hair bulb	Graying of the hair	Potential effect on self-esteem

Alternating hyperplasia and hypoplasia of nail matrix	Longitudinal ridges Thinner nails of the fingers Thickened, curled toenails	Nails prone to splitting Advise patient to wear gloves, keep nails short, avoid nail polish remover (causes dryness); refer to podiatrist May cause discomfort

Respiratory System

Decreased lung tissue elasticity	Decreased vital capacity Increased residual volume Decreased maximum breath capacity	Reduced overall efficiency of ventilatory exchange
Thoracic wall calcification	Increased anteroposterior diameter of chest	Obscuration of heart and lung sounds Displacement of apical impulse
Cilia atrophy	Change in mucociliary transport	Increased susceptibility to infection
Decreased respiratory muscle strength	Reduced ability to handle secretions and reduced effectiveness against noxious foreign particles Partial inflation of lungs at rest	Prone to atelectasis

Cardiovascular System

Heart valves fibrose and thicken	Reduced stroke volume, cardiac output; may be altered Slight left ventricular hypertrophy S_4 commonly heard Valve less dense; mitral leaflet stretches with intrathoracic pressure	Decreased responsiveness to stress Increased incidence of murmurs, *particularly aortic stenosis and mitral regurgitation*
Mucoid degeneration of mitral valve		
Fibroelastic thickening of the sinoatrial (SA) node; decreased number of pacemaker cells	Slower heart rate Irregular heart rate	Increased prevalence of arrhythmias
Increased subpericardial fat		
Collagen accumulation around heart muscle		
Elongation of tortuosity and calcification of arteries	Increased rigidity of arterial wall	Aneurysms may form

(continued)

Age-Related Change	Appearance or Functional Change	Implication
Cardiovascular System		
Elastin and collagen cause progressive thickening and loss of arterial wall resiliency	Increased peripheral vascular resistance	Decreased blood flow to body organs
Loss of elasticity of the aorta dilation		Altered distribution of blood flow
		Increased systolic blood pressure, contributing to coronary artery disease
Increased lipid content in artery wall	Lipid deposits form	Increased incidence of atherosclerotic events, such as *angina pectoris*, stroke, gangrene
Decreased baroreceptor sensitivity (stretch receptors)	Decreased sensitivity to change in blood pressure	Prone to loss of balance—potential for falls
	Decreased baroreceptor mediation to straining	Valsalva maneuver may cause sudden drop in blood pressure
Gastrointestinal System		
Liver becomes smaller	Decreased storage capacity	
Less efficient cholesterol stabilization absorption	Increased evidence of gall stones	
Dental enamel thins	Staining of tooth surface occurs	Tooth and gum decay; tooth loss
Gums recede	Teeth deprived of nutrients	
Fibrosis and atrophy of salivary glands	Prone to dry mucous membranes	Shift to mouth breathing is common
	Decreased salivary ptyalin	Membrane more susceptible to injury and infection
		May interfere with breakdown of starches
Atrophy and decrease in number of taste buds	Decreased taste sensation	Altered ability to taste sweet, sour, and bitter
		Change in nutritional intake
		Excessive seasoning of foods
Delay in esophageal emptying	Decline in esophageal peristalsis	Occasional discomfort as food stays in esophagus longer
	Esophagus slightly dilated	

Physiological Change	Implication
Decreased hydrochloric acid secretion Decrease in gastric acid secretion	Reduction in amount of iron and vitamin B_{12} that can be absorbed Possible delay in vitamin and drug absorption, *especially calcium and iron* Altered drug effect Fewer cases of gastric ulcers
Decreased muscle tone Atrophy of mucosal lining	Altered motility Decreased colonic peristalsis Prone to constipation, functional bowel syndrome, esophageal spasm, diverticular disease Decreased hunger sensations and emptying time
Decreased proportion of dietary calcium absorbed	Altered bone formation, muscle contractility, hormone activity, enzyme activation, clotting time, immune response Symptoms more marked in women than in men
Decreased basal metabolic rate (rate at which fuel is converted into energy)	May need fewer calories Possible effect on life span

Genitourinary and Reproductive Systems

Physiological Change	Implication
Reduced renal mass Loss of glomeruli	Decreased sodium conserving ability Decreased glomerular filtration rate Decreased creatinine clearance Increased blood urea nitrogen concentration
Histological changes in small vessel walls Sclerosis of supportive circulatory system Decline in number of functioning nephrons	Decreased renal blood flow Administration and dosage of drugs may need to be modified
	Decreased ability to dilute urine concentrate Altered response to reduced fluid load or increased fluid volume
Reduced bladder muscular tone	Decreased bladder capacity or increased residual urine Sensation of urge to urinate may not occur until bladder is full Urination at night may increase
Atrophy and fibrosis of cervical and uterine walls Reduced number and viability of oocytes in the aging ovary	Menopause; decline in fertility Narrowing of cervical canal
Decreased vaginal wall elasticity Narrowing of vaginal canal	Vaginal lining thin, pale, friable Potential for discomfort in sexual intercourse
Decreased levels of circulating hormones	Reduced lubrication during arousal state Increased frequency of sexual dysfunction

(continued)

Age-Related Change	Appearance or Functional Change	Implication
Genitourinary and Reproductive System		
Degeneration of seminiferous tubules	Decreased seminal fluid volume Decreased force of ejaculation Reduced elevation of testes	
Proliferation of stromal and glandular tissue	Prostatic hypertrophy	Potentially compromised genitourinary function; *urinary frequency, and increased risk of malignancy*
Involution of mammary gland tissue	Connective tissue replaced by adipose tissue	Easier to assess breast lesions
Neuromuscular System		
Decreased muscle mass	Decreased muscle strength Tendons shrink and sclerose	Decreased tendon jerks Increased muscle cramping
Decreased myosin adenosine triphosphatase (ADT) activity	Prolonged contraction time, latency period, relaxation period	Decreased motor function and overall strength
Deterioration of joint cartilage	Bone makes contact with bone	Potential for pain, crepitation, and limitation of movement
Loss of water from the cartilage	Narrowing of joint spaces	Loss of height
Decreased bone mass	Decreased bone formation and increased bone resorption, leading to osteoporosis	More rapid and earlier changes in women Greater risk of fractures
Decreased osteoblastic activity		
Osteoclasts resorb bone	Hormonal changes	Gait and posture accommodate to changes
Increased proportion of body fat	Centripetal distribution of fat and invasion of fat in large muscle groups	Anthropometric measurements required
Regional changes in fat distribution		Increased relative adiposity
Thickened leptomeninges in spinal cord	Loss of anterior horn cells in the lumbosacral area	Leg weakness may be correlated
Accumulation of lipofuscin	Altered RNA function and resultant cell death	
Loss of neurons and nerve fibers	Decreased processing speed and vibration sense Altered pain response	Increased time to perform and learn Possible postural hypotension Safety hazard
Decreased conduction of nerve fibers	Decreased deep tendon, Achilles tendon Decreased psychomotor performance	Alteration in pain response

Change	Finding	Implication
Few neuritic plaques		Possible cognitive and memory changes
Neurofibrillary tangles in hippocampal neurons		Heavy tangle formation and neuritic plaques in cortex of those with Alzheimer's
Changes in sleep-wake cycle		Increased or decreased time spent sleeping
		Increased nighttime awakenings
		Changed hormonal activity
		Decreased stage 4, stage 3, and rapid eye movement phases
		Deterioration of circadian organization
		Delayed reaction time
Slower stimulus identification and registration		Prone to falls
Decreased brain weight and volume		May be present in absence of mental impairments

Sensory System

Change	Finding	Implication
Morphological changes in choroid, epithelium, retina	Decreased visual acuity	Corrective lenses required
	Visual field narrows	Increased possibility of disorientation and social isolation
Decreased rod and cone function		Slower light and dark adaptation
Pigment accumulation		
Decreased speed of eye movements	Difficulty in gazing upward and maintaining convergence	
Sclerosis of pupil sphincter	Difficulty in adapting to lighting changes	Glare may pose an environmental hazard
	Increased threshold for light perception	Dark rooms may be hazardous
Increased intraocular pressure		Increased incidence of glaucoma
Distorted depth perception		Incorrect assessment of height of curbs and steps; potential for falls
Ciliary muscle atrophy	Altered refractive powers	Corrective lenses often required
Nuclear sclerosis (lens)	Presbyopia	Near work and reading may become difficult
Reduced accommodation	Hyperopia	
Increased lens size	Myopia	
Accumulation of lens fibers		
Lens yellows	Color vision may be impaired	Less able to differentiate lower color tones: blues, greens, violets
Diminished tear secretion	Dullness and dryness of the eyes	Irritation and discomfort may result
		Intactness of corneal surface jeopardized

(continued)

Age-Related Change	Appearance or Functional Change	Implication
Sensory System		
Loss of auditory neurons	Decreased tone discrimination and voice localization High frequency sounds lost first	Suspiciousness may be increased because of paranoid dimensions secondary to hearing loss Social isolation
Angiosclerosis calcification of inner ear membrane	Progressive hearing loss, especially at high frequency Presbycusis	Difficulty hearing, particularly under certain conditions such as *background noise, rapid speech, poor acoustics*
Decreased number of olfactory nerve fibers	Decreased sensitivity to odors	May not detect harmful odors Potential safety hazard
Alteration in taste sensation		Possible changes in food preferences and eating patterns
Reduced tactile sensation	Decreased ability to sense pressure, pain, temperature	Misperceptions of environment and safety risk
Endocrine System		
Decline in secretion of testosterone, growth hormone, insulin, adrenal androgens, aldosterone, thyroid hormone	Decreased hormone clearance rates	Increased mortality associated with certain stresses (burns, surgery)
Defects in thermoregulation	Shivering less intense Poor perceptions of changes in ambient temperature Reduced sweating; increased threshold for the onset of sweating	Susceptibility to temperature extremes *(hypothermia/hyperthermia)*
Reduction of febrile responses	Fever not always present with infectious process	Unrecognized infectious process operative

Change	Consequence	Clinical Implication
Alteration in tissue sensitivity to hormones	Decreased insulin response, glucose tolerance, and sensitivity of renal tubules to antidiuretic hormone (ADH)	
Enhanced sympathetic responsivity	Alteration in carbohydrate tolerance	
Increased nodularity and fibrosis of thyroid		Increased frequency of thyroid disease
Decreased basal metabolic rate		Increased incidence of obesity

Hematologic System

Change	Consequence	Clinical Implication
Decreased percentage of marrow space occupied by hematopoietic tissue	Ineffective erythropoiesis	Risky for patient who loses blood

Immune System

Change	Consequence	Clinical Implication
Thymic involution and decreased serum thymic hormone activity	Decreased number of T cells	Less vigorous and/or delayed hypersensitivity reactions
Decreased T-cell function	Production of antiself reactive T cells	Increased risk mortality
Appearance of autoantibodies	Impairment in cell-mediated immune responses	Increased incidence of infection
	Decreased cyclic adenosine monophosphate (AMP) and glucose monophosphate (GMP)	Reactivation of latent infectious diseases
	Decreased ability to reject foreign tissue	Increased prevalence of autoimmune disorders
	Increased laboratory autoimmune parameters	
Redistribution of lymphocytes	Impaired immune reactivity	
Changes in serum immunoglobulin	Increased immunoglobulin A (IgA) levels	Increased prevalence of infection
	Decreased immunoglobulin G (IgG) levels	

APPENDIX **B**

LABORATORY VALUES

IN THE OLDER ADULT

Laboratory Test	Normal Values	Changes with Age	Comments
Urinalysis			
Protein	0–5 mg/100 mL	Rises slightly	May be due to kidney changes with age, urinary tract infection, renal pathology
Glucose	0–15 mg/100 mL	Declines slightly	Glycosuria appears after high plasma level; unreliable
Specific gravity	1.005–1.020	Lower maximum in elderly 1.016–1.022	Decline in nephrons impairs ability to concentrate urine
Hematology			
Erythrocyte sedimentation rate	Men: 0–20 Women: 0–30	Significant increase	Neither sensitive or specific in aged
Iron	50–160 μg/dL	Slight decrease	
Iron binding	230–410 μg/dL	Decrease	
Hemoglobin	Men: 13–18 g/100 mL Women: 12–16 g/100 mL	Men: 10–17 g/mL Women: none noted	Anemia quite common in the elderly
Hematocrit	Men: 45–52% Women: 37–48%	Slight decrease speculated	Decline in hematopoiesis
Leukocytes	4300–10,800/mm^3	Drop to 3,100–9,000/mm^3	Decrease may be due to drugs or sepsis and should not be immediately attributed to age
Lymphocytes	500–2400 T cells/mm^3 50–200 B cells/mm^3	T-cell and B-cell levels fall	Infection risk higher; immunization encouraged
Platelets	150,000–350,000/mm^3	No change in number	

Blood Chemistry

Component	Normal value	Age-related change	Significance
Albumin	3.5–5.0/100 mL	Decline	Related to decrease in liver size and enzymes; protein energy malnutrition common
Globulin	2.3–3.5 g/100 mL	Slight increase	
Total serum protein	6.0–8.4 g/100 mL	No change	Decreases may indicate malnutrition, infection, liver disease
Blood urea nitrogen	Men: 10–25 mg/100 mL, Women: 8–20 mg/100 mL	Increases significantly up to 69 mg/100 mL	Decline in glomerular filtration rate; decreased cardiac output
Creatinine	0.6–1.5 mg/100 mL	Increases to 1.9 mg/100 mL seen	Related to lean body mass decrease
Creatinine clearance	104–124 mL/min	Decreases 10%/decade after 40 years of age	Used for prescribing medications for drugs excreted by kidney
Glucose tolerance	62–110 mg/dL after fasting; less than 120 mg/dL after 2 hours post-prandial	Slight increase of 10 mg/dL/decade after 30 years of age	Diabetes increasingly prevalent; drugs may cause glucose intolerance
Triglycerides	40–150 mg/100 mL	20–200 mg/100 mL	
Cholesterol	120–220 mg/100 mL	Men: increase to 50 mg/100 mL then decrease; Women: increase post-menopausally	Risk of cardiovascular disease
Thyroxine (T_4)	4.5–13.5 mcg/100 mL	No change	Changes suggest thyroid disease; may be seen in euthyroid patients with acute or chronic illness or caloric deficiencies
Triiodothyronine (T_3)	90–220 ng/100 mL	Decrease 25%	
Thyroid-stimulating hormone (TSH)	0.5–5.0 mcgu/mL	Slight increase	Sensitive indicator for diagnosing thyroid disease
Alkaline phosphatase	13–39 IU/L	Increase by 8–10 IU/L	Elevations greater than 20% usually due to disease; elevations may be found with bone abnormalities, drugs (e.g., narcotics), and eating a fatty meal

Data from Cavalieri et al. (1992); Davis (1993); Garner (1989); Kelso (1990); and Melillo (1993a, 1993b, 1993c).

APPENDIX C

COMMON TESTS AND
THEIR ASSOCIATIONS
WITH DISEASES AND
CONDITIONS

Laboratory Test	Increase	Decrease
Acid phosphatase	Prostate cancer, prostatic massage, prostatitis, myocardial infarction, excess platelet destruction, bone disease, liver disease	—
Alanine aminotransferase (ALT or SGPT)	Hepatitis, cirrhosis, liver metastases, obstructive jaundice, infectious mononucleosis, hepatic congestion, pancreatitis, renal disease, alcohol ingestion	Pyridoxine (vitamin B_6) deficiency
Albumin	Dehydration, diabetes insipidus	Overhydration, malnutrition, malabsorption, nephrosis, hepatic failure, burns, multiple myeloma, metastatic carcinomias, acute illness
Alkaline phosphatase	Bone growth, bone metastases, Paget's disease, osteomalacia, healing fracture, hyperparathyroidism, hepatic disease, obstructive jaundice, hepatic metastases, pulmonary infarction, heart failure	Pernicious anemia hypoparathyroidism, hypophosphatasia

(continued)

Laboratory Test	Increase	Decrease
α-Fetoprotein	Hepatoma, testicular tumor, hepatitis	—
Amylase	Pancreatitis, GI obstruction, mesenteric thrombosis and infarction, macroamylasemia, parotitis, renal disease, lung carcinoma, acute alcohol ingestion, after abdominal surgery	Massive pancreatic destruction
Aspartate aminotransferase (AST or SGOT)	Myocardial infarction, heart failure, myocarditis, pericarditis, myositis, trauma, hepatic disease, pancreatitis, renal infarction, neoplasia, cerebral damage, seizures, hemolysis, alcohol ingestion	Pyridoxine (vitamine B_6) deficiency, advanced stages of liver disease
Bilirubin	Hepatic disease, obstructive jaundice, hemolytic anemia, pulmonary infarction, Gilbert's disease, Dubin-Johnson syndrome	—
Calcium	Hyperparathyroidism, bone metastases, myeloma, sarcoidosis, hyperthyroidism, hypervitaminosis D, malignancy without bone metastases, milk-alkali syndrome	Hypoparathyroidism, renal failure, malabsorption, pancreatitis, hypoalbuminemia, vitamin D deficiency, overhydration
Cholesterol	Hypercholesterolemia, hypothyroidism, obstructive jaundice, nephrosis, diabetes mellitus, pancreatitis	Hyperthyroidism, infection, malnutrition, heart failure, malignancies, severe liver damage (due to chemicals, drugs, hepatitis)
High-density lipoprotein cholesterol	Vigorous exercise, increased clearance of triglyceride (VLDL), moderate alcohol consumption, exogenous intake of insulin or estrogens	Malnutrition, obesity, cigarette smoking, diabetes mellitus, hypothyroidism, liver disease, nephrosis, uremia
Creatine kinase	Myocardial infarction, muscle disease or injury, burns, chest trauma, collagen-vascular disease, meningitis, drug use (e.g., lovastatin), status epilepticus, brain infarction, hyperthermia, after surgery	—
Creatinine	Renal failure, urinary obstruction, dehydration, hyperthyroidism, muscle disease	Aging (decreases creatinine clearance but not serum creatinine concentration)

Laboratory Test	Increase	Decrease
Glucose	Diabetes mellitus, pheochromocytoma, hyperthyroidism, Cushing's syndrome, acromegaly, brain damage, hepatic disease, nephrosis, hemochromatosis, stress (e.g., from emotion, burns, shock, anesthesia), acute or chronic pancreatitis, Wernicke's encephalopathy (vitamin B_1 deficiency), chronic hypervitaminosis A, administration of thiazides, corticosteroids, epinephrine, estrogens, ethanol, phenytoin, propranolol, or IV glucose	Excess exogenous insulin, insulinoma, Addison's disease, myxedema, hepatic failure, malabsorption, pancreatitis, glucagon deficiency, extrapancreatic tumors, early diabetes mellitus, postgastrectomy, autonomic nervous system disorders, administration of oral hypoglycemic medications (factitious), malnutrition, alcoholism
Lactate dehydrogenase (LDH)	Myocardial infarction, pulmonary infarction, hemolytic anemia, pernicious anemia, leukemia, lymphoma, other malignancies, hepatic disease, renal infarction, seizures, cerebral damage, trauma, sprue	—
Lipase	Same as amylase (excluding parotitis and macroamylasemia)	—
Magnesium	Renal disease, excess exogenous magnesium	Diarrhea, malabsorption, renal tubular acidosis, acute tubular necrosis, chronic glomerulonephritis, aldosteronism, hyperthyroidism, hypercalcemia, uncontrolled diabetes, dietary deficit, administration of certain drugs (diuretics, antibiotics), alcoholism
Phosphorus	Renal failure, hypoparathyroidism, diabetic acidosis, acromegaly, hyperthyroidism, high phosphate intake (IV or PO), vitamin D intoxication, lactic acidosis, leukemia, volume contraction, hyperlipidemia, hyperbilirubinemia, dysproteinemia, heparin sodium contamination, spurious (prolonged refrigeration of sample)	Hyperparathyroidism, osteomalacia, hypokalemia, excess IV glucose, respiratory alkalosis, dietary deficit, ingestion of P-binding antacid, alcoholism, gout, hemodialysis, cirrhosis

(continued)

Laboratory Test	Increase	Decrease
Potassium	Hyperkalemic acidosis, diabetic acidosis, hypoadrenalism, hereditary hyperkalemia, hemolysis, myoglobulinuria, renal tubular defect, thrombocytosis, intake of K-retaining diuretic, ACE inhibitors, or large exogenous K load	Cirrhosis, malnutrition, vomiting, metabolic alkalosis, diarrhea, nephrosis, hyperadrenalism, ectopic adrenocorticotropic hormone excess, β-hydroxylase deficiency, administration of diuretics
Prostate-specific antigen (PSA)	Prostate cancer, benign prostatic hyperplasia, prostatic massage, prostatic abscess, prostatitis, cystoscopy	Administration of finasteride
Sodium	Dehydration, diabetes insipidus, excessive salt ingestion, diabetes mellitus with diuresis, diuretic phase of acute tubular necrosis, hypercalcemic nephropathy with diuresis, essential hypernatremia due to hypothalamic lesions	Excess exogenous antidiuretic hormone, nephrosis, hypoadrenalism, myxedema, heart failure, diarrhea, vomiting, diabetic acidosis, adrenocortical insufficiency, hyperlipidemia, hyperglycemia, hyperproteinemia (e.g., multiple myeloma), intake of diuretics or mannitol, spurious (serum osmolality is normal or increased—avoid by using direct-reading potentiometry with ion-selective electrode)
Total protein	Multiple myeloma, myxedema, lupus, sarcoidosis, diabetes insipidus, dehydration, collagen-vascular disease	Burns, cirrhosis, malnutrition, nephrosis, malabsorption, overhydration, GI protein loss

Laboratory Test	Increase	Decrease
Triglyceride	Nephrosis, cholestasis, pancreatitis, cirrhosis, diabetes mellitus, hepatitis, familial hypertriglyceridemia	Malnutrition
Urea nitrogen	Renal disease, dehydration, GI bleeding, leukemia, heart failure, shock, postrenal azotemia, obstruction of urinary tract, acute myocardial infarction	Hepatic failure, overhydration, acromegaly, dietary factors, prolonged IV feedings
Uric acid	Gout, renal failure, diuretic therapy, leukemia, lymphoma, polycythemia, acidosis, psoriasis, hypothyroidism, multiple myeloma, pernicious anemia, tissue necrosis, inflammation, 25% of relatives of patients with gout, cancer chemotherapy (e.g., nitrogen mustards, vincristine, mercaptopurine), hemolytic anemia, high-protein weight-reduction diet, lead poisoning, polycystic kidneys, calcinosis universalis and circumscripta, hypoparathyroidism, sarcoidosis, elevated serum triglyceride levels, use of low-dose aspirin	Administration of uricosuric drugs, allopurinol, or large doses of vitamin C; Wilson's disease

ACE = angiotensin converting enzyme; K = potassium; VLDL = very low density lipoprotein.

Based on material in *Interpretation of Diagnostic Tests*, ed. 4, by J Wallach. Boston, Little, Brown and Company, 1986, pp 41–96; used with permission.

APPENDIX **D**

MINIMUM

DATA SET

MINIMUM DATA SET (MDS) — *VERSION 2.0*
FOR NURSING HOME RESIDENT ASSESSMENT AND CARE SCREENING
BASIC ASSESSMENT TRACKING FORM

SECTION AA. IDENTIFICATION INFORMATION		GENERAL INSTRUCTIONS

SECTION AA. IDENTIFICATION INFORMATION

1.	RESIDENT NAME ⊛	a. (First) b. (Middle Initial) c. (Last) d. (Jr./Sr.)

GENERAL INSTRUCTIONS

Complete this information for submission with all full and quarterly assessments (Admission, Annual, Significant Change, State or Medicare required assessments, or Quarterly Reviews, etc.).

2.	GENDER ⊛	1. Male 2. Female

3.	BIRTHDATE ⊛	Month — Day — Year

4.	RACE/ ⊛ ETHNICITY	1. American Indian/Alaskan Native 4. Hispanic 2. Asian/Pacific Islander 5. White, not of 3. Black, not of Hispanic origin Hispanic origin

5.	SOCIAL ⊛ SECURITY AND ⊛ MEDICARE NUMBERS [C in 1st box if non Med. no.]	a. Social Security Number b. Medicare number (or comparable railroad insurance number)

6.	FACILITY PROVIDER NO. ⊛	a. State No. b. Federal No.

7.	MEDICAID NO. ["+" if pending, "N" if not a Medicaid ⊛ recipient]	

8.	REASONS FOR ASSESS- MENT	[Note—Other codes do not apply to this form]
		 a. Primary reason for assessment
		   1. Admission assessment (required by day 14)
		   2. Annual assessment
		   3. Significant change in status assessment
		   4. Significant correction of prior full assessment
		   5. Quarterly review assessment
		   10. Significant correction of prior quarterly assessment
		   0. *NONE OF ABOVE*
		 b. *Codes for assessments required for Medicare PPS or the State*
		   1. Medicare 5 day assessment
		   2. Medicare 30 day assessment
		   3. Medicare 60 day assessment
		   4. Medicare 90 day assessment
		   5. Medicare readmission/return assessment
		   6. Other state required assessment
		   7. Medicare 14 day assessment
		   8. Other Medicare required assessment

9.	SIGNATURES OF PERSONS COMPLETING THESE ITEMS:	

a. Signatures	Title	Date
b.		Date

⊛ = Key items for computerized resident tracking

☐ = When box blank, must enter number or letter

a. = When letter in box, check if condition applies

Code "NA" if information unavailable or unknown.

TRIGGER LEGEND

1	- Delirium	10A	- Activities (Revise)
2	- Cognitive Loss/Dementia	10B	- Activities (Review)
3	- Visual Function	11	- Falls
4	- Communication	12	- Nutritional Status
5A	- ADL-Rehabilitation	13	- Feeding Tubes
5B	- ADL-Maintenance	14	- Dehydration/Fluid Maintenance
6	- Urinary Incontinence and Indwelling Catheter	15	- Dental Care
7	- Psychosocial Well-Being	16	- Pressure Ulcers
8	- Mood State	17	- Psychotropic Drug Use
9	- Behavioral Symptoms	18	- Physical Restraints

MDS 2.0 1/30/98

MDS QUARTERLY ASSESSMENT FORM

Numeric Identifier

A1.	RESIDENT NAME	a. (First) b. (Middle Initial) c. (Last) d. (Jr/Sr)
A2.	ROOM NUMBER	
A3.	ASSESSMENT REFERENCE DATE	A. Last day of MDS observation period Month — Day — Year b. Original (0) or corrected copy of form (enter number of correction)
A4a.	DATE OF REENTRY	Date of reentry from most recent temporary discharge to a hospital in last 90 days (or since last assessment or admission if less than 90 days) Month — Day — Year
A6.	MEDICAL RECORD NO.	
B1.	COMATOSE	(Persistent vegetative state/no discernible consciousness) 0. No 1. Yes *(Skip to Section G)*
B2.	MEMORY	(Recall of what was learned or known) a. Short-term memory OK—seems/appears to recall after 5 minutes 0. Memory OK 1. Memory problem 8 b. Long-term memory OK—seems/appears to recall long past 0. Memory OK 1. Memory problem 9
B4.	COGNITIVE SKILLS FOR DAILY DECISION-MAKING	(Made decisions regarding tasks of daily life) 0. INDEPENDENT—decisions consistent/reasonable 1. MODIFIED INDEPENDENCE—some difficulty in new situations only 8 2. MODERATELY IMPAIRED—decisions poor; cues/ supervision required 9 3. SEVERELY IMPAIRED—never/rarely made decisions 9, 8日
B5.	INDICATORS OF DELIRIUM— PERIODIC DISORDERED THINKING/ AWARENESS	(Code for behavior in the *last 7 days*.) [Note: Accurate assessment requires conversations with staff and family who have direct knowledge of resident's behavior over this time.] 0. Behavior not present 1. Behavior present, not of recent onset 2. Behavior present, over last 7 days appears different from resident's usual functioning (e.g., new onset or worsening) a. EASILY DISTRACTED—(e.g., difficulty paying attention; gets sidetracked) 2 → 1, 17° b. PERIODS OF ALTERED PERCEPTION OR AWARENESS OF SURROUNDINGS—(e.g., moves lips or talks to someone not present; believes he/she is somewhere else; confuses night and day) 2 → 1, 17° c. EPISODES OF DISORGANIZED SPEECH—(e.g., speech is incoherent, nonsensical, irrelevant, or rambling from subject to subject; loses train of thought) 2 → 1, 17° d. PERIODS OF RESTLESSNESS—(e.g., fidgeting or picking at skin, clothing, napkins, etc; frequent position changes; repetitive physical movements or calling out) 2 → 1, 17° e. PERIODS OF LETHARGY—(e.g., sluggishness; staring into space; difficult to arouse; little body movement) 2 → 1, 17° f. MENTAL FUNCTION VARIES OVER THE COURSE OF THE DAY—(e.g., sometimes better, sometimes worse; behaviors sometimes present, sometimes not) 2 → 1, 17°
C4.	MAKING SELF UNDERSTOOD	(Expressing information content—however able) 0. UNDERSTOOD 1. USUALLY UNDERSTOOD—difficulty finding words or finishing thoughts 2. SOMETIMES UNDERSTOOD—ability is limited to making concrete requests 8 3. RARELY/NEVER UNDERSTOOD 9
C6.	ABILITY TO UNDERSTAND OTHERS	(Understanding verbal information content—however able) 0. UNDERSTANDS 1. USUALLY UNDERSTANDS—may miss some part/intent of message 8 2. SOMETIMES UNDERSTANDS—responds adequately to simple, direct communication 8, 9 3. RARELY/NEVER UNDERSTANDS 9
E1.	INDICATORS OF DEPRESSION, ANXIETY, SAD MOOD	(Code for indicators observed in last 30 days, irrespective of the assumed cause) 0. Indicator not exhibited in last 30 days 1. Indicator of this type exhibited up to five days a week 2. Indicator of this type exhibited daily or almost daily (6, 7 days a week)

VERBAL EXPRESSIONS OF DISTRESS
a. Resident made negative statements—e.g.:Nothing matters; Would rather be dead; What's the use; Regrets having lived so long; Let me die" 1 or 2 → 3
b. Repetitive questions—e.g. "Where do I go; What do I do?" 1 or 2 →

c. Repetitive verbalizations—e.g. calling out for help, ("God help me") 1 or 2 → 3
d. Persistent anger with self or others—e.g., easily annoyed, anger at placement in nursing home; anger at care received 1 or 2 → 8
e. Self deprecation—e.g. "I am nothing; I am of no use to anyone" 1 or 2 →

E1.	INDICATORS OF DEPRESSION, ANXIETY, SAD MOOD (cont.)	**VERBAL EXPRESSIONS OF DISTRESS** f. Expressions of what appear to be unrealistic fears—e.g., fear of being abandoned, left alone, being with others 1 or 2 → 8 g. Recurrent statements that something terrible is about to happen—e.g., believes he or she is about to die, have a heart attack 1 or 2 → 8 h. Repetitive health complaints—e.g., persistently seeks medical attention, obsessive concern with body functions 1 or 2 → 8 i. Repetitive anxious complaints/concerns (non-health related) e.g.: persistently seeks attention/reassurance regardingschedules,meals, laundry,clothing,relationship issues 1 or 2 → 8
		SLEEP-CYCLE ISSUES j. Unpleasant mood in morning 1 or 2 → 8 k. Insomnia/change in usual sleep pattern 1 or 2 → 8 **SAD, APATHETIC, ANXIOUS APPEARANCE** l. Sad, pained, worried facial expressions—e.g., furrowed brows m.Crying, tearfulness 1 or 2 → 8 n. Repetitive physical movements—e.g., pacing, hand wringing, restlessness, fidgeting, picking 1 or 2 → 8, 17° **LOSS OF INTEREST** o. Withdrawal from activities of interest—e.g.,no interest in long standing activities orbeingwithfamily/friends 1 or 2 → 8 p. Reduced social interaction 1 or 2 → 8
E2.	MOOD PERSISTENCE	One or more indicators of depressed, sad or anxious mood **were not easily altered by attempts to "cheer up", console, or reassure the resident over last 7 days** 0. No mood indicators 1. Indicators present, easily altered 8 2. Indicators present, not easily altered 8
E4.	BEHAVIORAL SYMPTOMS	(A) *Behavioral symptom frequency in last 7 days* 0. Behavior not exhibited in last 7 days 1. Behavior of this type occurred 1 to 3 days in last 7 days 2. Behavior of this type occurred 4 to 6 days, but less than daily 3. Behavior of this type occurred daily (B) *Behavioral symptom alterability in last 7 days* 0. Behavior not present OR behavior was easily altered 1. Behavior was not easily altered (A) (B) a. WANDERING (moving with no rational purpose, seemingly oblivious to needs or safety) A=1, 2, or 3 → 9, 17 b. VERBALLY ABUSIVE BEHAVIORAL SYMPTOMS (others were threatened, screamed at, cursed at) A=1, 2, or 3 → 9 c. PHYSICALLY ABUSIVE BEHAVIORAL SYMPTOMS (others were hit, shoved, scratched, sexually abused) A=1, 2, or 3 → 9 d. SOCIALLY INAPPROPRIATE/DISRUPTIVE BEHAVIORAL SYMPTOMS (made disruptive sounds, noisiness, screaming, self-abusive acts, sexual behavior or disrobing in public, smeared/threw food/feces, hoarding, rummaged through others' belongings) A=1, 2, or 3 → 9 e. RESISTS CARE (resisted taking medications/ injections, ADL assistance, or eating) A=1, 2, or 3 → 9

G1.	(A)	ADL SELF-PERFORMANCE—*(Code for resident's PERFORMANCE OVER ALL SHIFTS during last 7 days— Not including setup)* 0. INDEPENDENT—No help or oversight—OR—Help/oversight provided only 1 or 2 times during last 7 days 1. SUPERVISION—Oversight, encouragement or cueing provided 3 or more times during last 7 days —OR—Supervision (3 or more times) plus physical assistance provided only 1 or 2 times during last 7 days 2. LIMITED ASSISTANCE—Resident highly involved in activity; received physical help in guided maneuvering of limbs or other nonweight bearing assistance 3 or more times—OR—More help provided only 1 or 2 times during last 7 days 3. EXTENSIVE ASSISTANCE—While resident performed part of activity, over last 7-day period, help of the following type(s) provided 3 or more times: — Weight-bearing support — Full staff performance during part (but not all) of last 7 days 4. TOTAL DEPENDENCE—Full staff performance of activity during entire 7 days 8. ACTIVITY DID NOT OCCUR during entire 7 days (A)
a.	BED MOBILITY	How resident moves to and from lying position, turns side to side, and positions body while in bed. 1=8A, 2, 3, or 4 → 9A, 19, 8~18
b.	TRANSFER	How resident moves between surfaces—to/from: bed, chair, wheelchair, standing position (EXCLUDE to/from bath/toilet). 1, 2, 3, or 4 → 9A
c.	WALK IN ROOM	How resident walks between locations in his/her room. 1, 2, 3, or 4 → 9A
d.	WALK IN CORRIDOR	How resident walks in corridor on unit. 1, 2, 3, or 4 → 9A
e.	LOCOMOTION ON UNIT	How resident moves between locations in his/her room and adjacent corridor on same floor. If in wheelchair, self-sufficiency once in chair. 1, 2, 3, or 4 → 9A
f.	LOCOMOTION OFF UNIT	How resident moves to and returns from off unit locations (e.g., areas set aside for dining, activities, or treatments). If facility has only one floor, how resident moves to and from distant areas on the floor. If in wheelchair, self-sufficiency once in chair. 1, 2, 3, or 4 → 9A
g.	DRESSING	How resident puts on, fastens, and takes off all items of street clothing, including donning/removing prosthesis. 1, 2, 3, or 4 → 9A
h.	EATING	How resident eats and drinks (regardless of skill). Includes intake of nourishment by other means (e.g., tube feeding, total parenteral nutrition). 1, 2, 3, or 4 → 9A

Resident _____   Numeric Identifier _____

i.	TOILET USE	How resident uses the toilet room (or commode, bedpan, urinal); transfers on/off toilet, cleanses, changes pad, manages ostomy or catheter, adjusts clothes 1, 2, 3, or 4 = 5A
j.	PERSONAL HYGIENE	How resident maintains personal hygiene, including combing hair, brushing teeth, shaving, applying makeup, washing/drying face, hands, and perineum (EXCLUDE baths and showers) 1, 2, 3, or 4 = 5A
G2.	BATHING	How resident takes full-body bath/shower, sponge bath, and transfers in/out of tub/shower (EXCLUDE washing of back and hair.) *Code for most dependent in self-performance.* (A) BATHING SELF-PERFORMANCE codes appear below 0. Independent—No help provided 1. Supervision—Oversight help only 5A **(A)** 2. Physical help limited to transfer only 5A 3. Physical help in part of bathing activity 5A 4. Total dependence 6A 8. Activity itself did not occur during entire 7 days *1, 2, 3, or 4 = 6A*
G4.	FUNCTIONAL LIMITATION IN RANGE OF MOTION	*(Code for limitations during last 7 days that interfered with daily functions or placed residents at risk of injury)* (A) RANGE OF MOTION (B) VOLUNTARY MOVEMENT 0. No limitation 0. No loss 1. Limitation on one side 1. Partial loss 2. Limitation on both sides 2. Full loss **(A) (B)** a. Neck b. Arm—Including shoulder or elbow c. Hand—Including wrist or fingers d. Leg—Including hip or knee e. Foot—Including ankle or toes f. Other limitation or loss
G6.	MODES OF TRANSFER	*(Check all that apply during last 7 days)* Bedfast all or most of time 16 a. *NONE OF ABOVE* f. Bed rails used for bed mobility or transfer b.
H1.		CONTINENCE SELF-CONTROL CATEGORIES *(Code for resident's PERFORMANCE OVER ALL SHIFTS)* 0. *CONTINENT*—Complete control [includes use of indwelling urinary catheter or ostomy device that does not leak urine or stool] 1. *USUALLY CONTINENT*—BLADDER, incontinent episodes once a week or less; BOWEL, less than weekly 2. *OCCASIONALLY INCONTINENT*—BLADDER, 2 or more times a week but not daily; BOWEL, once a week 3. *FREQUENTLY INCONTINENT*—BLADDER, tended to be incontinent daily, but some control present (e.g., on day shift); BOWEL, 2-3 times a week 4. *INCONTINENT*—Had inadequate control. BLADDER, multiple daily episodes; BOWEL, all (or almost all) of the time
a.	BOWEL CONTINENCE	Control of bowel movement, with appliance or bowel continence programs, if employed 1, 2, 3, or 4 = 16
b.	BLADDER CONTINENCE	Control of urinary bladder function (if dribbles, volume insufficient to soak through underpants), with appliances (e.g., foley) or continence programs, if employed 2, 3, or 4 = 6
H2.	BOWEL ELIMINATION PATTERN	Fecal impaction 17* d. *NONE OF ABOVE* e.
H3.	APPLIANCES AND PROGRAMS	Any scheduled toileting plan a. Indwelling catheter 6 d. Bladder retraining program b. Ostomy present j. External (condom) catheter 6 c. *NONE OF ABOVE* m.
I2.	INFECTIONS	Urinary tract infection in last 30 days 14 j. *NONE OF ABOVE* e.
I3.	OTHER CURRENT DIAGNOSES AND ICD-9 CODES	*(Include only those diseases diagnosed in the last 90 days that have a relationship to current ADL status, behavior status, medical treatments, nursing monitoring, or risk of death)* Dehydration 276.5 = 14 a. [•] b. [•]
J1.	PROBLEM CONDITIONS	*(Check all problems present in last 7 days)* Hallucinations 17* i. Dehydrated; output exceeds input 16 c. *NONE OF ABOVE* p.
J2.	PAIN SYMPTOMS	*(Code the highest level of pain present in the last 7 days)* a. **FREQUENCY** with which resident complains or shows evidence of pain b. **INTENSITY** of pain 1. Mild pain 0. No pain *(skip to J4)* 2. Moderate pain 1. Pain less than daily 3. Times when pain is horrible or 2. Pain daily excruciating
J4.	ACCIDENTS	*(Check all that apply)* Fell in past 30 days 11, 17* a. Hip fracture in last 180 days 17* c. Fell in past 31-180 days 11, 17* b. Other fracture in last 180 days d. *NONE OF ABOVE* e.

J5.	STABILITY OF CONDITIONS	Conditions/diseases make resident's cognitive, ADL, mood or behavior status unstable—(fluctuating, precarious, or deteriorating) a. Resident experiencing an acute episode or a flare-up of a recurrent or chronic problem b. End-stage disease, 6 or fewer months to live c. *NONE OF ABOVE* d.

K3.	WEIGHT CHANGE	a. **Weight loss**—5% or more in **last 30 days**; or 10% or more in **last 180 days** b.
		    0. No 1. Yes 12
		b. **Weight gain**—5% or more in **last 30 days**; or 10% or more in **last 180 days** h.
		    0. No 1. Yes

K5.	NUTRITIONAL APPROACHES	Feeding tube 13, 14 b. On a planned weight change program h. *NONE OF ABOVE* i.
M1.	ULCERS (Due to any cause)	*(Record the number of ulcers at each ulcer stage—regardless of cause. If none present at a stage, record "0" (zero). Code all that apply during last 7 days. Code 9 = 9 or more.)* [*Requires full body exam.*] **Number at Stage** a. Stage 1. A persistent area of skin redness (without a break in the skin) that does not disappear when pressure is relieved. b. Stage 2. A partial thickness loss of skin layers that presents clinically as an abrasion, blister, or shallow crater. c. Stage 3. A full thickness of skin is lost, exposing the subcutaneous tissues-presents as a deep crater with or without undermining adjacent tissue. d. Stage 4. A full thickness of skin and subcutaneous tissue is lost, exposing muscle or bone.
M2.	TYPE OF ULCER	*(For each type of ulcer, code for the highest stage in the last 7 days using scale in item M1—i.e., 0=none; stages 1, 2, 3, 4)* a. Pressure ulcer—any lesion caused by pressure resulting in damage of underlying tissue 1 = 16; 2, 3, or 4 = 15, 16 b. Stasis ulcer—open lesion caused by poor circulation in the lower extremities

N1.	TIME AWAKE	*(Check appropriate time periods over last 7 days)*
		Resident awake all or most of time (i.e., naps no more than one hour per time period) in the:
		  N1a = 10B Morning 10B a. Evening c.
		  ONLY if
		  N2 = 0 Afternoon b. *NONE OF ABOVE* d.

(If resident comatose, skip to Section O)

N2.	AVERAGE TIME INVOLVED IN ACTIVITIES	(When awake and not receiving treatments or ADL care) N20 = 10B only if N1a = ✓ 0. Most—more than 2/3 of time 10B 2. Little—less than 1/3 of time 10A 1. Some—from 1/3 to 2/3 of time 3. None 10A
O1.	NUMBER OF MEDICATIONS	*(Record the number of different medications used in the last 7 days; enter "0" if none used)*
O4.	DAYS RECEIVED THE FOLLOWING MEDICATION	*(Record the number of DAYS during last 7 days; enter "0" if not used. Note—enter "1" for long-acting meds used less than weekly)* a. Antipsychotic 1-7=17 d. Hypnotic b. Antianxiety 1-7=11, 17 e. Diuretic 1-7=14 c. Antidepressant 1-7=11, 17
P4.	DEVICES AND RESTRAINTS	Use the following codes for last 7 days: 0. Not used 1. Used less than daily 2. Used daily Bed rails a. — Full bed rails on all open sides of bed b. — Other types of side rails used (e.g., half rail, one side) c. Trunk restraint 1 = 16; 2 = 11, 16, 18 d. Limb restraint 1, 2 = 18 e. Chair prevents rising 1, 2 = 18
Q2.	OVERALL CHANGE IN CARE NEEDS	Resident's overall level of self sufficiency has changed significantly as compared to status of 90 days ago (or since last assessment if less than 90 days) 0. No 1. Improved—receives fewer 2. Deteriorated—change supports, needs less receives restrictive level of care more support

R2. SIGNATURES OF PERSONS COMPLETING THE ASSESSMENT:

a. Signature of RN Assessment Coordinator (sign on above line)

b. Date RN Assessment Coordinator signed as complete   [   ] — [   ] — [   ]
                                  Month   Day   Year

c. Other Signatures	Title	Sections	Date
d.			Date
e.			Date
f.			Date
g.			Date

Form 1730RHH   © 1998 Briggs Corporation, Des Moines, IA 50306 (800) 247-2343   PRINTED IN U.S.A.
Copyright limited to addition of trigger system.
MDS 2.0 1/30/98   3 of 3

APPENDIX **E**

ORGANIZATION AND

SUPPORT GROUP

ADDRESSES AND

PHONE NUMBERS

Administration on Aging
330 Independence Avenue, SW
Suite 4760
Washington, DC 20201
202-619-0556

AIDS Hotline
Atlanta, Georgia
800-551-2728

Alzheimer's Disease Education and Referral
  Center
PO Box 8250
Silver Spring MD 20907
301-495-3311

American Association for International Aging
1900 L, NW Suite 510
Washington, DC 20036
202-833-8893

American Association of Homes and Services
  for the Aging (AAHSA)
901 E Street, NW
Suite 500
Washington, DC 20004-2837
202-783-2242

American Association of Retired Persons
  (AARP)
601 E Street, NW
Washington, DC 20049
202-434-2277

American Cancer Society (National Office)
Public Information Department
1599 Clifton Road, NE
Atlanta, GA 30329
404-320-3333

American Council of the Blind
1155 15th Street, NW
Suite 720
Washington, DC 20005
202-467-5081

American Dental Association
211 E. Chicago Avenue
Chicago, IL 60611-2678
312-440-2500

American Geriatrics Society, Inc.
770 Lexington Avenue
Suite 300
New York, NY 10021
212-308-1414

American Hospital Association (AHA)
One North Franklin Avenue
Chicago, IL 60606
312-422-3000

American Hospital Association (AHA)
325 7th St., NW
Washington, DC 20004
202-638-1100

American Lung Association
1740 Broadway
New York, NY 10019-4371
800-LUNG-USA
800-586-4872

American Medical Directors Association
(AMDA)
10480 Little Patuxent Parkway
Suite 760
Columbia, MD 21044

American Nurses Association (ANA)
600 Maryland Avenue, SW—Suite 100 West
Washington, DC 20024-2571
202-651-7000

American Parkinson's Disease Association
Staten Island, NY
800-223-2732

American Public Health Association
1015 15th Street, NW
Washington, DC 20005
202-789-5600

American Red Cross
National Headquarters
431 18th Street, NW
Washington, DC 20006
202-737-8300

American Sleep Disorder Association
1610 14th St., NW, Suite 300
Rochester, MN 55901
507-287-6006

American Society of Consultant Pharmacists
1321 Duke Street
Alexandria, VA 22314-3563
703-739-1300

American Society on Aging
833 Market Street, Suite 511
San Francisco, CA 94103
415-974-9600

American Speech-Language-Hearing Association
(ASHA)
10801 Rockville Pike, Dept MO
Rockville, MD 20852
800-638-8255

Arthritis Foundation
1330 W. Peachtree Street
Atlanta, GA 30309
404-872-7100

Association for Gerontology in Higher
Education
1001 Connecticut Avenue, NW
Suite 410
Washington, DC 20036
202-429-9277

Association of Hospital-Based Nursing Facilities
3501 Masons Mill Road—Suite 501A
Huntingdon Valley, PA 19006-3573
215-657-0228

Better Hearing Institute
PO Box 1840
Washington, DC 20013
800-424-8576

Better Vision Institute
1800 North Kent Street
Suite 904
Rosslyn, VA 22209
800-424-8422

Beverly Enterprises, Inc.
5111 Rogers Avenue
Suite 40A
Fort Smith, AR 72903
501-452-6712

Beverly Foundation
44 South Mentor Avenue
Pasadena, CA 91106-2902
818-792-2292

Department of Veterans Affairs
810 Vermont Avenue, NW
Washington, DC 20420
202-273-4800

Food and Drug Administration (FDA)
5600 Fishers Lane—Suite 1685
Parklawn Building
Rockville, MD 20857
301-443-3170

Food Allergy Network
4744 Holly Avenue
Fairfax, VA 22030-5647
800-929-4040

Geriatric Research and Training Center
  (GRTC)
3501 Masons Mill Road—Suite 501B
Huntingdon Valley, PA 19006
215-657-9989

Gerontological Nutritionists
678 Waller Street
San Francisco, CA 94117
415-749-4052

Gerontological Society of America
1275 K Street, NW—Suite 350
Washington, DC 20005-4006
202-842-1275

Guide Dog Foundation for the Blind, Inc.
371 East Jericho Turnpike
Smithtown, NY 11787
800-548-4337
516-265-2121 (in New York)

Healthcare Financial Management Association
1050 17th Street, NW—Suite 700
Washington, DC 20036
202-296-2920

Heart Information Service
Texas Heart Institute
PO Box 20345
Houston, TX 77225

Hospice Association of America (HAA)
228 Seventh Street, SE
Washington, DC 20003
202-546-4759

Medic Alert Foundation
Turlock, CA
800-344-3226

National Adult Day Services Association
c/o National Council on the Aging (NCOA)
409 Third Street, NW
Washington, DC 20024
202-479-6682

National Alzheimer's Association
919 North Michigan Avenue
Suite 1000
Chicago, IL 60611
313-335-8700
800-272-3900

National Association for Continence
800-252-3337

National Association of Area Agencies on Aging
1112 16th Street, NW—Suite 100
Washington, DC 20036
202-296-8130
(9 AM–11 PM EST Eldercare Locator)

National Association of Directors of Nursing
  Administration in Long-Term Care
(NADONA/LTC)
10999 Reed Hartman Highway—Suite 229
Cincinnati, OH 45242-8301
800-222-0539

National Association of Nutrition and Aging
  Services Programs
2675 44th Street, SW—Suite 305
Grand Rapids, MI 49509
800-999-6262

National Asthma Education Program
National Heart Lung/Blood Institute
PO Box 30105
Bethesda, MD 20834-0105
301-251-1222

National Conference of GNP's
PO Box 270101
Ft. Collins, CO 80527-0101
800-268-9678

National Council on the Aging, Inc.
409 3rd Street, SW—2nd Floor
Washington, DC 20024
202-479-1200

National Gerontological Nursing Association
7250 Parkway Drive—Suite 510
Hanover, MD 21076
800-723-0560

National Hearing Aid Helpline
20361 Middlebelt Road
Livonia, MD 48152
800-521-5247

National Herpes Hotline
919-361-8488

National Indian Council on Aging, Inc.
6400 Uptown Boulevard, NE
City Center—Suite 510 West
Albuquerque, NM 87110
505-888-3302

National Institute of Mental Health Aging
   Branch
5600 Fishers Lane, Room 18-101
Rockville, MD 20857
301-443-1185

National Institute of Senior Centers
c/o (NCOA) National Council on Aging
409 Third Street, SW
Washington, DC 20024
202-479-1200

National Institute on Community-Based Long-
   Term Care (NICLC)
c/o National Council on the Aging (NCOA)
409 Third Street, SW
Washington, DC 20024
202-479-6974

National Institute on Aging
Richard J. Hodes, MD
Director
301-496-9265

National League for Nursing
350 Hudson Street
New York, NY 10014
212-989-9393

National Parkinson's Foundation
1501 NW 9th Avenue
Bob Hope Road
Miami, FL 33136-1494
800-327-4545

National Pressure Ulcer Advisory Panel
SUNY at Buffalo, Beck Hall
3435 Main Street
Buffalo, NY 14214
716-881-3558

National STD Hotline
800-227-8922

National Stroke Association
96 Inverness Drive East, Suite 1
Englewood, CO 80112-5115
303-649-9299

Overeaters Anonymous
World Service Office
PO Box 44020
Rio Rancho, NM 87174-4020
505-891-2664

Parkinson's Disease Foundation
New York, NY
800-457-6676

Stuttering Foundation of America
P.O. Box 11749
Memphis, TN 38111-0749
800-992-9392

United Parkinson Foundation
Chicago, IL
312-733-1893

APPENDIX **F**

SUPPORT SYSTEMS

FOR ELDERS

State Elder Abuse Hot Line
Most states have instituted a 24-hour, toll-free number for receiving reports of abuse and neglect. Calls are confidential.

Adult Protective Services
This agency has legal responsibility and authority in most states to investigate reports of abuse and neglect in the home, community, and institutions and to provide services to elderly victims.

Accent on Information
A computerized retrieval system that offers access to information on problems. Issues of concern, products, and services available to the disabled.
309-378-2961

Administration on Aging
Information and referral service for home care needs. This agency will also provide support for elders in whatever area of assistance is needed.
202-619-0724

National Council on Aging
Promotes concerns for older people and develops resources and methods for meeting their needs. The organization holds conferences and workshops and provides a national information and consultation center.
202-479-1200

There is also a nationwide directory assistance service designed to help older adults and families locate resources. The number is 800-677-1116.

INDEX

An *f* following a page number indicates a figure; a *t* indicates a table.